AF411440

Applications of Crystal Engineering in Drug Delivery

Applications of Crystal Engineering in Drug Delivery

Editor

Hisham Al-Obaidi

MDPI • Basel • Beijing • Wuhan • Barcelona • Belgrade • Manchester • Tokyo • Cluj • Tianjin

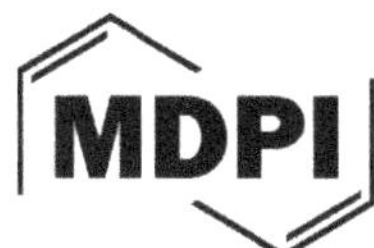

Editor
Hisham Al-Obaidi
University of Reading
Reading
UK

Editorial Office
MDPI
St. Alban-Anlage 66
4052 Basel, Switzerland

This is a reprint of articles from the Special Issue published online in the open access journal *Pharmaceutics* (ISSN 1999-4923) (available at: https://www.mdpi.com/journal/pharmaceutics/special_issues/crystal_drug).

For citation purposes, cite each article independently as indicated on the article page online and as indicated below:

LastName, A.A.; LastName, B.B.; LastName, C.C. Article Title. *Journal Name* **Year**, *Volume Number*, Page Range.

ISBN 978-3-0365-8094-4 (Hbk)
ISBN 978-3-0365-8095-1 (PDF)

Contents

About the Editor

Hisham Al-Obaidi

Hisham Al-Obaidi's research is focused on drug delivery and pharmaceutical sciences. He is currently based at the School of Pharmacy, University of Reading, United Kingdom, and has an extensive track record developing solid dispersions for oral and pulmonary drug delivery applications. His research interests include the assessment of drug–polymer compatibility using thermal analysis methods and developing particle engineering methods for novel applications, such as lung infections and cancer.

Preface to "Applications of Crystal Engineering in Drug Delivery"

Crystal engineering is a broad area of research that includes crystal habit modification, polymorphism, solid dispersions, and salt formation. All these pre-formulation and formulation techniques imply that the drug can be modified using methods such as solvent evaporation or mechanochemical activation. The drug properties can often be significantly altered when the crystalline structure is modified, such as in the case of amorphous form formation. The outcome of such modifications affects physical properties and can dramatically impact physiological properties, such as bioavailability and absorption. Recent advances in this area of research have shown the potential application of crystal engineering to achieve targeted drug delivery for novel molecules, such as anticancer drugs, antimicrobials, and vaccines. Drug delivery applications include various routes, such as oral, pulmonary, ophthalmic, buccal, vaginal, transdermal, and parenteral.

This reprint contains two reviews and eleven original research papers from different authors. The review articles focus on formulation approaches to modify polymorphism in carotenoids and the application of mechanical activation in modifying polymorphism. The research articles cover a breadth of different topics, such as metformin–NSAIDs salts, formation of hydrogel for prolonged release of curcumin, solubility improvement of spiro[cyclopropane-1,3′-oxindoles] (SCOs), in situ amorphization of olanzapine, crystal engineering of ionic co-crystals comprising azole functional groups, investigation of co-crystals and salts of tenoxicam, bulk properties of odanacatib prepared by jet milling or fast precipitation, crystallization thermodynamics of α-lactose monohydrate, preparation of glasdegib dimaleate form, utilization of tedizolid phosphate nanocrystals for ocular drug delivery, and preparation and characterization of co-crystals and salt forms of miconazole.

Hisham Al-Obaidi

Editor

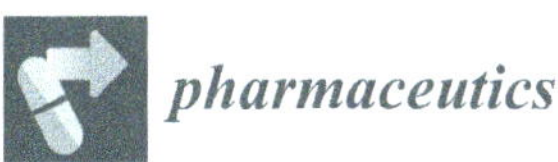

Review

Mechanical Activation by Ball Milling as a Strategy to Prepare Highly Soluble Pharmaceutical Formulations in the Form of Co-Amorphous, Co-Crystals, or Polymorphs

Luz María Martínez *, Jorge Cruz-Angeles, Mónica Vázquez-Dávila, Eduardo Martínez, Paulina Cabada, Columba Navarrete-Bernal and Flor Cortez

Tecnologico de Monterrey, School of Engineering and Sciences, Ave. Eugenio Garza Sada 2501 Sur, Monterrey 64849, NL, Mexico
* Correspondence: luzvidea@tec.mx; Tel.: +52-8183-581-400

Abstract: Almost half of orally administered active pharmaceutical ingredients (APIs) have low solubility, which affects their bioavailability. In the last two decades, several alternatives have been proposed to modify the crystalline structure of APIs to improve their solubility; these strategies consist of inducing supramolecular structural changes in the active pharmaceutical ingredients, such as the amorphization and preparation of co-crystals or polymorphs. Since many APIs are thermosensitive, non-thermal emerging alternative techniques, such as mechanical activation by milling, have become increasingly common as a preparation method for drug formulations. This review summarizes the recent research in preparing pharmaceutical formulations (co-amorphous, co-crystals, and polymorphs) through ball milling to enhance the physicochemical properties of active pharmaceutical ingredients. This report includes detailed experimental milling conditions (instrumentation, temperature, time, solvent, etc.), as well as solubility, bioavailability, structural, and thermal stability data. The results and description of characterization techniques to determine the structural modifications resulting from transforming a pure crystalline API into a co-crystal, polymorph, or co-amorphous system are presented. Additionally, the characterization methodologies and results of intermolecular interactions induced by mechanical activation are discussed to explain the properties of the pharmaceutical formulations obtained after the ball milling process.

Keywords: drug; amorphous; milling; co-crystals; polymorphs; mechanical activation

Citation: Martínez, L.M.; Cruz-Angeles, J.; Vázquez-Dávila, M.; Martínez, E.; Cabada, P.; Navarrete-Bernal, C.; Cortez, F. Mechanical Activation by Ball Milling as a Strategy to Prepare Highly Soluble Pharmaceutical Formulations in the Form of Co-Amorphous, Co-Crystals, or Polymorphs. *Pharmaceutics* **2022**, *14*, 2003. https://doi.org/10.3390/pharmaceutics14102003

Academic Editor: Korbinian Löbmann

Received: 22 August 2022
Accepted: 14 September 2022
Published: 21 September 2022

Publisher's Note: MDPI stays neutral with regard to jurisdictional claims in published maps and institutional affiliations.

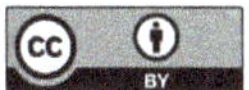

1. Introduction

Almost half of the oral administered commercial drugs have low solubility, which affects their bioavailability [1,2]. Several alternatives to modify the supramolecular structure of APIs have been proposed to overcome their low solubility; these strategies include amorphization [3–5], solid dispersion [6–9], preparation of co-crystals [10,11], and polymorphs [12–14], among others. These approaches to enhance solubility involve non-covalent interactions, such as the electrostatic or intermolecular interactions between API molecules and the components of pharmaceutical formulations. Non-covalent interactions are preferred because they do not alter the pharmacological activity of the APIs. The selection of each strategy to improve the drugs' properties depends on the particular API's chemical nature. Preparation methodologies of drug formulations also depend on API properties, such as structural and thermal stability. Considering that many APIs are thermosensitive, non-thermal emerging alternative techniques, such as mechanical activation or milling, have become an increasingly common preparation method for co-amorphous, co-crystals, and polymorph drugs.

Several publications present overviews of specific applications of milling for the development of pharmaceutical products. In 2013, Braga et al. [15] presented a summary of scientific literature on the preparation of only co-crystals, while Einfal et al. [16] published, in the same year, a summary of amorphization of APIs by milling. Furthermore, in 2015 an overview of different milling techniques for improving the solubility of poorly water-soluble drugs was published [17]; this last article covered different types of milling, but focused its analysis on particle size reduction. Although these reviews are complete within their specific scopes, the authors of the present work believe that ball milling is a technique that has become one of the most widely used methods to enhance a drug's physicochemical properties. For this reason, a summary of recent research in preparing and characterizing pharmaceutical formulations through ball milling to improve APIs' physical-chemical properties is worth an update on this topic.

The present review summarizes the most representative studies that applied ball milling to obtain different formulations with the enhanced properties of either co-crystal or co-amorphous systems, using low molecular weight components and polymorphs. First, a general description of these types of formulations is presented. Then, an analysis and comparison of the available information of milling conditions reported and their effects on improving drug properties are discussed. Unlike previously published reviews, this is the only work in which the solubility, phase transitions, structural stability, and characterization results of intermolecular interactions induced by mechanical activation are compared and presented together for co-crystals, co-amorphs, and polymorphs drugs.

2. Pharmaceutical Formulations Based on Structural Properties

2.1. Amorphous Pharmaceutical Formulations Prepared by Milling

An amorphous solid has no long-range order of molecular packing and lacks a well-defined molecular conformation. Amorphization has been introduced as a promising alternative to enhance drugs' solubility in the last two decades. It has been demonstrated that amorphous materials usually have a higher solubility and dissolution rate than their crystalline state [18,19]. The enhancement of solubility in amorphous materials can be explained, in terms of the ease of overcoming intermolecular forces [20–22]. One of the most common techniques to achieve amorphization is the process of melt quenching. This process consists of melting a crystalline sample and then proceeding to rapid cooling, thus obtaining the amorphous state [23–25]. This method presents disadvantages for thermosensitive drugs, since the high temperatures required to achieve melting may result in thermal decomposition. The study performed by Wlodarski et al. [26] is a clear example of the wide range of thermosensitive drugs that currently exist with low solubility that cannot be obtained in the amorphous state by melt quenching. Due to this drawback, mechanical stress is a non-thermal alternative introduced for amorphization. It has been proven that milling allows for the transformations of the solid crystalline state of matter, thus causing a shift from the crystalline form to the amorphous state [27,28]. The milling process consists of decreasing the compound particle size, thus promoting the accumulation of energy to such a degree that it goes over the critical value that causes a structural deformation of the crystalline structure, which results in the amorphization of the material [29]. However, due to having higher entropy and free energy than the corresponding crystals, the amorphous state is inherently unstable, and recrystallization may occur [30]. The preparation of binary systems forming intermolecular interactions has been reported to avoid recrystallization [30–33]. The selection of a co-former to obtain a co-amorphous system can be a second drug or an excipient, such as sugars, organic acids, amino acids, or surfactants [34–37]. For the reviewed studies in this work, the milling process for amorphization is solely reported under drying conditions. It has been observed that the addition of a solvent in the milling process tends to induce co-crystallization [38].

Besides amorphization, it is important to understand that ball milling is a technique that can lead to the formation of a microcrystalline (or nanocrystalline) state, where this last state involves particle size reduction without the deformation of the crystalline structure. Microcrystallinity results in an increased surface area, higher drug solubility, and increased dissolution rate [39].

There are multiple techniques, such as X-ray diffraction, dynamic light scattering, infrared and Raman spectroscopy, differential scanning calorimetry, and scanning electron microscopy, that are useful techniques for differentiating the microcrystalline and analysis of amorphous states. The following section presents drug formulations in the form of co-crystals.

2.2. Drug Co-Crystals Prepared by Mechanical Activation

Another strategy to enhance solubility with the mixtures of two components is the formation of co-crystals. Co-crystals have acquired different definitions over the years; generally, a co-crystal is a solid material composed of two or more molecules in the same crystal lattice.

Pharmaceutical co-crystals are crystalline single-phase materials composed of two or more compounds. Co-crystals typically consist of an API and one or more additional molecular or ionic compounds called "co-formers" that are kept together via hydrogen bond or electrostatic interactions [10,40–42]. A cocrystal has a different crystal structure to either of the starting materials and, as a result, different physicochemical properties [43]. Figure 1 shows a schematic representation of a co-crystal structure, compared with a co-amorphous system and polymorph. Co-crystals are prepared by different methods, such as the supercritical anti-solvent (SAS) process [44], extrusion [45], freeze-drying [46], spray drying [47], and laser radiation [48]. However, chemical integrity is not always maintained with these preparation methodologies. Some limitations are sometimes encountered, like solubility of the components in a given solvent or solvent mixture and thermal degradation. As a counterpart, mechanochemical methods have also proven effective for co-crystal formation; the preparation of co-crystal by mechanical activation can be achieved by dry and liquid-assisted grinding [49–51]. Several studies report the preparation of co-crystals by grinding with a mortar [52,53]. However, those results are not included in this review.

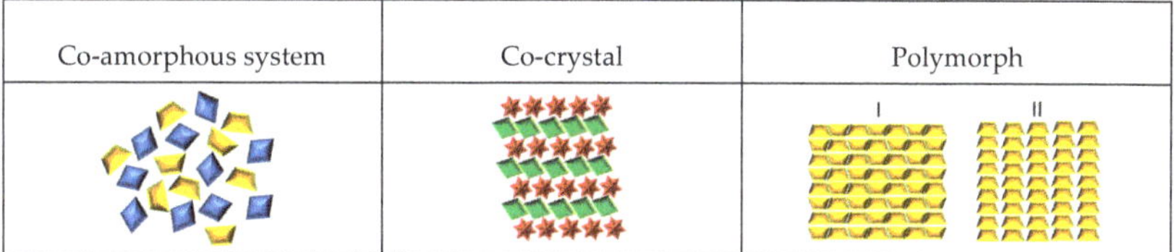

Co-amorphous system	Co-crystal	Polymorph

Figure 1. Schematic representation of API formulations: co-amorphous system, co-crystal, and polymorph.

2.3. Drug Polymorphs as a Result of the Milling Process

It is estimated that about 80–90% of organic compounds are polymorphic [54]. Polymorphic solids exist in multiple crystalline solid forms [55–58]. It is well-known that changing the arrangement of atoms, molecules, or ions within a crystalline lattice raises the differences in physicochemical properties, including the solubility and bioavailability [59]. Therapeutic efficacy is also affected by structural arrangements [54]. One example of a polymorphism affecting drug properties is when a drug interconverts into more and less soluble forms, thus limiting its absorption and bioavailability [12]. There is a wide range of methodologies to prepare polymorphs: crystallization from a single or mixed solvent [60], exposure to organic vapor [61], dehydration of solvates by heat or by slurry [62], seeding [63], laser-induced [64], or supercritical fluid crystallization [65] are some of these preparation methods. However, this review is focused on the obtention of polymorphic forms using ball milling. The occurrence of polymorphism is not limited to single component formulations, but its existence has also been documented in multicomponent systems, such as co-crystals, salts, solvates, and hydrates [57]. Some examples are addressed later in this review.

Below are some of the schematic representations of the previously described systems (see Figure 1).

Various factors can individually change and influence the final characteristics of an active pharmaceutical ingredient after milling. Therefore, it is necessary to identify the prevailing conditions under which amorphous systems, co-crystals, and polymorphs are obtained using griding or milling. In the following sections, the analyses of each experimental condition are presented.

3. Factors Affecting Drug Formulations during the Mechanical Activation Process

Tables 1–3 present an overview of the experimental milling conditions, such as the instrument (type of mill), solvent, time, and temperature, which are reported for each type of drug formulation. The first column contains a code with one number and a letter identifying each drug formulation in all tables. In each code, the number refers to a consecutive numeration of the article reviewed, and the letter stands for the following criteria: A, amorphous; C, co-crystal; and P, polymorph.

3.1. Ball Milling Instruments

After reviewing the information presented in Tables 1–3, it can be inferred that a planetary ball mill is the type of mill most commonly used in all three types of drug formulations. Planetary instruments have vessels placed inside a rotating disk and can induce high energy to the powder to prompt changes. Zirconium oxide (ZrO_2) and stainless-steel milling jars are the most common cells used for polymorphs and amorphous, whereas stainless steel alone is the most used for co-crystals. In most cases, the milling jar material is the same as the milling balls, except for the work of co-crystals reported by Stolar et al. [66], who use a different material: polymethylmethacrylate for the milling jar and stainless steel for the balls. Only Manin et al. [67] report the use of agate. For oscillatory/vibrational mills, the milling speed ranges from 10 to 30 Hz for all drug formulations. The most common speed for amorphous and co-crystals is 30 Hz. No trend is observed for polymorphs. In planetary mills, values reported ranges from 4.2 to 10.8 Hz for amorphous, with 6.7 Hz being the most common value for all formulations (amorphous, polymorphs, and co-crystals).

3.2. Temperature during the Milling Process

From Table 1, it was observed that, for amorphous systems, most milling processes were carried out in cold conditions (4–6 °C) or cryogenic temperatures (cell dips in liquid nitrogen), whereas for co-crystals, the temperature commonly used for grinding was room temperature. For polymorphs, the milling temperatures reported range from cryogenic temperature to 130 °C, although room temperature was the most common condition (see Tables 2 and 3).

3.3. Phase Transformation Mechanism by Ball Milling and Temperature Effect

The process of amorphization by milling can be explained from different perspectives. One of them indicates that, when a crystalline material is milled under direct collision, the first thing that is caused is the reduction of the material's particle size, which is accompanied by changes in morphology and crystallinity. Understanding that if this milling process is carried out below the glass transition temperature (Tg) of the material (because, at this point, the molecular mobility decreases), amorphization is facilitated [16,17,27,68,69].

For co-crystallization there are three accepted mechanisms using grinding methods, i.e., molecular diffusion, and eutectic formation, which are mediated by an amorphous phase. The molecular diffusion mechanism is representative of the solvent/liquid-assisted grinding method. When drops of solvent are used for a mixture with components that are similar, in terms of solubility, the liquid solvent serves as a medium for promoting molecular diffusion and facilitating the interaction between the drug and co-former [15]. Moreover, the eutectic co-crystallization mechanism suggests that, when two solids are in physical contact by grinding at the eutectic temperature, there is a liquid phase formation, where the solid remains from both original crystals work as seeds for the co-crystallization process. [70–72]. Lastly, grinding can also induce enough disorder in solid mixtures to promote an amorphous phase formation. Storage or milling conditions, such as solvents and water presence, can increase molecular mobility and promote the co-crystallization of previously formed amorphous phases [73].

The polymorph formation mechanism upon milling is strongly related to several factors induced by the mechanical stress of high-energy milling. The main factors are temperature and microstructural changes, such as the size of crystallites, crystalline defects, and lattice distortions; these factors are believed to work collectively.

As previously mentioned in the mechanism for amorphization by milling, when milling occurs below the glass transition temperature, the material leads to amorphization; however, when milling occurs at a temperature above Tg, the material leads to polymorphic transformations, whereby in the formation of polymorphs by grinding the amorphous state is an intermediate state [74,75].

In addition to temperature, experimental work shows that a certain extent of defects in the system are necessary to trigger the polymorphic transformation. For most crystalline compounds, the stress applied during mechanical milling can create new defects in their crystal lattices and contribute to lattice disorder. The nucleation and growth of the new lattice defects formed within the structure may result in solid-state polymorphic interconversion upon milling [75,76]. Evidence of these factors affecting the formation of polymorphs is the study of the conversion of ranitidine hydrochloride from form 1 into form 2 [74]. Grinding of form 1 generates large amounts of heat and vibrational energy, giving rise to grinding-induced crystal lattice disruption or process-induced disorder. The formation of an amorphous intermediate follows the elimination of form 1 crystals. Finally, through continuous milling, form 2 nuclei are produced.

An analysis of experimental data related to the temperature effect during phase transformation by milling is shown in Table 1. It was observed that, for amorphous systems, most milling processes were carried out in cold conditions (4–6 °C) or cryogenic temperatures (cell dips in liquid nitrogen). This is consistent with the mechanism proposed, in which it was established that amorphization occurs at a temperature below the glass transition temperature. For co-crystals, the temperature commonly used for grinding was room temperature. This could be explained because mechanical activation generates heat during milling, and the sample is exposed to temperatures near or above the glass transition temperature. For polymorphs, the milling temperatures reported ranges from cryogenic temperature to 130 °C, although room temperature was the most common condition (see Tables 2 and 3).

3.4. Solvent Effect

Dry ball milling (DBM) is when a sample is subjected to the milling procedure under dry conditions. Terms such as "wet grinding", "solvent-drop grinding", "liquid assisted grinding", and "kneading" all imply that a solvent is involved, whether by intention or not (air humidity) [15]. In 2006, Friscić et al. changed the solvent drop grinding term into liquid-assisted grinding (LAG) [77], which became the most frequently used expression to indicate a grinding process with a tiny amount of solvent [15]. According to Tables 1–3, most studies prepared the formulation by adding a solvent to induce co-crystallization. In contrast, co-amorphous and polymorphs were mainly obtained under dry conditions. Additionally, it has been observed that the addition of a small amount of solvent increases the rate of co-crystallization [51] by a process called solution-mediated phase transformation [78]. Therefore, most co-crystals require adding a particular solvent to improve the miscibility of the drug and co-formers. Whereas, for polymorphs, adding a solvent also allows for accessibility to new metastable forms and a shorter experimental time to obtain new polymorphs [79]. It has been shown that the chemical properties of the solvent can lead to a specific polymorph [79–83].

3.5. Effect Changing Composition

Most of the co-crystals prepared by milling use the 1:1 molar ratio; from all the articles reviewed, just five studies prepared co-crystals using molar ratios of 2:1 or 1:2. A similar situation was observed for co-amorphous formulations, although it was common to find studies with molar ratios 1:1, 1:2, and 2:1. Just one study reported a formulation with a molar ratio 1:4 and 1:5 (see Table 1).

3.6. Milling Time

Tables 1–3 show that adequate milling time to produce an intended structural change varies between studies. When a thermosensitive drug is subjected to milling, it is necessary to program pauses at specific times to maintain low temperatures. Nonetheless, there are studies with no thermosensitive drugs that have reported milling times between 30 to 180 min with no breaks.

For the preparation of co-crystals, short periods between 20 to 60 min are reported, although one study reported 5 h [44]. Milling time for polymorphs is longer than for co-crystals; usually, the required time is longer than one hour, and one study even lasted 10 h [34]. Moreover, when there are more than two polymorphic structures of the compound, the increase in milling time can lead to several transformations or what is called two-step polymorphisms.

For co-amorphous, the milling time varies, depending on the type of mill and milling temperature; however, the most common time range is between 60 and 180 min.

In all drug formulations studied here, a difficulty emerges in characterizing all of the properties of the drug formulations obtained by milling with one single analytical method. As a result, in an effort to study their enhanced properties, a wide number of characterization techniques are used to study them. The most used techniques for characterization in all drug formulations (amorphs, co-crystals, and polymorphs) are XRD and thermal techniques, followed by FT-IR. That is the main reason why this review focuses on a detailed analysis of characterization results and the primary information that can be obtained from each characterization method.

Table 1. Conditions of preparation of co-amorphs by ball milling method.

#	Drug 1	Drug 2 Molar-Ratio	Amorphous Stability (Storage-Conditions)	Mill Type	Volume Cell Material	Balls-Num. Material and Sample Weight	Milling Frequency	Milling Temp. (°C)	Milling Time	Ref.
1A	Mebendazole Carvedilol Carbamazepine Simvastatin Indomethacin Furosemide	Twenty different amino acids 1:1	Not reported	Oscillatory ball mill	25 mL Jar	2 (d = 12 mm) stainless steel balls 1000 mg	30 Hz	Not specified	1, 5, 15, 30, and 60 min	[84]
2A	Furosemide Nitrofurantoin Cimetidine Mebendazole	Arginine Citrulline	Dry conditions at 25 °C or 40 °C for 15 months of storage	Oscillatory ball mill	25 mL Jar	2 (d = 12 mm) stainless steel balls 750 mg	30 Hz	5 °C	180 min	[85]
3A	Sulfathiazole Sulfadimidine	Polyvinylpyrrolidone Xpvp: 0.6 and 0.7	Storage at 4 °C over a year	Planetary mill	50 cm³ ZrO₂ milling jars	3 balls (d = 20 mm) ZrO₂. 2.5 g	6.6 Hz	Room temperature	10 h (15 h total) 10 min pauses after every 20 min	[86]
4A	Naproxen	Cimetidine 1:2, 1:1, 2:1	Dry conditions at 4, 25 and 40 °C for up to 33 days or further extended to 186 days	Oscillatory ball mill	25 mL stainless steel milling jar	2 (d = 12 mm) stainless steel balls 1 g of sample per grinding cell	30 Hz	4 °C ± 2 °C	60 min	[87]
5A	γ-Indomethacin	Ranitidine hydrochloride 2:1, 1:1, 1:2	Dry conditions at 4, 25, and 40 °C up to 30 days	Oscillatory ball mill	25 mL stainless steel milling jar	2 (d = 12 mm) stainless steel balls 1 g of sample per grinding cell	30 Hz	4 °C ± 2 °C	60 min	[28]
6A	γ-Indomethacin α-Indomethacin	None	Not reported Not reported	Oscillatory ball mill	25 mL stainless steel milling jar	6 (d = 9 mm) stainless steel balls 1 g of sample per grinding cell	30 Hz	4 °C ± 2 °C immersion in liquid nitrogen	6 h	[88]
7A	Tadalafil	None	Not reported Not reported	6770 SPEX freezer/mill Planetary ball mill	Stainless steel vessel 250 mL zirconium jar	Stainless steel rod (no balls) 1 g of sample per grinding cell 6 zirconia balls (d = 20 mm) 16 g of sample per grinding cell	15 Hz 6.6 Hz	Cryogenic temperature (liquid nitrogen) Room temperature	10 min grinding, 3 min cool-down (2 h total) 15 min cycles, 5 min breaks (24 h total)	[26]
8A	Glibenclamide	None	Not reported	6770 SPEX freezer/mill	Stainless steel vessel	Stainless steel rod (no balls) 1 g	15 Hz	Cryogenic temperature (liquid nitrogen)	6 min grinding, 3 min cool-down (3 h total)	[89]
9A	Trehalose dihydrate	None	Not reported	Spex SamplePrep 6870 freezer/mill	Polycarbonate vials (23.9 cm³) with steel end caps	Magnetic rod (no balls) 1 g	15 cycles per second	Cryogenic temperature (liquid nitrogen)	2 min milling, 1 min of cool-down (30 min total)	[90]

Table 1. *Cont.*

#	Drug 1	Drug 2 Molar-Ratio	Amorphous Stability (Storage-Conditions)	Mill Type	Volume Cell Material	Balls-Num. Material and Sample Weight	Milling Frequency	Milling Temp. (°C)	Milling Time	Ref.
10A	Atenolol	Hydrochlorothiazide 1:1, 1:2, and 2:1	Stored in desiccators at 4 °C and 25 °C for 30 days	6770 SPEX freezer/mill	Airtight tube	1 g	10 Hz	Cryogenic temperature (liquid nitrogen)	2 min milling, 2 min cool down (48 min total)	[91]
11A	Furosemide / Indomethacin	Tryptophan 1:1 / Arginine	Not reported	Oscillatory ball mill	25 mL jars	2 stainless steel balls (d = 12 mm) 500 mg	30 Hz	6 °C	90 min	[92]
12A	Dexamethasone	None	Not reported	High-energy planetary mill	43 cm³ ZrO₂ milling jars	7 ZrO₂ balls (d = 15 mm) 1.1 g	6.6 Hz	Room temperature	15 min milling, 5 min cool down (12 h total)	[27]
13A	α-Lactose	None	Not reported	Planetary ball mill	12 cm³ stainless steel jar	50 stainless steel balls (d = 5 mm) 1 g	6.6 Hz	30 ± 5% relative humidity and 22 ± 3 °C	20 min milling, 5 min cool down (1–20 h total)	[93]
14A	α-D-Glucose	None	Not reported	High-energy planetary mill	45 cm³ ZrO₂ milling jar	7 ZrO₂ balls (d = 1.5 cm) 1 g	5 Hz	−15 °C / 25 °C	20 min milling 10 min cool down (1 and 14 h total)	[58]
15A	Mebendazole / Tadalafil / Piroxicam	Aspartame 1:1/1:1:1 / Phenylalanine 1:1/1:1:1	Stored in desiccators at 40 °C and 25 °C up to 4 months	Oscillatory ball mill	25 mL ball milling jars	2 stainless steel balls (d = 12 mm) 500 mg	30 Hz	5 °C (cold room)	90 min	[94]
16A	α-D-Glucose / β-Glucose	None	Not reported / Not reported	High-energy planetary mill	45 cm³ ZrO₂ milling jar	7 ZrO₂ balls (d = 1.5 cm) 1 g	5 Hz	−15 °C / 25 °C	20 min milling, 10 min cool down (1, 14 h total)	[95]
17A	Carvedilol / Carbamazepine / Furosemide / Indomethacin / Mebendazole / Simvastatin	11 different amino acids 1:1	Stored at 25 °C under dry conditions for up to 2 years	Mixer mill MM400	25 mL stainless steel jars	2 stainless steel balls (d = 12 mm) 1000 mg	30 Hz	6 °C (cold room)	90 min	[31]
18A	Salts of indomethacin	Lysine 1:1	Stored at 25 °C, and 40 °C under dry conditions up to 36 weeks	Vibrational ball mill	25 mL milling jars	2 stainless steel balls (d = 12 mm) 1000 mg	30 Hz	6 °C (cold room)	60 min	[96]
19A	Mebendazole	Tryptophan Xdrug = 0.1, 0.3, and 0.5	Not reported	Vibrational ball mill	50 mL stainless steel jars	2 stainless steel balls (d = 12 mm)	30 Hz	Room temperature	60, 120, and 150 min	[97] unpublished data

Table 1. *Cont.*

#	Drug 1	Drug 2 Molar-Ratio	Amorphous Stability (Storage-Conditions)	Mill Type	Volume Cell Material	Balls-Num. Material and Sample Weight	Milling Frequency	Milling Temp. (°C)	Milling Time	Ref.
20A	18 different drugs	NaTC natural bile acid surfactant sodium taurocholate 1:1	Stored at 22 ± 2 °C	Oscillatory ball mill	25 mL stainless steel jar	1 stainless steel ball (d = 15-mm) 1 g	25 Hz	Room temperature and −10 ± 2 °C	180 min. total time, with 10 min. break every 30 min; 120 min, with 7.5 min breaks cooled in liquid nitrogen	[37]
21A	Carbamazepine; Indomethacin	Arginine; Phenylalanine; Tryptophan	Not reported	Oscillatory ball mill	25 mL stainless steel jar	2 stainless steel ball (d = 12 mm) 500 mg	30 Hz	6 °C	90 min	[98]
22A	(S)-Naproxen	L-arginine	Stored at 25 °C, and 40 °C under dry conditions	Oscillatory ball mill	25 mL stainless steel jar	2 stainless steel ball (d = 12 mm) 1 g	30 Hz	6 °C	60 min	[99]
23A	Griseofulvin	Aspartic Ac; Lysine; Methionine; Valine; Tryptophan	Stored at 23–28 °C under dry conditions up to 12 months	High-energy planetary ball mill	Stainless steel crucible	3 stainless steel balls 2.5 g	9.3 Hz	Not specified	6 h, with 0.5 min pauses every 30 min	[100]
24A	Naproxen	Tryptophan and proline	Stored at 40 °C under dry conditions up to 332 days	Oscillatory ball mill	25 mL stainless steel jar	2 stainless steel ball (d = 12 mm) 1 g	30 Hz	6 °C	90 min	[101]
25A	Mebendazole	None; Dipeptide 1:1; Aminoacid mixtures 1:1:1	Stored at 40 °C under dry conditions up 4 weeks or 3 months	Oscillatory ball mill	25 mL stainless steel jar	2 stainless steel ball (d = 12 mm) 500 mg	30 Hz	5 °C	90–180 min	[102]
26A	Oxaprozin	RameβCD 1:1; RameβCD-Arg. 1:1:1	Not reported	High-energy vibrational micro mill	Not specified	Not specified	24 Hz	Not specified	30 min	[103]
27A	Furosemide; γ-Indomethacin; γ-Indomethacin + CA	Arginine 1:1	Not reported	Vibrational ball milling	25 mL stainless steel jar	2 stainless steel ball (d = 9 mm) 500 mg	25 Hz	6 °C	99 min	[104]
28A	Indomethacin; Furosemide	L-tryptophan 1:1	Not reported	Oscillatory ball mill	25 mL stainless steel jar	2 stainless steel ball (d = 12 mm) 1500 mg	30 Hz	6 °C	0, 5, 15, 30, 45, 60, and 90 min. 3 or 6 h	[105]

Table 1. *Cont.*

#	Drug 1	Drug 2 Molar-Ratio	Amorphous Stability (Storage-Conditions)	Mill Type	Volume Cell Material	Balls-Num. Material and Sample Weight	Milling Frequency	Milling Temp. (°C)	Milling Time	Ref.
29A	Naproxen	Naproxen sodium 2:1, 1:1, and 1:2	Stored at 40 °C under dry conditions up to 2 weeks or 2 months	Oscillatory ball mill	25 mL stainless steel jar	2 stainless steel ball (d = 12 mm) 500 mg	30 Hz	4 °C	90 min	[106]
30A	Carvedilol	Glutamic Ac / Aspartic Ac	Not reported	Vibrational ball mill	25 mL stainless steel jar	2 stainless steel ball (d = 12 mm) 700 mg	30 Hz	6 °C	60 min	[107]
31A	Indomethacine	Arginine / Phenylalanine / Tryptophan	Stored in refrigerator (≈5 °C)	Mixer mill MM400	25 mL stainless steel jar	2 stainless steel ball (d = 12 mm) 500 mg	30 Hz	Not specified	60 min, with 10 min pauses; cell would be in liquid nitrogen for 2 min	[6]
32A	Simvastatin / Glibenclamide	Lysine / Serine / Threonine / Aspartic acid	Stored in desiccators at 4 °C	Oscillatory ball mill	25 mL stainless steel jar	2 stainless steel ball (d = 15 mm) 500 mg	30 Hz	Not specified	60 min. with 10 min. pauses cell would be in liquid nitrogen for 2 min	[108]
33A	Indomethacin / Carbamazepine	Arginine / Tryptophan / Tyrosine / Phenylalanine	Stored at 40 °C under dry conditions	Oscillatory ball mill	25 mL stainless steel jar	2 stainless steel ball (d = 12 mm) 500 mg	30 Hz	6 °C	90 min	[98]
34A	Indomethacin	Tryptophan	-	Oscillatory mill	12 mL Stainless steel jar	2 stainless steel ball (d = 10 mm) 1.2 g	10.83 Hz	Not specified	360 min	[109]
35A	Carbamazepine	Citric acid	Stored at 40 °C under dry conditions up to 2 months	Oscillatory ball mill	25 mL stainless steel jar	2 stainless steel ball (d = 12 mm) 500 mg	30 Hz	4 °C	90–180 min	[10]
36A	Arginine / Serine / Quercetin	Glibenclamide 1:1	Stored at 4 °C, room temperature, and 40 °C up to 13 months	Oscillatory ball mill	25 mL milling chambers	2 stainless steel balls (d = 12 mm) 500 mg	30 HZ	Not specified	60 min, chambers were cooled in liquid nitrogen	[11]
37A	Glutamic ac / L-arginine / Glutamic Ac-Arginine / Arginine-glutamic ac / Glutamic-arginine	Mebendazole 1:1 and 1:1:1	Stored at 40 °C and 25 °C in desiccators under dry conditions up to 6 months	Oscillatory ball mill	25 mL stainless steel jar	2 stainless steel ball (d = 1.2 cm) 500 mg	30 Hz	5 °C (cold room)	30, 60, and 90 min	[12]

Table 1. *Cont.*

#	Drug 1	Drug 2 Molar-Ratio	Amorphous Stability (Storage-Conditions)	Mill Type	Volume Cell Material	Balls-Num. Material and Sample Weight	Milling Frequency	Milling Temp. (°C)	Milling Time	Ref.
38A	Mefenamic acid	Meglumine 1:1, 1:2, and 1:4	Not reported	Planetary ball mill	Not specified	5 stainless steel balls (d = 10 mm)	4.16 Hz	Not specified	20 min	[113]
	Indomethacin	PVP 1:1, 1:2, and 1:4								
39A	L-methionine	Rutin 1:1, 1:2, 2:1	Not reported	Planetary ball mill	45 mL zirconia jar	8 YTZ balls (d = 10 mm)	10 Hz	Room temperature	12 h with a break every 10 min	[114]
	Naringin hydrate									
	Quercetin dihydrate									
	Hesperidin Chlorothiazide Indapamide Triamterene Nifedipine									
40A	Benzamidine	Gliclazide 1:1, 1:5, or 5:1	Stored in a desiccator at 22 ± 2 °C, and 40 °C under relative humidity up to 180 days	Oscillatory ball mill	25 mL stainless steel milling jar	Stainless steel ball (d = 15 mm) 0.25 g	25 Hz	Cromilling inmersing jars in liquid nitrogen for 5 min prior to milling. 7.5 min milling	180 min, with a cool down period of 15 min after every 30 min	[38]
41A	Arginine	Quercetin 1:1, 1:2	Not reported	Not specified	25 mL stainless steel	1–3 stainless steel ball (d = 18, 15, and 12 mm)	Not specified	2 h	Not specified	[115]
	Glutamic acid									
	Aspartic acid									
	Tryptophan									
	Glycin									
42A	Candesartan cilexetil	Hydrochlorothiazide	Stored at 4 °C, 30 °C, and 40 °C under dry conditions up to 90 days	Planetary ball mill	125 mL stainless steel grinding jars	3 stainless steel grinding balls (d = 10-mm) 2 g	9.3 Hz	Room temperature	2.5 h	[116]
		Hydroxypropyl methylcellulose								
		Acetate succinate (HPMCAS) type M								

Table 2. Conditions of preparation of co-crystals by grinding method.

#	Sample	Molar Ratio	Method of Preparation	Milling Type	Instrument Brand	Milling Jar	Balls (# and Material)	Milling Frequency	Milling Temp	Milling Time	Ref.
1C	Nicotinamide: L-(+)-Ascorbic acid	1:1	Assisted by solvent	Vibrational	Mixer Mill (IST 500) InSolido Technologies	Polymethylmetacrylate	Two stainless steel balls	30 Hz	NR	60 min	[66]
2C	Salicylic acid:2-pyridone Salicylic acid: 4-Pyridone	1:1	NR	Vibrational	Mixer Mill (IST 500) InSolido Technologies	Polymethylmetacrylate	Two stainless steel balls	30 Hz	NR	50 min	[117]
3C	Ciprofloxacin-thymol	1:2	Assisted by solvent (EtOH)	NR	Retsch MM200 ball miller,	NR	NR	20 Hz	NR	30 min	[118]
4C	Urea-caffeine	1:1	NR	Oscillatory ball	Mixer Mill MM400-Retsch GmbH, Haan	Stainless steel jar	One 15 mm stainless steel ball	25 Hz	Room temperature	60 min	[119]
5C	Brexpiprazol-Catechol Brexpiprazol-Succinic acid	1:1	NR	NR	Nano Ball Mill (Fritsch Premium Line, FRITSCH GmbH, Idar-Oberstein, Germany) using	NR	Stainless steel balls	8.3 Hz	NR	120 min	[120]
6C	Quercetin-malonic acid	1:1 and 1:2	Solvent drop grinding	NR	NR	NR	NR	NR	NR	30 min.	[121]
7C	Paracetamol-trimethylglycine	1:1	NA	Planetary ball	QM-3SP2, Nanjing NTU Instrument Co.	NR	NR	6.6 Hz	NR	5 h	[44]
8C	Meloxicam-benzoic acid	1:1	LAG	NR	Retsch CryoMill	NR	NR	25 Hz	Room temperature	30 min	[122]
9C	Acetazolamide and 4-hydroxybenzoic acid	1:1	LAG	Planetary ball	QM-3SP04, gear type	25 mL stainless steel milling jars	NR	25 Hz	NR	30 min	[123]
10C	Furosemide-urea and carbamazepine-indomethacin	1:1	LAG	NR	Retsch MM400 ball mill	50 mL jar, with two 5 mm stainless steel balls and drops of acetone.	NR	NR	NR	60 min	[51]
11C	Ciprofloxacin-nicotinic and isonicotinic acids	1:1	Assisted or not by solvent (EtOH)	NR	Retsch MM 400 mixer mill	10 mL stainless-steel jars	1 stainless steel ball of 7 mm diameter, 100, 500 mg sample	30 and 15 Hz	NR	30 min	[124]
12C	Pyrazinamide-diflunisal	1:1	LAG	Oscillatory ball mill	Mixer Mill MM400	25 mL stainless steel milling jars	NR	15 Hz	Room temperature	60 min	[125]
13C	Acetazolamide-4-aminobenzoic acid	1:1	With solvent	Planetary ball	Fritsch micro mill model Pulverisette 7	12 mL agate grinding jars	Ten 5 mm agate balls	8.3 Hz	NR	30 min	[67]
14C	Acetazolamide-nicotinamide-2-pyridone	1:1:1	LAG with ethyl acetate and tetrahydrofuran solvents	Planetary ball	QM-3SP04, gear type	25 mL stainless steel milling jars	NR	15 Hz	NR	60 min	[126]

Table 2. *Cont.*

#	Sample	Molar Ratio	Method of Preparation	Milling Type	Instrument Brand	Milling Jar	Balls (# and Material)	Milling Frequency	Milling Temp	Milling Time	Ref.
15C	β-Lapachone-resorcinol	1:1	LAG	NR	Retsh Mixer Mill (Model MW 200)	Stainless steel jar together	A stainless steel ball	20 Hz	NR	20 min	[127]
16C	Norfloxacin-nicotinic acid	NR	NT and LAG	Ocillatory ball system	Mixer Mill MM 400, Retsch GmbH and Co	Stainless steel jars	7 mm diameter stainless steel ball	15 Hz	NR	30 min	[128]
17C	Chlorothiazide, D-proline, L-proline	1:1	NT and LAG	Oscillatory ball	Retsch (MM400, Retsch)	NR	NR	30 Hz	NR	30 min	[129]
18C	Praziquantel, poloxamer F-127, and sucrose stearate	20:1, 10:1, 10:2, and 10:3	NT	High-energy vibrational ball	Mixer Mill MM 200, Retch, GmbH	10 mL volume stainless steel grinding jars	Two 7 mm stainless steel grinding balls	25 Hz	28.10–30.34 °C	30 or 90 min	[130]
19C	Ferulic acid, urea, nicotinamide, and isonicotinamide (INA)	1:1 and 1:2	LAG	NR	Retsch Mixer Mill (model MM301)	Stainless steel grinding jar	One 7 mm stainless steel ball	20 Hz	NR	20 min	[131]
20C	Ketoconazole, fumaric acid, and succinic acid	1:1.1 and 1:1	NT and LAG	Oscillatory ball	Retsch MM 400	25 mL stainless steel jars	One stainless steel ball	19 Hz	NR	60 min	[132]
21C	Itraconazole: 4-aminobenzoic acid Itraconazole: 4-hydroxybenzamide	1:1 2:1 1:2	LAG	Planetary micro	Fritsch planetary micro mill, Pulverisette 7	12 mL agate grinding jars	Ten 5 mm agate balls	8.3 Hz	NR	40 min	[133]
22C	S-ibuprofen: nicotinamide	1:1	N.R	Oscillatory ball	MM400—Retsch	10 mL ZrO$_2$ milling jars	One ball, 10 mm	30 Hz	NR	60 and 10 min and 5 min pauses	[134]
23C	Pyrazinamide: 4-aminosalicylic acid	1:1	LAG	Planetary ball	QM3SP04, gear type, Nanjing University Instrument Factory	20 mL stainless steel grinding tank	N.R	20 Hz	Room temperature	40 min	[135]
24C	Theophylline: 4-aminobenzoic acid	1:1	N.R	N.R	MM 400, Retsch, Germany	10 mL jar 25 mL jar	One ball, 8.74 mm, One ball, 13.72 mm	30 Hz	N.R	Period times: 2,5,10, 15, 20, and 25 min	[136]
25C	Betulin-terephthalic acid	1:1 2:1	Assisted by solvent	NR	SPEX 8000 mixer mill (CertiPrep Inc., Metuchen, NJ, USA)	60 mL steel jar	Steel balls 6 mm	NR	NR	Pre-milled: 5 min After solvent: 10 min	[137]
26C	5-Fluorocytosine:5-fluorouracil	1:1	NT SDG	Oscillatory	Mixer Mill MM400 RETSCH	25-mL stainless steel milling jar	Two 7 mm stainless steel balls	25 Hz	Room temperature	90 min SDG: 60 min	[138]
27C	Nicotinamide:adipic acid (polymorph, form 2)	1:1	Assisted by solvent (acetonitrile)	NR	Retsch MM400 mill (in-house modified)	Stainless steel milling jar	Two 7 mm stainless steel balls	30 Hz	NR	60–90 min	[139]

LAG: liquid assisted grinding; NT: neat grinding, SDG: solvent drop-grinding; NR: not reported.

Table 3. Conditions of preparation of polymorphs by mechanical activation.

#	Sample	Obtained Polymorph	Mill Type	Milling Cell	Ball (#, Material) Sample Weight	Milling Frequency	Milling Temperature	Milling Time and Solvent	Ref.
1P	Ranitidine hydrochloride	Ranitidine hydrochloride, form 2	Oscillatory ball mill (mixer mill MM301, Retsch GmbH and Co., Weinheim, Germany)	25 mL Stainless steel	2 stainless steel balls ($d = 12$ mm) 1 g s	30 Hz	$12 \pm 3\,^{\circ}\mathrm{C}$	180 min, stop every 30 min to scrape and remix powder	[74]
		Ranitidine, form 2 (with traces of form 1)					$35\,^{\circ}\mathrm{C}$	120 min, stop every 30 min to scrape and remix powder	
		Ranitidine, form 2						240 min, stop every 30 min to scrape and remix powder	
2P	Chlorhexidine dihydrochloride	2-step polymorphism produces ChxHC form 2 as a precursor of form 3	High-energy planetary mill (Pulverisette 7; Fritsch, Idar-Oberstein)	43 cm^3 ZrO$_2$	7 ZrO$_2$ balls ($d = 15$ mm) 1 g	6.6 Hz	Room temperature	12 h (15 min milling periods with 5 min rests)	[140]
3P	Γ-sorbitol	A form sorbitol	High-energy planetary micro-mill (Pulverisette 7; Fritsch, Idar-Oberstein)	45 cm^3 zirconium	7 zirconium balls ($d = 15$ mm) 1 g of sample	6.6 Hz	Room temperature	10 h	[34]
4P	Rivastigmine (RHT form 2)	RHT form I	Retsch planetary ball mill PM100	50 mL stainless steel	3 stainless steel balls ($d = 20$ mm) 1 g	6.6 Hz	Room temperature	3 h (stopping at 15 min, 30 min, 1 h and 2 h)	[141]
5P	o-Aminobenzoic acid (mixture of FII and FIII forms)	FIII form	Oscillatory ball mill (Mixer mill MM400, Retsch GmbH and Co., Germany)	25 mL stainless steel	One stainless steel ball ($d = 15$ mm) 0.5 g 30 µL of solvent	25 Hz	Room temperature	2.5 h (30 min milling periods with 15 min pauses) Solvent: valeric acid (FIV and FIII)	[54]
		FII form							
	m-Aminobenzoic acid (FIII form)	FIV form							
		FIV and FIII							
	Carbamazepine	FIV form							
	p-aminobenzoic acid	β-PABA							
	o-Aminobenzoic acid (mixture of FII and FIII forms)	FI form (FII converts to FIII and subsequently FIII converts to FI.)			1 stainless steel ball ($d = 15$ mm) 0.5 g 30 µL of solvent		Cryogenic temperature (immersed in liquid N$_2$ for 5 min prior to miling every 7.5 min)	2.5 h (7.5 min milling and 2.5 min pauses in liquid nitrogen) Solvent: valeric acid, 10% acetamide or ethanol. (FI)	
		FI form							
6P	Dexamethasone	DEX form A and B	High-energy planetary mill (Pulverisette 7, Fritsch, Idar-Oberstein)	43 cm^3 ZrO$_2$	7 ZrO$_2$ balls ($d = 15$ mm) 1.1 g	6.6 Hz	Room temperature	12 h (15 min milling periods, with 5 min rests)	[27]

Table 3. *Cont.*

#	Sample	Obtained Polymorph	Mill Type	Milling Cell	Ball (#, Material) Sample Weight	Milling Frequency	Milling Temperature	Milling Time and Solvent	Ref.
7P	Sofosbuvir (anhydrous form 1)	Form A or B	Vibrational ball mill (MM400, RETSCH)	5 mL stainless steel	2 stainless steel balls (d = 5 mm) 50 mg 10 µL of Solvent	25 Hz	Room temperature	30 min Solvent: water or methanol	[79]
		Form A						30 min Solvent: anisole, n-butyl acetate, or ethyl acetate	
		Form A (form 1 changes to form V)						30 min Solvent: anisole	
		Form A						60 min, solvent: tetrahydrofuran	
		Form A (form 1 changes into form B and then forms A)						20 min, solvent: butyl acetate or ethyl acetate	
8P	Sulindac (form II)	Form II and form I	High-energy planetary mill (Pulverisette 7eFritsch)	43 cm^3 ZrO$_2$	7 ZrO$_2$ balls (d = 15 mm) 1 g	6.6 Hz	Room temperature	5 min	[69]
		Form I						600 min (10 min milling, with 5 min pauses)	
		Mixture of form II and form I						20 min (10 min milling periods, with 5 min pauses)	
9P	Γ-sorbitol	A form sorbitol	High-energy planetary mill (Pulverisette 7-Fritsch)	43 cm^3 ZrO$_2$	7 ZrO$_2$ balls (d = 15 mm)	6.6 Hz	Room temperature (dry nitrogen atmosphere)	10 h	[75]
	Mannitol (β)	α Mannitol							
	Mannitol (δ)	α Mannitol							
10P	Famotidine (form B)	Form A (form B to A transformation ratio increased with milling time)	Oscillatory ball mill (Mixer Mill MM301, Retsch GmbH and Co., Germany)	25 mL stainless steel	2 stainless steel balls (d = 12 mm) 0.2 g	15 Hz	130 °C	10 min	[142]
							110 °C	20 min	
							110 °C	30 min	
11P	Gabapentin (GBP) form I	GBP form II	Oscillatory ball mill (Mixer Mill MM301, Retsch GmbH and Co., Germany)	25 mL stainless steel	2 stainless steel balls (d = 15 mm) 0.2 g of sample	20 Hz	Room temperature	120 min	[76]
	GBP form II	GBP form III						105 min	
		GBP form IV						120 min	
	GBP form III	GBP form II						15 min	
		GBP form III (produced by the coexistence of form I and II after 15 min milling)						60 min	
		GBP form IV						105 min	
	GBP form IV	GBP form II						2 min	
		GBP form III						30 min	
		GBP form IV						105 min	

Table 3. *Cont.*

#	Sample	Obtained Polymorph	Mill Type	Milling Cell	Ball (#, Material) Sample Weight	Milling Frequency	Milling Temperature	Milling Time and Solvent	Ref.
12P	Ciprofloxacin salicylate (monohydrate)	Form I (after 4 min of neat grinding) From 2 (after 9.5 min of neat grinding)	Fritsch planetary micro mill, model Pulverisette 7	12 mL agate	10 agate balls (d = 5 mm) 0.1 g 60 µL of solvent	8.3 Hz	NR	50 min, solvent: water, and the use of water/organic solvents decreases the time of existence for form I	[143]
	Ciprofloxacin salicylate (3.67 hydrate)	Form II (after 17 min of neat grinding)							
	Anhydrous ciprofloxacin salicylate	From I							
13P	γ-sorbitol	Form α (complete transformation)	High-energy planetary mill (Pulverisette, 7-Fritsch)	43 cm^3 ZrO$_2$	7 ZrO$_2$ balls (d = 15 mm)	6.6 Hz	Room temperature	180 min (10 min milling periods, with 5 min rests)	[144]
14P	Ethenzamide: ethylmalonic acid (Co-crystal)	Form I (SDG with n-hexane) Form II (after neat grinding or SDG with toluene or cyclohexane)	Oscillatory ball mill (Mixer Mill MM301, Retsch GmbH and Co., Germany)	10 mL stainless steel	1 stainless steel ball (d = 7 mm) 0.1 g of EA and 0.0799 g of EMA (1:1 molar ratio) 0.05 mL of solvent	20 Hz	Room temperature	15 min, solvent: toluene, cyclohexane or n-hexane	[145]
15P	Caffeine: glutaric acid (co-crystal)	Form I (after neat grinding and SDG with n-hexane, cyclohexane or heptane)	Oscillatory ball mill (Mixer Mill, Retsch GmbH and Co., Germany)	Stainless steel (volume NR)	2 stainless stell balls (d = NR) 0.75 g (1:1 molar ratio)	30 Hz	Room temperature	60 min Solvent: n-hexane, cyclohexane, or heptane	[146]

NR: not reported; SDG: solvent drop grinding.

4. Evaluation of Physicochemical Properties of Co-Amorphous, Co-Crystals, and Polymorphs Induced by Mechanical Activation

With the purpose of evaluating the outcomes of the milling process, different characterization techniques are applied to determine structural changes and their effects on the properties of the final pharmaceutical formulation. This section is divided into solubility evaluation, intermolecular interactions by spectroscopic techniques, such as Raman, Infrared, and ss-NMR, phase transitions by thermal analysis techniques, and structural characterization by X-ray diffraction. An overview of results for each kind of drug formulation (amorphous, co-crystal, or polymorph) is presented for each characterization technique. An additional section on characterization techniques by microscopy is included. This last section refers to the methods that have been used little, until the moment of elaboration of this review but that provide relevant information, regarding the formulation's characteristics.

4.1. Evaluation of Solubility Enhancements as an Effect of the Milling Process

Solubility enhancement is an essential property for developing novel drugs. Solubility evaluation results may be expressed in different ways, for example, powder dissolution and intrinsic dissolution rate (IDR); however, both studies compare the solubility enhancement of the crystalline materials and formulation after milling. In the case of powder dissolution, analyses are performed using only the systems in powder. In contrast, the intrinsic dissolution rate (IDR) can be defined as the dissolution of a drug substance under specific conditions, such as a constant surface area and agitation speed [91].

Tables 4 and 5 provide an overview of the solubility results reported for amorphous, co-amorphous, and co-crystals. As mentioned before, in the first column of the tables, a code with a number and letter is used to identify each drug formulation. In each code, the letter stands for the following criteria: A—amorphous, C—co-crystal, and P—polymorph. Note that in Tables 4–6, the codes in the column are not consecutive numbers because not all articles analyzed their formulations with all the characterization techniques. Therefore, data are only exhibited in the tables when the articles performed those studies. All the articles report solubility enhancements in diverse ways, such as folds, solubility value, or dissolution rate, using various units. The articles that did not report folds have been marked with an asterisk (*); to simplify the analysis, those values were converted to folds using the formula:

$$\text{Folds Increase} = \frac{\text{Increased solubility value}}{\text{Solubility value of crystalline or unprocessed material}} \tag{1}$$

It is important to mention that no information of solubility regarding polymorphs (obtained by milling) was found.

(a)   Solubility for co-amorphous systems after ball milling

As seen in Table 4, it is relevant to note that a constant dissolution rate verifies that the drug in the co-milled sample does not recrystallize during dissolution. The steady behavior shows that the interaction between two drugs or drug–excipient in the amorphous binary system is strong and stable enough to prevent structural rearrangement during dissolution. Moreover, extended times in intrinsic dissolution studies (where no changes in rate are observed) show that bioavailability would not be decreased due to recrystallization in in vivo conditions [87]. Except from the LAG sample reported by Kasten et al. [96], the articles typically show a decrease in dissolution rate.

Table 4. Overview of solubility enhancement of amorphous systems prepared by ball milling.

#	Solubility Evaluation (UV, HPLC)	Sample	Ratio/Composition	Solubility Increment (Folds)	Ref.
2A	HPLC (IDR)	Furosemide-arginine	1:1	38	[85]
		Nitrofurantoin-arginine		20	
3A	UV (IDR)	Sulfathiazole-polyvinylpyrrolidone	Xpvp = 0.7	5.2	[86]
		Sulfadimidine-polyvinylpyrrolidone		26.5	
4A	UV (IDR)	Co-milled naproxen	1:1	4	[87]
		Co-milled cimetidine		2	
7A	HPLC (Solubility)	Tadalafil *	N/A	1.25 (in H2O)	[26]
				0.79 (in 0.1 M HCl)	
				1.35 (Buffer pH = 6.8)	
				1.83 (in water)	
10A	UV (IDR)	Atenolol-hydrochlorothiazide	1:1	12.5	[91]
15A	HPLC (Powder dissolution studies)	Mebendazole-ASPA	1:1	8.13	[94]
		Tadalafil-ASPA		Similar increase to MEB but less pronounced	
		Piroxicam-ASPA		32.1–35	
17A	HPLC (IDR)	Fur-Phe, Fur-Pro, Fur-Trp	1:1	0.9–1.0	[31]
		Fur-Ile, Fur-Leu, Fur-Met, Fur-Val, Ind-Ile, Ind-Leu, Ind-Met, Ind-Phe, Ind-Pro, Ind-Trp, Ind-Val, Meb-Met, Cbz-Trp		1.1–3.0	
		Fur-Arg, Fur-His, Fur-Lys, Ind-Arg, Ind-Lys, Car-Ile, Car-Leu, Car-Met, Car-Phe, Car-Trp, Car-Val, Meb-Ile, Meb-Leu, Meb-Phe, Meb-Trp		3.1–431.8	
18A	HPLC (IDR)	Indomethacin-lysine	1:1	90 / 14	[96]
23A	HPLC (Kinetic solubility studies)	Griseofulvin-tryptophan	1:1	1.19	[100]
25A	HPLC (Dissolution tests)	Mebendazole-histidine-glycine	1:1:1	19	[102]
		Mebendazole-tryptophan-phenylalanine	1:1:1	46	
		Mebendazole-proline-tryptophan	1:1:1	4.3	
29A	UV	Naproxen-NAP(Na)	1:1	2.9	[106]
30A	UV (IDR)	Carvedilol-L-glutamic acid	1:1	12	[107]
		Carvedilol-L-aspartic acid		13	
		Carvedilol-L-glutamic acid		14	
		Carvedilol-L-aspartic acid		2	
31A	Dissolution studies	Indomethacin-arginine	1:1	1.4	[36]
		Indomethacin-phenylalanine		1	
		Indomethacin-tryptophan		1	
33A	HPLC (IDR)	Carbamazepine-arginine-tryptophan *	1:1:1	1.38	[98]
		Carbamazepine-phenylalanine-tryptophan *	1:1:1	1.2	
		Carbamazepine-tryptophan *	1:1	1.08	
		Indomethacin-L-arginine *	1:1	306	
		Indomethacin-L-phenylalanine *	1:1	4.3	
		Indomethacin-L-tryptophan *	1:1	2.4	
		Indomethacin-L-phenylalanine-L-tryptophan *	1:1:1	3.35	
35A	UV	Carbamazepine-citric acid	1:1	2.2	[110]
		Carbamazepine-citric acid-arginine	1:1:1	2.68	
		Carbamazepine-citric acid-arginine	1:1:2	3.28	
		Carbamazepine-citric acid-arginine	1:1:3	3.4	

Table 4. *Cont.*

#	Solubility Evaluation (UV, HPLC)	Sample	Ratio/Composition	Solubilty Increment (Folds)	Ref.
36A	HPLC	Glibenclamide-serine	1:1	10	[111]
		Glibenclamide-quercetin	1:1	20	
		Glibenclamide-arginine	1:1	19	
		Glibenclamide-arginine-sls	1:1	21	
37A	HPLC	Mebendazole (Meb)-glutamate-arginine (crystalline salt) *	1:1:1	5.2	[112]
		Meb-glutamate-arginine (amorphous salt) *	1:1:1	3.5	
		Meb-arginineglutamate *	1:1	5.16	
		Meb-glutamatearginine *	1:1	4.9	
38A	HPLC	Indomethacin-meglumine *	1:1	18.56	[113]
			1:2	25.39	
			1:4	28	
		Mefenamic acid-meglumine *	1:1	81	
			1:2	108.6	
			1:4	394.3	
		Indomethacin-polyvinylpyrrolidone *	1:1	0.3	
			1:2	0.3	
			1:4	0.48	
		Mefenamic acid-polyvinylpyrrolidone *	1:1	1.6	
			1:2	4	
			1:4	10.6	
41A	UV	Quercetin-arginine *	1:2	21	[115]

Acronym: IDR: intrinsic dissolution rate.

There are many co-amorphous formulations prepared by milling, in which acidic and basic excipients were used to form salts. The article that shows the highest increase in solubility was published by Kasten et al. [31], using both DBM and LAG as preparation methods. They found that the co-amorphous salt formulations of basic AAs and acidic drugs had the most significant increase in dissolution rate. The use of amino acids, particularly arginine (a basic amino acid)-based salts, showed substantial dissolution enhancement, combined with acid drugs, approximately 140–431.8-fold, when compared to the amorphous drug, possibly due to strong molecular interactions attributed to salt formation. Therefore, the salt formation of an acid-basic system could be a meaningful approach to enhancing solubility properties in drug formulations. Other milling conditions were also analyzed for amorphs and co-crystals to determine if milling conditions directly affect the solubility of the obtained system. Apparently, long milling times do not affect the increase of solubility. Caron et al. [86] measured 15 h, in total, of effective milling, and sulfadimidine-polyvinylpyrrolidone had an increase of 26.5 times its solubility. Whereas Kasten et al. [31] milled a wide variety of samples for a total of 90 min and showed that increases in solubility ranged from 0.9 to 431.8 times.

For co-amorphous, milling time is relevant to obtaining the new drug formulation; nevertheless, once amorphization is achieved, longer milling times do not enhance solubility. This demonstrates that properties and possible interactions between drug–drug or drug–excipient are more important than long milling times to increase solubility. Finally, in Table 4, no trend is observed, regarding the type of mill or milling cell material towards affecting solubility enhancement. These milling conditions are relevant for the obtention of the amorphous and co-amorphous systems. Still, they do not seem to have an impact on the increase of the solubility of the sample. There is a possibility that 30 Hz might be the optimal milling frequency, as the highest increase in solubility was observed at this speed (at 1:1 molar ratio), but it should also be noticed that all these articles [31,85,94,96,102] used amino acids for the experiments, which could be a relevant factor influencing the solubility.

Table 5. Overview of solubility enhancement reported for co-crystal drugs.

#	Solubility Evaluation (UV, HPLC)	Sample	Folds	Ref.
3C	In vitro	Ciprofloxacin-thymol (1:2)	4	[118]
5C	UV	Brexpiprazol-catechol (1:1)	2.5	[120]
		Brexpiprazol-succinic acid (1:1)	2.5	
6C	UV	Quercetin-malonic acid (1:2)	1.056	[121]
7C	UV	Paracetamol-trimethylglycine * (1:1)	0.82	[44]
11C	UV	Ciprofloxacin-nicotinic acid (1:1)	20 (in water)	[124]
			1.5	
		Ciprofloxacin-isonicotinic acid (1:1)	20	
			2.5	
13C	HPLC	Acetazolamide-4-aminobenzoic acid * (1:1)	2.5	[67]
			2.17	
15C	IDR	β-lapachone-resorcinol (1:1)	2	[127]
16C	UV	Norfloxacin-nicotinic acid (with EtOH) pH = 3	No change	[128]
		Norfloxacin-nicotinic acid (with EtOH) pH = 6.1	2	
		Norfloxacin-nicotinic acid (with EtOH) pH = 8.5	<2	
17C	UV (Powder dissolution)	Chlorothiazide-DL-proline (w/acetonitrile-water)	1.05	[129]
		Chlorothiazide-L-proline hydrate (w/acetonitrile-water)	Lower value than the initial drug	
		Chlorothiazide-D-proline hydrate (w/acetonitrile-water)		
19C	HPLC (In vitro release test)	Ferulic acid-nicotinamide	2.4	[131]
		Ferulic acid-isonicotinamide	3.1	
		Ferulic acid-urea	1.1	
21C	HPLC	Itraconazole-4-hydroxybenzamide form II (1:2)	225	[133]
		Itraconazole-4-aminobenzoic acid (1:1)	64	

(b) Solubility of co-crystals after grinding

Comparing results from Tables 4 and 5, the co-crystals' primary preparation method is solvent-assisted, and solubility enhancement ranges from less than 1-fold to a maximum of 20 times. The works of Arabiani et al. [120] and Zhao et al. [44] have shown that it is possible to obtain co-crystals under dry conditions. Still, solubility was respectively little (1.056-fold) or not enhanced at all (0.86-fold, compared to paracetamol alone) (see Table 5). On the other hand, independently of the API, studies with amorphous systems clearly show a higher increase in solubility than co-crystals, as shown in Tables 4 and 5. Several authors have suggested that the physicochemical properties (melting temperature, solvation, etc.) of all the components of the co-crystal, as well as the solution properties of the medium (pH, surfactant, etc.), can significantly influence the solubility and dissolution of the co-crystals [127,147,148]. Other authors have mentioned that this induced improvement in solubility could possibly be the effect of the co-former being drawn out of the crystal lattice and into the aqueous medium [149]. For hydrophilic co-formers of co-crystals [121,124] interactions might be developed with -OH groups from water molecules by new hydrogen bonding, resulting in an enhancement of drug solubility. This theory is valid for a hydrophilic co-formers [44,127]; however, depending on the properties of the co-former, other factors, such as pH, could be more suitable to increase solubility, such as low pH for acid co-formers [124]. To sum up, it is necessary to release co-crystals in a suitable medium to improve dissolution behavior.

Table 6. Overview of structural characterization by spectroscopy of amorphous/co-amorphous drugs obtained by milling.

#	Sample	Analytical Technique	Wavenumber (cm^{-1})/δ (ppm)		Interpretation	Ref.
			Crystalline	**Co-Amorphous**		
4A	Naproxen–cimetidine	Raman	670 (C-S-C str)	666 cm^{-1}	Shift → unknown mechanism of interaction	[87]
			1601 (ring str)	1604 cm^{-1}	Shift → solid-state interaction of imidazole ring with naproxen	
5A	γ-Indomethacin–ranitidine hydrochloride	DRIFTS (FT-IR)	1717 and 1692 (C=O)	1723 and 1679	Broadening and shift	[28]
			N/A	1735 cm^{-1}	Shoulder appearance	
			N/A	1723 (C=O)	Peak formation → conjugated carbonyl acid system	
			1692 (C=N)	1679 cm^{-1}	Shift → larger C=N double bond character or interaction at benzoyl C=O ocurred	
			1620 (aci-nitro C=N str)	1610	Shift → nitro group forming a bond with indomethacin and indirectly reducing the C=N double bond character	
			N/A	1579	Small peak formation → interaction at the amidine moiety	
6A	γ/α-Indomethacin	Raman	N/A	1540 to 1700 and 2930 to 3100 cm^{-1}	Large spectral differences → variations in molecular conformation and intermolecular bonding of amorphous forms	[88]
8A	Glibenclamide	FT-IR	3315 (N-H str)	N/A	Absence of band upon cryomilling	[89]
			1714 (C=O str)	N/A	Loss in intensity but clearly apparent	
			N/A	1637 (C=N str)	New band → conversion of the amide to the imidic acid form	
9A	Trehalose dihydrate	Raman	30–400 (several peaks)	N/A	Presence of only a broad peak (boson) → amorphous material	[90]
			443, 835, 906, and 1449	433, 843, 912, and 1455 cm^{-1}	Shift → amorphous transformation	
10A	Atenolol-hydrochlorothiazide	FT-IR	3361 (N-H str) and 3169 (OH str)	3464 and 3357 cm^{-1}	Shift	[91]
			1636 (C=O str)	1664 cm^{-1}	Shift → formation of intermolecular interactions	
			1317 (-SO2 str)	1327 cm^{-1}	Shift → involvement of -SO$_2$ in intermolecular hydrogen bonding	
11A	Indomethacin-arginine	FT-IR	1613 (guanidine group)	1603 cm^{-1}	Reduction of signal → possibly extremely weak interactions	[92]
			1709 and 1738 cm−1 (C=O)	N/A	Disappearance of peaks → possibly extremely weak interactions	
		ssNMR	159 ppm (guanidine resonance) and 157 ppm (C5)	N/A	Overlap → not easy to identify salt formation	
	Furosemide-arginine	FT-IR	1670 (C=O)	N/A	Decrease of peak → salt formation	
		ssNMR	169 and 173 ppm (C=O)	175 ppm	One broad resonance → similar environments in the mixture. π-π interactions involved	
15A	Piroxicam-ASPA	FT-IR	1377	1392 cm^{-1}	Shift → possible interaction between components	[94]
16A	α-D-glucose	Raman	769.2 and 838	N/A	Presence of only the respective vibrational broadened bands → samples free of mutarotation and show anomeric purity	[95]
	β-glucose		896.4	N/A		
18A	Indomethacin-lysine	FT-IR	1713 (C=O str)	N/A	Disappearance of band → suggests ionization and salt formation	[96]
			N/A	1586 and 1561 cm^{-1} (COO-)	Broad peak → ionized carboxyl group for DMB and LAG, respectively	
19A	Mebendazole-tryptophan	FT-IR	1717 (C=O)	1727 cm^{-1}	Shift → loss of hydrogen bonds	[97]
	Pioglitazona-tryptophan		2930 (N-H)	1924 cm^{-1}	Shift → formation of hydrogen bonds	

Table 6. *Cont.*

#	Sample	Analytical Technique	Wavenumber (cm^{-1})/δ (ppm)		Interpretation	Ref.
			Crystalline	**Co-Amorphous**		
20A	Mefenamic acid-NaTC	FT-IR	754 and 776	747 and 769 cm^{-1}	Broadening and shift → loss of long-range order	[37]
			888	N/A	Intensity of strong, sharp band decreases	
			1256	1219 cm^{-1}	Shift and overlapping with band at 1193 cm^{-1} → changes in the hydrogen bonding network of mefenamic acid on amorphization	
			1329	1319 cm^{-1}	Shift → changes in the hydrogen bonding network of mefenamic acid on amorphization	
			1509/1502	1507 cm^{-1}	Split peak becomes a broad centered band	
			1648 and 1196	1662 and 1193 cm^{-1}	Shift → no evidence for specific API-NaTC interactions; hydrogen bonding interactions can be ruled out	
21A	Indomethacin-arginine	FT-IR	N/A	1590 cm^{-1} (indol)	Peak structure of individual compounds transformed into a broad plateau with a small peak	[98]
			1707 and 1734	N/A	Disappearance of peaks → carboxylic acid vibrations	
			1314 and 1219	1319 and 1222 cm^{-1}	Shift (chlorobenzene and indol, respectively) → changes in molecular environment	
22A	(S)-naproxen-L-arginine	FT-IR	N/A	1568 cm^{-1} (C=O)	New broad peak for the LAG sample → carboxyl group ionized	[99]
			N/A	1708 cm^{-1}	New band appearance	
			N/A	1543 cm^{-1} (C=O)	New peak with lower intensity compared to LAG sample (DBM formulation)	
			N/A	1679 cm^{-1}	Broad shoulder (DMB)	
23A	Griseofulvin-tryptophan	FT-IR	3401 (NH and OH str), 3011 (CH str)	N/A	Enlargement and broadening of bands	[100]
			N/A	3227 cm^{-1}	New band appearance	
			1663 (QC, C=O)	1648 cm^{-1}	Small displacement → formation of hydrogen bonding interaction	
24A	Naproxen-tryptophan	FT-IR	1369	N/A	Decrease of C=O band due to interactions with NAP	[101]
			1659	1664 cm^{-1}	Band transformed into a peak with decreased intensity → interactions involving CO_2^-	
	Naproxen-tryptophan-proline		1650–1750	1699 cm^{-1}	Transformation into a broad peak	
			1581	1577 cm^{-1} (amide)	Shift of small shoulder	
	Naproxen-arginine		1679 and 1728 cm^{-1}	N/A	Disappearance → indicates salt formation	
			1540, 1600–1700	N/A	Reduction of bands (amide and guanidyl) → Supports salt formation	
	Naproxen-arginine-proline		1550 (amide)	1556 cm^{-1}	Shift → co-amorphous system	
			1610		Disappearance of band → co-amorphous blend	
26A	Oxaprozin-randomly-methylated-βCD systems	FT-IR	1725	1718 cm^{-1} (OXA carbonyl)	Reduction of intensity and shift → strong solid-state interactions between the components	[103]
27A	Furosemide-arginine	FT-IR	1672 and 1562	N/A	Transformation of bands into shoulders → Salt formation upon co-amorphization	[104]
			1591	1602 cm^{-1}	Shift → salt formation upon co-amorphization	
			1714 and 1689	N/A	Disappearance of bands → salt formation	
	Indomethacin-arginine		N/A	1680 and 1500 cm^{-1}	Simultaneous formation of a band plateau → Salt formation	
			N/A	1589 cm^{-1}	Formation of a small peak → salt formation	

Table 6. *Cont.*

#	Sample	Analytical Technique	Wavenumber (cm^{-1})/δ (ppm)		Interpretation	Ref.
			Crystalline	Co-Amorphous		
29A	Naproxen-NAP(Na)	FT-IR	1638–1682	1639 cm^{-1}	Disappearance of peaks and formation of a broaden single peak	[106]
			1603	1605 cm^{-1}	Shift	
			1585–1574	N/A	Peaks weakened and broadened → formation of intermolecular interactions involving carbonyl groups	
		Raman	N/A	747 cm^{-1}	Peak broadened and then disappeared → crystallization of NAP and NAP(Na)	
			N/A	742 cm^{-1}	Appearance and increase in peak → presence of NAP indicates increasing presence of crystalline NAP	
			N/A	1383 cm^{-1}	Small shoulder peak after 10 min → decreased presence of NAP(Na)	
31A	Arginine-indomethacin	FT-IR	N/A	1500–1750 cm^{-1}	Formation of a plateau	[36]
				1321 cm^{-1}	Presence of peak	
32A	Simvastatin-L-lysine	FT-IR	3442	3350 cm^{-1} (OH)	Broadening → no clear evidence of strong intermolecular interactions between the components	[108]
			1356 and 1319	1350 and 1312 cm^{-1}	Shift (aliphatic) → no clear evidence of strong intermolecular interactions between the components	
	Glibenclamide-L-serine		1519	1534 cm^{-1}	Shift (NH urea group) → intermolecular interaction	
			1584 (C=O)	1595 cm^{-1}	Shift and merging → intermolecular interaction	
34A	L-tryptophan-indomethacin	Raman	N/A	1680 cm^{-1} (C=O)	Appearance and increase in intensity of a broad band → loss of crystalline forms due to changed intermolecular environment	[109]
		FT-IR	1661 and 1582	1609 cm^{-1}	Loss of initial bands and formation of broad band	
			495	532 cm^{-1}	Peak shift	
35A	Carbamazepine-citric acid-arginine (1:1:1)	FT-IR	1725, 1659, and 1628, 1568 (C=N)	1724, 1659, 1630, and 1573 cm^{-1}	Shift of bands. C=O peak weakened and became a shoulder peak → formation of intermolecular interactions between components	[110]
			1659	1678 cm^{-1}	Peak strengthened and shifted → intermolecular interactions	
	Carbamazepine-citric acid-arginine (1:1:2)		1659 and 1630	1678 and 1682 cm^{-1}	Shift (guanidyl)	
			1568 (C=N)	N/A	Broadening of peak	
	Carbamazepine-citric acid-arginine (1:1:3)		1659 and 1630	1634 and 1636 cm^{-1}	Shift (guanidyl) → formation of a stronger interaction with the amide group and/or aromatic ring	
			1568 (C=N)	1559 and 1589 cm^{-1}	Formation of a doublet → formation of a stronger interaction with the amide group and/or aromatic ring	
36A	Glibenclamide-quercetin	FT-IR	1713 and 1649 (C=O)	1680 and 1650 cm^{-1}	Broadening and shift of peaks → amorphization	[111]
38A	Mefenamic acid-meglumine	FT-IR	N/A	1375 cm^{-1}	Formation of a new band → chemical interaction between carbonyl group and secondary amino group of the components	[113]
40A	Gliclazide-triamterene	FT-IR	N/A	3290 (N-H) cm^{-1}	Formation of new H bonds	[38]
			1565 and 1530 (NH2)	1570 and 1536 cm^{-1}	Shift → formation of new H bonds	
41A	Quercetin-arginine	FT-IR	3400–3200 (OH) cm^{-1}	N/A	Loss of intensity → weak intermolecular bonding with the amino acid	[115]
			1645 (C=O)	1654 cm^{-1}	Shift → intermolecular H-bonding	
42A	Candesartan cilexetil-hydrochlorothiazide	FT-IR	N/A	1732 cm^{-1}	Visualization of band → occurrence of hydrogen bonds between the components	[116]

The results are similar to co-amorphous, in terms of the milling conditions to obtain co-crystals. As mentioned before, long milling times do not affect the increase of solubility. In fact, the longest milling time was performed by Zhao et al. [44] under dry conditions of paracetamol-trimethylglycine, and the solubility of the ball-milled co-crystals turned out to be lower than the paracetamol alone; the authors argue that supramolecular interactions, such as hydrogen bonding, might have caused this decrease in solubility. Anyway, only Shemchuk et al. [118] and Setyawan et al. [121] performed solubility studies at molar ratios different than 1:1. Still, no relation was observed to conclude that a specific molar ratio might render a higher increase in solubility. As previously mentioned for amorphs, in Table 5, no trend is observed regarding the type of mill, milling cell material, or milling speed towards affecting solubility enhancement.

To the authors' knowledge, the solubility of polymorphs has not been studied in vitro or in vivo. Still, it would be worth analyzing whether there are significant differences in solubility between one form and the other, as one form of the crystalline drug could show better properties and, therefore, novel applications for therapeutics. A parameter related to improving properties, such as solubility or stability of a system, is the formation of the interaction between the formulation components. Therefore, the most widely used techniques for structurally analyzing co-amorphous, co-crystal, or polymorphous systems will be described then.

4.2. FT-IR Spectroscopic Evaluation of Intermolecular Interactions Induced by Ball Milling

Fourier transform infrared spectroscopy (FT-IR), Raman, and solid-state nuclear magnetic resonance (ss-NMR) are the primary intramolecular methods of probing the sample at the molecular level [16]. Tables 6–8 show an overview of the main spectroscopic results (FT-IR, DRIFTS, ATR-FT-IR Raman, and ss-NMR) reported to identify and study the structural rearrangement and possibility of recognizing new interactions in the formulation. Changes in the spectra from the initial crystalline materials to another form of the drug formulation (call it amorphous or co-amorphous system, co-crystal, or polymorph) might be expressed in different forms, such as peak formation, reduction of signal, the disappearance of peaks, and the merging of bands. The overall changes in each drug formulation will be explained in detail in the following subsections. Tables 6–8 show the analytical technique used, characteristic signals, and interpretation of each API change.

Table 7. Overview of structural characterization by spectroscopy of drug co-crystals obtained by milling.

#	Sample	Analytical Technique	Wavenumber (cm^{-1})		Interpretation	Ref.
			Crystalline	**Co-Crystal**		
1C	Nicotinamide: L-(+)-ascorbic acid	Raman	104, 146, 666, 1329	93, 133, 631, 1292 cm^{-1}	Change form I → form II	[66]
4C	Urea-caffeine	ATR-FTIR	1682 (C=O)	1707	Shift → hydrogen bonding	[119]
			3341 (N-H)	3185	Shift → hydrogen bonding	
			N/A	809	Appearance of a new peak → co-crystal	
5C	Brexpiprazol-catechol (1:1)	Raman	1320.8, 1375.7, 1469.6, 1650.4	1223.4, 1284.1, 1321.47, 1375.2, 1495.4, 1668.3	Shift, decrease in C=O str → hydrogen bonding	[120]
	Brexpiprazol-succinic acid (1:1)		1320.8, 1375.7, 1469.6, 1650.4	1226.8, 1292.2, 1332.6, 1381.6, 1497.4, 1665.7	Shift, decrease in C=O str → hydrogen bonding	
6C	Quercetin-malonic acid	FT-IR	3411 (O-H)	3427 (1:1) and to 3466 cm^{-1} (1:2)	Shift → co-crystal formation	[121]
			1667 and 1612 (C=O)	1638 cm^{-1} (1:2)	Disappearance and shift → co-crystal formation	

Table 7. Cont.

#	Sample	Analytical Technique	Wavenumber (cm^{-1})		Interpretation	Ref.
			Crystalline	Co-Crystal		
7C	Paracetamol-trimethylglycine	FT-IR	1647 (-CONH$_2$), 1595, 1506, 1452 (C$_6$H$_6$), and 804 (-C$_6$H$_4$-) for PCA. 1400 cm^{-1} (C-N str) and 1323 (-COO-) for TMG.	N/A	No obvious difference in spectra of sample and co-crystal → proton transfer does not occur, no chemical reaction, this confirms co-crystal formation	[44]
		Raman	1643 (C=O), 1605 (C=C), 1364 (C-H), 1229 (-OH, aryl), 1161 (N-H), 850 (C$_6$H$_6$, aryl), and 789 (C-O)	1629, 1607, 1591, 1371, 1224, 1159, 858, and 774 cm^{-1}	Shift and reduction of band intensities → molecular complex is a co-crystal	
			1454 (C-N) and 882 (-COO-)	1443 and 886 cm^{-1}	Shift and reduction of band intensities → molecular complex is a co-crystal	
9C	Acetazolamide-4-hydroxybenzoic acid	Raman	N/A	251 (NH, OH), 1694 and 1738 (sci of, CNH and tor -CH3, and C=O, oop bend of ring)	Appearance of peaks → hydrogen bonding interaction leads to co-crystal formation	[123]
			1081 and 1120	N/A	Weak broad peaks → co-crystal	
			910, 1383	947 (N-H, -CH$_3$) and 1372 (HC=CH, O-H, C-N) cm^{-1}	Shift → co-crystal formation	
			1284		Disappearance → co-crystal formation	
11C	Ciprofloxacin-nicotinic acid/EtOH	FT-IR	N/A	1729 (COOH), 1627 (C=(ketone)), and 3200–2000 (OH)	Presence of bands and OH superimposed by C-H vib, abscence of H bonding → co-crystal formation	[124]
			1589 (asym COO-) and 1375 (sym COO-)	N/A	Stretches of COO → co-crystal formation	
			1705 (C=O)	1728 cm^{-1}	Displacement and increase in intensity	
	Ciprofloxacin-isonicotinic acid		1589 (asym COO-)	N/A	Lower intensity and absence of bands attributed to vibrations of H bond → formation of new supramolecular synthons	
12C	Pyrazinamide-diflunisal	Raman	N/A	244 (benzene ring, C-F), 1185 (O-H, HC-CH), 1370 (OH, O=C-O, C-H), 1406 (COH, C-H) and 1750 (C=O, C-O, C-N, C=O, C-C)	Appearance of peaks → hydrogen bonding in COOH-pyridine hetero-synthon leads to co-crystal formation	[125]
			807	N/A	Disappearance → co-crystal formation	
			458 and 1620	449 and 1612 cm^{-1} (C=O, C-O, C-C, O-H, C=OH)	Shift → co-crystal formation	
14C	Acetazolamide, nicotinamide-2-pyridone	Raman	N/A	475, 857 (CH, NH), 928 and 1716 (C=O, N-H, HO-C=O)	Appearance of bands → hydrogen bonding interaction leads to co-crystal formation	[126]
			1014	N/A	Disappearance → co-crystal formation	
			1242, 1456 and 1542	1260 (O=C-N-H, HC=CH), 1466 (-CH3, O=CNH, N-C-H) and 1559 (C-CH, HC=CH, NCH) cm^{-1}	Shift → hydrogen bonding interaction leads to co-crystal formation	

Table 7. *Cont.*

#	Sample	Analytical Technique	Wavenumber (cm^{-1})		Interpretation	Ref.
			Crystalline	Co-Crystal		
16C	Norfloxacin-nicotinic acid	FT-IR	1716 (C=O)	1728 and 1707 cm^{-1}	Displacement → New intermolecular interactions	[128]
			N/A	365–2492 cm^{-1}	Presence of a broad band → interactions through carboxyl and aromatic nitrogen groups of Nicotinic acid molecules	
17C	Chlorothiazide-L-proline hydrate	FT-IR	N/A	3337 (NH) cm^{-1}	Broad peaks → hydrogen bonding	[129]
	Chlorothiazide-D-proline hydrate			1332 cm^{-1}	Shift → formation of hydrogen bond O-H water -Osulfonamide	
18C	Praziquantel-poloxamer F-127 and sucrose stearate	ATR-FTIR	1625	1621 cm^{-1}	Shift → hydrogen bond formation	[130]
20C	Ketoconazole-fumaric acid	FT-IR	1645 (C=O)	1700 cm^{-1}	Shift → strong hydrogen bonding	[132]
	Ketoconazole-succinic acid			1714 cm^{-1}		
21C	Itraconazole-4-hydroxybenzamide (1:2)	FT-IR	1697 (C=O)	1690 cm^{-1}	Shift → participation in hydrogen bonding	[133]
			N/A	3469 (N-H) cm^{-1}	More prominent band of form II → higher involvement in hydrogen bonds than form I	
				3111 (C-H) cm^{-1}	Sharp peak of form I → asymmetric stretching in both molecules	
	Itraconazole-4-aminobenzoic acid (1:1)			1689 cm^{-1}	Shift → participation in hydrogen bonding	
23C	Pyrazinamide-4-aminosalicylic acid	Raman	416, 781, 1055, 1662	366, 893, 1000, 1552, 1637 cm^{-1}	New peaks → formation of a co-crystal	[135]
25C	Betulin-terephthalic acid (w/acetone or isopropanol)	ATR-FTIR	NR	3300–3600 (OH) and 1020 (C-O) cm^{-1}	Shift → intermolecular hydrogen bonding	[137]

N/A = not applicable, NR = not reported.

(c)   Structural characterization of amorphous systems by spectroscopy techniques

Among the articles analyzed for amorphous and co-amorphous systems, the technique mainly used for spectroscopic characterization is FT-IR and Raman. For the infrared spectroscopy results, band shifting indicates that the system is suffering changes in the internal structure. It is important to notice is that a relation between the shifts and hydrogen bonding has been found, as shifts towards a higher wave number may be linked to the loss of hydrogen bonds [24], while a shift to a lower wavenumber is related to the formation of hydrogen bonding. A more stable amorphous state would be expected [97].

In the case of studies that performed Raman spectroscopy, all of them reported shifts in the spectra or band broadening, which conclude the possible formation of interactions between the components at a molecular level. It is essential to mention that both bathochromic and hypsochromic shifts happen due to variations in molecular conformation and intermolecular bonding of amorphous forms [88]. Due to the fact that Raman is not affected by the polarizability of water molecules, another meaningful use of this technique, along with UV imaging, is to study dissolution behavior, as it reveals potential changes in the physicochemical properties of the crystalline and amorphous drugs, as well as solid-state changes during dissolution; case in point, the co-amorphous systems prepared by Ueda et al. showed changes in the spectra of the samples, which were clear indicators of recrystallization [106]. Finally, from all the papers analyzed, it was observed that another application of Raman is to quantify the amorphous content of a drug as milling time increases; this is called apparent amorphicity (%) and has been studied to observe rising levels of amorphizing material [93,150].

Table 8. Overview of structural characterization by spectroscopy of drug polymorphs obtained by milling.

#	Sample	Analytical Technique	Wavenumber (cm^{-1})/δ (ppm)		Interpretation	Ref.
			Polymorph I	Polymorph II		
1P	Ranitidine hydrochloride form 1	DRIFTS	1551 (form 1)	1046 (form 2)	Identification of each band → presence of polymorph	[74]
4P	Rivastigmine (RHT form II)	ATR-FTIR	1694 (carbamate, form II)	1725 cm^{-1}	Band broadening and shift → form II to I	[141]
6P	Dexamethasone	ssNMR	14–155 ppm (form B)	N/A	Disappearance at high temperatures → change in conformational properties of the molecules and coarsening process.	[27]
10P	Famotidine (form B)	Raman	3406 (N-H str) and 2897 (C-H sym str) (form B)	3455 (N-H str), 3422, 2997 cm^{-1}	Clear observation of bands → polymorphic conversion to form A	[142]
			2920 cm^{-1} (form A)	N/A	Increase in peak intensity → presence of form A	
			2897 cm^{-1}	N/A	Decrease in peak intensity → form B dropped off	
11P	Gabapentin (GBP) form I, II, III, and IV	FT-IR	3300 (OH str, form I)	N/A	Disappearance → dehydration	[76]
			1660 (C=O, form I)	N/A	Decrease in peak intensity → decrease in hydrogen bonding due to dehydration and polymorphic transformation to II	
			1624 (carboxylate, form I)	1620 cm−1 and then to 1615 cm^{-1}	Shift and decrease in peak intensity → decrease in hydrogen bonding due to dehydration and polymorphic transformation to II	
			N/A	1301, 709, 2930, 2153, 1615, 1547, and 1165 (form II)	Appearance of peaks → presence of form II	
			N/A	1699 and 1677 (GBP-lactam)	Appearance of peaks → formation of traces of GBP-lactam due to heating effect	
			N/A	1644, 1584, 1510, 1462, 1400, 1231, 1160, 1512, 2926, and 2200 (form III)	Appearance of specific peaks → presence of form III	
			N/A	3150, 1523, 1397, 1377, 1087, 2121, 1621, 1576, and 1431 (form IV)	Appearance of peaks → presence of form IV	

N/A = not applicable.

Finally, in Table 6, the usefulness of NMR in amorphous systems is that it gives information regarding the thermal degradation of samples after milling. For example, Oliveira et al. [27] concluded during their study that the NMR spectrum of the milled dexamethasone was totally similar to that of the initial one, as it showed that a high-energy mechanical action is capable of amorphizing the sample without inducing chemical degradation, contrary to the spectra obtained from melt quenching, where the method of preparation may cause degradation.

(d)   Structural characterization of co-crystals by spectroscopy techniques

FT-IR and Raman are the analytical techniques commonly used for co-crystal identification. As can be observed in Table 7, Raman spectroscopy is an advantageous technique for the analysis of co-crystals, particularly when the samples are hydrated because monitoring of water presents low Raman scattering [151], in comparison to FT-IR, which can have an uptake of humidity from the air and show the presence of a broad -OH band. Analysis from Table 7 shows that FT-IR does not seem to be the most common technique for interpreting co-crystal formation prepared by ball milling. However, there are some studies where FT-IR has been successfully used for identifying co-crystals [152,153]. In these cases, co-crystals were prepared by methods other than grinding, such as solvent evaporation or sublimation.

In Raman, it has been suggested that the shift in the conformer to lower or higher wavenumbers with the corresponding reduction in the band intensities affect the distribution of the electron cloud and suggests the formation of a co-crystal and not simply a physical mixture [44]. Several studies argue that the spectra confirm the effect of hydrogen bonding interaction in the complex formed, which is key to co-formation, rather than a simple mixture of the two starting reactants [123].

A study performed by Elsei et al. [140] supports the idea of Oliveira et al. (mentioned in the spectroscopic techniques for amorphs section)—that when no changes are observed between the ^{1}H NMR milled and non-milled spectra, it allows for confirmation that the samples can be safely ball-milled without inducing thermal degradation, compared to other techniques, such as melt quenching. This has been confirmed by ^{1}H NMR, ^{13}C, and ^{15}N spectroscopy [154].

(e)   Spectroscopic studies reported for polymorphs obtained by ball milling

Table 8 summarizes several authors' interpretations, regarding the analysis of polymorphic transformations by spectroscopic techniques. During mechanochemical milling, certain forms of drugs can be produced; however, due to the low glass transition temperature of the drug (further discussed in the phase transition by thermal techniques section), they are not necessarily stable, which results in reversion into a more stable crystalline form. Therefore, identifying polymorphs is imperative for formulation developments and complying with the regulatory authorities [141]. As shown in Table 8, each polymorph of a drug exhibits specific bands that allow a clear identification in FT-IR and Raman. After polymorphic transformation, some bands may disappear (due to conversion from one form to another), and new peaks with increased intensity now show up, thus allowing for the identification of the new polymorph. Less common, but also seen, is the shift of bands, which also indicates polymorphism. Finally, regarding polymorphism, an example is presented here to make this section clearer: in the spectra of a ball-milled sample that shows peaks from two different forms, form A and form B, this would be an indicator that the mixture contains both polymorphs; this indicates that more milling time is necessary to reach full conversion into a specific form (from A → B or vice-versa), where only the peaks of one specific form will be noticeable.

ssNMR has been little used, but it is useful to observe that the disappearance of bands indicates a change in conformational properties, such as the arrangement of molecules in the unit cell and coarsening process [27]. The ^{1}H NMR proton spin-lattice relaxation time measured at various temperatures may be used to differentiate between various polymorphic forms of a drug [155].

Contrary to amorphous systems and co-crystals, to the author's knowledge, ^{1}H NMR cannot be used in these cases to observe if the polymorph suffers thermal degradation, because proton NMR signals change as a new polymorphic form develop, but further investigation needs to be performed in this field.

4.3. Thermal Analysis Techniques to Study Phase Transitions Induced by Grinding

Regarding the thermal analysis of samples, the most commonly used technique reported for the study of milled formulations is differential scanning calorimetry (DSC). This technique identifies phase transitions as a function of a heating process (melting, crystallization, decomposition, and glass transition temperatures). Another technique is thermogravimetry (TGA), which measures the loss of mass as a function of the temperature, due to loss of water [44] or volatile samples [124], respectively. The most common rate used is 10 °C/min, but the smaller heating ramps of 5 °C/min [68,95,100] and 2 °C/min in several articles have also been used (see Table 9). It is well-known that many transitions, such as crystallization, decomposition, evaporation, etc., are kinetic events, as functions of time and temperature. Therefore, the transition will shift to a higher temperature when heated at a higher rate. Another transition that can also be affected by the heating speed is the glass transition temperature; its shift is the result of some events. First, the temperature of the center of the sample lags the temperature of the surface. The temperature lag increases with the heating rate and causes the glass transition to shift to a slightly higher temperature. Secondly, the glass transition is associated with a change in molecular mobility, and this mobility has a small time-dependent or kinetic contribution [156].

Table 9. Overview of thermal characterization (DSC) of amorphous samples obtained by ball milling.

#	Sample	Molar Ratio/Composition	Glass Transition Temperature (Tg)/($^\circ$C)	Milling Temperature	Conditions	Ref.
2A	Furosemide-arginine	1:1	127 ± 0.5	5 $^\circ$C	2 $^\circ$C/min, -10 $^\circ$C to 180 $^\circ$C, 50 mL/min	[85]
	Furosemide-citrulline	1:1	77.1 ± 5.6			
	Nitrofurantoin-arginine	1:1	139.1 ± 0.2			
	Nitrofurantoin-citrulline	1:1	$49.3 \pm 2.1/108.5 \pm 0.3$			
	Cimetidine-arginine	1:1	40.4 ± 3.1			
	Cimetidine-citrulline	1:1	39.5 ± 1.5			
	Mebendazole-arginine	1:1	$53.5 \pm 3.3/112.2 \pm 0.4$			
	Mebendazole-citrulline	1:1	$43.6 \pm 1.2/112.1 \pm 0.2$			
3A	Sulfathiazole-polyvinylpyrrolidone	STZ/PVP Xpvp = 0.4	173.2	Room temperature	10 $^\circ$C/min	[86]
	Sulfadimidine-polyvinylpyrrolidone	SDM/PVP Xpvp = 0.6	146.7			
4A	Naproxen-cimetidine	1:1	34.5	4 ± 2 $^\circ$C	10 K min^{-1}	[87]
		2:1	31.5			
		1:2	40.2			
5A	γ-indomethacin–ranitidine hydrochloride	1:1	32.5	4 ± 2 $^\circ$C	10 K per min from 0 to 160 $^\circ$C	[28]
		2:1	34.3			
		1:2	29.3			
6A	γ-indomethacin	N/A	39.23	4 ± 2 $^\circ$C	10 K min^{-1} from 0 to 180 $^\circ$C under nitrogen gas flow 50 mL min^{-1}	[88]
	α-indomethacin	N/A	37.92			
7A	Tadafil	N/A	147	Cryogenic temperature (liquid nitrogen)	10 $^\circ$C/min under nitrogen atmosphere (60 mL/min)	[26]
8A	Glibenclamide	N/A	65	Cryogenic temperature (samples immersed in liquid nitrogen)	10 K/min from 20 to 190 $^\circ$C	[89]
9A	Trehalose dihydrate	N/A	21	Cryogenic temperature (samples immersed in liquid nitrogen)	10 $^\circ$C/min from 0 to 150 $^\circ$C	[90]
10A	Atenolol-hydrochlorothiazide	1:1	311.44	Cryogenic temperature (samples immersed in liquid nitrogen)	10 $^\circ$C/min, starting at -20 $^\circ$C	[91]
		1:2	315.82			
		2:1	Not determined due to fast recrystallization			
11A	Indomethacin-tryptophan	1:1	Tg ranges from 120 to 45 $^\circ$C, decreasing as mol% of Ind increases	6 $^\circ$C	2 K/min from -20 to 180 $^\circ$C	[92]
	Furosemide-tryptophan	1:1	Tg ranges from 138 to 80 $^\circ$C, decreasing as mol% of Fur increases			
12A	Dexamethasone	N/A	115 < Tg < 120	Room temperature	0.663 $^\circ$C and 50 S, "Heat only" conditions	[27]
13A	α-lactose	N/A	70	30 $\pm$ 5% relative humidity and 22 ± 3 $^\circ$C	From 0 to 240°, 10 $^\circ$C/min under N2 flow of 50 mL/min	[93]

Table 9. *Cont.*

#	Sample	Molar Ratio/Composition	Glass Transition Temperature (Tg)/(°C)	Milling Temperature	Conditions	Ref.
14A	α-D-glucose	N/A	38	−15 °C and 0% relative humidity	5 °C/min, flushed with highly pure nitrogen gas	[68]
15A	Mebendazole-ASPA	1:1	91	5 °C, cold room	−10 °C to 180 °C, 2 °C/min, nitrogen flow was 50 mL/min	[94]
	Tadalafil-ASPA	1:1	102.9			
	Piroxicam-ASPA	1:1	76			
16A	α-D-glucose	N/A	38	−15 °C and 0% relative humidity	5 °C/min	[95]
	β-D-glucose	N/A	39		5 °C/min	
17A	Carvedilol, carbamazepine, furosemide, indomethacin, mebendazole-amino acids	1:1	A single Tg for each formulation	Cold room (+6 °C)	Nitrogen flow of 50 mL/min, 2 °C/min heated to 180 °C	[31]
18A	Indomethacin-lysine	1:1	100 (DMB)	Cold room (+6 °C)	Nitrogen flow of 50 mL/min, 2 °C/min heated to 180 °C	[96]
19A	Mebendazole-tryptophan	Xmeb = 0.1	53.5	Room temperature	−5 °C to 210 °C at 10 °C/min	[97]
	Pioglitazona-tryptophan	Xpgz = 0.1, 150 min	44.9			
22A	(S)-naproxen-L-arginine	1:1	91.9 ± 0.2	6 °C	Nitrogen flow of 50 mL/min, 2 °C/min from −10 °C to 180 °C	[99]
23A	Griseofulvin-tryptophan	1:1	113.46	NR	25 to 300 °C, 5 °C/min	[100]
24A	Naproxen-tryptophan-proline	1:1:1	55.1 ± 3.1	6 °C	Nitrogen flow of 20 mL/min, 10 K/min, from −20 to 170 °C	[101]
	Naproxen-tryptophan	1:1	58.2 ± 0.5			
	Tryptophan-proline	1:1	67.2 ± 6.8			
25A	Mebendazole-tryptophanphenylalanine	1:1:1	107.5 ± 0.2	5 °C	2 °C/min, heating to 180 °C	[102]
	Mebendazole-phenylalaninetryptophan	1:1:1	104.6 ± 0.2			
	Mebendazole-aspartatetyrosine	1:1:1	61.2 ± 0.9			
	Mebendazole-histidineglycine	1:1:1	34.9 ± 1.2/89 ± 0.6			
	Mebendazole-prolinetryptophan	1:1:1	6.5 ± 0.2			
	Mebendazole-tryptophan	1:1	128.7 ± 0.2			
	Mebendazole-proline	1:1	96.9 ± 0.1			
	Mebendazole-proline-tryptophan	1:1:1	56.3 ± 0.2			
	Mebendazole-tryptophan-phenylalanine	1:1:1	119 ± 0.1			
27A	Indomethacin-arginine	1:1	117 ± 4	6 °C	Nitrogen gas flow of 50 mL/min, 2 °C/min, from −10 to 180 °C, 0.212 °C and a period of 40 s	[104]
29A	Naproxen-NAP(Na)	2:1	55.8	4 °C	2 °C/min, 0.2120 °C with a period of 40 s	[106]
		1:1	40			
		1:2	NR			
31A	Indomethacin-arginine	1:1	62.9 ± 0.8	NR	Nitrogen gas flow of 50 mL/min, 10 °C/min to 180 °C	[36]
	Indomethacin-phenylalanine		55.3 ± 0.4			
	Indomethacin-tryptophan		62.7 ± 7.0			
32A	Simvastatin-lysine	1:1	33.2 ± 0.9	6″C	Nitrogen flow of 50 mL/min, 10 °C/min, from −50 °C to 280 °C (depending on the sample)	[108]
	Glibenclamide-serine	1:1	70.1 ± 1.3			
	Glibenclamide-threonine	1:1	58.4 ± 1.3			
	Glibenclamide-serine-threonine	1:1:1	62.5 ± 4.5			

Table 9. *Cont.*

#	Sample	Molar Ratio/Composition	Glass Transition Temperature $(T_g)/(^{\circ}C)$	Milling Temperature	Conditions	Ref.
33A	Indomethacin-arginine	1:1	36.7 ± 0.8	6 °C	Nitrogen gas flow, 20 mL/min, from −20 to 180 °C, 10 K/min	[98]
	Indomethacin-phenylalanine	1:1	64.1 ± 1.4			
	Indomethacin-tryptophan	1:1	47.8 ± 2.9			
	Indomethacin-phenylalanine-tryptophan	1:1:1	68.7 ± 2.6			
	Indomethacin-arginine-phenylalanine	1:1:1	63.1 ± 0.8			
	Carbamazepine-tryptophan	1:1	81 ± 0.6		Nitrogen gas flow, 20 mL/min, from −20 to 200 °C, 10 K/min	
	Carbamazepine-phenylalanine-tryptophan	1:1:1	75.1 ± 1.1			
	Carbamazepine-arginine-tryptophan	1:1:1	65.4 ± 1.1			
35A	Carbamazepine-citric acid	1:1	38.8 ± 2.7	4 °C	Nitrogen gas at 50 mL/min, 2 °C/min from 0 to 150 °C, 0.212 °C with a period of 40 s	[110]
	Citric acid-arginine	1:1	56.2 ± 0.7			
	Citric acid-arginine	1:2	106 ± 0.3			
	Citric acid-arginine	1:3	130.5 ± 0.1			
	Citric acid-arginine	1:4	119 ± 0.1			
	Carbamazepine-citric acid-arginine	1:1:1	77.8 ± 1.8			
	Carbamazepine-citric acid-arginine	1:1:2	105.3 ± 0.2			
	Carbamazepine-citric acid-arginine	1:1:3	127.8 ± 0.8			
36A	Glibenclamide-quercetin	1:1	85.97 ± 0.29	Cryomilled	Nitrogen glow of 50 mL/min, 1 °C/min	[111]
37A	Mebendazole-glutamate-arginine (crystalline salt)	1:1:1	37.8	Cold rooms (5 °C)	Nitrogen gas flow of 50 mL/min, 2 °C/min, 0.212 °C (amplitude), 40 s (period)	[112]
	Mebendazole-glutamate-arginine (amorphous salt)	1:1:1	37.3			
	Meb-glutamatearginine	1:1	36.5/77			
	Meb-arginineglutamate	1:1	36.3/76.3			
42A	Candesartan cilexetil-hydrochlorothiazide	NA	110	Room temperature	Nitrogen gas flow, 100 mL/min, 10 °C/min, from 30 to 300 °C	[116]

Tables 9–11 show all the thermal characterization and phase transitions of co-amorphous, co-crystals, and polymorphs. The following sections discuss specific results for each kind of formulation.

(f)   Thermal analysis of ball-milled co-amorphous systems

After analyzing the thermal characterization results of the amorphous and co-amorphous samples obtained by milling (shown in Table 9), it can be concluded that the determination of glass transition temperature (Tg) is a very useful tool to reach conclusions of amorphization of the material. For binary systems, detecting a single Tg is a clear indication of a homogeneous, single-phase, co-amorphous mixture [94]. Most of the co-amorphous system reported a single Tg, except Wu et al. [102], who prepared a total of nine co-amorphous systems and found two Tgs in the mebendazole-histidine-glycine ternary system; the rest showed only one Tg.

Table 10. Overview of thermal characterization (DSC) of drug co-crystals obtained by ball milling.

#	Sample	Tm Parent Drug 1 (°C) *	Tm Parent Drug 2 (°C)	Tm of Co-Crystal (°C)	Ref.
4C	Urea-caffeine	135.3	235.9	132.7	[119]
5C	Brexpiprazol-catechol	184.8	106.3	161.3	[120]
	Brexpiprazol-succinic acid	184.8	156.1	156.1	
6C	Quercetin-malonic acid	321.92	135.07	283.02 (1:1)	[121]
				266.61 (1:2)	
7C	Paracetamol-trimethylglycine	170.2	320.7	Endo peak = 174.5 °C and 177.4 °C	[44]
11C	Ciprofloxacin-nicotinic acid	254.8	235.1	241	[124]
	Ciprofloxacin-isonicotinic acid	268.3	267.94	242	
13C	Acetazolamide (polymorph I)-4-aminobenzoic acid	269.4	190.5	208.9	[67]
15C	β-lapachone-resorcinol	156	110	131	[127]
16C	Norfloxacin-nicotinic acid (Neat grinding)	222.8	237.1	230.5	[128]
	Norfloxacin-nicotinic acid (LAG)			236.1	
17C	Chlorothiazide-DL-proline	NR	NR	212.9	[129]
18C	Praziquantel-F-127 2B (20:1)	140.23	56.22	133.06	[130]
	Praziquantel-F-127 4B (10:2)			135.97	
19C	Ferulic acid-nicotinamide	172.8	NR	124.6	[131]
	Ferulic acid-isonicotinamide			143.9	
	Ferulic acid-urea			158.1	
20C	Ketoconazole-fumaric acid	151	294	168	[132]
	Ketoconazole-succinic acid		188	164	
21C	Itraconazole-4-aminobenzoic acid *	167	188.5	163.4	[133]
22C	Ibuprofen-nicotinamide	NR	NR	80.5	[134]
24C	Theophylline-4-aminobenzoic acid	274	187	Endos = 161.2 and 168.2	[136]

* Parent drug 1 is the left in the column Sample. Thus, drug parent 2 is on the right.

Several articles report the values of Tg at different molar ratios, namely 1:1, 1:2, and 2:1. In some cases, the determination of Tg is not possible, due to fast recrystallization or because it is not reported, but the rest of the articles reported the value of Tg at each molar ratio. In most cases, Tg's value at 1:1 ratio tends to be between the values at ratios of 1:2 and 2:1. When the composition is different than 1:1, the newly observed Tg tends to be closer to the Tg of the component present in excess within the mix [87,157]. This is because the excess components in a mixture show a tendency to recrystallize [158]. These shifts in the value of Tg give clear information regarding the development of new interactions of the components in the sample, and this is where the Gordon–Taylor equation is very relevant. The theoretical Tg for a co-amorphous system containing two amorphous components can be calculated with this equation [159]

$$T_{g1,2} = \frac{w_1 T_{g1} + K w_2 T_{g2}}{w_1 + K w_2} \tag{2}$$

where $Tg_{1,2}$ is the glass transition temperature of the co-amorphous mixture, w_1, w_2, Tg_1, and Tg_2 are the weight fractions and glass transition temperatures for the two amorphous components, and K is a constant expressed as:

$$K = \frac{T_{g1} \times \rho_{g1}}{T_{g2} \times \rho_{g2}} \tag{3}$$

where ρ_1 and ρ_2 are the densities of each of the two components [92].

The Gordon–Taylor equation assumes no interaction between the molecules in the mixture; therefore, large deviations could suggest that the two components interact at the molecular level [87]. A negative deviation from the predicted value of Tg by the Gordon–Taylor equation indicates a non-ideal mixing [158,160,161]. In this sense, free volume additivity, interactions between components, and loss of hydrogen bonding during mixing could account for this non-ideal mixing and negative deviations [160]. On the other hand, it has been mentioned that, when the Tgs of the co-amorphous systems are higher than the Tgs (a positive deviation) calculated by the Gordon–Taylor equation, it suggests strong molecular interactions between the components [92,96]; such interactions can be hydrogen bonding [162], π–π interactions [98], and salt formation [163] between the drug and co-former, thus leading, again, to a rise in the value of the experimental Tg over the theoretical Tg [94]. This deviation between theoretical and experimental Tg strongly depends on the drug–drug or drug–co-former selected for study. It is worth mentioning that Kasten et al. [31] concluded that the highest increase in Tgs occurred in the acidic drug basic AAs combinations (See Table 9), due to interactions resulting in salt formation. As was mentioned in Section 3.2, amorphization for milling requires to be performed at temperatures far below from the glass transition temperature; as shown in the data from Table 9, all reported experimental conditions agreed with this statement.

(g)   Phase transitions reported for co-crystals prepared by milling

After analyzing the data presented in Table 10, it was concluded that DSC can identify the melting point of co-crystals, as it is, in general, remarkably different from the pure melting temperatures of APIs and pure co-former [44]. Identifying new endothermic peaks between the melting points of both components indicates the formation of the co-crystal phase [121,124,127].

According to Stoler et al. [70], identifying a eutectic mixture in a phase diagram will result in a classic V shape (where the minimum point represents the eutectic point). By contrast, the binary-phase diagram for a co-crystal exhibits two eutectic points and a region of co-crystal at the maximum between the two eutectic points, resulting in a W-shaped phase diagram for co-crystals [71,72,164] (See Figure 2 for a representation of these diagrams).

In conclusion, for co-crystals ball-milled samples, endothermic peaks usually are located between the melting points of the parent compounds to proof the co-crystal formation (See Table 10); except, Nugrahani et al. [165] and Macfhionnghaile et al. [119] found values of Tm of the co-crystal lower than the parent drug, and Zhao et al. [44] found two endothermic peaks in the sample analyzed.

(h)   Phase transitions of polymorphs resulting from mechanical activation

After reviewing the results of the thermal analysis presented in Table 11, it can be concluded that DSC is a valuable technique to identify phase transitions. With DSC, it is also possible to observe reminiscence of residual solvents [79] and melting temperature (Tm) to identify polymorphs. Between two polymorphs, a higher melting point would indicate a more stable form of the drug.

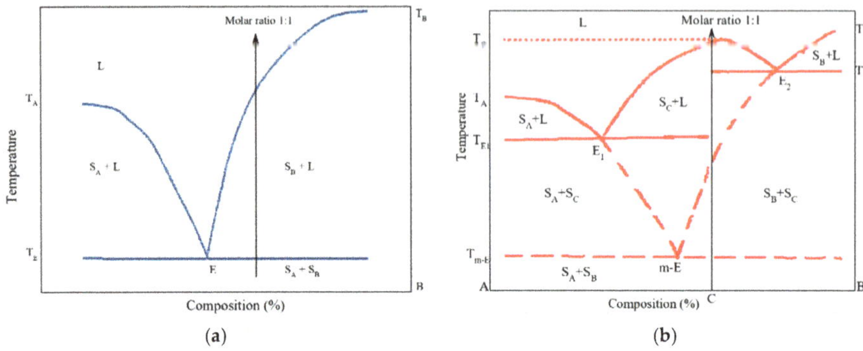

Figure 2. (**a**) Binary phase diagram of a combination incapable of co-crystal formation. (**b**) Binary phase diagrams of co-crystal formation. L, liquid; S_A, solid of component A; S_B, solid of component B; T_E, eutectic temperature; S_C, co-crystal; E, eutectic point; m-E, metastable eutectic point; $T_{m\text{-}E}$ metastable eutectic temperature; T_A, melting temperature of component A; T_B, melting temperature of component B; T_C, melting temperature of co-crystal. Obtained and replotted from [71,72].

Other transitions, such as crystallization temperature (Tc) and other endothermic signals, are also reported (along with the articles) and summarized in Table 11. For example, Elisei et al. (Elisei et al., 2018) determined two different crystallization temperatures, one for form 2 (Tc = 124 °C) and another for form 3 (Tc = 157 °C). Finally, a melting temperature of form 3 (Tm = 256 °C) from chlorohexidine dihydrochloride polymorph. In conclusion, endothermic peaks, such as melting temperatures, are very important because higher values lead to more stable polymorphic forms, and lower values lead to metastable forms.

As mentioned in Section 3.2, crystallization and polymorphic transformations occurred during the milling process at temperatures above the glass transition temperatures; however, most of the studies of co-crystals or polymorphs do not report Tg values of the materials.

Table 11. Overview of thermal characterization (DSC) of drug polymorphs obtained by ball milling.

#	Sample	Polymorph Identified	Transition Temperature (°C)	Milling Temperature	Conditions and Milling Time	Ref.
1P	Ranitidine hydrochloride	Form 1	Tm = 142.73	12 ± 3 °C and 35 °C	0 to 160 °C, 10 K/min	[74]
		Form 2	Tm = 145.01			
2P	Chlorhexidine dihydrochloride	Form 2	Tc$_2$ = 124	Room temperature	5 °C/min	[140]
		Form 3	Tc$_3$ = 157			
		Form 3	Tm$_3$ = 256			
3P	Γ-sorbitol	Form A	Decrease in melting temperature (value not reported)	Room temperature	NR	[34]
4P	Rivastigmine (RHT form II)	Form II	Tm$_1$ = 97.5, Tm$_2$ = 124.5	Room temperature	10 °C/min from 0 to 150 °C	[141]
		Form II	Exo peak = 105.5			
		Form I	Tm = 123.5			
6P	Dexamethasone	Form A	Tm = 242	Room temperature	5 °C/min	[27]
		Form B	Tm = 250			
7P	Sofosbuvir (anhydrous form 1)	Form 1	Tm = 96.57	Room temperature	0 to 300 °C, 5 °C/min	[79]
		Form A	Tm = 117.90			
		Form B	Tm = 124.83			
		Form V	Tm = 71.54			
8P	Sulindac (form II)	II → I	Endo peak = 160	Room temperature	5 °C/min	[69]
9P	Γ-sorbitol	Γ-sorbitol	Tm = 98.5	Room temperature with dry nitrogen atmosphere	5 °C/min	[75]
		A-form	Tm = 85			
12P	Sulfamerazine	Form I	Tm = 236	Room temperature	100 mL/min	[166]
		Form II	Tm = 212–214			

4.4. Identification of Amorphous and Crystalline Phases by Powder X-ray Diffraction (PXRD)

X-ray diffraction patterns show specific features, depending on the sample analyzed, and allow identification of amorphous and co-amorphous systems, co-crystals, and polymorphs. In this sense, a diffused halo is a clear indicator of the amorphous state (See Figure 3). In addition, XRD allows for identifying specific peaks in co-crystals, differentiation between polymorphs, and degree of crystallinity. In the following, Tables 12 and 13, the diffraction peaks were directly taken from the articles; when values were not reported, the diffractograms were analyzed in WebPlotDigitizer-3.8 to obtain the accurate values. The samples are marked with an asterisk (*) when data were obtained using this program.

XRD is a technique that can also be useful to identify changes in the crystal system and space groups. Anyway, it allows for the identification of specific peaks that correspond to a particular co-crystal form. From Table 12, it was observed that peaks might vary slightly, depending on the molar ratio [121], and they might even be solvent-dependent [124]. It is worth mentioning that a co-crystal with two polymorphic forms was obtained by Stolar et al. [66] upon the use of mechanochemical preparation (See Row 1 Table 12), but these results will not be further discussed, as they exceed the objectives set out in this review.

Finally, Table 12 also shows that all the articles that reported measurement conditions used a voltage of 40 kV, and the main current used was 40 mA, with step sizes ranging from 0.01 to 0.4, when reported.

A similar analysis can be performed for polymorphs. Each polymorph of a drug shows characteristic diffraction peaks, which enable the accurate identification of the form. It is important to know that milling might cause the disappearance of certain peaks, and new peaks might grow and increase in intensity; this is a clear indicator of the presence of a certain form of the drug (see Table 13).

Besides the information previously discussed, this technique allows analysis of the stability over time of pharmaceutical formulations, which will be discussed below.

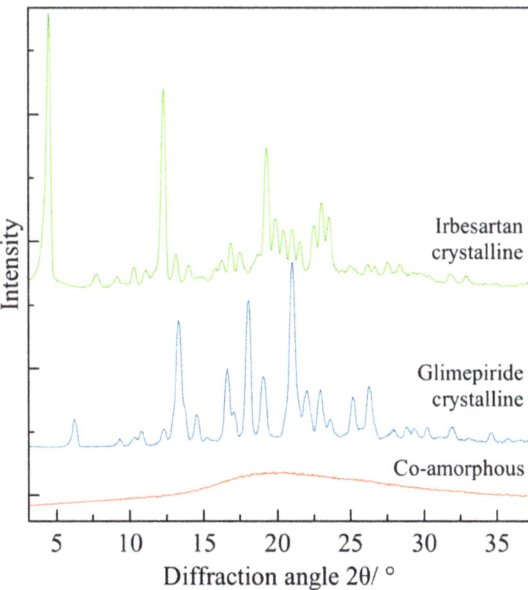

Figure 3. Example of diffractogram of the crystalline pure drug (irbesartan and glimepiride) and co-amorphous form of the binary system.

Table 12. Overview of identification of diffraction peaks and measurement conditions for co-crystals.

#	Sample	Co Crystal	Characteristic Peaks (° 2θ)	Conditions: Current (mA), Voltage (kV), etc.	Ref.
1C	Nicotinamide-L-(+)-ascorbic acid *	Form I polymorph	1.2, 1.5, 1.9, 2.1, 2.8, 3.2, 3.3	7.5 mA, 40 kV	[66]
		Form II polymorph	1.5, 1.8, 2.1, 2.7, 3.1, 3.2		
2C	Salicylic acid-2-pyridone *	sal2hyp	7.8, 11.02, 15.2, 15.8, 16.7, 24.1, 26.8, 28.7	Exposure time 9 s, time separation between patterns 10 s	[117]
	Salicylic acid-3-hydroxypiridine *	sal3hyp	9.2, 20.3, 23.2, 27.5, 31.6		
	Salicylic acid-4-pyridone *	sal4hyp	1.6, 1.9, 2.0, 2.1, 2.8, 3		
3C	Ciprofloxacin-thymol *	N/A	5.3, 7.1, 7.8, 11.4, 13.2, 15.7, 17.51, 19.4, 20.9	40 kV, 40 mA, step size 0.0130°	[118]
4C	Urea-caffeine	N/A	8.64, 10.82, 13.89, 24.30, 25.08, 25.46	35 kV, 25 mA	[119]
5C	Brexpiprazol-catechol	N/A	8.42, 8.88, 11.83, 12.15, 15.75, 16.22	40 kV, 30 mA, step 0.03°	[120]
	Brexpiprazol-succinic acid	N/A	3.67, 9.94, 18.47, 22.25, 22.53, 23.98, 24.3		
6C	Quercetin-malonic acid	CC1 (1:1)	16.21, 19.87, 28.88	40 kV, 40 mA	[121]
		CC2 (1:2)	16.18, 19.86, 28.83		
7C	Paracetamol-trimethylglycine	N/A	17.50, 23.03	40 mA, 40 kV	[44]
8C	Meloxicam-benzoic acid *	N/A	9.2, 12.9, 15.5, 16.7, 20.2, 25.9, 27.3, 28.7, 29.4, 33.1, 35.0	40 kV, 40 mA	[122]
10C	Furosemide-urea *	N/A	7.9, 10.7, 21.1, 26.1, 30.7	Step size 0.017°, collection time 18 h	[51]
11C	Ciprofloxacin-nicotinic acid	CIP-NCA/EtOH (1:1)	9.2, 11.5, 18.5, 19.5, 22.9, 23.4, 26.4, 28.5, 29.4	40 kv, 15 mA, 5–50°, step 0.04°, speed 4°/min	[124]
	Ciprofloxacin-isonicotinic acid	CIP-INCA (without EtOH)	5.4, 10.6, 19.2, 21.4, 28.4		
		CIP-INCA/EtOH	5.4, 10.6		
13C	Acetazolamide-4-aminobenzoic acid *	N/A	6.4, 10.1, 12.1, 12.9, 13.4, 14.1, 15.6, 16.7, 17.2, 17.6, 18.2, 18.3, 19.6, 20.1, 21.4, 22, 23.3, 24.9, 25.6, 26.2, 26.6, 27.8, 29.1	Ambient conditions	[67]
15C	β-Lapachone-resorcinol *	N/A	9.9, 10.5, 11.9, 12.9, 16.8, 18.1, 19.1, 21.4, 21.8, 24.9, 28.8	Speed 1°/min, step size 0.01°	[127]
16C	Norfloxacin-nicotinic acid (with EtOH)	N/A	5.4, 14.5, 25.4	Room temperature, 40 kV, 40 mA	[128]
17C	Chlorothiazide-DL-proline * (w/acetonitrile-water)	N/A	7.3, 20.1, 22.8, 24.12, 25.01	Ambient temperature, 40 kV, 100 mA, 8°/min	[129]
	Chlorothiazide-L-proline hydrate * (w/acetonitrile-water)		8.02, 11.42, 16.4, 23.47, 23.83, 24.95, 25.3		
	Chlorothiazide-D-proline hydrate* (w/acetonitrile-water)		8.2, 11.7, 16.2, 16.7, 17.5, 24.03, 25.2, 26.5, 29.2, 30.9		
18C	Praziquantel-F-127 2B (20:1) *	N/A	8.06, 15.2, 16.4, 16.9, 19.9	40 mA, 40 kV, scan rate 0.02°/s	[130]
	Praziquantel-F-127 4B (10:2) *		6.08, 7.9, 11.9, 12.5, 15.1, 18.8, 19.8, 22.8, 25.3		
20C	Ketoconazole-fumaric acid *	N/A	8.03, 12.2, 16.9, 19.3, 20.3, 21.6, 23.9, 25.7, 28.8	40 kV, 40 mA, step size 0.02°, counting time set 0.2 s/step	[132]
	Ketoconazole-succinic acid *		6.7, 7.9, 12.1, 17.1, 17.7, 19.3, 20.1, 21.2, 23.3, 23.8, 24.3		
21C	Itraconazole-4-hydroxybenzamide form I (1:2) *	N/A	7.3, 9.4, 9.7, 10.3, 11.1, 12.3, 12.7, 16.2, 16.6, 19.3, 20.4, 21.6, 26, 26.3	Ambient conditions, rotated at 15 rpm	[133]
	Itraconazole-4-hydroxybenzamide form II (1:2) *		5.7, 11.4, 12.9, 18.7, 19.04, 21.01, 22.3, 23.8, 25.2		
	Itraconazole-4-aminobenzoic acid (1:1) *		6.1, 10.8, 11.4, 11.9, 13.5, 14, 16.4, 18.8, 19.2, 20.4, 21.2, 21.5, 22, 22.5, 24		
23C	Pyrazinamide-4-aminosalicylic acid	N/A	5.95, 11.91, 13.06, 13.54, 28.25	NR	[135]
24C	Theophylline-4-aminobenzoic acid	N/A	12.3, 14, 15.5, 26.4, 27.5, 28.6	40 kV, 40 mV, step size 0.026° and step time of 56 s	[136]
25C	Betulin-rerephthalic acid (w/acetone) *	N/A	5.08, 8.6, 10.2, 12.8, 14, 14.7, 16, 18.8, 21.3	Range from 5 to 70°	[137]
	Betulin-Terephthalic acid (w/isopropanol) *	N/A	5.1, 8.7, 9.4, 10.2, 12.9, 14.2, 14.6, 16.1, 17.3, 17.9, 18.9, 19.3		

Table 13. Overview of identification of diffraction peaks for polymorphs.

#	Sample	Polymorph Identification	Characteristic Peaks (° 2θ)	Ref.
1P	Ranitidine hydrochloride *	Form 1	17, 21.8, 24.9	[74]
		Form 2	20.40, 23.7	
2P	Chlorhexidine dihydrochloride *	Form 1 → initial spectrum	13.9, 18.5, 23.7	[140]
		Form 2 → few peaks	5.2	
		Form 3 → many Bragg peaks	14.9, 28.3	
3P	γ-Sorbitol *	A phase → Sharp peaks, increased milling time	16.6, 30.9	[34]
		γ phase	11.6, 25.5	
4P	Rivastigmine	Form II	9.5, 11.3, 14.2, 15.5, 19.1, 20	[141]
		Form I → Broadeneing of peaks	5.1, 14.7, 16.5, 17.6, 18.6, 20.4, 21.1	
5P	o-Aminobenzoic acid	FI	10.7, 13.7, 14.35, 16.4, 18.6, 23.5, 24.3, 24.9, 26.2, 27.6, 30.5	[54]
		FII	11.2, 15.4, 22.2, 26.7	
	m-Aminobenzoic acid (FIII form)	FI	8.6, 17.2, 24.9	
		FIII	8.3, 16.8, 17.9, 23.7, 23.7, 24.2, 25.9, 26.6, 27.8	
	p-aminobenzoic acid	β-form	17.2, 17.6, 20, 21.9, 25.5, 27.9	
		α-PABA	17.1, 19.9, 21.8, 25.3, 27.8	
6P	Dexamethasone *	Form A	7.9, 13.5, 16.0, 17.6	[27]
		Form B	7.5, 16.8, 18.4	
7P	Sofosbuvir *	Form I	5.3, 7.6, 9.0, 9.8, 10.3	[79]
		Form A	6.2, 8.4, 10.5, 12.8, 17.4, 17.9, 18.2, 20.3, 21.1	
		Form B	7.9, 10.3, 12.3, 16.7, 17.1, 19.3, 20, 20.9	
		Form V	5.6, 6.9, 7.5, 10, 10.8, 13.8, 16.4, 19.7, 25.4	
8P	Sulindac *	Form I	10.8, 17.6	[69]
		Form II	9.3, 16.1	
9P	Γ-sorbitol *	Γ-form	11.7, 25.6	[75]
		A-Form	16.7, 31.1	
12P	Sulfamerazine	I	12.6, 14.8, 16.3, 17.4, 20.5, 22.7, 23, 24.6, 31.2, 32.7	[166]
		II	14.5, 17.0, 19.2, 21.5, 26.6, 27.4, 27.9	

(i)   Measurement of structural stability on co-amorphous systems during storage by XRD

It is well-known that amorphous samples are not necessarily stable and can recrystallize upon environmental conditions such as high humidity and temperature modification. Table 14 summarizes the information found on articles regarding structural stability, which has been measured under different temperatures ranging from 4 °C to 40 °C, under dry (silica gel and P_2O_5) and other humidity conditions (5, 10, and 75% RH) and storage days from 2 to 730 days observing if recrystallization occurred.

More than half of the articles studied structural stability at 25 °C and 40 °C, whereas fewer articles kept the samples at 4 °C or below for further analysis. This stability may depend on the properties of each drug alone, as well as the storage under dry conditions. Note that highly unstable compounds recrystallize immediately after the end of the milling process, even at very low temperatures, such as −15 °C, and a relatively long milling time (14 h) [68]. The reason is that the amorphous state of single drugs is usually less stable (see trehalose dihydrate and α-D-glucose in Table 14) than a co-amorphous system. Therefore, they tend to recrystallize. Nonetheless, other individual drugs studied, such as tadalafil [26] and glibenclamide [89], did not crystallize after 365 and 210 days of storage and 25 °C, respectively. A low percentage of relative humidity rendered amorphous samples for more extended periods.

Badal Tejedor et al. suggest that amorphization is a phenomenon that begins at the surface and propagates to the bulk, thus disrupting the crystalline structure of the material, where additional changes clearly occur at the surface during prolonged milling times [93]. They noticed that other factors can affect the amorphous state's physical stability once amorphization is reached. These are: (1) remanence of nuclei during milling [167]; (2) different local order in the milled material changes nucleation and growth properties of the crystalline form [95]; and (3) larger specific surface of the milled material can also promote crystallization because the molecular mobility is higher at the surface than in bulk [168].

Table 14. Overview of structural stability of amorphous systems upon storage in diverse conditions.

#	Sample	XRD Interpretation	Storage Time (Days)	Storage Conditions *	Ref.
2A	Furosemide-arginine, furosemide-citrulline nitrofurantoin-arginine, nitrofurantoin-citrulline (1:1)	Remained amorphous	450	25 °C, (dry conditions, silica gel)	[85]
	Furosemide-arginine, furosemide-citrulline, nitrofurantoin-arginine	Remained amorphous	450	40 °C, (dry conditions, silica gel)	
	Nitrofurantoin-citrulline	Recrystallization of Nitrofurantoin	450	40 °C, (dry conditions, silica gel)	
3A	Sulfathiazole-polyvinylpyrrolidone sulfadimidine-polyvinylpyrrolidone	Diffused halo → amorphous state	365	4 °C with desiccant	[86]
4A	Naproxen-cimetidine (1:1)	Halo, most stable sample	186	4 °C, 25 °C and 40 °C, dry conditions (silica gel)	[87]
	Naproxen-cimetidine (2:1)	Halo, stable	33	4 °C, dry conditions (silica gel)	
	Naproxen-cimetidine (2:1)	Crystalline naproxen (in excess) peaks	33	25 °C and 40 °C, dry conditions (silica gel)	
	Naproxen-cimetidine (1:2)	Traces of crystalline cimetidine	33	4 °C, 25 °C and 40 °C, dry conditions (silica gel)	
5A	γ-indomethacin–ranitidine hydrochloride (1:1)	Halo, highest stability	30	4 °C and 25 °C, dry conditions (silica gel)	[28]
	γ-indomethacin–ranitidine hydrochloride (2:1)	Small crystalline peaks of indomethacin (indo in excess)	30	25 °C and 40 °C, dry conditions (silica gel)	
	γ-indomethacin–ranitidine hydrochloride (1:2)	Progressive increase in peak intensity as temperature increased.	30	4 °C, 25 °C and 40 °C, dry conditions (silica gel)	
6A	γ-indomethacin	γ-form, crystallized	<1	22 °C over P_2O_5	[88]
	α-indomethacin	α-form crystallized to γ-form	4		
7A	Tadafil	Amorphous	365	4 °C with desiccant	[26]
8A	Glibenclamide (GCM)	Broad halo, amorphous state	210	25 °C, 10% RH, dry conditions	[89]
9A	Trehalose dihydrate	Recrystallised material is trehalose dihydrate	2	25 °C	[90]
10A	Atenolol-hydrochlorothiazide (1:1)	Amorphous, stable	30	4 °C and 25 °C, in desiccator	[91]
	Atenolol-hydrochlorothiazide (1:2)	Amorphous, stable	30	4 °C, in desiccator	
	Atenolol-hydrochlorothiazide (1:2)	Traces of crystals	30	25 °C, in desiccator	
12A	Dexamethasone	Form A converts to form B	7	150 °C	[27]
14A	α-D-glucose	Absence of Bragg peaks → amorphization	Immediate analysis after 14 hrs of milling	−15 °C	[68]
		Well-defined Bragg peaks → crystalline state	Immediate analysis after 14 hrs of milling	25 °C	
15A	Mebendazole-ASPA	Amorphous	120 days	25 °C and 40 °C (silica gel)	[94]
	Tadalafil-ASPA	Amorphous	120 days	25 °C and 40 °C (silica gel)	
	Piroxicam-ASPA	Amorphous	120 days	25 °C and 40 °C (silica gel)	
16A	β-D-Glucose	Bragg peaks restore immediately after the end of the milling process	1 h	25 °C	[95]

Table 14. *Cont.*

#	Sample	XRD Interpretation	Storage Time (Days)	Storage Conditions *	Ref.
17A	Carvedilol, carbamazepine, furosemide, indomethacin, mebendazole-amino acids	Recrystallization → Meb-Lys, Meb-Ile, Meb-Leu, Car-Val, Sim-Lys, Ind-Ile, Ind-Val	140	25 °C, 5% RH (P_2O_5)	[31]
		Recrystallization peaks → Fur-Met, Fur-Val, Ind-Leu	140–365		
		Amorphous → Arg-Fur, Arg-Ind, His-Fur, Lys-Fur, Lys-Ind, Car-Ile, Car-Leu, Car-Met, Car-Phe, Car-Trp, Meb-Met, Meb-Phe, Meb-Trp, Sim-Phe, Cbz-Trp, Sim-Trp	365–730		
18A	Indomethacin-lysine	Amorphous halo	252 days	DMB, 25 °C (P_2O_5) and 40 °C (silica gel), dry conditions	[96]
		Recrystallization → within 25 days it turned into same crystalline form of LAG	10 days	DMB, 25 °C, 75% RH	
		Crystalline form	252 days	LAG, 25° and 40 °C	
23A	Griseofulvin-tryptophan	Amorphous state, no recrystalization detected	365	Silica gel (13–32% RH), vacuum, 23–28 °C	[100]
25A	Mebendazole-tryptophan-phenylalanine	Remained amorphous	90	40 °C, 2% RH (silica gel)	[102]
	Mebendazole-tryptophanphenylalanine	Remained amorphous			
	Mebendazole-phenylalanine-tryptophan	Remained amorphous			
	Mebendazole-aspartate-tyrosine	Remained amorphous			
	Mebendazole-histidine-glycine	Remained amorphous			
	Mebendazole-proline-tryptophan	Remained amorphous			
	Mebendazole-prolinetryptophan	Remained amorphous			
	Mebendazole-tryptophan	Remained amorphous			
	Mebendazole-proline	Recrystallized			
	All samples	Remained amorphous	90	25 °C, 2% RH (silica gel)	
29A	Naproxen-NAP(Na) (2:1)	Recrystallization peaks are visible	7	40 °C, silica gel	[106]
	Naproxen-NAP(Na) (1:1)	Remained amorphous	60		
32A	Simvastatin-lysine	Amorphous	150	4 °C and 0% RH	[108]
		Recrystallization	90	40 °C and 0% RH	
		Recrystallization	56	Ambient temperature and 60% RH	
	Glibenclamide-threonine	Recrystallization	40	40 °C and 0% RH	
	Glibenclamide-serine-threonine	Recrystallization	90		
	Glibenclamide-serine	Amorphous	180		
	Glibenclamide-serine	Amorphous	180		
	Glibenclamide-threonine	Recrystallization	44	4 °C and 0% RH	
	Glibenclamide-serine-threonine	Recrystallization	90		
	Glibenclamide-serine	Recrystallization	150	Ambient temperature and 60% RH	
	Glibenclamide-threonine	Recrystallization	26		
	Glibenclamide-serine-threonine	Recrystallization	90		
33A	Indomethacin, carbamazepine, L-arginine, L-phenylalanine, L-tryptophan and L-tyrosine	Remained amorphous (halo)	180	40 °C, dry conditions (silica gel)	[169]
35A	Carbamazepine-arginine (1:1, 1:2, 1:3, 1:4) carbamazepine-Citric acid-arginine (1:1:1, 1:1:2, 1:1:3)	Amorphous	60	40 °C, silica gel	[110]

Table 14. *Cont.*

#	Sample	XRD Interpretation	Storage Time (Days)	Storage Conditions *	Ref.
36A	Mebendazole (Meb)-glutamate-arginine (crystalline salt), meb-arginine-glutamate (amorphous salt), meb-glutamatearginine, meb-arginineglutamate (dipeptide)	Remained amorphous	180	25 °C, dry conditions (silica gel), 2% RH	[112]
	Meb-glutamate-arginine meb-arginine-glutamate	Recrystallization	180	40 °C, dry conditions (silica gel), 2% RH	
	Meb-glutamatearginine meb-arginineglutamate	Remained amorphous	180		
38A	Glibenclamide-serine glibenclamide-arginine	Samples after storage were similar to the patterns exhibited before the test	180	40 °C and 75% RH	[170]
39A	Rutin-naringin hydrate (all molar ratios), rutin-hesperidin (all molar ratios), rutin-methionine (1:1), rutin-quercetin dihydrate (1:1, 2:1)	Remained amorphous	12 h	Dry and wet conditions	[114]
	Rutin-methionine (1:2 and 2:1)	Small peaks	12 h	Dry conditions	
	Rutin-quercetin dihydrate (1:2)	Small peaks	12 h	Dry and wet conditions	
40A	Gliclazide (Glz)-nifedipine	Crystallized to a physical mixture	3	Ambient temperature, 56% RH	[38]
	Glz-indapamide, Glz-triamterene, Glz-hydrochlorothiazide	Remained amorphous	180		
	Glz-chlorothiazide	Recrystallized	30		
	Glz-indapamide, Glz-triamterene, Glz-hydrochlorothiazide	Remained amorphous	120		
	Glz-hydrochlorothiazide	New peaks	30	Ambient temperature, 98% RH	
	Glz-triamterene	Small peaks	120		
	Glz-benzamidine	New pattern assigned to the salt	30		
42C	Cilexetil-hydrochlorothiazide	Recrystallization	30	4 °C, 0% RH	[116]
	Cilexetil-hydrochlorothiazide-hydroxypropylmethylcellulose acetate succinate type M (HPMCAS)		60		
	Cilexetil-hydrochlorothiazide		15	40 °C, 75% RH	
	Cilexetil-hydrochlorothiazide-HPMCAS (CH50)	Small reflections	90		
	Cilexetil-hydrochlorothiazide-HPMCAS (CH70)		30		
43C	Glibenclamide-quercetin	Remained amorphous	120	4 °C, 0% RH	[111]
		Recrystallization	390		
			10	Room temperature, 60% RH	
			120	40 °C, 0% RH	

* Acronyms: DMB: dry ball milling, LAG: liquid-assisted grinding, RH: relative humidity.

In this sense, several authors prepared the amorphous systems at different molar ratios (see Table 14), and it was clearly observed that the 1:1 preparation allows for the obtention of the structurally most stable ball-milled mixtures from 30 to 186 days, compared to 2:1 and 1:2 molar ratios.

It has been argued that recrystallization prevails at high temperatures, while amorphization prevails at low temperatures due to low molecular mobility [95] in amorphous systems. For preparations that involve molar ratios different than 1:1, the amorphous state stable is maintained at low temperatures (4 °C). However, as the temperature rises in the sample, recrystallization occurs in the form of a progressive increase in peak intensity, where the excess compound is the one that recrystallizes first [28,87,91]. This observation is supported by thermal behavior, as the samples shift the Tg towards the compound present in excess (See Table 9).

Finally, it is important to mention the results obtained by Kasten et al. (2017), as they analyzed two methods of preparation: DMB and LAG. Interestingly, DMB, whether at 25 or 40 °C, under dry conditions, resulted in a stable amorphous form for 252 days of the amorphous salts prepared. On the other hand, increasing relative humidity at 75% and maintaining the temperature at 25 °C caused recrystallization in the sample after 10 days; surprisingly, not into the crystalline form of the initial compounds, instead they transform into LAG peaks of the crystalline salt. This article is relevant for developing novel drugs because it indicates that although recrystallization of the DBM sample might occur, the recrystallization process will not lead to the initial material. Instead, a crystalline salt will be obtained (the same salt as the one prepared by LAG process). This means enhanced solubility over the crystalline drug will be obtained, even after recrystallization. To put this in perspective, 14-fold (crystalline salt), compared to 90-fold, of the co-amorphous salt.

(j)   Measurement of structural stability on co-crystals after milling by XRD

Co-crystals have been little studied, compared to amorphous systems. Only a few articles have subjected the samples to stability tests. The reports showed that the storage time ranged from hours to 180 days, where relative humidity conditions higher than 80% caused the partial dissociation of co-crystals [165] (for further details, see Table 15). More articles are needed to reach conclusions regarding the structural stability of co-crystals, but these drug formulations are stable at high relative humidity values (75% RH) and relatively high temperatures (40 °C).

Table 15. Overview of structural stability of co-crystals upon storage in diverse conditions.

#	Co-Crystal	XRD Interpretation	Storage Time (Days)	Storage Conditions *	Ref.
1C	Nicotinamide-L-(+)-ascorbic acid	Without changes in peaks → chemically stable	180	At shelf	[66]
3C	Ciprofloxacin-thymol	Stable, no changes of crystalline phase	50	Open air	[118]
4C	Urea-caffeine	Formation of co-crystal	Within hours	25 °C, 30% RH	[119]
7C	Paracetamol-trimethylglycine	Physically stable	90	40 and 75% RH	[44]

* Acronym: RH: relative humidity.

(k)   Structural stability on polymorphs after mechanical activation by XRD

The structural stability of polymorphs has been little studied, as well. Only a few articles were found that performed structural stability tests (see Table 16). The range of temperatures was wide, from 25 °C and heating up to 150 °C, where only Kamali et al. [54] reported humidity with a value of 85% RH. The storage time varied from immediate analysis to 150 days, which allowed for studying the transformations from one polymorph to another. In principle, these changes between forms happen due to the metastable states of the drugs because the system looks for the state with the lowest energy and, therefore, changes into a more stable crystalline form.

These results conclude that a wide field in co-crystals and polymorphs, regarding the structural stability of systems, is yet to be studied and understood. It would be worth researching, in more detail, the shelf life of co-crystals and polymorphs with improved solubility and higher stability. These drug formulations could be used in the pharmaceutical industry, due to their superior properties and therapeutic effects.

Table 16. Overview of structural stability of polymorphs upon storage in diverse conditions.

#	Sample	Polymorph Identification	XRD Interpretation	Storage Time (Days)	Storage Conditions	Ref.
5P	o-aminobenzoic acid	Polymorphs: I, II, III, and IV	FII → reappearance of FII	9	25 °C, 40% and 85% RH	[54]
			FII → reappearance of FIII	150	25 °C, 85% RH	
			FI → FII	150	25 °C, 85% RH	
	m-aminobenzoic acid	Polymorphs: I, II, III, IV, and V	FIV	150	25 °C, 85% RH	
			FI → reappearance of FIII	3	25 °C, 85% RH	
	p-aminobenzoic acid	Polymorphs: α and β	β polymorph	150	25 °C, 85% RH	
6P	Dexamethasone	Form A	Broaden Bragg peaks, characteristic of form A	Immediate	Freshly milled samples	[27]
		Form B	Predominantly peaks of form B, peaks of form A decrease	7	Heating up to 150 °C	
7P	Sofosbuvir	Form V	V → transformation to A	120	NR	[79]

Acronym: RH: Relative humidity.

5. Characterization by Microscopy

Finally, other techniques, although rarely mentioned, are also important for the characterization of drug formulations prepared by milling. For instance, scanning electron microscopy is a well-known technique for analyzing the morphologies of the particles. For pharmaceutical compounds, shape, size, and agglomeration are important characteristics for evaluation. According to Badal Tejedor et al. [93], topographical changes at the particle surface after short and longer milling times suggest changes of the particles' mechanical properties. It would be worth investigating how size and shape affect the stability and behavior of the compound. Amaro et al. used SEM to analyze polymorphs of rivastigmine hydrogen and found different morphologies for forms I (plate-like shape) and II (elongated tetrahedral/needle-like shape). This technique is useful for reinforcing the information obtained from other techniques for the identification of polymorphs [141].

Another common technique for studing the surface mechanical properties, topography, and energy dissipation [171] of a sample is atomic force microscopy (AFM). Badal Tejedor et al. [93] have concluded that crystalline materials show less deformation under an applied pressure with low energy dissipation in AFM, contrary to an amorphous material, which will be more viscous and show higher dissipation, possibly due to the disorder of the atoms in the structure. The presence of both low and high dissipation values across the map would indicate a partially induced surface amorphization [93].

Finally, ultraperformance liquid chromatography (UPLC) is a little used method, but it used to observe the purity of the sample. In this sense, impurities would be present as major or minor intensity peaks in a chromatogram [89], depending on the drug formulation analyzed.

6. Concluding Remarks and Future Works

This review focused on characterization results, in order to study different drug formulations, i.e., co-amorphs, co-crystals, and polymorphs, upon milling.

The analyses of experimental milling conditions showed that, in most cases, the milling method is in dry conditions and low or cryogenic temperatures for co-amorphous. Processing times for this kind of formulation ranged from 60 to 180 min. While, for co-crystals, the grinding time reported was shorter, around 30 min, and required solvent-assisted milling at room temperature. For polymorphs, prolonged periods, longer than one hour, were needed to induce structural rearrangement; milling was performed at room temperature in most cases to obtain a polymorph. It is important to note that this information regarding milling times is just an observation of the range of minimum and maximum periods of milling, based on the experimental data reported in the tables. However, parameters such as time, temperature, frequency, and the number of balls are inherent to the material or system, so the effect of milling parameters on the structure change is multifactorial.

Co-amorphous and co-crystal systems that were successfully prepared by milling with enhanced solubility have been widely studied, thus demonstrating the potential of ball milling as a preparation method for drug formulations. Despite the achievements in increases in its solubility, future work is still needed to improve the stability of co-amorphous; additionally, a wide field, regarding the shelf life of polymorphs and co-crystals, is yet to be researched and understood.

Finally, although scaling ball milling to industrial capacities is still a challenge to address, this preparation method represents a non-thermal and advantageous alternative, as it results in drug formulations with enhanced properties.

Author Contributions: Conceptualization, L.M.M. and J.C.-A.; writing—original draft preparation: M.V.-D., E.M., L.M.M. and J.C.-A.; data curation: L.M.M., J.C.-A., M.V.-D., E.M., P.C., C.N.-B. and F.C.; writing—review and editing: L.M.M., J.C.-A., M.V.-D., E.M., P.C., C.N.-B. and F.C.; supervision: L.M.M. and J.C.-A. All authors have read and agreed to the published version of the manuscript.

Funding: This research received no external funding.

Institutional Review Board Statement: Not applicable.

Informed Consent Statement: Not applicable.

Data Availability Statement: Data is contained within the article.

Acknowledgments: In memory of our beloved Javier Rivas, to whom we owe so much. Rest in peace. The authors would like to thank the School of Engineering and Sciences and the Bioprocess Research Group.

References

1. Takagi, T.; Ramachandran, C.; Bermejo, M.; Yamashita, S.; Yu, L.X.; Amidon, G.L. A Provisional Biopharmaceutical Classification of the Top 200 Oral Drug Products in the United States, Great Britain, Spain, and Japan. *Mol. Pharm.* **2006**, *3*, 631–643. [CrossRef] [PubMed]
2. Thayer, A.M. Finding Solutions. *Chem. Eng. News* **2010**, *88*, 13–18. [CrossRef]
3. Kalepu, S.; Nekkanti, V. Insoluble Drug Delivery Strategies: Review of Recent Advances and Business Prospects. *Acta Pharm. Sin. B* **2015**, *5*, 442–453. [CrossRef]
4. Dengale, S.J.; Grohganz, H.; Rades, T.; Löbmann, K. Recent Advances in Co-Amorphous Drug Formulations. *Adv. Drug Deliv. Rev.* **2016**, *100*, 116–125. [CrossRef] [PubMed]
5. Mizoguchi, R.; Waraya, H.; Hirakura, Y. Application of Co-Amorphous Technology for Improving the Physicochemical Properties of Amorphous Formulations. *Mol. Pharm.* **2019**, *16*, 2142–2152. [CrossRef]
6. Martínez, L.M.; Videa, M.; López Silva, T.; Castro, S.; Caballero, A.; Lara-Díaz, V.J.; Castorena-Torres, F. Two-Phase Amorphous-Amorphous Solid Drug Dispersion with Enhanced Stability, Solubility and Bioavailability Resulting from Ultrasonic Dispersion of an Immiscible System. *Eur. J. Pharm. Biopharm.* **2017**, *119*, 243–252. [CrossRef]
7. Vo, C.L.N.; Park, C.; Lee, B.J. Current Trends and Future Perspectives of Solid Dispersions Containing Poorly Water-Soluble Drugs. *Eur. J. Pharm. Biopharm.* **2013**, *85*, 799–813. [CrossRef]
8. Zhang, X.; Xing, H.; Zhao, Y.; Ma, Z. Pharmaceutical Dispersion Techniques for Dissolution and Bioavailability Enhancement of Poorly Water-Soluble Drugs. *Pharmaceutics* **2018**, *10*, 74. [CrossRef]
9. Tran, P.H.L.; Tran, T.T.D. Nano-Sized Solid Dispersions for Improving the Bioavailability of Poorly Water-Soluble Drugs. *Curr. Pharm. Des.* **2020**, *26*, 4917–4924. [CrossRef]
10. Dutt, B.; Choudhary, M.; Vikaas, B. Cocrystallization: An Innovative Route toward Better Medication. *J. Rep. Pharm. Sci.* **2020**, *9*, 256–270. [CrossRef]
11. Berry, D.J.; Steed, J.W. Pharmaceutical Cocrystals, Salts and Multicomponent Systems; Intermolecular Interactions and Property Based Design. *Adv. Drug Deliv. Rev.* **2017**, *117*, 3–24. [CrossRef] [PubMed]
12. Blagden, N.; de Matas, M.; Gavan, P.T.; York, P. Crystal Engineering of Active Pharmaceutical Ingredients to Improve Solubility and Dissolution Rates. *Adv. Drug Deliv. Rev.* **2007**, *59*, 617–630. [CrossRef] [PubMed]
13. Llinàs, A.; Goodman, J.M. Polymorph Control: Past, Present and Future. *Drug Discov. Today* **2008**, *13*, 198–210. [CrossRef] [PubMed]
14. Douroumis, D.; Ross, S.A.; Nokhodchi, A. Advanced Methodologies for Cocrystal Synthesis. *Adv. Drug Deliv. Rev.* **2017**, *117*, 178–195. [CrossRef]
15. Braga, D.; Maini, L.; Grepioni, F. Mechanochemical Preparation of Co-Crystals. *Chem. Soc. Rev.* **2013**, *42*, 7638–7648. [CrossRef] [PubMed]

16. Einfal, T.; Planinšek, O.; Hrovat, K. Methods of Amorphization and Investigation of the Amorphous State. *Acta Pharm.* **2013**, *63*, 305–334. [CrossRef]
17. Loh, Z.H.; Samanta, A.K.; Sia Heng, P.W. Overview of Milling Techniques for Improving the Solubility of Poorly Water-Soluble Drugs. *Asian J. Pharm. Sci.* **2015**, *10*, 255–274. [CrossRef]
18. Korhonen, O.; Pajula, K.; Laitinen, R. Rational Excipient Selection for Co-Amorphous Formulations. *Expert Opin. Drug Deliv.* **2017**, *14*, 551–569. [CrossRef]
19. Han, J.; Wei, Y.; Lu, Y.; Wang, R.; Zhang, J.; Gao, Y.; Qian, S. Co-Amorphous Systems for the Delivery of Poorly Water-Soluble Drugs: Recent Advances and an Update. *Expert Opin. Drug Deliv.* **2020**, *17*, 1411–1436. [CrossRef]
20. Kanaujia, P.; Poovizhi, P.; Ng, W.K.; Tan, R.B.H. Amorphous Formulations for Dissolution and Bioavailability Enhancement of Poorly Soluble APIs. *Powder Technol.* **2015**, *285*, 2–15. [CrossRef]
21. Martínez-Jiménez, C.; Cruz-Angeles, J.; Videa, M.; Martínez, L.M. Co-Amorphous Simvastatin-Nifedipine with Enhanced Solubility for Possible Use in Combination Therapy of Hypertension and Hypercholesterolemia. *Molecules* **2018**, *23*, 2161. [CrossRef] [PubMed]
22. Cruz-Angeles, J.; Videa, M.; Martínez, L.M. Highly Soluble Glimepiride and Irbesartan Co-Amorphous Formulation with Potential Application in Combination Therapy. *AAPS PharmSciTech* **2019**, *20*, 144. [CrossRef] [PubMed]
23. Martínez, L.M.; Videa, M.; López-Silva, G.A.; de los Reyes, C.A.; Cruz-Angeles, J.; González, N. Stabilization of Amorphous Paracetamol Based Systems Using Traditional and Novel Strategies. *Int. J. Pharm.* **2014**, *477*, 294–305. [CrossRef]
24. Martínez, L.M.; Videa, M.; Sosa, N.G.; Ramírez, J.H.; Castro, S. Long-Term Stability of New Co-Amorphous Drug Binary Systems: Study of Glass Transitions as a Function of Composition and Shelf Time. *Molecules* **2016**, *21*, 1712. [CrossRef] [PubMed]
25. Chavan, R.B.; Thipparaboina, R.; Kumar, D.; Shastri, N.R. Co Amorphous Systems: A Product Development Perspective. *Int. J. Pharm.* **2016**, *515*, 403–415. [CrossRef] [PubMed]
26. Wlodarski, K.; Sawicki, W.; Paluch, K.J.; Tajber, L.; Grembecka, M.; Hawelek, L.; Wojnarowska, Z.; Grzybowska, K.; Talik, E.; Paluch, M. The Influence of Amorphization Methods on the Apparent Solubility and Dissolution Rate of Tadalafil. *Eur. J. Pharm. Sci.* **2014**, *62*, 132–140. [CrossRef]
27. Oliveira, P.F.M.; Willart, J.-F.; Siepmann, J.; Siepmann, F.; Descamps, M. Using Milling To Explore Physical States: The Amorphous and Polymorphic Forms of Dexamethasone. *Cryst. Growth Des.* **2018**, *18*, 1748–1757. [CrossRef]
28. Chieng, N.; Aaltonen, J.; Saville, D.; Rades, T. Physical Characterization and Stability of Amorphous Indomethacin and Ranitidine Hydrochloride Binary Systems Prepared by Mechanical Activation. *Eur. J. Pharm. Biopharm.* **2009**, *71*, 47–54. [CrossRef]
29. Baláž, P.; Achimovičová, M.; Baláž, M.; Billik, P.; Cherkezova-Zheleva, Z.; Criado, J.M.; Delogu, F.; Dutková, E.; Gaffet, E.; Gotor, F.J.; et al. Hallmarks of Mechanochemistry: From Nanoparticles to Technology. *Chem. Soc. Rev.* **2013**, *42*, 7571. [CrossRef]
30. Yu, L. Amorphous Pharmaceutical Solids: Preparation, Characterization and Stabilization. *Adv. Drug Deliv. Rev.* **2001**, *48*, 27–42. [CrossRef]
31. Kasten, G.; Löbmann, K.; Grohganz, H.; Rades, T. Co-Former Selection for Co-Amorphous Drug-Amino Acid Formulations. *Int. J. Pharm.* **2019**, *557*, 366–373. [CrossRef] [PubMed]
32. Huang, Y.; Zhang, Q.; Wang, J.R.; Lin, K.L.; Mei, X. Amino Acids as Co-Amorphous Excipients for Tackling the Poor Aqueous Solubility of Valsartan. *Pharm. Dev. Technol.* **2017**, *22*, 69–76. [CrossRef] [PubMed]
33. Zhu, S.; Gao, H.; Babu, S.; Garad, S. Co-Amorphous Formation of High-Dose Zwitterionic Compounds with Amino Acids to Improve Solubility and Enable Parenteral Delivery. *Mol. Pharm.* **2018**, *15*, 97–107. [CrossRef] [PubMed]
34. Descamps, M.; Willart, J.F.; Dudognon, E.; Caron, V. Transformation of Pharmaceutical Compounds upon Milling and Comilling: The Role of Tg. *J. Pharm. Sci.* **2006**, *96*, 1398–1407. [CrossRef]
35. Wu, W.; Ueda, H.; Löbmann, K.; Rades, T.; Grohganz, H. Organic Acids as Co-Formers for Co-Amorphous Systems—Influence of Variation in Molar Ratio on the Physicochemical Properties of the Co-Amorphous Systems. *Eur. J. Pharm. Biopharm.* **2018**, *131*, 25–32. [CrossRef] [PubMed]
36. Ojarinta, R.; Heikkinen, A.T.; Sievänen, E.; Laitinen, R. Dissolution Behavior of Co-Amorphous Amino Acid-Indomethacin Mixtures: The Ability of Amino Acids to Stabilize the Supersaturated State of Indomethacin. *Eur. J. Pharm. Biopharm.* **2017**, *112*, 85–95. [CrossRef]
37. Gniado, K.; MacFhionnghaile, P.; McArdle, P.; Erxleben, A. The Natural Bile Acid Surfactant Sodium Taurocholate (NaTC) as a Coformer in Coamorphous Systems: Enhanced Physical Stability and Dissolution Behavior of Coamorphous Drug-NaTc Systems. *Int. J. Pharm.* **2018**, *535*, 132–139. [CrossRef]
38. Aljohani, M.; MacFhionnghaile, P.; McArdle, P.; Erxleben, A. Investigation of the Formation of Drug-Drug Cocrystals and Coamorphous Systems of the Antidiabetic Drug Gliclazide. *Int. J. Pharm.* **2019**, *561*, 35–42. [CrossRef]
39. Bansal, S.; Bansal, M.; Kumria, R. Nanocrystals: Current Strategies and Trends. *Int. J. Res. Pharm. Biomed. Sci.* **2012**, *4*, 10.
40. Babu, N.J.; Nangia, A. Solubility Advantage of Amorphous Drugs and Pharmaceutical Cocrystals. *Cryst. Growth Des.* **2011**, *11*, 2662–2679. [CrossRef]
41. Kumari, N.; Ghosh, A. Cocrystallization: Cutting Edge Tool for Physicochemical Modulation of Active Pharmaceutical Ingredients. *Curr. Pharm. Des.* **2020**, *26*, 4858–4882. [CrossRef] [PubMed]
42. Elder, D.P.; Holm, R.; De Diego, H.L. Use of Pharmaceutical Salts and Cocrystals to Address the Issue of Poor Solubility. *Int. J. Pharm.* **2013**, *453*, 88–100. [CrossRef] [PubMed]
43. Karimi-Jafari, M.; Padrela, L.; Walker, G.M.; Croker, D.M. Creating Cocrystals: A Review of Pharmaceutical Cocrystal Preparation Routes and Applications. *Cryst. Growth Des.* **2018**, *18*, 6370–6387. [CrossRef]

44. Zhao, Z.; Liu, G.; Lin, Q.; Jiang, Y. Co-Crystal of Paracetamol and Trimethylglycine Prepared by a Supercritical CO_2 Anti-Solvent Process. *Chem. Eng. Technol.* **2018**, *41*, 1122–1131. [CrossRef]
45. Koide, T.; Takeuchi, Y.; Otaki, T.; Yamamoto, K.; Shimamura, R.; Ohashi, R.; Inoue, M.; Fukami, T.; Izutsu, K. ichi Quantification of a Cocrystal and Its Dissociated Compounds in Solid Dosage Form Using Transmission Raman Spectroscopy. *J. Pharm. Biomed. Anal.* **2020**, *177*, 112886. [CrossRef]
46. Neurohr, C.; Revelli, A.L.; Billot, P.; Marchivie, M.; Lecomte, S.; Laugier, S.; Massip, S.; Subra-Paternault, P. Naproxen-Nicotinamide Cocrystals Produced by CO_2 Antisolvent. *J. Supercrit. Fluids* **2013**, *83*, 78–85. [CrossRef]
47. Müllers, K.C.; Paisana, M.; Wahl, M.A. Simultaneous Formation and Micronization of Pharmaceutical Cocrystals by Rapid Expansion of Supercritical Solutions (RESS). *Pharm. Res.* **2015**, *32*, 702–713. [CrossRef]
48. Kudo, S.; Takiyama, H. Production Method of Carbamazepine/Saccharin Cocrystal Particles by Using Two Solution Mixing Based on the Ternary Phase Diagram. *J. Cryst. Growth* **2014**, *392*, 87–91. [CrossRef]
49. Zhou, J.; Li, L.; Zhang, H.; Xu, J.; Huang, D.; Gong, N.; Han, W.; Yang, X.; Zhou, Z. Crystal Structures, Dissolution and Pharmacokinetic Study on a Novel Phosphodiesterase-4 Inhibitor Chlorbipram Cocrystals. *Int. J. Pharm.* **2020**, *576*, 118984. [CrossRef]
50. Merah, A.; Abidi, A.; Chaffai, N.; Bataille, B.; Gherraf, N. Role of Hydroxypropylmethylcellulose (HPMC 4000) in the Protection of the Polymorphs of Piroxicam Extended Release Tablets. *Arab. J. Chem.* **2017**, *10*, S1243–S1253. [CrossRef]
51. Al Rahal, O.; Majumder, M.; Spillman, M.J.; van de Streek, J.; Shankland, K. Co-Crystal Structures of Furosemide: Urea and Carbamazepine: Indomethacin determined from powder X-ray diffraction data. *Crystals* **2020**, *10*, 42. [CrossRef]
52. Nugrahani, I.; Utami, D.; Ayuningtyas, L.; Garmana, A.N.; Oktaviary, R. New Preparation Method Using Microwave, Kinetics, In Vitro Dissolution-Diffusion, and Anti-Inflammatory Study of Diclofenac- Proline Co–Crystal. *ChemistrySelect* **2019**, *4*, 13396–13403. [CrossRef]
53. Kuang, W.; Ji, S.; Wang, X.; Zhang, J.; Lan, P. Relationship between Crystal Structures and Physicochemical Properties of Lamotrigine Cocrystal. *Powder Technol.* **2021**, *380*, 18–25. [CrossRef]
54. Kamali, N.; Gniado, K.; McArdle, P.; Erxleben, A. Application of Ball Milling for Highly Selective Mechanochemical Polymorph Transformations. *Org. Process Res. Dev.* **2018**, *22*, 796–802. [CrossRef]
55. Chieng, N.; Rades, T.; Aaltonen, J. An Overview of Recent Studies on the Analysis of Pharmaceutical Polymorphs. *J. Pharm. Biomed. Anal.* **2011**, *55*, 618–644. [CrossRef]
56. Cruz-Cabeza, A.J.; Bernstein, J. Conformational Polymorphism. *Chem. Rev.* **2014**, *114*, 2170–2191. [CrossRef]
57. Cruz-Cabeza, A.J.; Reutzel-Edens, S.M.; Bernstein, J. Facts and Fictions about Polymorphism. *Chem. Soc. Rev.* **2015**, *44*, 8619–8635. [CrossRef]
58. Zvoníček, V.; Skořepová, E.; Dušek, M.; Žvátora, P.; Šoóš, M. Ibrutinib Polymorphs: Crystallographic Study. *Cryst. Growth Des.* **2018**, *18*, 1315–1326. [CrossRef]
59. Stahly, G.P. Diversity in Single- and Multiple-Component Crystals. the Search for and Prevalence of Polymorphs and Cocrystals. *Cryst. Growth Des.* **2007**, *7*, 1007–1026. [CrossRef]
60. Morissette, S.L.; Soukasene, S.; Levinson, D.; Cima, M.J.; Almarsson, Ö. Elucidation of Crystal Form Diversity of the HIV Protease Inhibitor Ritonavir by High-Throughput Crystallization. *Proc. Natl. Acad. Sci. USA* **2003**, *100*, 2180–2184. [CrossRef]
61. Lee, J.; Boerrigter, S.X.M.; Jung, Y.W.; Byun, Y.; Yuk, S.H.; Byrn, S.R.; Lee, E.H. Organic Vapor Sorption Method of Isostructural Solvates and Polymorph of Tenofovir Disoproxil Fumarate. *Eur. J. Pharm. Sci.* **2013**, *50*, 253–262. [CrossRef] [PubMed]
62. Campeta, A.M.; Chekal, B.P.; Abramov, Y.A.; Meenan, P.A.; Henson, M.J.; Shi, B.; Singer, R.A.; Horspool, K.R. Development of a Targeted Polymorph Screening Approach for a Complex Polymorphic and Highly Solvating API. *J. Pharm. Sci.* **2010**, *99*, 3874–3886. [CrossRef] [PubMed]
63. Beckmann, W.; Nickisch, K.; Budde, U. Development of a Seeding Technique for the Crystallization of the Metastable a Modification of Abecarnil. *Org. Process Res. Dev.* **1998**, *2*, 298–304. [CrossRef]
64. Zaccaro, J.; Matic, J.; Myerson, A.S.; Garetz, B.A. Nonphotochemical, Laser-Induced Nucleation of Supersaturated Aqueous Glycine Produces Unexpected γ-Polymorph. *Cryst. Growth Des.* **2001**, *1*, 5–8. [CrossRef]
65. Pasquali, I.; Bettini, R.; Giordano, F. Supercritical Fluid Technologies: An Innovative Approach for Manipulating the Solid-State of Pharmaceuticals. *Adv. Drug Deliv. Rev.* **2008**, *60*, 399–410. [CrossRef]
66. Stolar, T.; Lukin, S.; Tireli, M.; Sović, I.; Karadeniz, B.; Kereković, I.; Matijašić, G.; Gretić, M.; Katančić, Z.; Dejanović, I.; et al. Control of Pharmaceutical Cocrystal Polymorphism on Various Scales by Mechanochemistry: Transfer from the Laboratory Batch to the Large-Scale Extrusion Processing. *ACS Sustain. Chem. Eng.* **2019**, *7*, 7102–7110. [CrossRef]
67. Manin, A.N.; Drozd, K.V.; Surov, A.O.; Churakov, A.V.; Volkova, T.V.; Perlovich, G.L. Identification of a Previously Unreported Co-Crystal Form of Acetazolamide: A Combination of Multiple Experimental and Virtual Screening Methods. *Phys. Chem. Chem. Phys.* **2020**, *22*, 20867–20879. [CrossRef]
68. Dujardin, N.; Willart, J.F.; Dudognon, E.; Danède, F.; Descamps, M. Mechanism of Solid State Amorphization of Glucose upon Milling. *J. Phys. Chem. B* **2013**, *117*, 1437–1443. [CrossRef]
69. Latreche, M.; Willart, J.F.; Guerain, M.; Hédoux, A.; Danède, F. Using Milling to Explore Physical States: The Amorphous and Polymorphic Forms of Sulindac. *J. Pharm. Sci.* **2019**, *108*, 2635–2642. [CrossRef]
70. Stoler, E.; Warner, J.C. Non-Covalent Derivatives: Cocrystals and Eutectics. *Molecules* **2015**, *20*, 14833–14848. [CrossRef]

71. Yamashita, H.; Hirakura, Y.; Yuda, M.; Teramura, T.; Terada, K. Detection of Cocrystal Formation Based on Binary Phase Diagrams Using Thermal Analysis. *Pharm. Res.* **2013**, *30*, 70–80. [CrossRef] [PubMed]
72. Yamashita, H.; Hirakura, Y.; Yuda, M.; Terada, K. Coformer Screening Using Thermal Analysis Based on Binary Phase Diagrams. *Pharm. Res.* **2014**, *31*, 1946–1957. [CrossRef] [PubMed]
73. Ren, R.; Yang, Z.; Shaw, L.L. Polymorphic Transformation and Powder Characteristics of TiO_2 during High Energy Milling. *J. Mater. Sci.* **2000**, *35*, 6015–6026. [CrossRef]
74. Chieng, N.; Zujovic, Z.; Bowmaker, G.; Rades, T.; Saville, D. Effect of Milling Conditions on the Solid-State Conversion of Ranitidine Hydrochloride Form 1. *Int. J. Pharm.* **2006**, *327*, 36–44. [CrossRef] [PubMed]
75. Willart, J.F.; Lefebvre, J.; Danède, F.; Comini, S.; Looten, P.; Descamps, M. Polymorphic Transformation of the Γ-Form of D-Sorbitol upon Milling: Structural and Nanostructural Analyses. *Solid State Commun.* **2005**, *135*, 519–524. [CrossRef]
76. Lin, S.Y.; Hsu, C.H.; Ke, W.T. Solid-State Transformation of Different Gabapentin Polymorphs upon Milling and Co-Milling. *Int. J. Pharm.* **2010**, *396*, 83–90. [CrossRef]
77. Friščić, T.; Trask, A.V.; Jones, W.; Motherwell, W.D.S. Screening for Inclusion Compounds and Systematic Construction of Three-Component Solids by Liquid-Assisted Grinding. *Angew. Chemie—Int. Ed.* **2006**, *45*, 7546–7550. [CrossRef]
78. Greco, K.; Bogner, R. Solution-Mediated Phase Transformation: Significance During Dissolution and Implications for Bioavailability. *J. Pharm. Sci.* **2012**, *101*, 2996–3018. [CrossRef]
79. Chatziadi, A.; Skořepová, E.; Rohlíček, J.; Dušek, M.; Ridvan, L.; Šoóš, M. Mechanochemically Induced Polymorphic Transformations of Sofosbuvir. *Cryst. Growth Des.* **2020**, *20*, 139–147. [CrossRef]
80. Trask, A.V.; Shan, N.; Motherwell, W.D.S.; Jones, W.; Feng, S.; Tan, R.B.H.; Carpenter, K.J. Selective Polymorph Transformation via Solvent-Drop Grinding. *Chem. Commun.* **2005**, 880–882. [CrossRef]
81. Bouvart, N.; Palix, R.M.; Arkhipov, S.G.; Tumanov, I.A.; Michalchuk, A.A.L.; Boldyreva, E.V. Polymorphism of Chlorpropamide on Liquid-Assisted Mechanical Treatment: Choice of Liquid and Type of Mechanical Treatment Matter. *CrystEngComm* **2018**, *20*, 1797–1803. [CrossRef]
82. Fischer, F.; Heidrich, A.; Greiser, S.; Benemann, S.; Rademann, K.; Emmerling, F. Polymorphism of Mechanochemically Synthesized Cocrystals: A Case Study. *Cryst. Growth Des.* **2016**, *16*, 1701–1707. [CrossRef]
83. Gu, C.H.; Li, H.; Gandhi, R.B.; Raghavan, K. Grouping Solvents by Statistical Analysis of Solvent Property Parameters: Implication to Polymorph Screening. *Int. J. Pharm.* **2004**, *283*, 117–125. [CrossRef] [PubMed]
84. Kasten, G.; Grohganz, H.; Rades, T.; Löbmann, K. Development of a Screening Method for Co-Amorphous Formulations of Drugs and Amino Acids. *Eur. J. Pharm. Sci.* **2016**, *95*, 28–35. [CrossRef]
85. Wu, W.; Löbmann, K.; Rades, T.; Grohganz, H. On the Role of Salt Formation and Structural Similarity of Co-Formers in Co-Amorphous Drug Delivery Systems. *Int. J. Pharm.* **2018**, *535*, 86–94. [CrossRef]
86. Caron, V.; Tajber, L.; Corrigan, O.I.; Healy, A.M. A Comparison of Spray Drying and Milling in the Production of Amorphous Dispersions of Sulfathiazole/Polyvinylpyrrolidone and Sulfadimidine/Polyvinylpyrrolidone. *Mol. Pharm.* **2011**, *8*, 532–542. [CrossRef]
87. Allesø, M.; Chieng, N.; Rehder, S.; Rantanen, J.; Rades, T.; Aaltonen, J. Enhanced Dissolution Rate and Synchronized Release of Drugs in Binary Systems through Formulation: Amorphous Naproxen-Cimetidine Mixtures Prepared by Mechanical Activation. *J. Control. Release* **2009**, *136*, 45–53. [CrossRef]
88. Karmwar, P.; Graeser, K.; Gordon, K.C.; Strachan, C.J.; Rades, T. Investigation of Properties and Recrystallisation Behaviour of Amorphous Indomethacin Samples Prepared by Different Methods. *Int. J. Pharm.* **2011**, *417*, 94–100. [CrossRef]
89. Wojnarowska, Z.; Grzybowska, K.; Adrjanowicz, K.; Kaminski, K.; Paluch, M.; Hawelek, L.; Wrzalik, R.; Dulski, M.; Sawicki, W.; Mazgalski, J.; et al. Study of the Amorphous Glibenclamide Drug: Analysis of the Molecular Dynamics of Quenched and Cryomilled Material. *Mol. Pharm.* **2010**, *7*, 1692–1707. [CrossRef]
90. Megarry, A.J.; Booth, J.; Burley, J. Amorphous Trehalose Dihydrate by Cryogenic Milling. *Carbohydr. Res.* **2011**, *346*, 1061–1064. [CrossRef]
91. Moinuddin, S.M.; Ruan, S.; Huang, Y.; Gao, Q.; Shi, Q.; Cai, B.; Cai, T. Facile Formation of Co-Amorphous Atenolol and Hydrochlorothiazide Mixtures via Cryogenic-Milling: Enhanced Physical Stability, Dissolution and Pharmacokinetic Profile. *Int. J. Pharm.* **2017**, *532*, 393–400. [CrossRef]
92. Jensen, K.T.; Larsen, F.H.; Löbmann, K.; Rades, T.; Grohganz, H. Influence of Variation in Molar Ratio on Co-Amorphous Drug-Amino Acid Systems. *Eur. J. Pharm. Biopharm.* **2016**, *107*, 32–39. [CrossRef] [PubMed]
93. Badal Tejedor, M.; Pazesh, S.; Nordgren, N.; Schuleit, M.; Rutland, M.W.; Alderborn, G.; Millqvist-Fureby, A. Milling Induced Amorphisation and Recrystallization of α-Lactose Monohydrate. *Int. J. Pharm.* **2018**, *537*, 140–147. [CrossRef]
94. Wu, W.; Löbmann, K.; Schnitzkewitz, J.; Knuhtsen, A.; Pedersen, D.S.; Grohganz, H.; Rades, T. Aspartame as a Co-Former in Co-Amorphous Systems. *Int. J. Pharm.* **2018**, *549*, 380–387. [CrossRef] [PubMed]
95. Dujardin, N.; Willart, J.F.; Dudognon, E.; Hédoux, A.; Guinet, Y.; Paccou, L.; Chazallon, B.; Descamps, M. Solid State Vitrification of Crystalline α and β-D-Glucose by Mechanical Milling. *Solid State Commun.* **2008**, *148*, 78–82. [CrossRef]
96. Kasten, G.; Nouri, K.; Grohganz, H.; Rades, T.; Löbmann, K. Performance Comparison between Crystalline and Co-Amorphous Salts of Indomethacin-Lysine. *Int. J. Pharm.* **2017**, *533*, 138–144. [CrossRef] [PubMed]

97. Martinez, L.M.; Cruz, J. Preparación de Formulaciones Farmacéuticas Amorfas Usando Metodologías Alternativas Emergentes de Amorfización. 2018. Available online: https://www.researchgate.net/publication/363611674_PREPARACION_DE_FORMULACIONES_FARMACEUTICAS_AMORFAS_USANDO_METODOLOGIAS_ALTERNATIVAS_EMERGENTES_DE_AMORFIZACION (accessed on 1 March 2021).
98. Löbmann, K.; Laitinen, R.; Strachan, C.; Rades, T.; Grohganz, H. Amino Acids as Co-Amorphous Stabilizers for Poorly Water-Soluble Drugs—Part 2: Molecular Interactions. *Eur. J. Pharm. Biopharm.* **2013**, *85*, 882–888. [CrossRef]
99. Kasten, G.; Lobo, L.; Dengale, S.; Grohganz, H.; Rades, T.; Löbmann, K. In Vitro and in Vivo Comparison between Crystalline and Co-Amorphous Salts of Naproxen-Arginine. *Eur. J. Pharm. Biopharm.* **2018**, *132*, 192–199. [CrossRef]
100. França, M.T.; Marcos, T.M.; Pereira, R.N.; Stulzer, H.K. Could the Small Molecules Such as Amino Acids Improve Aqueous Solubility and Stabilize Amorphous Systems Containing Griseofulvin? *Eur. J. Pharm. Sci.* **2020**, *143*, 105178. [CrossRef]
101. Jensen, K.T.; Löbmann, K.; Rades, T.; Grohganz, H. Improving Co-Amorphous Drug Formulations by the Addition of the Highly Water Soluble Amino Acid, Proline. *Pharmaceutics* **2014**, *6*, 416–435. [CrossRef]
102. Wu, W.; Löbmann, K.; Schnitzkewitz, J.; Knuhtsen, A.; Pedersen, D.S.; Rades, T.; Grohganz, H. Dipeptides as Co-Formers in Co-Amorphous Systems. *Eur. J. Pharm. Biopharm.* **2019**, *134*, 68–76. [CrossRef] [PubMed]
103. Mennini, N.; Maestrelli, F.; Cirri, M.; Mura, P. Analysis of Physicochemical Properties of Ternary Systems of Oxaprozin with Randomly Methylated-ß-Cyclodextrin and L-Arginine Aimed to Improve the Drug Solubility. *J. Pharm. Biomed. Anal.* **2016**, *129*, 350–358. [CrossRef] [PubMed]
104. Petry, I.; Löbmann, K.; Grohganz, H.; Rades, T.; Leopold, C.S. In Situ Co-Amorphisation of Arginine with Indomethacin or Furosemide during Immersion in an Acidic Medium—A Proof of Concept Study. *Eur. J. Pharm. Biopharm.* **2018**, *133*, 151–160. [CrossRef] [PubMed]
105. Jensen, K.T.; Larsen, F.H.; Cornett, C.; Löbmann, K.; Grohganz, H.; Rades, T. Formation Mechanism of Coamorphous Drug-Amino Acid Mixtures. *Mol. Pharm.* **2015**, *12*, 2484–2492. [CrossRef] [PubMed]
106. Ueda, H.; Peter Bøtker, J.; Edinger, M.; Löbmann, K.; Grohganz, H.; Müllertz, A.; Rades, T.; Østergaard, J. Formulation of Co-Amorphous Systems from Naproxen and Naproxen Sodium and in Situ Monitoring of Physicochemical State Changes during Dissolution Testing by Raman Spectroscopy. *Int. J. Pharm.* **2020**, *587*, 119662. [CrossRef] [PubMed]
107. Mishra, J.; Löbmann, K.; Grohganz, H.; Rades, T. Influence of Preparation Technique on Co-Amorphization of Carvedilol with Acidic Amino Acids. *Int. J. Pharm.* **2018**, *552*, 407–413. [CrossRef] [PubMed]
108. Laitinen, R.; Löbmann, K.; Grohganz, H.; Strachan, C.; Rades, T. Amino Acids as Co-Amorphous Excipients for Simvastatin and Glibenclamide: Physical Properties and Stability. *Mol. Pharm.* **2014**, *11*, 2381–2389. [CrossRef]
109. Walker, G.; Römann, P.; Poller, B.; Löbmann, K.; Grohganz, H.; Rooney, J.S.; Huff, G.S.; Smith, G.P.S.; Rades, T.; Gordon, K.C.; et al. Probing Pharmaceutical Mixtures during Milling: The Potency of Low-Frequency Raman Spectroscopy in Identifying Disorder. *Mol. Pharm.* **2017**, *14*, 4675–4684. [CrossRef]
110. Ueda, H.; Wu, W.; Löbmann, K.; Grohganz, H.; Müllertz, A.; Rades, T. Application of a Salt Coformer in a Co-Amorphous Drug System Dramatically Enhances the Glass Transition Temperature: A Case Study of the Ternary System Carbamazepine, Citric Acid, and l-Arginine. *Mol. Pharm.* **2018**, *15*, 2036–2044. [CrossRef]
111. Sormunen, H.; Ruponen, M.; Laitinen, R. The Effect of Co-Amorphization of Glibenclamide on Its Dissolution Properties and Permeability through an MDCKII-MDR1 Cell Layer. *Int. J. Pharm.* **2019**, *570*, 118653. [CrossRef]
112. Wu, W.; Grohganz, H.; Rades, T.; Löbmann, K. Comparison of Co-Former Performance in Co-Amorphous Formulations: Single Amino Acids, Amino Acid Physical Mixtures, Amino Acid Salts and Dipeptides as Co-Formers. *Eur. J. Pharm. Sci.* **2021**, *156*, 105582. [CrossRef] [PubMed]
113. Slámová, M.; Prausová, K.; Epikaridisová, J.; Brokešová, J.; Kuentz, M.; Patera, J.; Zámostný, P. Effect of Co-Milling on Dissolution Rate of Poorly Soluble Drugs. *Int. J. Pharm.* **2021**, *597*, 120312. [CrossRef] [PubMed]
114. Fujioka, S.; Kadota, K.; Yoshida, M.; Shirakawa, Y. Improvement in the Elution Behavior of Rutin via Binary Amorphous Solid with Flavonoid Using a Mechanochemical Process. *Food Bioprod. Process.* **2020**, *123*, 274–283. [CrossRef]
115. Hatwar, P.; Pathan, I.B.; Chishti, N.A.H.; Ambekar, W. Pellets Containing Quercetin Amino Acid Co-Amorphous Mixture for the Treatment of Pain: Formulation, Optimization, In-Vitro and In-Vivo Study. *J. Drug Deliv. Sci. Technol.* **2021**, *62*, 102350. [CrossRef]
116. Pinto, J.M.O.; Leão, A.F.; Bazzo, G.C.; Mendes, C.; Madureira, L.M.P.; Caramori, G.F.; Parreira, R.L.T.; Stulzer, H.K. Supersaturating Drug Delivery Systems Containing Fixed-Dose Combination of Two Antihypertensive Drugs: Formulation, in Vitro Evaluation and Molecular Metadynamics Simulations. *Eur. J. Pharm. Sci.* **2021**, *163*, 105860. [CrossRef] [PubMed]
117. Lukin, S.; Stolar, T.; Tireli, M.; Barišić, D.; di Michiel, M.; Užarević, K.; Halasz, I. Solid-State Supramolecular Assembly of Salicylic Acid and 2-Pyridone, 3-Hydroxypyridine or 4-Pyridone. *Croat. Chem. Acta* **2017**, *90*, 707–710. [CrossRef]
118. Shemchuk, O.; Agostino, S.; Fiore, C.; Zannoli, S.; Grepioni, F.; Braga, D. Natural Antimicrobials Meet a Synthetic Antibiotic: Carvacrol/Thymol and Ciprofloxacin Cocrystals as a Promising Solid-State Route to Activity Enhancement. *Cryst. Growth Des.* **2020**, *20*, 6796–6803. [CrossRef]
119. Macfhionnghaile, P.; Crowley, C.M.; McArdle, P.; Erxleben, A. Spontaneous Solid-State Cocrystallization of Caffeine and Urea. *Cryst. Growth Des.* **2020**, *20*, 736–745. [CrossRef]
120. Arabiani, M.R.; Lodagekar, A.; Yadav, B.; Chavan, R.B.; Shastri, N.R.; Purohit, P.Y.; Shelat, P.; Dave, D. Mechanochemical Synthesis of Brexpiprazole Cocrystals to Improve Its Pharmaceutical Attributes. *CrystEngComm* **2019**, *21*, 800–806. [CrossRef]

121. Setyawan, D.; Jovita, R.O.; Iqbal, M.; Paramanandana, A.; Yusuf, H.; Lestari, M.L.A.D. Co-Crystalization of Quercetin and Malonic Acid Using Solvent-Drop Grinding Method. *Trop. J. Pharm. Res.* **2018**, *17*, 997–1002. [CrossRef]

122. Tantardini, C.; Arkipov, S.G.; Cherkashina, K.A.; Kil'met'ev, A.S.; Boldyreva, E.V. Synthesis and Crystal Structure of a Meloxicam Co-Crystal with Benzoic Acid. *Struct. Chem.* **2018**, *29*, 1867–1874. [CrossRef]

123. Wang, Y.; Xue, J.; Qin, J.; Liu, J.; Du, Y. Structure and Spectroscopic Characterization of Pharmaceutical Co-Crystal Formation between Acetazolamide and 4-Hydroxybenzoic Acid. *Spectrochim. Acta—Part A Mol. Biomol. Spectrosc.* **2019**, *219*, 419–426. [CrossRef] [PubMed]

124. De Almeida, A.C.; Torquetti, C.; Ferreira, P.O.; Fernandes, R.P.; dos Santos, E.C.; Kogawa, A.C.; Caires, F.J. Cocrystals of Ciprofloxacin with Nicotinic and Isonicotinic Acids: Mechanochemical Synthesis, Characterization, Thermal and Solubility Study. *Thermochim. Acta* **2020**, *685*, 178346. [CrossRef]

125. Wu, X.; Wang, Y.; Xue, J.; Liu, J.; Qin, J.; Hong, Z.; Du, Y. Solid Phase Drug-Drug Pharmaceutical Co-Crystal Formed between Pyrazinamide and Diflunisal: Structural Characterization Based on Terahertz/Raman Spectroscopy Combining with DFT Calculation. *Spectrochim. Acta—Part A Mol. Biomol. Spectrosc.* **2020**, *234*, 118265. [CrossRef]

126. Fang, J.; Zhang, Z.; Bo, Y.; Xue, J.; Wang, Y.; Liu, J.; Qin, J.; Hong, Z.; Du, Y. Vibrational Spectral and Structural Characterization of Multicomponent Ternary Co-Crystal Formation within Acetazolamide, Nicotinamide and 2-Pyridone. *Spectrochim. Acta—Part A Mol. Biomol. Spectrosc.* **2021**, *245*, 118885. [CrossRef]

127. Liu, C.; Liu, Z.; Chen, Y.; Chen, Z.; Chen, H.; Pui, Y.; Qian, F. Oral Bioavailability Enhancement of β-Lapachone, a Poorly Soluble Fast Crystallizer, by Cocrystal, Amorphous Solid Dispersion, and Crystalline Solid Dispersion. *Eur. J. Pharm. Biopharm.* **2018**, *124*, 73–81. [CrossRef] [PubMed]

128. Ferreira, P.O.; de Almeida, A.C.; dos Santos, É.C.; Droppa, R.; Ferreira, F.F.; Kogawa, A.C.; Caires, F.J. A Norfloxacin-Nicotinic Acid Cocrystal: Mechanochemical Synthesis, Thermal and Structural Characterization and Solubility Assays. *Thermochim. Acta* **2020**, *694*, 178782. [CrossRef]

129. Teng, R.; Wang, L.; Chen, M.; Fang, W.; Gao, Z.; Chai, Y.; Zhao, P.; Bao, Y. Amino Acid Based Pharmaceutical Cocrystals and Hydrate Cocrystals of the Chlorothiazide: Structural Studies and Physicochemical Properties. *J. Mol. Struct.* **2020**, *1217*, 128432. [CrossRef]

130. Gaggero, A.; Jurišić Dukovski, B.; Radić, I.; Šagud, I.; Škorić, I.; Cinčić, D.; Jug, M. Co-Grinding with Surfactants as a New Approach to Enhance in Vitro Dissolution of Praziquantel. *J. Pharm. Biomed. Anal.* **2020**, *189*, 113494. [CrossRef]

131. Aitipamula, S.; Das, S. Cocrystal Formulations: A Case Study of Topical Formulations Consisting of Ferulic Acid Cocrystals. *Eur. J. Pharm. Biopharm.* **2020**, *149*, 95–104. [CrossRef]

132. Hossain Mithu, M.S.; Ross, S.A.; Hurt, A.P.; Douroumis, D. Effect of Mechanochemical Grinding Conditions on the Formation of Pharmaceutical Cocrystals and Co-Amorphous Solid Forms of Ketoconazole—Dicarboxylic Acid. *J. Drug Deliv. Sci. Technol.* **2021**, *63*, 102508. [CrossRef]

133. Vasilev, N.A.; Surov, A.O.; Voronin, A.P.; Drozd, K.V.; Perlovich, G.L. Novel Cocrystals of Itraconazole: Insights from Phase Diagrams, Formation Thermodynamics and Solubility. *Int. J. Pharm.* **2021**, *599*, 120441. [CrossRef] [PubMed]

134. Guerain, M.; Guinet, Y.; Correia, N.T.; Paccou, L.; Danède, F.; Hédoux, A. Polymorphism and Stability of Ibuprofen/Nicotinamide Cocrystal: The Effect of the Crystalline Synthesis Method. *Int. J. Pharm.* **2020**, *584*, 119454. [CrossRef]

135. Zhang, Z.; Fang, J.; Bo, Y.; Xue, J.; Liu, J.; Hong, Z.; Du, Y. Terahertz and Raman Spectroscopic Investigation of Anti-Tuberculosis Drug-Drug Cocrystallization Involving 4-Aminosalicylic Acid and Pyrazinamide. *J. Mol. Struct.* **2021**, *1227*, 129547. [CrossRef]

136. Shaikh, R.; Shirazian, S.; Guerin, S.; Sheehan, E.; Thompson, D.; Walker, G.M.; Croker, D.M. Understanding Solid-State Processing of Pharmaceutical Cocrystals via Milling: Role of Tablet Excipients. *Int. J. Pharm.* **2021**, *601*, 120514. [CrossRef] [PubMed]

137. Mikhailovskaya, A.V.; Myz, S.A.; Bulina, N.V.; Gerasimov, K.B.; Kuznetsova, S.A.; Shakhtshneider, T.P. Screening and Characterization of Cocrystal Formation between Betulin and Terephthalic Acid. *Mater. Today Proc.* **2019**, *25*, 381–383. [CrossRef]

138. Da Silva, C.C.P.; de Melo, C.C.; Souza, M.S.; Diniz, L.F.; Carneiro, R.L.; Ellena, J. 5-Fluorocytosine/5-Fluorouracil Drug-Drug Cocrystal: A New Development Route Based on Mechanochemical Synthesis. *J. Pharm. Innov.* **2019**, *14*, 50–56. [CrossRef]

139. Germann, L.S.; Arhangelskis, M.; Etter, M.; Dinnebier, R.E.; Friščić, T. Challenging the Ostwald Rule of Stages in Mechanochemical Cocrystallisation. *Chem. Sci.* **2020**, *11*, 10092–10100. [CrossRef]

140. Elisei, E.; Willart, J.F.; Danède, F.; Siepmann, J.; Siepmann, F.; Descamps, M. Crystalline Polymorphism Emerging From a Milling-Induced Amorphous Form: The Case of Chlorhexidine Dihydrochloride. *J. Pharm. Sci.* **2018**, *107*, 121–126. [CrossRef]

141. Amaro, M.I.; Simon, A.; Cabral, L.M.; De Sousa, V.P.; Healy, A.M. Rivastigmine Hydrogen Tartrate Polymorphs: Solid-State Characterisation of Transition and Polymorphic Conversion via Milling. *Solid State Sci.* **2018**, *49*, 29–36. [CrossRef]

142. Cheng, W.T.; Lin, S.Y.; Li, M.J. Raman Microspectroscopic Mapping or Thermal System Used to Investigate Milling-Induced Solid-State Conversion of Famotidine Polymorphs. *J. Raman Spectrosc.* **2007**, *38*, 1595–1601. [CrossRef]

143. Surov, A.O.; Vasilev, N.A.; Churakov, A.V.; Stroh, J.; Emmerling, F.; Perlovich, G.L. Solid Forms of Ciprofloxacin Salicylate: Polymorphism, Formation Pathways, and Thermodynamic Stability. *Cryst. Growth Des.* **2019**, *19*, 2979–2990. [CrossRef]

144. Dupont, A.; Guerain, M.; Danède, F.; Paccou, L.; Guinet, Y.; Hédoux, A.; Willart, J.-F. Kinetics and Mechanism of Polymorphic Transformation of Sorbitol under Mechanical Milling. *Int. J. Pharm.* **2020**, *590*, 119902. [CrossRef]

145. Aitipamula, S.; Chow, P.S.; Tan, R.B.H. Conformational and Enantiotropic Polymorphism of a 1:1 Cocrystal Involving Ethenzamide and Ethylmalonic Acid. *CrystEngComm* **2010**, *12*, 3691–3697. [CrossRef]

146. Trask, A.V.; Motherwell, W.D.S.; Jones, W. Solvent-Drop Grinding: Green Polymorph Control of Cocrystallisation. *Chem. Commun.* **2004**, *4*, 890–891. [CrossRef] [PubMed]
147. Good, D.J.; Naír, R.H. Solubility Advantage of Pharmaceutical Cocrystals. *Cryst. Growth Des.* **2009**, *9*, 2252–2264. [CrossRef]
148. Alhalaweh, A.; Roy, L.; Rodríguez-Hornedo, N.; Velaga, S.P. PH-Dependent Solubility of Indomethacin-Saccharin and Carbamazepine-Saccharin Cocrystals in Aqueous Media. *Mol. Pharm.* **2012**, *9*, 2605–2612. [CrossRef]
149. Bavishi, D.D.; Borkhataria, C.H. Spring and Parachute: How Cocrystals Enhance Solubility. *Prog. Cryst. Growth Charact. Mater.* **2016**, *62*, 1–8. [CrossRef]
150. Pazesh, S.; Lazorova, L.; Berggren, J.; Alderborn, G.; Gråsjö, J. Considerations on the Quantitative Analysis of Apparent Amorphicity of Milled Lactose by Raman Spectroscopy. *Int. J. Pharm.* **2016**, *511*, 488–504. [CrossRef]
151. Soares, F.L.F.; Carneiro, R.L. Green Synthesis of Ibuprofen-Nicotinamide Cocrystals and in-Line Evaluation by Raman Spectroscopy. *Cryst. Growth Des.* **2013**, *13*, 1510–1517. [CrossRef]
152. Mukherjee, A.; Tothadi, S.; Chakraborty, S.; Ganguly, S.; Desiraju, G.R. Synthon Identification in Co-Crystals and Polymorphs with IR Spectroscopy. Primary Amides as a Case Study. *CrystEngComm* **2013**, *15*, 4640–4654. [CrossRef]
153. Saha, S.; Rajput, L.; Joseph, S.; Mishra, M.K.; Ganguly, S.; Desiraju, G.R. IR Spectroscopy as a Probe for C-H···X Hydrogen Bonded Supramolecular Synthons. *CrystEngComm* **2015**, *17*, 1273–1290. [CrossRef]
154. Skorupska, E.; Kaźmierski, S.; Potrzebowski, M.J. Solid State NMR Characterization of Ibuprofen:Nicotinamide Cocrystals and New Idea for Controlling Release of Drugs Embedded into Mesoporous Silica Particles. *Mol. Pharm.* **2017**, *14*, 1800–1810. [CrossRef] [PubMed]
155. Apih, T.; Žagar, V.; Seliger, J. NMR and NQR Study of Polymorphism in Carbamazepine. *Solid State Nucl. Magn. Reson.* **2020**, *107*, 101653. [CrossRef]
156. Thomas, L.C. Use of Multiple Heating Rate DSC and Modulated Temperature DSC to Detect and Analyze Temperature-Time-Dependent Transitions in Materials. *Am. Lab.* **2001**, *33*, 26–31. Available online: https://www.researchgate.net/publication/28 6909193_Use_of_multiple_heating_rate_DSC_and_modulated_temperature_DSC_to_detect_and_analyze_temperature-time-dependent_transitions_in_materials (accessed on 1 March 2021).
157. Kissi, E.O.; Kasten, G.; Löbmann, K.; Rades, T.; Grohganz, H. The Role of Glass Transition Temperatures in Coamorphous Drug-Amino Acid Formulations. *Mol. Pharm.* **2018**, *15*, 4247–4256. [CrossRef] [PubMed]
158. Löbmann, K.; Laitinen, R.; Grohganz, H.; Gordon, K.C.; Strachan, C.; Rades, T. Coamorphous Drug Systems: Enhanced Physical Stability and Dissolution Rate of Indomethacin and Naproxen. *Mol. Pharm.* **2011**, *8*, 1919–1928. [CrossRef]
159. Gordon, M.; Taylor, J. Ideal Copolymers and the Second-Order Transition of Rubbers. *J. Appl. Chem.* **1952**, *2*, 493–500. [CrossRef]
160. Shamblin, S.L.; Huang, E.Y.; Zografi, G. The Effects of Co-Lyophilized Polymeric Additives on the Glass Transition Temperature and Crystallization of Amorphous Sucrose. *J. Therm. Anal.* **1996**, *47*, 1567–1579. [CrossRef]
161. Taylor, L.S.; Zografi, G. Sugar-Polymer Hydrogen Bond Interactions in Lyophilized Amorphous Mixtures. *J. Pharm. Sci.* **1998**, *87*, 1615–1621. [CrossRef]
162. Masuda, T.; Yoshihashi, Y.; Yonemochi, E.; Fujii, K.; Uekusa, H.; Terada, K. Cocrystallization and Amorphization Induced by Drug-Excipient Interaction Improves the Physical Properties of Acyclovir. *Int. J. Pharm.* **2012**, *422*, 160–169. [CrossRef] [PubMed]
163. Yamamura, S.; Gotoh, H.; Sakamoto, Y.; Momose, Y. Physicochemical Properties of Amorphous Salt of Cimetidine and Diflunisal System. *Int. J. Pharm.* **2002**, *241*, 213–221. [CrossRef]
164. Warner, J.C. Entropic Control in Chemistry and Design. *Pure Appl. Chem.* **2006**, *78*, 2035–2041. [CrossRef]
165. Nugrahani, I.; Utami, D.; Ibrahim, S.; Nugraha, Y.P.; Uekusa, H. Zwitterionic Cocrystal of Diclofenac and L-Proline: Structure Determination, Solubility, Kinetics of Cocrystallization, and Stability Study. *Eur. J. Pharm. Sci.* **2018**, *117*, 168–176. [CrossRef] [PubMed]
166. Zhang, G.G.Z.; Gu, C.; Zell, M.T.; Todd Burkhardt, R.; Munson, E.J.; Grant, D.J.W. Crystallization and Transitions of Sulfamerazine Polymorphs. *J. Pharm. Sci.* **2002**, *91*, 1089–1100. [CrossRef] [PubMed]
167. Willart, J.F.; De Gusseme, A.; Hemon, S.; Odou, G.; Danede, F.; Descamps, M. Direct Crystal to Glass Transformation of Trehalose Induced by Ball Milling. *Solid State Commun.* **2001**, *119*, 501–505. [CrossRef]
168. Desprez, S.; Descamps, M. Transformations of Glassy Indomethacin Induced by Ball-Milling. *J. Non. Cryst. Solids* **2006**, *352*, 4480–4485. [CrossRef]
169. Löbmann, K.; Grohganz, H.; Laitinen, R.; Strachan, C.; Rades, T. Amino Acids as Co-Amorphous Stabilizers for Poorly Water Soluble Drugs—Part 1: Preparation, Stability and Dissolution Enhancement. *Eur. J. Pharm. Biopharm.* **2013**, *85*, 873–881. [CrossRef]
170. Sterren, V.B.; Zoppi, A.; Abraham-Miranda, J.; Longhi, M.R. Enhanced Dissolution Profiles of Glibenclamide with Amino Acids Using a Cogrinding Method. *Mater. Today Commun.* **2021**, *26*, 102126. [CrossRef]
171. Tejedor, M.B.; Nordgren, N.; Schuleit, M.; Pazesh, S.; Alderborn, G.; Millqvist-Fureby, A.; Rutland, M.W. Determination of Interfacial Amorphicity in Functional Powders. *Langmuir* **2017**, *33*, 920–926. [CrossRef]

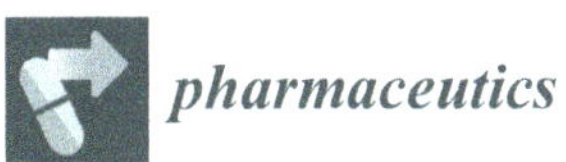 *pharmaceutics*

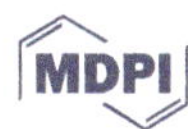

Review

Formulation Approaches to Crystalline Status Modification for Carotenoids: Impacts on Dissolution, Stability, Bioavailability, and Bioactivities

Wan-Yi Liu [1,†], Yun-Shan Hsieh [1,†], Horng-Huey Ko [1,2,3,4,*] and Yu-Tse Wu [1,5,*]

1   School of Pharmacy, College of Pharmacy, Kaohsiung Medical University, Kaohsiung 80708, Taiwan
2   Department of Fragrance and Cosmetic Science, College of Pharmacy, Kaohsiung Medical University, Kaohsiung 80708, Taiwan
3   Department of Medical Research, Kaohsiung Medical University Hospital, Kaohsiung Medical University, Kaohsiung 80708, Taiwan
4   Drug Development and Value Creation Center, Kaohsiung Medical University, Kaohsiung 80708, Taiwan
5   Center for Cancer Research, Kaohsiung Medical University, Kaohsiung 80708, Taiwan
*   Correspondence: hhko@kmu.edu.tw (H.-H.K.); ytwu@kmu.edu.tw (Y.-T.W.);
    Tel.: +886-7-3121101 (ext. 2643) (H.-H.K.); +886-7-3121101 (ext. 2254) (Y.-T.W.)
†   These authors contributed equally to this work.

Abstract: Carotenoids, including carotenes and xanthophylls, have been identified as bioactive ingredients in foods and are considered to possess health-promoting effects. From a biopharmaceutical perspective, several physicochemical characteristics, such as scanty water solubility, restricted dissolution, and susceptibility to oxidation may influence their oral bioavailability and eventually, their effectiveness. In this review, we have summarized various formulation approaches that deal with the modification of crystalline status for carotenoids, which may improve their physicochemical properties, oral absorption, and biological effects. The mechanisms involving crystalline alteration and the typical methods for examining crystalline states in the pharmaceutical field have been included, and representative formulation approaches are introduced to unriddle the mechanisms and effects more clearly.

Keywords: carotenoids; crystallization status modification; formulation approaches

Citation: Liu, W.-Y.; Hsieh, Y.-S.; Ko, H.-H.; Wu, Y.-T. Formulation Approaches to Crystalline Status Modification for Carotenoids: Impacts on Dissolution, Stability, Bioavailability, and Bioactivities. *Pharmaceutics* **2023**, *15*, 485. https://doi.org/10.3390/pharmaceutics15020485

Academic Editors: Anne Marie Healy and Hisham Al-Obaidi

Received: 16 December 2022
Revised: 30 January 2023
Accepted: 30 January 2023
Published: 1 February 2023

1. Introduction

Carotenoids are composed of compounds containing typically 40 carbon atoms and are synthesized by plants or microorganisms. The structure of carotenoids commonly includes a central carbon chain with several conjugated double bonds and they partially have different cyclic or acyclic end groups [1]. Carotenoids are divided into carotenes and xanthophylls depending on the chemical structure as presented in Figure 1. Carotenes, such as α-carotene, β-carotene, and lycopene, only contain carbon and hydrogen in their structure without oxygen atoms. Xanthophylls, such as astaxanthin, β-cryptoxanthin, lutein, and zeaxanthin, are the other type; they are carotenoids containing one or more oxygen atoms in their structure. The bioactivities of carotenoids have been demonstrated to be associated with chemical structures, such as the number of conjugated double bonds and the types of functional groups at the ends [2].

Carotenoids exhibit well-known anti-oxidative activities and are most likely involved in scavenging the singlet oxygen and peroxy radicals [3]. Reactive oxygen species (ROS) are generated during normal metabolism and engaged in enzymatic reactions, mitochondrial electron transport and signal transduction. Excessive ROS would damage biologically essential factors and elevate the risk of degenerative diseases [4]. Therefore, carotenoids are considered excellent antioxidants that benefit various diseases associated with oxidative stress. The bioactivities of carotenoids have been reported in previous studies and are listed in Table 1.

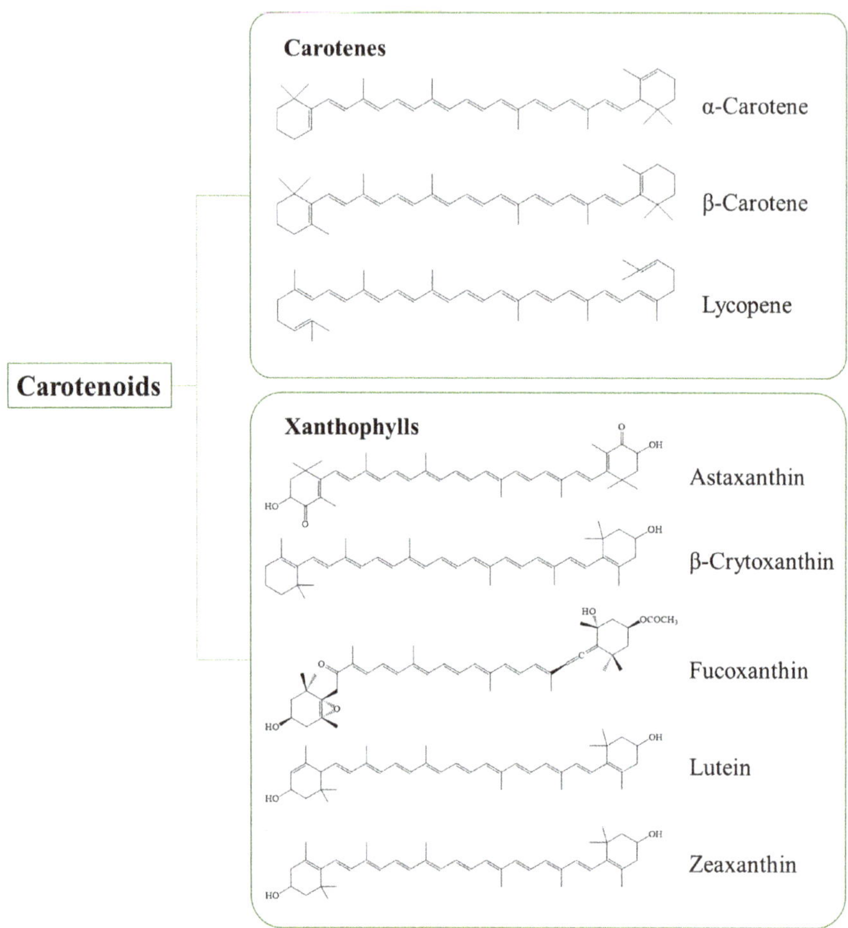

Figure 1. The structure of carotenes and xanthophylls.

Carotenoids commonly exist in crystalline states and exhibit an ordered intermolecular arrangement in the solid state. Various intermolecular interactions, such as hydrogen bonding and π-π stacking interactions, maintain the structure integrity and crystalline status of carotenoids [5,6]. The crystalline status of carotenoids contributes to the scant solubility and dissolution, which further restricts their oral bioavailability and health-promoting effects. Therefore, improving the solubility of carotenoids is a critical issue for achieving the desired plasma concentration in systemic circulation to attain the expected biological effects [7]. The higher lattice energy of crystalline compounds usually correlates with their poor solubilities, because the energy has to be overcome before the compound can be dissolved in the medium [8]. Carotenoids have poor aqueous solubility owing to the higher lattice energy. Thus, the crystalline status is a crucial factor for the application of carotenoids.

Table 1. The bioactivities of carotenoids that have been reported in previous studies.

Carotenoids	Dose	Model	Bioactivities	Reference
Astaxanthin	1.0 mg/mouse/day	Diabetic C57BL/KsJ-db/db mice	Anti-diabetic (Blood glucose↓ and preservation of -cell function)	[9]
Astaxanthin	2 mg	Healthy women	Immune response improvement (Mitogen-induced lymphoproliferation↑ Natural killer cell, total T and B cell↑ DNA damage biomarker↓)	[10]
Astaxanthin	5 μM	Primary hippocampal neurons	Treatment of Hcy-mediated neurological disorders (ROS and superoxide anion↓)	[11]
β-Carotene	45 mg/day	Healthy older adults	Immunostimulant (Total T cells and NK cell↑)	[12]
β-Carotene	200 mg/Kg	Male albino mice	Anticonvulsant activity (Duration of general tonic–clonic seizures↓ General tonic–clonic seizures latency↑)	[13]
β-Carotene	30 μM	Human prostate cancer cell line (PC-3 cell)	Anticancer (cell viability: 51.4%)	[14]
β-Carotene	2.05 mg/Kg	Male albino mice	Treatment of Alzheimer's disease (Acetylcholinesterase and amyloid β-protein↓)	[15]
β-Cryptoxanthin	0.8 mg/Kg/day	Male mice	Anti-obesity (Adipocyte hypertrophy↓)	[16]
Fucoxanthin	5 μM	Human fibroblast	Protection against UVB radiation-induced oxidative stress (ROS↓)	[17]
Fucoxanthin	1.06-2.22%	C57BL/6J mice	Anti-obesity and anti-diabetic effects (Body weight and white adipose tissue↓ MCP-1 expression↓ and Adrb3 and GLUT4↑)	[18]
Fucoxanthin	0.2%	C57BL/6N mice	Anti-obesity (Fatty acid β-oxidation activity and lipogenic enzyme activities ↓)	[19]
Lutein and Zeaxanthin	Oral: lutein 100 ppm zeaxanthin 6 ppm Topical: lutein 10 ppm zeaxanthin 0.6 ppm	Healthy women	Photoprotective (Lipid peroxidation↓ skin lipid, skin hydration and skin elasticity↑)	[20]
Lutein and Zeaxanthin	Lutein: 5% zeaxanthin: 0.2%	β5−/− mice	Prevention of age-related retinal pigment epithelium actin damage (4-hydroxynonenal-adduct formation, age-related cone and rod photoreceptor dysfunction ↓)	[21]
Lutein and Zeaxanthin	Lutein:10 mg Zeaxanthin: 2 mg	Healthy older adults	Improvement of cognitive function (Macular pigment optical density, complex attention and cognitive flexibility domains↑)	[22]

Table 1. *Cont.*

Carotenoids	Dose	Model	Bioactivities	Reference
Lycopene	5 µg/mL	Fungal cell (*Candida albicans*)	Antifungi (Destruction of fungi membrane and inhibition of the normal budding process)	[23]
Lycopene	2 µM	Rat cortical neurons	Treatment of Alzheimer's disease (Intracellular ROS and superoxide production↓)	[24]
Lycopene	0.2 or 0.5 µM	Neuronal SH-SY5Y cells	Neuron protection (ROS↓ and mitochondrial dysfunction ↓)	[25]
Lycopene	0.03% (*w/w*, mixed into normal chow)	Male C57BL/6J mice	Treatment of Alzheimer's disease (Memory loss behavior, amyloid plaques, amyloid precursor protein, neuronal β-secretase BACE1, inflammatory mediators and oxidative stress↓, α-secretase ADAM10↑)	[26]
Lycopene	2 µM	Mice cerebral cortical neurons	Neuron protection (Nerve growth factor, brain-derived neurotrophic factor, and vascular endothelial growth factor excretion↑ and anti-apoptosis)	[27]
Lycopene	100 mg/Kg	Female Sprague-Dawley rats	Treatment of vascular dementia (Oxidative stress in hippocampus↓)	[28]

↑: enhancement. ↓: reduction. ROS: reactive oxygen species. Adrb3: β3-adrenergic receptor. GLUT4: glucose transporter 4.

2. Effects of Crystalline Status Modification on the Physicochemical Properties of Carotenoids

The chemical structures of carotenoids possess many chiral centers, which result in a variety of conformations. The *cis*-form (Z-form) and *trans*-form (E-form) have been demonstrated to affect the crystalline state and further have an impact on the physicochemical properties. In general, the all-*trans* carotenoid isomers are the most stable ones owing to their different Gibbs free energies and exist commonly in nature. Only 5-*cis*-lycopene was found to be more stable than all-*trans*-isomers [29]. The *cis*-form isomers display diverse properties compared to the *trans*-form isomers, such as a shallower color caused by the shorter maximum absorption wavelength and smaller extinction coefficient [30], reduction in the crystalline ratio, lower melting point, and poor stability [31]. Taking β-carotene as an example, Figure 2 shows the isomers of β-carotene and the maximum absorption wavelength of these compounds [32]. A previous study reported the transformation method and different properties of the E-form and Z-form carotenoids. The Z-form lycopene has been discovered to have a 4000-fold higher solubility compared to the E-form in ethanol [6]. The lower degree of crystallinity leads to higher solubility in bile acid micelles, and the higher solubility would further result in greater bioaccessibility. Interestingly, the ideal bioaccessibility cannot completely correlate with bioavailability [6]. The cellular uptake efficiency is a critical factor that influences bioavailability, and the efficiency depends on the molecular structure and hydrophobic properties. In previous studies, Yang et al. [33,34] found that the *trans*-lutein had better passive diffusion into enterocytes due to the linear structure, and the affinity to transporters in the intestine changed the cellular uptake efficiency as well because the relatively higher solubility of 9Z-astaxanthin caused poorer affinity to the transporter compared with 13Z-astaxanthin and the *trans*-isomer. This theory can also be applied to β-carotene. E-β-carotene was also reported to exhibit higher absorption than the Z-form in both in vitro [35] and in vivo studies [36]. Therefore, modification of the crystalline conformation impacts the solubility, dissolution, intestinal absorption, and further bioavailability of carotenoids, together with the bioactivity.

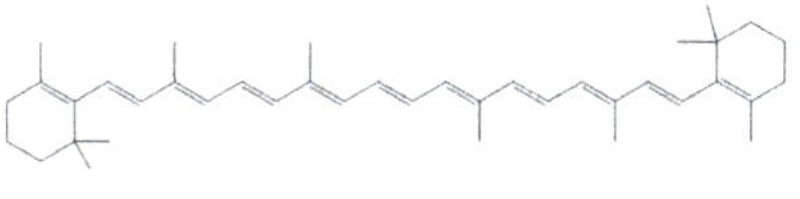

All-trans-β-carotene (λ_{max}: 451.4 nm)

Isomers

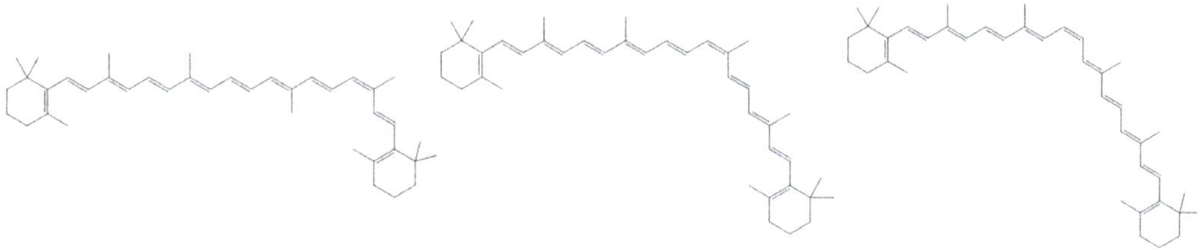

9-cis-isomer (λ_{max}: 446.4 nm)   13-cis-isomer (λ_{max}: 439.1 nm)   15-cis-isomer (λ_{max}: 443.8 nm)

Figure 2. The structures of E (*trans*)- and Z (*cis*)- forms of β-carotene.

Micronized crystalline lutein has been prepared to improve its dissolution and oral bioavailability [37]. A wet-jet milling method with high mechanical force was applied to reduce the particle size, and the procedures also converted the crystalline form into the polymorphic state, which belonged to a metastable situation with higher energy. The effects of size reduction and crystalline transformation are beneficial to dissolution and oral absorption. Though the solubility may have effects on the transporter affinity, the absorption still requires the transition from solid form to solution [38]. In order to improve the aqueous solubility of active crystalline compounds, the alternation of the crystalline condition is the simplest method. Crystalline states can be classified into three types—polymorphic state, pseudo-polymorphic state, and amorphous state—the difference among the three states is shown in Figure 3. Polymorphs are the same constituents with different crystalline arrangements, and they often benefit solubility. Notably, the improvement is small due to the small energy difference between the polymorphs [39]. Pseudo-polymorphs include hydrates or solvates, and they are usually unwanted crystalline forms. In the case of solvates, this depends on the characteristics of solvents. On the other hand, water forms hydrogen bonds with the active compounds in hydrates, and the lattice enthalpy would escalate to decrease the solubility, accompanied by a lower bioavailability [5]. The amorphous state lacks the ordered arrangement of molecules, causing amorphs to have poor thermodynamic stability, and it is usually the first choice to greatly enhance the aqueous solubility [40]. The amorphous state is divided into molecularly pure, which only transfers the crystalline state of the active compounds and formulation. Both of them may increase the solubility; however, the stability and scale-up of the molecularly pure type are hard to achieve [41]. Therefore, preparing a formulation to transfer the crystal to another state is quite an important technique to enhance the solubility and oral absorption, and then exhibit the expected bioactivities. To distinguish the crystalline status in the formulation, detection methods have been introduced.

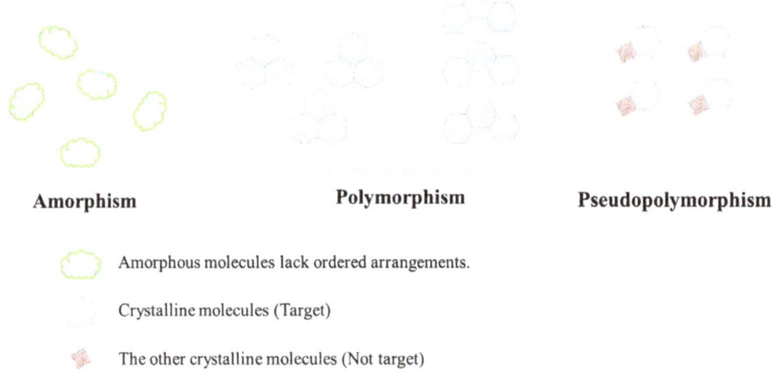

Figure 3. The difference among amorphism, polymorphism, and pseudo-polymorphism.

3. Methods for Examining the Crystalline Status

Powder X-ray diffraction (PXRD), differential scanning calorimetry (DSC), thermogravimetric analysis (TGA), transmission electron microscopy (TEM), and scanning electron microscopy (SEM) are fundamental methods to determine the characterization of the crystal in pharmaceutical formulations; usually, more than two methods are adopted to reveal more reliable results.

3.1. PXRD

PXRD is a well-known method to qualify the crystalline state and quantify the crystallinity as well as crystal size in a formulation. Fingerprint data of APIs can be obtained by PXRD, and possible polymorphs can be identified. The intensities of diffraction peaks are positively related to crystallinity, and we can use them to calculate the percentage of amorphization. However, nanocrystals and amorphism are hard to differentiate because the low crystallinity leads to broad peaks (i.e., Scherrer broadening) [42]. The nanocrystal size can be calculated using the Scherrer equation (Equation (1)), and the formula is only viable for nanocrystals around 100–200 nm [43].

$$\tau = k\lambda/(\beta \cos\theta) \tag{1}$$

where τ is the average size of the crystal; k is the shape factor; λ is the wavelength of the X-ray; β is the line broadening at half the maximum intensity in radians; θ is the Bragg angle.

Figure 4 shows the PXRD profiles of β-carotene and nanoformulations, where the API group presents sharp and strong peaks compared with the nanoformulation groups, indicating the API has been encapsulated in the formulations in an amorphous state.

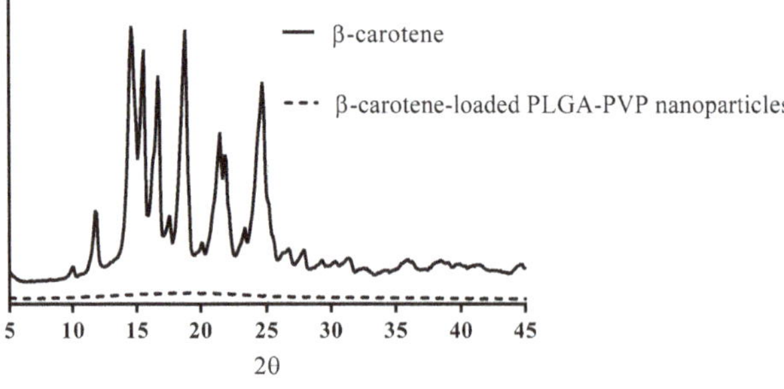

Figure 4. PXRD profiles of β-carotene and its nanoformulations.

3.2. Electron Microscopy—TEM and SEM

For nanoscale crystals, electron microscopy is applied to visualize the lattice. The crystal size and the structure of the lattice are provided by TEM. The sizes calculated using TEM may be larger than those from the Scherrer equation as particles seen in the TEM images are possibly not crystals, and the crystalline imperfections broaden the peaks in PXRD, causing calculation bias [44]. SEM is a technology suitable for morphology observation, and the relationship between phases such as erosion can be further acquired compared with TEM [45]. However, the two technologies are limited by the samples "seen" by the microscope, and only unilateral information may be obtained. Thus, more significant sample sizes and observed angles are needed to avoid sampling errors and to obtain the whole morphology.

3.3. Thermal Methods—DSC and TGA

Thermal methods detect the thermal behavior of the whole sample, and they will not encounter issues with the difference between the surface and the core or the sampling bias [46]. DSC measures the heat required for the temperature increase in the samples; the heat absorption from melt formation or release due to the crystallization will be detected [42], and T_m (melting point), T_g (glass transition temperature), T_c (crystallization temperature), and T_d (degradation temperature) can be obtained [47]. The endothermic T_m peak disappears once the crystals convert into amorphs, and the concept can be applied to confirm the encapsulation of amorphous APIs in formulations [48]. Taking DSC thermograms (Figure 5) as an example, the peak standing for the melting point of β-carotene at 186 °C was observed in the crystalline API and physical mixture, and the peak disappeared in the formulation group. However, it is hard to distinguish the amorph merely from the thermogram when the degree of crystallization is relatively high, and a simple formula (Equation (2)) can be used to calculate the amorphous content [49].

$$\text{Amorphous content} = \frac{\Delta H_f^{\text{amorphous}}}{\Delta H_f^{\text{crystal}}} \tag{2}$$

where $\Delta H_f^{\text{amorphous}}$ represents the enthalpy of the fusion of the amorphous fraction, and $\Delta H_f^{\text{crystal}}$ represents the enthalpy of the fusion of the crystalline fraction.

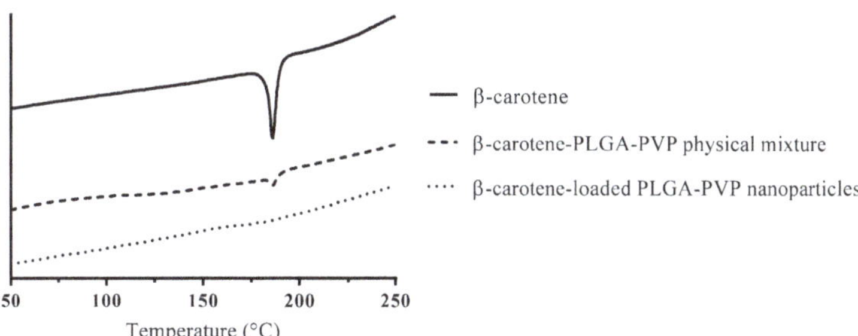

Figure 5. DSC thermograms of β-carotene, a β-carotene-PLGA-PVP physical mixture, and β-carotene-loaded PLGA-PVP nanoparticles.

TGA measures the weight loss resulting from heating, and this technology can be used to investigate crystals containing volatile substances [5]. It is also often conducted combined with DSC to further confirm the thermal behavior. The crystal and amorph can be distinguished by the different weight loss under the same temperature [50], which can be used to prove the complex formation [51].

4. Effects of Preparation Factors on Crystalline Status of Active Pharmaceutical Ingredients

Turning active pharmaceutical ingredients (APIs) into amorphous or polymorph states is expected to change their biopharmaceutical properties, including their dissolution rate and bioavailability, which can be accomplished using various manufacturing processes. Major preparation factors that affect the crystalline status are summarized in Figure 6.

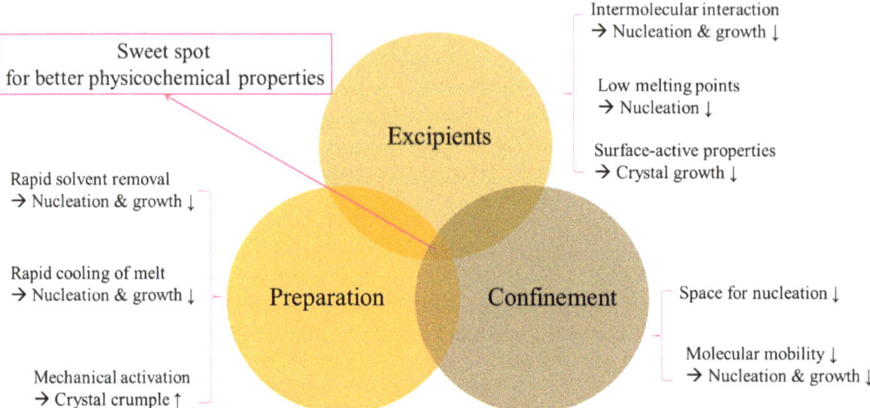

Figure 6. Formulation conditions affecting crystallization.

4.1. Excipients

Crystallization often includes two major steps, namely, nucleation and growth; the addition of excipients can manipulate the crystallization of APIs. The rate of nucleation is usually positively related to molecular mobility, suggesting that the restriction of molecular mobility through intermolecular interaction between excipients and APIs can also affect the crystallization of APIs.

Poly(ethylene oxide) as a plasticizer increases the nucleation rate due to its water-absorbing properties [52]. Amphiphilic polymers are preferred for hydrophobic carotenoids because the hydrophobic substituents of the excipients increase the interaction with carotenoids, and the hydrophilic substituents interact with water to enhance the dissolution [53]. In addition, lipids act as inhibitors or promoters of crystallization. The choice of lipids is based on three principles: hydrocarbon chain lengths, unsaturated degrees, and esterification degrees [54]. Saturated fatty acids with high polarity and a short chain length (e.g., butyric acid) have lower melting points, and the lower melting point prevents the molecule from forming crystalline nuclei. Meanwhile, fatty acids can adsorb on the interface of the liquid—solid nucleus to inhibit crystalline growth because of their surface-active properties [55].

Moisture also plays an essential role in crystalline formation. When water and APIs form crystals together, hydrates are produced, and the hydrogen bonding between water and APIs leads to higher lattice enthalpy and poorer bioavailability [5]. Hydroxyl groups of hydroxypropyl methylcellulose (HPMC) inhibit hydrate formation by occupying the sites where APIs and water have hydrogen bindings. The higher molecular weight of the excipients provides more functional groups for interactions and the full surface coverage of APIs [56]. Excipients with charges, such as dextran, alginate, and chitosan, can form ionic interactions with APIs possessing opposite charges, therefore, preventing the ongoing crystallization of APIs [56]. As excipients have great impacts on the stabilization of amorph conditions, excipient screening is an essential step for developing optimal formulations.

4.2. Preparation

Dissolution followed by rapid precipitation, melting followed by rapid cooling, and direct solid conversion are major methods to change the crystalline status of APIs. For the technique of dissolution followed by rapid precipitation, excipients dissolved in organic solvents loosen their structure, having interactions with the solvents. Meanwhile, APIs dissolved in organic solvents (i.e., amorphous states of APIs) enter the structure of the excipients and integrate into loosened excipients. With the rapid removal of solvents, the excipient and the amorphous APIs do not have enough time for ordinary crystallization and finally form a compact structure [57].

For the method of melting followed by rapid cooling, excipients and APIs are melted via heating. In the melt phase, the heat loosens the structure of the excipients, allowing APIs to occupy the space inside the excipients. Thereafter, fast cooling of the melt dramatically increases the viscosity and decreases the volume in a short time, resulting in much slower molecular mobility and molecule arrangement to prevent nucleation and crystalline growth [58].

Direct solid conversion refers to mechanical activation by milling. During the milling process, local heat accompanied by cooling results in amorphization, and the procedure increases static disorder and intrinsic dynamic disorder to the threshold value of the lattice, leading to the crumpling of the crystals. A limitation of this method, which should be taken into consideration, is the possibility of incomplete crystalline disorder [59]. The milling processing only renders the surface of the ingredients amorphized and may lead to inconsistent results in the physicochemical characterization [46].

In fact, for APIs, different manufacturing processes will produce varying degrees of amorphous forms, which cause diverse profiles in solubility, dissolution, and bioavailability [60].

4.3. Confinement (Change in Particle Sizes)

Confinement in the pharmaceutical field represents the physical restriction of APIs at the indicated scale. Under confinement, a different polymorph or amorph may appear, and confinement represents a practical handle to control or stabilize crystalline growth, as shown in Figure 7. The reasons why confinement affects the crystalline behavior remain unclear, but there are some proposed mechanisms: (i) When the size of the confinement is smaller than the critical nucleus size of the most stable crystals, the crystalline growth will be inhibited and a new polymorph or amorph will possibly form [61]. However, all polymorph forms of acetaminophen can grow under nanoconfinement [62]. The opposite result may relate to the chosen size for the confinement. Several pore sizes have been studied for the crystalline behavior of nifedipine, and McKenna and his colleague found a new polymorph presented at a certain pore size [63]. (ii) APIs in each compartment have to nucleate independently. As long as the compartment walls are not nucleated, homogeneous nucleation will dominate, which takes longer for crystallization. (iii) A thickness of 1 nm immobilizes the surface layer with high surface energy possibly forming at the compartment walls, and the immobilized layer slows the crystallization kinetics significantly [63,64]. The nanocompartments of the liposome truly inhibit crystalline growth [65]. Praziquantel occurs in its amorphous form under nanoconfinement because of its larger crystalline lattice, and amorphous praziquantel was found to increase the dissolution rate by five-fold [66]. This strategy can also be applied to hydrophobic carotenoids. Next, the application of these theories in carotenoid formulations will be introduced based on different types of formulations.

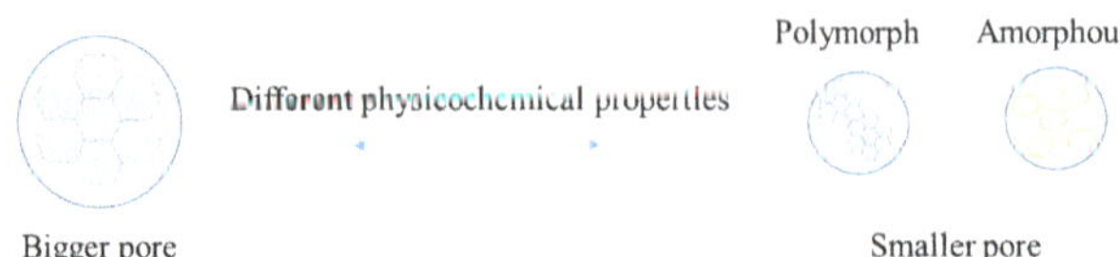

- The confinement size is smaller than the critical nucleus size of the substance → amorphous
- The confinement inhibits the nucleation → amorphous or polymorph substance

Figure 7. The concept of confinement and the relationship between confinement and crystals.

5. Approaches for the Crystalline Status Modification of Carotenoids

5.1. Co-Crystallization

Co-crystallization is defined as a single structurally homogeneous crystallization containing at least two neutral units (API and excipients) existing in solid and definite stoichiometric amounts [67]. This method is usually accomplished via supersaturation, which refers to slow cooling until the solubility limit is reached. Usually, the solubility of products prepared using this approach may not be significantly increased owing to the existence of a crystalline lattice structure, but it may provide several advantages, such as ease of preparation, lower hygroscopicity, and greater chemical stability of the products [68]. The commonly used excipients for co-crystallization systems should contain specific functional groups, including carboxylic acids (e.g., acetic acid and salicylic acid), amides (e.g., nicotinamide, saccharin, and urea), and alcohols (e.g., mannitol and sorbitol) to form intermolecular bonds with APIs [69].

The utilization of a supersaturated sucrose solution has been proposed for the preparation of carotenoid-rich extracts via the co-crystallization method [70], which aims to improve the dispersibility, hygroscopicity, and thermal stability of β-carotene. The ordered crystal of sucrose is transformed into an irregular and porous structure after the incorporation of β-carotene during the cooling and recrystallization processes. The crystalline status of co-crystallization can be evidenced by DSC and XRD examination. Though the technique of preparing pharmaceutical co-crystals with sucrose is believed to improve the solubility, dissolution, and other physicochemical properties of the encapsulated materials [71], merely the dissolution kinetics of sucrose have been determined in the current literature. One possible reason might be that the true solubility of the cocrystal products is not readily determined because API tends to transform into the most stable form in solution [72]. Few studies on carotenoid-loaded co-crystallization have discussed the crystalline state. Therefore, it may be an unexplored frontier and require more investigation for further discussion.

5.2. Solid Dispersion

Solid dispersion is a commonly used technology for crystalline state alternation and is defined as the dispersion of APIs in an inert carrier, such as sugars, polymers, and surfactants (Figure 8). Solvent evaporation and hot-melt methods are commonly operated, and the amorphous state may be produced during solvent removal or cooling [41]. The interaction between polymers and APIs generally results from the occurrence of hydrogen bonds and hydrophobic interaction. When solid dispersions are placed into an aqueous medium, such as simulated gastric fluid or simulated intestinal fluid, they would rapidly dissolve and exist in the supersaturation state owing to the amorphous state occurrence. Therefore, this may increase the aqueous solubility of poorly soluble APIs. Some polymers have been reported to retard crystalline growth in several ways: polyvinylpyrrolidone (PVP) suppresses the nucleation process and HPMC adsorbs on the surface of the crystal to prevent the formation of crystals [73]. In addition, the nucleation and growth procedures may be retarded via hydrogen bonding between APIs and excipients, which further inhibits crystalline formation [74].

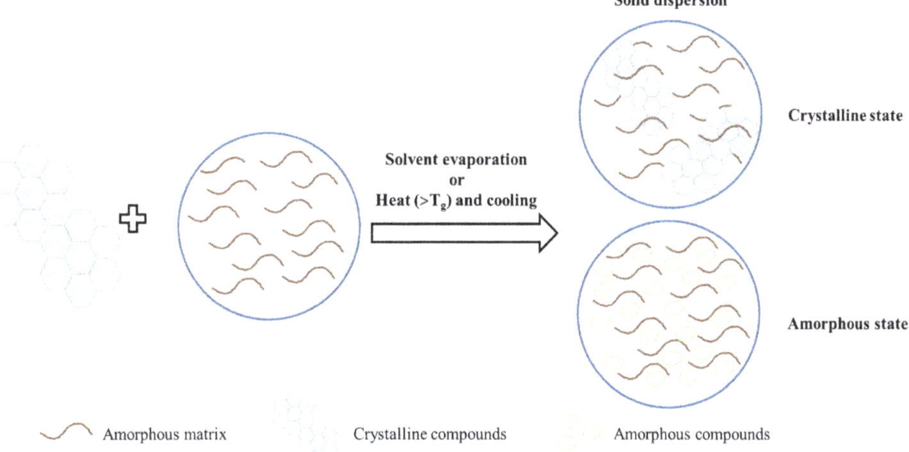

Figure 8. The scheme of solid dispersions.

It has been reported that β-carotene containing a solid dispersion composed of PVP and sucrose fatty acid ester (S-1670) was prepared by hot-melt extrusion and was found to be in an amorphous state via DSC and XRD. It was also proved to enhance solubility by about 390-fold, dissolution behavior, and also oral bioavailability [75–77]. A solid dispersion prepared using cyclic amylopectin has been used to protect β-carotene from light, heat and oxidation. The crystalline state of the solid dispersion was hard to detect using XRD owing to the uniform distribution in cyclic amylopectin. Starch was reported to inhibit the crystallization of a water-insoluble compound, β-carotene, and the composite was formed in an amorphous state. Cyclic amylopectin with a hydrophobic internal core could bind with β-carotene and hydrophobic compounds via intermolecular forces to generate a more amorphous formation [78].

Chang et al. [79] prepared lycopene dripping pills consisting of PEG 6000, Cremophor EL, and Tween 80 to improve the release behavior and oral bioavailability by approximately six-fold. The dripping pills were determined to be in an amorphous form via SEM and DSC. In this study, it was demonstrated that the lower viscosity caused by excessive emulsifiers may facilitate recrystallization.

5.3. Inclusion Complex

A complex is defined as the combination of APIs and ligands through hydrogen bonding, van der Waals forces, or hydrophobic effects [80]. Only a few compounds can be used as ligands to encapsulate hydrophobic carotenoids such as β-cyclodextrin, β-lactoglobulin, and amylose. The interaction of inclusion is shown in Figure 9.

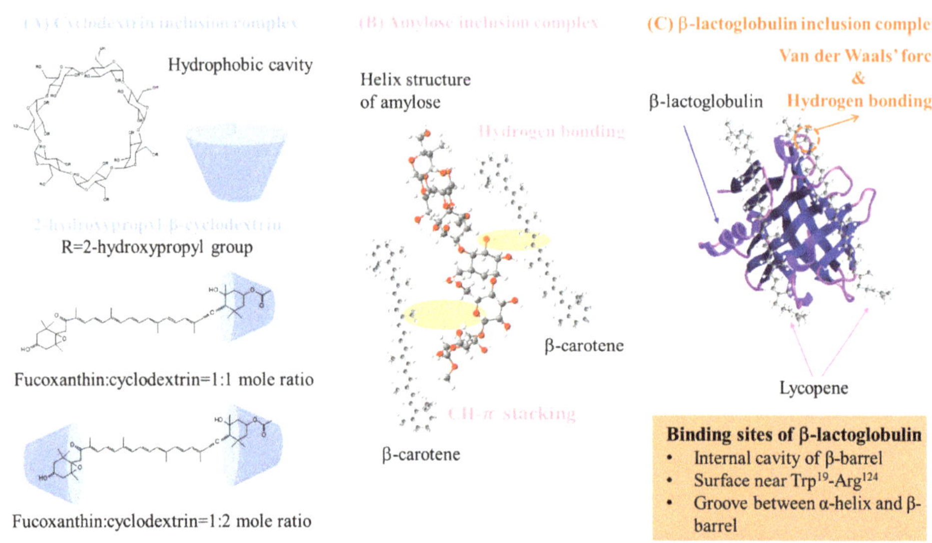

Figure 9. Scheme diagrams of (**A**) cyclodextrin, (**B**) amylose, and (**C**) β-lactoglobulin inclusion complexes [81–83].

Cyclodextrin is a cyclic oligosaccharide and is classified into different types based on the number of glucose residues, and it is the most well-studied complex ligand involving encapsulated carotenoids. Carotenoids can be encapsulated in the hydrophobic cavity of cyclodextrin through non-covalent interactions to stabilize the carotenoids with a random transformation from a crystalline to an amorphous state [84], and the hydrophilic outer surface of cyclodextrin helps the dissolution of carotenoids. Encapsulation in α-, β-, and γ-cyclodextrin was studied in tomato oil, which contained a lot of carotenoids. The complex presented as the microcrystalline in the emulsion form, and the complex powder was obtained with lyophilization to remove the solvent, accompanied by higher encapsulation and higher antioxidant capability [85]. The β-carotene/β-cyclodextrin complex was proposed, and β-carotene existed as an amorphous state in the complex, as shown in the results of DSC and XRD, leading to a 10- and 40-fold higher solubility and stability, respectively. Moreover, the antitumor activity was also improved [86]. The β-carotene/2-hydroxylproply-β-cyclodextrin/carrageenan/soy protein complex was also proposed and presented as an amorphous state in the DSC thermogram; it showed excellent bioaccessibility (78%) [87]. Astaxanthin has been prepared as a complex as well. The hexatomic side ring of astaxanthin was incorporated into the cavity of methyl-β-cyclodextrin to form a complex in an amorphous state, which was proved by the DSC thermogram, and the product exhibited 54-fold higher solubility, a 10-fold dissolution rate, and better bioaccessibility [88]. Sun et al. [81] proposed fucoxanthin (FX)/2-hydroxylpropyl-β-cyclodextrin via sonication and spray drying. The results of FTIR revealed that the characteristic peaks of FX disappeared, indicating that FX may have been successfully encapsulated, and the molecular docking suggested hydrogen bonding between FX and 2-hydroxylpropyl-β-cyclodextrin. XRD analysis also confirmed the amorphous state of FX. The FX/2-hydroxylpropyl-β-cyclodextrin complex showed better stability and antitumor activities toward HCT-116 and Caco-2 cells compared with free FX.

Amylose is also a food polymer that can accommodate hydrophobic carotenoids via V-amylose crystalline formation, and whether complexes are formed depends on the size, shape, and hydrophobicity of APIs. V-amylose is produced by the addition of ethanol as a precipitant; however, ethanol cannot incorporate into the hydrophobic cavity, and a hydrophobic carotenoid will be trapped by a nonspecific or specific interaction and stabilized with amylose polycrystals [89–91] which may be why APIs exist as amorphs in the amylose complex. However, among carotenoids, only β-carotene has been studied in the starch-complex system; the major finding was improved stability.

β-lactoglobulin is also regarded as a complex ligand for carotenoids, existing as the principal protein in whey protein. It can possibly bind hydrophobic carotenoids via the internal cavity of the β-barrel, the surface near Trp^{19}-Arg^{124}, and the groove between the α-helix and β-barrel of β-lactoglobulin [83,92]; the interaction may lower the molecular mobility to prevent recrystallization [93]. The binding mechanism has been studied in lycopene [94], but the effects on the bioactivity and physicochemical properties caused by the crystalline alteration still need to be further studied.

5.4. Micro/Nano Particles

Microparticle preparation includes spray drying, hot-melt extrusion, and phase separation [95], and the removal of solvents in spray drying as well as the cooling of the melt in extrusion causes APIs to remain in an amorphous state. In terms of phase separation, it works in a way similar to that of nanoprecipitation, which is the most common method used for nanoparticle preparation. The main concept of nanoprecipitation is solvent shifting, namely, the ouzo process. The schematic diagram of nanoprecipitation is shown in Figure 10, where hydrophobic APIs and polymers are dissolved in an organic solvent, and the organic solvent is added dropwise into an antisolvent (typically water). The solvent in the droplets moves toward the antisolvent, and the antisolvent does the reverse, causing a supersaturated state. This supersaturated state will further lead to the coprecipitation of hydrophobic APIs and the hydrophobic moiety of polymers forming nanoparticles with the surface coverage of the hydrophilic moiety of the polymers. The precipitated APIs remain amorphous as they do not have enough time to recrystallize in such a quick solvent replacement [96,97].

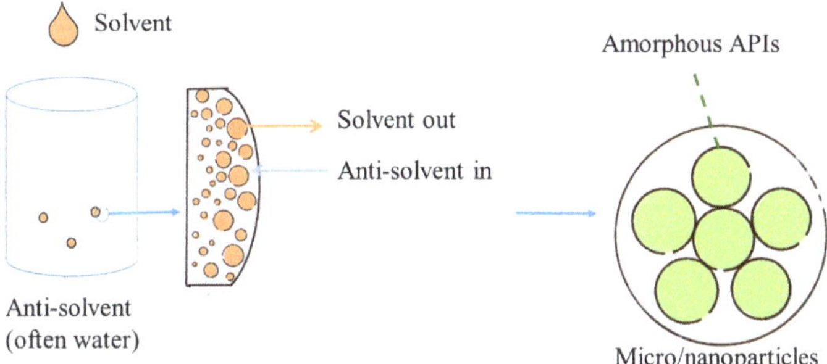

Figure 10. The mechanism of trapping amorphous APIs in nanoparticles via nanoprecipitation [96].

In our previous study about carotenoid nanoparticles [98], β-carotene-loaded PLGA-PVP nanoparticles were proposed, where amorphous β-carotene may benefit the solubility and oral absorption. Better oral absorption may result from nanoparticle morphology. Hu et al. [99] found that smooth and globular nanoparticles without irregularly lumpy astaxanthin crystals penetrate more easily into the cell. The theory has been applied in the micro-scale dimension, where astaxanthin-loaded hydrophilic microcapsules were obtained by spray drying. XRD analysis indicated that astaxanthin was encapsulated in an amorphous state, and the HepG2 cell growth inhibition activity was boosted [100]. Lutein and PVP have been prepared as particles to increase solubility and stability. PVP can inhibit crystallization by reducing molecular mobility, and the hydrogen bonding with lutein stabilizes the amorphous lutein, accompanied by higher stability against heat, light, and oxygen [101]. Lutein was also incorporated in zein nanoparticles and exhibited 80-fold higher water solubility. No crystalline peaks of lutein were found in XRD analysis as the nanoconfinement restricted the crystallization [102] and resulted in higher cellular uptake. Without excipients, the optical properties of β-carotene, lycopene, astaxanthin, and lutein nanoparticles obtained via nanoprecipitation were compared. With this preparation, the shell of the nanoparticles remained amorphous, and the core was still crystallized, as shown in cryo-TEM images. Moreover, the effective conjugation length of amorphous molecules was shorter than that of bulk crystals, and the absorption wavelength of amorphous molecules was blue-shifted. As a result, the color of the nanoparticles and crystals was rendered yellow and red, respectively [103]. In addition to the amorphous form, a new crystal may appear in the formulation. Ling et al. [104] proposed astaxanthin colloidal particles, and the decreased crystallinity led to a higher dissolution rate. Notably, astaxanthin has two common crystalline forms: polymorph I and polymorph II. A different polymorph was observed within the colloidal nanoparticle in the XRD analysis.

5.5. Lipid-Based Formulations

Lipid-based formulations, including emulsions, solid lipid nanoparticles (SLNs), nanostructured lipid carriers (NLCs), and self-emulsifying drug delivery systems (SEDDSs), are suitable for developing active lipid-soluble compounds, such as carotenoids, for oral bioavailability improvement. Emulsions, SLNs, and NLCs are composed of an aqueous phase and a lipid phase, with a surfactant for stabilization. The lipids used in these formulations are liquid, solid, and a mixture of liquid and solid oil, respectively (Figure 11). SEDDSs contain only oil and surfactants without water. Crystalline APIs would first be dissolved or melted to disperse in the oil to maintain the liquid state during the preparation procedure, so the APIs may be a solution type. Crystallization may occur after homogenization, cooling, or the storage period. In addition, supersaturation also causes the crystalline condition; therefore, the solubility of crystalline APIs in the solvent (solid lipid and liquid lipid) is crucial for crystallization. The general solubility equation (Equation (3)) is always utilized to calculate the solubility of crystalline APIs in a solvent using easily measurable properties [105].

$$\text{Log } S_W = 0.5 - 0.01 \, (T_m - 25) - \log K_{OW} \tag{3}$$

where S_W is the molar water solubility, T_m is the melting point, and K_{OW} is the oil–water partition coefficient of the solute.

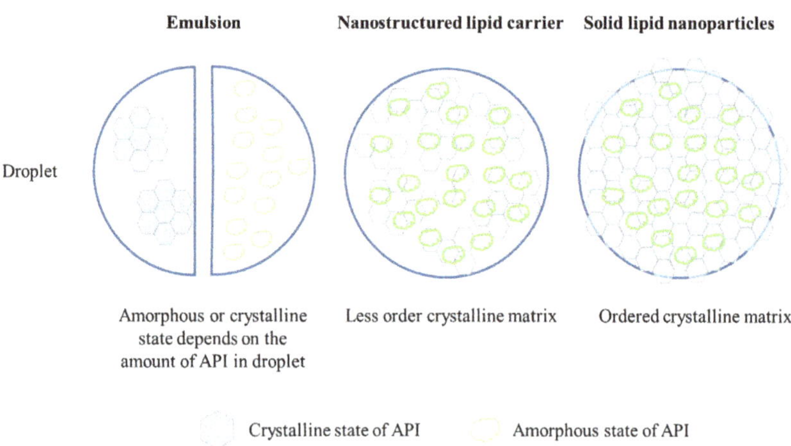

Figure 11. Illustration of a lipid-based formulation.

For crystallization suppression, there are two main strategies: (i) enhancement of the saturated solubility to impede nucleation, and (ii) slowing down the diffusion for the prevention of crystalline growth (Figure 12). For the enhancement of the saturated solubility, the addition of surfactants, phospholipids, or high polarity, short-length saturated fatty acids could form micelles to reduce the driving force of nucleation and prevent crystal formation. Furthermore, the addition of non-polar agents, such as globular proteins or cyclodextrins, on their surfaces for incorporation with hydrophobic active compounds could also enhance the saturated solubility [55,105]. In order to slow down diffusion, viscosity changes and size reductions are often used. In a previous study, the addition of sugars enhanced the viscosity of the continuous phase to block the APIs' diffusion, and the growth was retarded [105]. A previous study demonstrated that heterogeneous nucleations are confined when the average diameter of the drops is reduced and the crystallization is limited [54].

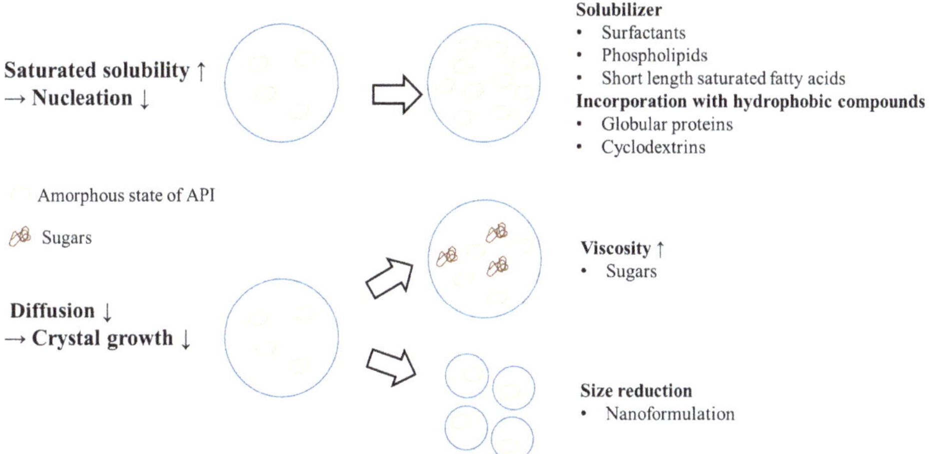

Figure 12. The mechanism of crystallization suppression in a lipid-based formulation.

Apart from these strategies to prevent crystallization, the selection of lipids may affect the crystallization of imperfect crystalline or amorphous states and have different drug loadings, sizes, charges, and release behaviors [106]. The commonly used solid lipids in this formulation preparation contain triglycerides, waxes, fatty acids, and fatty alcohols and the lipid composition may have an influence on the crystalline state of SLNs/SLMs [107]. Taking the commonly used solid lipids, triglycerides as an example, these exhibit polymorphism upon cooling and possibly form the crystalline structure of α, β′, and β crystals with hexagonal, orthorhombic, and triclinic unit structures, respectively. The α-form is the most unstable structure, and spherical particles have been observed when triglycerides are in this form. During storage, the prepared formulation may spontaneously transfer the crystalline structure to a lower-energy state. Some lipids with higher polarity and amphiphilic properties, such as phospholipids, sterols, and di- and mono-acylglycerols, have been regarded as crystallization modifiers and affect the crystallization process [108]. In addition, the type of emulsifier may also affect the crystallization of lipid-based formulations [109]. The longer alkyl chain length of the surfactants has been shown to enhance the crystallinity of lipid-based formulations [107]. Thus, both the lipids and surfactants used in the formulation play a vital role in the modulation of the crystallization process. More research on each formulation is discussed as follows.

5.5.1. Solid Lipid Nanoparticles/Microparticles

The composition of solid lipid nanoparticles/microparticles (SLNs/SLMs) is similar to that of emulsions, but solid lipids are applied in the oil phase to have controlled release behavior or particle stability. The encapsulated drug may be prevented from crystallization and then form a solid solution. The distribution of carotenoids in SLNs may be uniform due to the high hydrophobicity and crystallization temperature [110]. High-energy-state α-crystals were found in the lipids of initial SLNs owing to rapid cooling, and the α-crystals may transfer to β-forms during storage [111]. Compared to α crystals, highly lipophilic compounds such as carotenoids tend to be expelled under the β-crystalline state and the drug content may be reduced to affect the therapeutic effect. Therefore, the stability of SLNs is usually mentioned as a concern [112].

Some research has been reported about carotenoids containing SLNs/SLMs. β-carotene has been developed as an SLM using stearic acid and sunflower oil to prevent degradation during 7-month storage. The addition of sunflower oil resulted in less ordered crystals and induced an amorphous state, indicating the mixture of long-chained solid lipids and liquid lipids was suitable for the preparation of stable SLMs to prevent β-carotene degradation and exhibit excellent bioactivities [113]. Chen et al. [114] used both palm stearin and cholesterol as the solid lipid carrier of fucoxanthin to avoid the highly ordered crystalline structure of single solid lipids. The results showed that the SLN-microcapsules exist in an amorphous state owing to anti-solvent precipitation and ultrasonic treatment to form micelles easily and are capable of absorption by intestinal epithelial cells, indicating that the solubility of carotenoids could be enhanced to reduce the driving force of nucleation. The higher glass transition temperature indicated that the formulation has better temperature resistance [115]. Zeaxanthin was also prepared for SLNs using glycerol monostearate or glycerol distearate to resolve the problem of lipophilicity and instability. The crystallinity was determined to decrease in the formulation via the examination of DSC with the melting enthalpy decrease manner. The crystals of lipids preferred to form α-crystals with the high-energy state during the rapid cooling procedure [116]. Glycerol distearate is a mixture of C16 and C18 fatty acids and has a relatively low melting point and enthalpy compared to glycerol monostearate, indicating it has a poor crystalline structure. Therefore, SLNs prepared using glycerol distearate have the irregularity of the lipid crystals and display greater dissolution behavior [116].

5.5.2. Nanostructured Lipid Carrier

Nanostructured lipid carriers (NLCs) are similar to nanoemulsions and SLNs, but the lipids in NLCs include not only solid lipids but also liquid lipids. The incorporation of liquid lipids can allow the internal lipid phase to have a less-ordered crystalline arrangement to obviate the condition of active compound leakage and load more active compounds. Owing to the composition of both solid and liquid lipids, crystallinity is always considered. The crystalline index (CI) was reported to determine the crystalline state of APIs loaded in NLCs and it is calculated using Equation (4). A higher CI indicates that the encapsulation efficiency of NLCs may be higher owing to the less-ordered crystalline arrangement [106].

$$\text{CI } (\%) = \frac{M_s}{M_p \times \gamma} \times 100 \tag{4}$$

where M_s indicates the melting enthalpy of NLCs, M_p indicates the melting enthalpy of pure solid lipids, and γ indicates the solid lipid concentration (%) in NLCs.

Astaxanthin-loaded NLCs have been developed to improve the physicochemical characteristics and storage stability. Glyceryl behenate and oleic acid were selected as solid and liquid lipids and lecithin and Tween 80 were chosen as surfactants in the oil phase and water phase, respectively. The authors evaluated the properties of NLCs prepared via lecithin removal, replacing Tween 80 with Tween 20 or replacing oleic acid with triacylglycerols, and the results showed that there is no improvement in the stability of the NLCs due to the chemically homogenous structure of the lipid mixture. In these formulations, β-crystals were formed and the aggregation, which contributed to the hydrophobic interaction, partial coalescence, or the penetration of lipid crystals, made the NLCs unstable. Among these solid lipids, NLCs prepared using glyceryl behenate were reported to have a more imperfect crystalline lattice and lead to high stability and entrapment. The crystal was demonstrated to be a metastable β' polymorph, and the reduction in crystallinity compared to glyceryl behenate was determined by the broader and lower intensities in the XRD patterns and DSC thermogram. The incorporation of bioactive compounds may also make more imperfect crystals, leading to better encapsulation efficiency. The melting point of astaxanthin disappeared in the NLC group, indicating that astaxanthin is not in the crystalline state at this temperature and can be considered to be physically stable at high temperatures [115]. Oleic acid has been reported as a crystallization inhibitor. Oleic acid can adsorb and crystallize at the surface in the beginning so the crystallization may be hindered [54].

Glycerol monostearate or glycerol distearate as a solid lipid, medium-chain triglycerides as a liquid lipid, and soy lecithin and Tween 80 as surfactants were used to prepare NLCs to load zeaxanthin. The enthalpy reduction was observed in the NLC group compared to SLNs, indicating the crystallinity decrease in the lipid matrix. The lower enthalpy and crystallinity are capable of encapsulating more APIs and displaying better release behavior. Similar to the results of SLNs, NLCs prepared using glycerol distearate also had better properties. The results showed that the incorporation of liquid lipids and the selection of lipids have an influence on the crystallinity, and further improve the physicochemical characteristics of active compounds and formulations [116].

5.5.3. Microemulsion/Nanoemulsion

An emulsion is a mixture of two immiscible phases (aqueous phase and liquid oil phase) supported by a surfactant to reduce surface tension under thermodynamically unstable conditions. Solubilized and crystallized β-carotene nanoemulsions have been prepared to compare the influence of physical properties on bioaccessibility. The crystalline state was examined while passing through the stimulated digestion process, and no crystal was observed during digestion in the solubilized β-carotene nanoemulsion group. In the crystallized β-carotene nanoemulsion group, the initial crystals gradually disappeared and possibly contributed to the dilution by digestive juice in each step. The free fatty acid release profiles in the in vitro digestion study indicated that the physical state of β-carotene has no influence on lipid digestion. The bioaccessibility results showed that the solubilized β-carotene nanoemulsions had an 11.7- and 46-fold enhancement compared to crystallized β-carotene nanoemulsions and crystallized β-carotene in phosphate buffer saline, respectively, suggesting that the solubilization state without crystals is the suitable delivery strategy [117]. A previous study developed a lutein-loaded whey protein emulsion, which is similar to a Pickering emulsion. The crystalline form of the formulation containing only whey protein and phospholipids could be observed using a microscope, and the situation could be improved after the addition of mono- and di-glycerides. The mono- and di-glycerides benefited the solubility of lutein crystals and were demonstrated to be physical barriers in the crystalline growth process to prevent the carotenoids from crystallization, as well as improve the stability [118].

5.5.4. Self-Emulsifying Drug Delivery System

A self-emulsifying drug delivery system (SEDDS) is a mixture of active compounds, oils, surfactants, and co-surfactants through a gentle stirring procedure and the o/w emulsion is obtained by contact with digestion fluids and digestive motility. SEDDSs can be divided into two groups according to the droplet size. The droplet size of self-microemulsifying drug delivery systems and self-nanoemulsifying drug delivery systems is 100–250 nm and less than 100 nm, respectively [119]. A SEDDS is often in an amorphous state owing to being dissolved in lipids and surfactants. The crystallization always occurs during digestion due to the supersaturation to make excess active compounds precipitate or crystallize. In order to prevent supersaturation, some precipitation inhibitors have been reported, including cellulose (HPMC and hydroxypropyl cellulose), polymers (PVP and Soluplus®), surfactants (Tween, Cremophor, and D-α-Tocopherol polyethylene glycol 1000 succinate), and cyclodextrins [120,121]. The mechanism of the commonly used precipitation inhibitor HPMC, is to adsorb onto the surface to inhibit the nucleation and growth and to form intramolecular and intermolecular hydrogen bonds between the active compounds and itself via the hydroxyl groups in the structure. In addition, the "Spring and Parachute" is also observed in formulations with these excipients. Supersaturation may be rapidly reached, displaying spring behavior and the nucleation or crystalline growth may be restrained to stabilize the metastable supersaturated samples, witnessing the parachute phenomenon (Figure 13). In this way, the precipitation is inhibited, and there is a longer time for absorption in the expected regions [121]. The degree of supersaturation (S) is driven to precipitate, and it can be calculated using Equation (5) [122].

$$S = \frac{\text{total drug concentration}}{\text{saturation concentration of the drug in the solvent}} \tag{5}$$

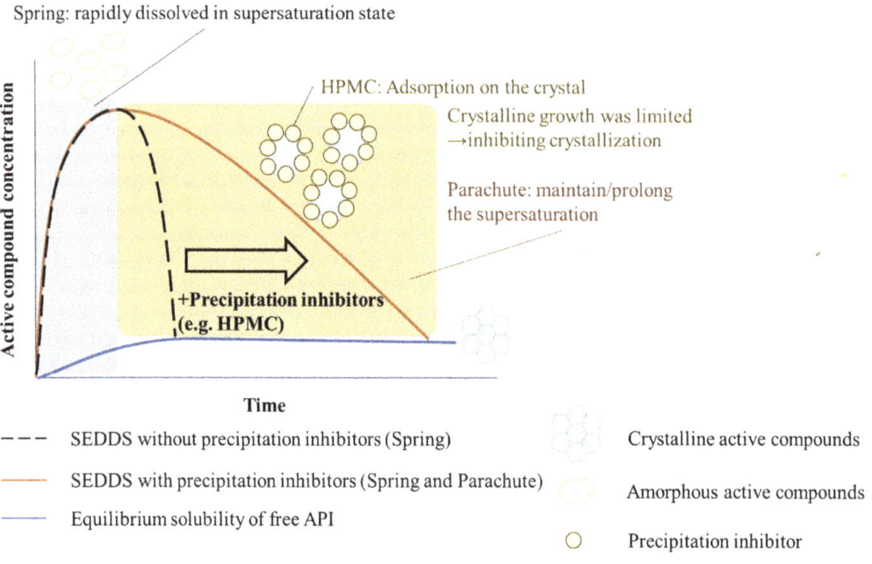

Figure 13. The mechanism of the "Spring and Parachute".

A SEDDS was incorporated with a solid dispersion, named a lipid-based solid dispersion (LBSD), to load lycopene to enhance the dissolution characteristics and oral absorption of lycopene. The results of XRD and DSC indicated that new signals appeared in the LBSD and that it had a lower melting point. The release behavior of the amorphous marketed product, Lycovit®, was significantly increased compared to the lycopene crystals, suggesting the benefit of crystalline transition. Although no obvious enhancement was observed in the LBSD owing to the non-amorphous state, the pharmacokinetic study demonstrated a significant improvement in oral absorption compared to Lycovit® due to the long-chained triglyceride for lymphatic transportation, suggesting the crystalline state did not fully affect the oral absorption in this study [123]. Aung et al. [124] prepared astaxanthin-loaded SMEDDS tablets containing SMEDDS, hydrophilic polymers as precipitation inhibitors, and microcrystalline cellulose for tableting. The SMEDDS, composed of rice bran oil, Kolliphor® RH 40, Span® 20, and two polymers, HPMC and polyvinyl alcohol, was used to obtain the supersaturation state and enhance the release of astaxanthin. The crystallinity was determined by PXRD and transferred from a crystalline to amorphous state after preparing the supersaturable SMEDDS. The SMEDDS with or without precipitation inhibitors enhanced the release behavior, antioxidant activity, and cellular uptake. The precipitation inhibitors in the SMEDDS could hinder the nucleation and precipitation and thus maintain astaxanthin in the solubilized form.

5.6. Liposome

The liposome is composed of a hydrophobic phospholipid bilayer shell and a hydrophilic core to form a spherical structure. Active lipophilic compounds tend to be encapsulated within the lipid bilayer and not precipitate in a crystalline form. Regarding the active hydrophilic compounds, they were loaded in the aqueous core with the crystalline precipitate, amorphous precipitate, or solution state depending on the properties of the active compounds and preparation process (Figure 14) [125]. Carotenoids are lipophilic compounds with high octanol–water partition coefficients; therefore, they are usually encapsulated within the phospholipid bilayer. Astaxanthin has been prepared for the liposome using the film dispersion-ultrasonic technique. XRD was conducted to examine the crystalline state of astaxanthin, soybean phosphatidylcholine (excipient), and the liposome. Pure astaxanthin was determined to be in a crystalline state owing to the existence of many peaks. The pattern of liposomes was different from that of astaxanthin and soybean phosphatidylcholine, implying that astaxanthin was successfully encapsulated in the liposomes with hydrogen bonds between astaxanthin and the phospholipid bilayer. The aqueous solubility of astaxanthin was observed to be enhanced 17-fold compared to pure astaxanthin, which may be attributed to the crystalline alternation of astaxanthin after liposome encapsulation [126].

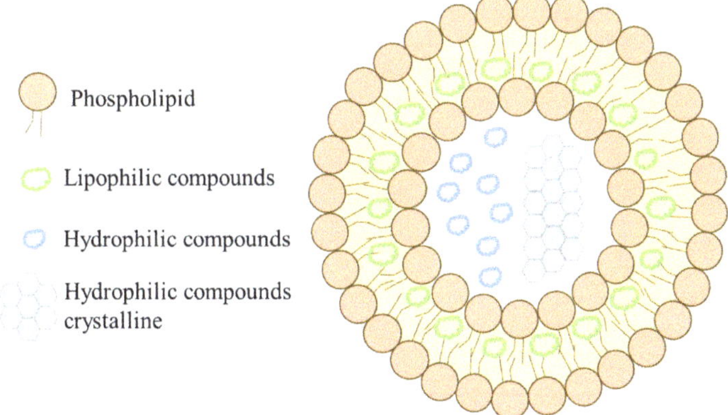

Figure 14. Schematic of the hydrophilic and lipophilic compounds within a liposome. The right indicates that the hydrophilic compounds in the core may undergo crystallization and precipitation.

Although there are some studies illustrating other factors majorly affecting oral absorption, such as intestine-specific transporters or lymphatic transport, solubility enhancement was mainly discussed and proved to efficiently improve oral bioavailability. The simplest way to enhance solubility is to alter the crystalline state from crystals to amorphs or polymorphs. The limitation is the instability of crystals owing to the high-energy state. To overcome this problem, there are many strategies and principles for crystallization suppression discussed in this article. To summarize, carotenoid formulations involved in the change of crystallinity are listed in Table 2. This article included various carotenoid-containing formulations, including those prepared using polymers or lipids, and the discussion of crystalline alternation. It may provide information to develop carotenoid-loaded formulations to deal with the problem of solubility and stability and exhibit outstanding bioactivities.

Table 2. The summary of carotenoid formulations involved in the crystalline change.

Carotenoids	Formulation	Composition	Crystalline Status	Results	Reference
Carotenoids	Co-crystal	Sucrose	Crystals	Thermal stability↑	[70]
β-carotene	Solid dispersion	Poly (vinyl pyrrolidone) Sucrose fatty acid ester (S-1670)	Amorphs	Solubility↑ Dissolution↑ Bioavailability↑	[75–77]
β-carotene	Solid dispersion	Cyclic amylopection	Amorphs	Stability↑	[78]
β-carotγene	Inclusion complex	Amylose (Amylomaize starch)	Both Amorphs and crystals	Stability↑	[89]
β-carotene	Inclusion complex	Amylose (Corn starch)	Both Amorphs and crystals	Stability↑	[91]
β-carotene	Inclusion complex	Amylose (High-amylose corn starch)	Amorphs	Stability↑	[90]
β-carotene	Inclusion complex	2-hydroxylproply-β-cyclodextrin Carrageenan Soy protein	Amorphs	Bioaccessibility↑	[87]
β-carotene	Nanoparticles	Poly (lactic-co-glycolic) acid Poly (vinyl pyrrolidone)	Amorphs	Bioavailability↑	[98]
β-carotene	Nanoemulsion	Corn oil	Amorphs	Bioaccessibility↑	[117]
β-carotene	Solid lipid microparticles	Stearic acid Sunflower oil	Amorphs or Less ordered crystals	Stability↑	[113]
Lycopene	Solid dispersion (Dripping pills)	PEG 6000 Cremophor® EL Tween® 80	Amorphs	Dissolution↑ Bioavailability↑	[79]
Lycopene (Tomato oil)	Inclusion complex	α, β, γ-cyclodextrin	Microcrystals	Color change Stability↑ Antioxidation↑	[85]
Lycopene	Lipid based solid dispersion	Gelucire 44/14	Polymorphs	Dissolution↑ Bioavailability↑	[123]
Astaxanthin	Inclusion complex	Methyl-β-cyclodextrin	Amorphs	Solubility↑ Dissolution↑ Bioaccessibility↑	[88]
Astaxanthin	Colloidal particles	Tween® 20 Sodium caseinate Gum arabic Povidone K30 Copovidone	Polymorphs	Dissolution↑ Cellular uptake↑	[104]
Astaxanthin	Microparticles	PEG 6000 Poloxamer 188 Tocopherol Colloidal silicon dioxide	Amorphs	HepG2 cell growth inhibition activity↑	[100]
Astaxanthin	Nanoparticles	Poly(lactic-co-glycolic acid)	Amorphs	Cellular uptake↑ Photoprotection↑	[99]
Astaxanthin	Liposome	Soybean phosphatidyl choline Cholesterol	Both Amorphs and crystals	Solubility↑ Stability↑	[126]
Astaxanthin	Nanostructured lipid carrier	Glyceryl behenate Oleic acid Lecithin Tween® 80	Amorphs	Stability↑	[115]
Astaxanthin	Self-microemulsifying drug delivery system	Rice bran oil Kolliphor® RH 40 Span® 20 HPMC Polyvinyl alcohol	Amorphs	Dissolution↑ Antioxidation↑ Cellular uptake↑	[124]

Table 2. *Cont.*

Carotenoids	Formulation	Composition	Crystalline Status	Results	Reference
Fucoxanthin	Inclusion complex	2-hydroxylpropyl-β-cyclodextrin	Amorphs	Solubility↑ Stability↑ Anti-tumor activity↑	[81]
Fucoxanthin	Solid lipid nanoparticle-microcapsules	Palm stearin Cholesterol	Amorphs	Solubility↑ Stability↑ Bioavailability↑	[114]
Lutein	Particles	Polyvinylpyrrolidone Tween® 80	Amorphs	Stability↑	[101]
Lutein	Nanoparticles	Zein Sophorolipid	Amorphs	Solubility↑ Bioaccessibility↑	[102]
Lutein	Nanoemulsion	Blending plant oil Mono- and di-glycerides Lecithin Whey protein	Amorphs	Dissolution↑ Stability↑	[118]
Zeaxanthin	Solid lipid nanoparticles	Glycerol monostearate Glycerol distearate	Possible amorphs	Dissolution↑	[116]
Zeaxanthin	Nanostructured lipid carrier	Glycerol monostearate Glycerol distearate Medium-chain triglyceride Soy lecithin Tween® 80	Possible amorphs	Dissolution↑	[116]

↑: enhancement. ↓: reduction.

6. Conclusions

This review deals with the mechanisms of converting crystals into amorphs and stabilizing the amorphs in terms of polymer- and lipid-based formulations. Factors such as the types of excipients, manufacturing processes, and changes in particle size can transform the crystalline forms of APIs into other polymorph or amorph statuses. This review also provides representative and practical strategies for the delivery of carotenoids. These pharmaceutical technologies related to crystalline status modification efficiently improve the physicochemical properties of carotenoids, which amends their oral bioavailability and biological effects.

Author Contributions: Conceptualization, W.-Y.L., Y.-S.H., H.-H.K. and Y.-T.W.; methodology, W.-Y.L., Y.-S.H., H.-H.K. and Y.-T.W.; investigation, W.-Y.L. and Y.-S.H.; resources, W.-Y.L. and Y.-S.H.; writing—original draft preparation, W.-Y.L. and Y.-S.H.; writing—review and editing, W.-Y.L., Y.-S.H., H.-H.K. and Y.-T.W.; visualization, W.-Y.L. and Y.-S.H.; supervision, H.-H.K. and Y.-T.W.; project administration, H.-H.K. and Y.-T.W.; funding acquisition, Y.-T.W. W.-Y.L., H.-H.K. and Y.-S.H. contributed equally to this work. All authors have read and agreed to the published version of the manuscript.

Funding: This research was funded by Ministry of Science and Technology, Taiwan, R.O.C., under grant no. MOST110-2410-H-037-008-MY2. This study is supported partially by Kaohsiung Medical University Research Center Grant (KMU-TC111A04).

Institutional Review Board Statement: Not applicable.

Informed Consent Statement: Not applicable.

Data Availability Statement: Not applicable.

Acknowledgments: Thank Ting-An Liang for the image support.

Conflicts of Interest: The authors declare no conflict of interest.

References

1. Gary Williamson, A.G.M.; Graham, A.B.; Catherine, S.B. *Food Chemistry, Function and Analysis*, Gary Williamson, A.G.M., Graham, A.B., Catherine, S.B., Eds.; RSC Publishing: Cambridge, UK, 2019; pp. 15–20. [CrossRef]
2. Sridhar, K.; Inbaraj, B.S.; Chen, B.-H. Recent advances on nanoparticle based strategies for improving carotenoid stability and biological activity. *Antioxidants* **2021**, *10*, 713. [CrossRef] [PubMed]
3. Stahl, W.; Sies, H. Bioactivity and protective effects of natural carotenoids. *Biochim. Biophys. Acta* **2005**, *1740*, 101–107. [CrossRef] [PubMed]
4. Bayr, H. Reactive oxygen species. *Crit. Care Med.* **2005**, *33*, S498–S501. [CrossRef]
5. Adejare, A. *Remington: The Science and Practice of Pharmacy*; Academic Press: Cambridge, MA, USA, 2020.
6. Honda, M.; Kageyama, H.; Hibino, T.; Zhang, Y.; Diono, W.; Kanda, H.; Yamaguchi, R.; Takemura, R.; Fukaya, T.; Goto, M. Improved carotenoid processing with sustainable solvents utilizing Z-isomerization-induced alteration in physicochemical properties: A review and future directions. *Molecules* **2019**, *24*, 2149. [CrossRef] [PubMed]
7. Stegemann, S.; Leveiller, F.; Franchi, D.; De Jong, H.; Lindén, H. When poor solubility becomes an issue: From early stage to proof of concept. *Eur. J. Pharm. Sci.* **2007**, *31*, 249–261. [CrossRef]
8. Van den Mooter, G. The use of amorphous solid dispersions: A formulation strategy to overcome poor solubility and dissolution rate. *Drug Discov. Today Technol.* **2012**, *9*, e79–e85. [CrossRef]
9. Uchiyama, K.; Naito, Y.; Hasegawa, G.; Nakamura, N.; Takahashi, J.; Yoshikawa, T. Astaxanthin protects β-cells against glucose toxicity in diabetic db/db mice. *Redox Rep.* **2002**, *7*, 290–293. [CrossRef]
10. Park, J.S.; Chyun, J.H.; Kim, Y.K.; Line, L.L.; Chew, B.P. Astaxanthin decreased oxidative stress and inflammation and enhanced immune response in humans. *Nutr. Metab.* **2010**, *7*, 1–10. [CrossRef]
11. Wang, X.-j.; Chen, W.; Fu, X.-t.; Ma, J.-k.; Wang, M.-h.; Hou, Y.-j.; Tian, D.-c.; Fu, X.-y.; Fan, C.-d. Reversal of homocysteine-induced neurotoxicity in rat hippocampal neurons by astaxanthin: Evidences for mitochondrial dysfunction and signaling crosstalk. *Cell Death Discov.* **2018**, *4*, 1–11. [CrossRef]
12. Wood, S.M.; Beckham, C.; Yosioka, A.; Darban, H.; Watson, R.R. β-Carotene and selenium supplementation enhances immune response in aged humans. *Integr. Med. Int.* **2000**, *2*, 85–92. [CrossRef]
13. Yusuf, M.; Khan, R.A.; Khan, M.; Ahmed, B. Plausible antioxidant biomechanics and anticonvulsant pharmacological activity of brain-targeted β-carotene nanoparticles. *Int. J. Nanomed.* **2012**, *7*, 4311.
14. Jayappriyan, K.; Rajkumar, R.; Venkatakrishnan, V.; Nagaraj, S.; Rengasamy, R. In vitro anticancer activity of natural β-carotene from Dunaliella salina EU5891199 in PC-3 cells. *Biomed. Prev. Nutr.* **2013**, *3*, 99–105. [CrossRef]
15. Hira, S.; Saleem, U.; Anwar, F.; Sohail, M.F.; Raza, Z.; Ahmad, B. β-Carotene: A natural compound improves cognitive impairment and oxidative stress in a mouse model of streptozotocin-induced Alzheimer's disease. *Biomolecules* **2019**, *9*, 441. [CrossRef]
16. Takayanagi, K.; Morimoto, S.-i.; Shirakura, Y.; Mukai, K.; Sugiyama, T.; Tokuji, Y.; Ohnishi, M. Mechanism of visceral fat reduction in Tsumura Suzuki obese, diabetes (TSOD) mice orally administered β-cryptoxanthin from Satsuma mandarin oranges (Citrus unshiu Marc). *J. Agric. Food Chem.* **2011**, *59*, 12342–12351. [CrossRef]
17. Heo, S.-J.; Jeon, Y.-J. Protective effect of fucoxanthin isolated from Sargassum siliquastrum on UV-B induced cell damage. *J. Photochem. Photobiol. B Biol.* **2009**, *95*, 101–107. [CrossRef]
18. Maeda, H.; Hosokawa, M.; Sashima, T.; Murakami-Funayama, K.; Miyashita, K. Anti-obesity and anti-diabetic effects of fucoxanthin on diet-induced obesity conditions in a murine model. *Mol. Med. Rep.* **2009**, *2*, 897–902. [CrossRef] [PubMed]
19. Woo, M.N.; Jeon, S.M.; Shin, Y.C.; Lee, M.K.; Kang, M.A.; Choi, M.S. Anti-obese property of fucoxanthin is partly mediated by altering lipid-regulating enzymes and uncoupling proteins of visceral adipose tissue in mice. *Mol. Nutr. Food Res.* **2009**, *53*, 1603–1611. [CrossRef]
20. Palombo, P.; Fabrizi, G.; Ruocco, V.; Ruocco, E.; Fluhr, J.; Roberts, R.; Morganti, P. Beneficial long-term effects of combined oral/topical antioxidant treatment with the carotenoids lutein and zeaxanthin on human skin: A double-blind, placebo-controlled study. *Ski. Pharmacol. Physiol.* **2007**, *20*, 199–210. [CrossRef]
21. Yu, C.-C.; Nandrot, E.F.; Dun, Y.; Finnemann, S.C. Dietary antioxidants prevent age-related retinal pigment epithelium actin damage and blindness in mice lacking αvβ5 integrin. *Free Radic. Biol. Med.* **2012**, *52*, 660–670. [CrossRef]
22. Hammond Jr, B.R.; Miller, L.S.; Bello, M.O.; Lindbergh, C.A.; Mewborn, C.; Renzi-Hammond, L.M. Effects of lutein/zeaxanthin supplementation on the cognitive function of community dwelling older adults: A randomized, double-masked, placebo-controlled trial. *Front. Aging Neurosci.* **2017**, *9*, 254. [CrossRef]
23. Sung, W.-S.; Lee, I.-S.; Lee, D.-G. Damage to the cytoplasmic membrane and cell death caused by lycopene in Candida albicans. *J. Microbiol. Biotechnol.* **2007**, *17*, 1797–1804.
24. Qu, M.; Jiang, Z.; Liao, Y.; Song, Z.; Nan, X. Lycopene prevents amyloid [beta]-induced mitochondrial oxidative stress and dysfunctions in cultured rat cortical neurons. *Neurochem. Res.* **2016**, *41*, 1354–1364. [CrossRef]
25. Hwang, S.; Lim, J.W.; Kim, H. Inhibitory effect of lycopene on amyloid-β-induced apoptosis in neuronal cells. *Nutrients* **2017**, *9*, 883. [CrossRef] [PubMed]
26. Wang, J.; Li, L.; Wang, Z.; Cui, Y.; Tan, X.; Yuan, T.; Liu, Q.; Liu, Z.; Liu, X. Supplementation of lycopene attenuates lipopolysaccharide-induced amyloidogenesis and cognitive impairments via mediating neuroinflammation and oxidative stress. *J. Nutr. Biochem.* **2018**, *56*, 16–25. [CrossRef] [PubMed]

27. Huang, C.; Gan, D.; Fan, C.; Wen, C.; Li, A.; Li, Q.; Zhao, J.; Wang, Z.; Zhu, L.; Lu, D. The secretion from neural stem cells pretreated with lycopene protects against tert-butyl hydroperoxide-induced neuron oxidative damage. *Oxid. Med. Cell. Longev.* **2018**, *2018*, 1–14. [CrossRef] [PubMed]
28. Zhu, N.-W.; Yin, X.-L.; Lin, R.; Fan, X.-L.; Chen, S.-J.; Zhu, Y.-M.; Zhao, X.-Z. Possible mechanisms of lycopene amelioration of learning and memory impairment in rats with vascular dementia. *Neural Regen. Res.* **2020**, *15*, 332. [CrossRef]
29. Chasse, G.A.; Chasse, K.P.; Kucsman, A.; Torday, L.L.; Papp, J.G. Conformational potential energy surfaces of a lycopene model. *J. Mol. Struct.: THEOCHEM* **2001**, *571*, 7–26. [CrossRef]
30. Khoo, H.-E.; Prasad, K.N.; Kong, K.-W.; Jiang, Y.; Ismail, A. Carotenoids and their isomers: Color pigments in fruits and vegetables. *Molecules* **2011**, *16*, 1710–1738. [CrossRef]
31. Zia-Ul-Haq, M.; Dewanjee, S.; Riaz, M. *Carotenoids: Structure and Function in the Human Body*; Springer: Berlin/Heidelberg, Germany, 2021.
32. Jing, C.; Qun, X.; Rohrer, J. HPLC separation of all-trans-β-carotene and its iodine-induced isomers using a C30 column. *Thermo Sci.* **2012**, *391*, 2–6.
33. Yang, C.; Fischer, M.; Kirby, C.; Liu, R.; Zhu, H.; Zhang, H.; Chen, Y.; Sun, Y.; Zhang, L.; Tsao, R. Bioaccessibility, cellular uptake and transport of luteins and assessment of their antioxidant activities. *Food Chem.* **2018**, *249*, 66–76. [CrossRef]
34. Yang, C.; Hassan, Y.I.; Liu, R.; Zhang, H.; Chen, Y.; Zhang, L.; Tsao, R. Anti-inflammatory effects of different astaxanthin isomers and the roles of lipid transporters in the cellular transport of astaxanthin isomers in Caco-2 cell monolayers. *J. Agric. Food Chem.* **2019**, *67*, 6222–6231. [CrossRef] [PubMed]
35. During, A.; Hussain, M.M.; Morel, D.W.; Harrison, E.H. Carotenoid uptake and secretion by CaCo-2 cells: β-carotene isomer selectivity and carotenoid interactions1. *J. Lipid Res.* **2002**, *43*, 1086–1095. [CrossRef] [PubMed]
36. Furr, H.C.; Clark, R.M. Intestinal absorption and tissue distribution of carotenoids. *J. Nutr. Biochem.* **1997**, *8*, 364–377. [CrossRef]
37. Sato, H.; Matsushita, T.; Ueno, K.; Kikuchi, H.; Yamada, K.; Onoue, S. Oily Suspension of Micronized Crystalline Lutein for the Improvement of Dissolution and Oral Bioavailability. *Food Sci. Technol.* **2022**, *2*, 272–279. [CrossRef]
38. Faller, B.; Desrayaud, S.; Berghausen, J.; Laisney, M.; Dodd, S. 4 How solubility influences bioavailability. *Solubility Pharm. Chem.* **2020**, *113*, 113–132.
39. Pudipeddi, M.; Serajuddin, A.T. Trends in solubility of polymorphs. *J. Pharm. Sci.* **2005**, *94*, 929–939. [CrossRef]
40. Kaushal, A.M.; Gupta, P.; Bansal, A.K. Amorphous drug delivery systems: Molecular aspects, design, and performance. *Crit. Rev. Ther. Drug Carr. Syst.* **2004**, *21*, 133–193. [CrossRef]
41. Vasconcelos, T.; Marques, S.; das Neves, J.; Sarmento, B. Amorphous solid dispersions: Rational selection of a manufacturing process. *Adv. Drug. Deliv. Rev.* **2016**, *100*, 85–101. [CrossRef]
42. Healy, A.M.; Worku, Z.A.; Kumar, D.; Madi, A.M. Pharmaceutical solvates, hydrates and amorphous forms: A special emphasis on cocrystals. *Adv. Drug. Deliv. Rev.* **2017**, *117*, 25–46. [CrossRef]
43. Zhou, W.; Greer, H.F. What can electron microscopy tell us beyond crystal structures? *Eur. J. Inorg. Chem.* **2016**, *2016*, 941–950. [CrossRef]
44. Stevenson, H.P.; Makhov, A.M.; Calero, M.; Edwards, A.L.; Zeldin, O.B.; Mathews, I.I.; Lin, G.; Barnes, C.O.; Santamaria, H.; Ross, T.M. Use of transmission electron microscopy to identify nanocrystals of challenging protein targets. *Proc. Natl. Acad. Sci. USA* **2014**, *111*, 8470–8475. [CrossRef]
45. Nurit, T.-G. Minerals Observed by Scanning Electron Microscopy (SEM), Transmission Electron Microscopy (TEM) and High Resolution Transmission Electron Microscopy (HRTEM). In *Electron Microscopy*; IntechOpen: London, UK, 2022.
46. Bruni, G.; Berbenni, V.; Sartor, F.; Milanese, C.; Girella, A.; Franchi, D.; Marini, A. Quantification methods of amorphous/crystalline fractions in high-energy ball milled pharmaceutical products. *J. Therm. Anal. Calorim.* **2012**, *108*, 235–241. [CrossRef]
47. Leyva-Porras, C.; Cruz-Alcantar, P.; Espinosa-Solís, V.; Martínez-Guerra, E.; Piñón-Balderrama, C.I.; Compean Martínez, I.; Saavedra-Leos, M.Z. Application of differential scanning calorimetry (DSC) and modulated differential scanning calorimetry (MDSC) in food and drug industries. *Polymers* **2019**, *12*, 5. [CrossRef] [PubMed]
48. Yu, D.G.; Branford-White, C.; Li, L.; Wu, X.M.; Zhu, L.M. The compatibility of acyclovir with polyacrylonitrile in the electrospun drug-loaded nanofibers. *J. Appl. Polym. Sci.* **2010**, *117*, 1509–1515. [CrossRef]
49. Shah, B.; Kakumanu, V.K.; Bansal, A.K. Analytical techniques for quantification of amorphous/crystalline phases in pharmaceutical solids. *J. Pharm. Sci.* **2006**, *95*, 1641–1665. [CrossRef]
50. Kumar, S.; Rao, R. Analytical tools for cyclodextrin nanosponges in pharmaceutical field: A review. *J. Incl. Phenom. Macrocycl. Chem.* **2019**, *94*, 11–30. [CrossRef]
51. Mura, P. Analytical techniques for characterization of cyclodextrin complexes in the solid state: A review. *J. Pharm. Biomed. Anal.* **2015**, *113*, 226–238. [CrossRef] [PubMed]
52. Zhang, J.; Liu, Z.; Wu, H.; Cai, T. Effect of polymeric excipients on nucleation and crystal growth kinetics of amorphous fluconazole. *Biomater. Sci.* **2021**, *9*, 4308–4316. [CrossRef]
53. Wilson, V.R.; Lou, X.; Osterling, D.J.; Stolarik, D.F.; Jenkins, G.J.; Nichols, B.L.; Dong, Y.; Edgar, K.J.; Zhang, G.G.; Taylor, L.S. Amorphous solid dispersions of enzalutamide and novel polysaccharide derivatives: Investigation of relationships between polymer structure and performance. *Sci. Rep.* **2020**, *10*, 1–12. [CrossRef]

54. Bayard, M.; Cansell, M.; Leal-Calderon, F. Crystallization of emulsified anhydrous milk fat: The role of confinement and of minor compounds. *A DSC Study. Food Chem.* **2022**, *373*, 131605. [CrossRef]
55. Bayard, M.; Kauffmann, B.; Vauvre, J.-M.; Leal-Calderon, F.; Cansell, M. Isothermal crystallization of anhydrous milk fat in presence of free fatty acids and their esters: From nanostructure to textural properties. *Food Chem.* **2022**, *366*, 130533. [CrossRef] [PubMed]
56. Gift, A.D.; Southard, L.A.; Riesberg, A.L. Influence of polymeric excipient properties on crystal hydrate formation kinetics of caffeine in aqueous slurries. *J. Pharm. Sci.* **2012**, *101*, 1755–1762. [CrossRef] [PubMed]
57. Teja, S.B.; Patil, S.P.; Shete, G.; Patel, S.; Bansal, A.K. Drug-excipient behavior in polymeric amorphous solid dispersions. *J. Excip. Food Chem.* **2016**, *4*, 1048.
58. Iyer, R.; Petrovska Jovanovska, V.; Berginc, K.; Jaklič, M.; Fabiani, F.; Harlacher, C.; Huzjak, T.; Sanchez-Felix, M.V. Amorphous Solid Dispersions (ASDs): The Influence of Material Properties, Manufacturing Processes and Analytical Technologies in Drug Product Development. *Pharmaceutics* **2021**, *13*, 1682. [CrossRef] [PubMed]
59. Einfalt, T.; Planinšek, O.; Hrovat, K. Methods of amorphization and investigation of the amorphous state. *Acta Pharm.* **2013**, *63*, 305–334. [CrossRef] [PubMed]
60. Noonan, T.J.; Chibale, K.; Cheuka, P.M.; Kumar, M.; Bourne, S.A.; Caira, M.R. Five solid forms of a potent imidazopyridazine antimalarial drug lead: A preformulation study. *Cryst. Growth Des.* **2019**, *19*, 4683–4697. [CrossRef]
61. Diao, Y.; Whaley, K.E.; Helgeson, M.E.; Woldeyes, M.A.; Doyle, P.S.; Myerson, A.S.; Hatton, T.A.; Trout, B.L. Gel-induced selective crystallization of polymorphs. *J. Am. Chem. Soc.* **2012**, *134*, 673–684. [CrossRef] [PubMed]
62. Beiner, M.; Rengarajan, G.; Pankaj, S.; Enke, D.; Steinhart, M. Manipulating the crystalline state of pharmaceuticals by nanoconfinement. *Nano Lett.* **2007**, *7*, 1381–1385. [CrossRef]
63. Cheng, S.; McKenna, G.B. Nanoconfinement effects on the glass transition and crystallization behaviors of nifedipine. *Mol. Pharm.* **2019**, *16*, 856–866. [CrossRef]
64. Rengarajan, G.; Enke, D.; Steinhart, M.; Beiner, M. Stabilization of the amorphous state of pharmaceuticals in nanopores. *J. Mater. Chem.* **2008**, *18*, 2537–2539. [CrossRef]
65. Cipolla, D.; Wu, H.; Salentinig, S.; Boyd, B.; Rades, T.; Vanhecke, D.; Petri-Fink, A.; Rothin-Rutishauser, B.; Eastman, S.; Redelmeier, T. Formation of drug nanocrystals under nanoconfinement afforded by liposomes. *RSC Adv.* **2016**, *6*, 6223–6233. [CrossRef]
66. Salas-Zúñiga, R.; Mondragón-Vásquez, K.; Alcalá-Alcalá, S.; Lima, E.; Höpfl, H.; Herrera-Ruiz, D.; Morales-Rojas, H. Nanoconfinement of a Pharmaceutical Cocrystal with Praziquantel in Mesoporous Silica: The Influence of the Solid Form on Dissolution Enhancement. *Mol. Pharm.* **2021**, *19*, 414–431. [CrossRef] [PubMed]
67. Aakeröy, C.B.; Salmon, D.J. Building co-crystals with molecular sense and supramolecular sensibility. *CrystEngComm* **2005**, *7*, 439–448. [CrossRef]
68. Steed, J.W. The role of co-crystals in pharmaceutical design. *Trends Pharmacol. Sci.* **2013**, *34*, 185–193. [CrossRef] [PubMed]
69. Miroshnyk, I.; Mirza, S.; Sandler, N. Pharmaceutical co-crystals–an opportunity for drug product enhancement. *Expert Opin. Drug Deliv.* **2009**, *6*, 333–341. [CrossRef] [PubMed]
70. Kaur, P.; Elsayed, A.; Subramanian, J.; Singh, A. Encapsulation of carotenoids with sucrose by co-crystallization: Physicochemical properties, characterization and thermal stability of pigments. *LWT* **2021**, *140*, 110810. [CrossRef]
71. Chezanoglou, E.; Goula, A.M. Co-crystallization in sucrose: A promising method for encapsulation of food bioactive components. *Trends Food Sci. Technol.* **2021**, *114*, 262–274. [CrossRef]
72. Good, D.J.; Rodriguez-Hornedo, N. Solubility advantage of pharmaceutical cocrystals. *Cryst. Growth Des.* **2009**, *9*, 2252–2264. [CrossRef]
73. Huang, Y.; Dai, W.-G. Fundamental aspects of solid dispersion technology for poorly soluble drugs. *Acta Pharm. Sin. B.* **2014**, *4*, 18–25. [CrossRef]
74. Newman, A.; Knipp, G.; Zografi, G. Assessing the performance of amorphous solid dispersions. *J. Pharm. Sci.* **2012**, *101*, 1355–1377. [CrossRef]
75. Ishimoto, K.; Miki, S.; Ohno, A.; Nakamura, Y.; Otani, S.; Nakamura, M.; Nakagawa, S. β-Carotene solid dispersion prepared by hot-melt technology improves its solubility in water. *J. Food Sci. Technol.* **2019**, *56*, 3540–3546. [CrossRef] [PubMed]
76. Otani, S.; Miki, S.; Nakamura, Y.; Ishimoto, K.; Ago, Y.; Nakagawa, S. Improved bioavailability of β-carotene by amorphous solid dispersion technology in rats. *J. Nutr. Sci. Vitaminol.* **2020**, *66*, 207–210. [CrossRef] [PubMed]
77. Ishimoto, K.; Nakamura, Y.; Otani, S.; Miki, S.; Maeda, S.; Iwamoto, T.; Konishi, Y.; Ago, Y.; Nakagawa, S. Examination of dissolution ratio of β-carotene in water for practical application of β-carotene amorphous solid dispersion. *J. Food Sci. Technol.* **2022**, *59*, 114–122. [CrossRef] [PubMed]
78. Wang, Y.; Chen, C.; Hu, X.; Campanella, O.H.; Miao, M. Fabrication and characterizations of cyclic amylopectin-based delivery system incorporated with β-carotene. *Food Hydrocoll.* **2022**, *130*, 107680. [CrossRef]
79. Chang, C.-W.; Wang, C.-Y.; Wu, Y.-T.; Hsu, M.-C. Enhanced solubility, dissolution, and absorption of lycopene by a solid dispersion technique: The dripping pill delivery system. *Powder Technol.* **2016**, *301*, 641–648. [CrossRef]
80. Fuenmayor, C.A.; Baron-Cangrejo, O.G.; Salgado-Rivera, P.A. Encapsulation of carotenoids as food colorants via formation of cyclodextrin inclusion complexes: A review. *Polysaccharides* **2021**, *2*, 454–476. [CrossRef]

81. Sun, X.; Zhu, J.; Liu, C.; Wang, D.; Wang, C.-Y. Fabrication of fucoxanthin/2-hydroxypropyl-β-cyclodextrin inclusion complex assisted by ultrasound procedure to enhance aqueous solubility, stability and antitumor effect of fucoxanthin. *Ultrason. Sonochem.* **2022**, *90*, 106215. [CrossRef] [PubMed]

82. Escobar-Puentes, A.A.; Reyes-López, S.Y.; Baltazar, Á.d.J.R.; López-Teros, V.; Wall-Medrano, A. Molecular interaction of β-carotene with sweet potato starch: A bleaching-restitution assay. *Food Hydrocoll.* **2022**, *127*, 107522. [CrossRef]

83. Gheonea, I.; Aprodu, I.; Râpeanu, G.; Stănciuc, N. Binding mechanisms between lycopene extracted from tomato peels and bovine β-lactoglobulin. *J. Lumin.* **2018**, *203*, 582–589.

84. Kaur, M.; Bawa, M.; Singh, M. β-Carotene-β-cyclodextrin inclusion complex: Towards enhanced aqueous solubility. *J. Glob. Biosci.* **2016**, *5*, 3665–3675.

85. Durante, M.; Milano, F.; De Caroli, M.; Giotta, L.; Piro, G.; Mita, G.; Frigione, M.; Lenucci, M.S. Tomato oil encapsulation by α-, β-, and γ-Cyclodextrins: A comparative study on the formation of supramolecular structures, antioxidant activity, and carotenoid stability. *Foods* **2020**, *9*, 1553. [CrossRef] [PubMed]

86. Yazdani, M.; Tavakoli, O.; Khoobi, M.; Wu, Y.S.; Faramarzi, M.A.; Gholibegloo, E.; Farkhondeh, S. Beta-carotene/cyclodextrin-based inclusion complex: Improved loading, solubility, stability, and cytotoxicity. *J. Incl. Phenom. Macrocycl. Chem.* **2022**, *102*, 55–64. [CrossRef]

87. Lakshmanan, M.; Moses, J.A.; Chinnaswamy, A. Encapsulation of β-carotene in 2-hydroxypropyl-β-cyclodextrin/carrageenan/soy protein using a modified spray drying process. *Int. J. Food Sci. Technol.* **2022**, *57*, 2680–2688. [CrossRef]

88. Nalawade, P.; Gajjar, A. Assessment of in-vitro bio accessibility and characterization of spray dried complex of astaxanthin with methylated betacyclodextrin. *J. Incl. Phenom. Macrocycl. Chem.* **2015**, *83*, 63–75. [CrossRef]

89. Kim, J.-Y.; Seo, T.-R.; Lim, S.-T. Preparation of aqueous dispersion of β-carotene nano-composites through complex formation with starch dextrin. *Food Hydrocoll.* **2013**, *33*, 256–263. [CrossRef]

90. Kong, L.; Bhosale, R.; Ziegler, G.R. Encapsulation and stabilization of β-carotene by amylose inclusion complexes. *Food Res. Int.* **2018**, *105*, 446–452. [CrossRef]

91. Kim, J.-Y.; Huber, K.C. Preparation and characterization of corn starch-β-carotene composites. *Carbohydr. Polym.* **2016**, *136*, 394–401. [CrossRef]

92. Allahdad, Z.; Khammari, A.; Karami, L.; Ghasemi, A.; Sirotkin, V.A.; Haertlé, T.; Saboury, A.A. Binding studies of crocin to β-Lactoglobulin and its impacts on both components. *Food Hydrocoll.* **2020**, *108*, 106003. [CrossRef]

93. Buszewski, B.; Rodzik, A.; Railean-Plugaru, V.; Sprynskyy, M.; Pomastowski, P. A study of zinc ions immobilization by β-lactoglobulin. *Colloids. Surf., A. Physicochem. Eng. Asp.* **2020**, *591*, 124443. [CrossRef]

94. Wang, C.; Chen, L.; Lu, Y.; Liu, J.; Zhao, R.; Sun, Y.; Sun, B.; Cuina, W. pH-Dependent complexation between β-lactoglobulin and lycopene: Multi-spectroscopy, molecular docking and dynamic simulation study. *Food Chem.* **2021**, *362*, 130230. [CrossRef]

95. Thakur, S.; Sharma, R.; Garg, T. A review on microparticles: Preparation techniques and evaluation. *Pharma Innov. J.* **2022**, *11*, 837–840.

96. Zhu, Z. Effects of amphiphilic diblock copolymer on drug nanoparticle formation and stability. *Biomaterials* **2013**, *34*, 10238–10248. [CrossRef] [PubMed]

97. Cordt, C.; Meckel, T.; Geissler, A.; Biesalski, M. Entrapment of hydrophobic biocides into cellulose acetate nanoparticles by nanoprecipitation. *Nanomaterials* **2020**, *10*, 2447. [CrossRef] [PubMed]

98. Liu, W.-Y.; Hsieh, Y.-S.; Wu, Y.-T. Poly (Lactic-Co-Glycolic) Acid–Poly (Vinyl Pyrrolidone) Hybrid Nanoparticles to Improve the Efficiency of Oral Delivery of β-Carotene. *Pharmaceutics* **2022**, *14*, 637. [CrossRef] [PubMed]

99. Hu, F.; Liu, W.; Yan, L.; Kong, F.; Wei, K. Optimization and characterization of poly (lactic-co-glycolic acid) nanoparticles loaded with astaxanthin and evaluation of anti-photodamage effect in vitro. *R. Soc. Open Sci.* **2019**, *6*, 191184. [CrossRef]

100. Nalawade, P.; Gajjar, A. Optimization of astaxanthin microencapsulation in hydrophilic carriers using response surface methodology. *Arch. Pharm. Res.* **2015**, 1–17. [CrossRef]

101. Zhao, C.; Cheng, H.; Jiang, P.; Yao, Y.; Han, J. Preparation of lutein-loaded particles for improving solubility and stability by Polyvinylpyrrolidone (PVP) as an emulsion-stabilizer. *Food Chem.* **2014**, *156*, 123–128. [CrossRef]

102. Yuan, Y.; Li, H.; Liu, C.; Zhang, S.; Xu, Y.; Wang, D. Fabrication and characterization of lutein-loaded nanoparticles based on zein and sophorolipid: Enhancement of water solubility, stability, and bioaccessibility. *J. Agric. Food Chem.* **2019**, *67*, 11977–11985. [CrossRef]

103. Suzuki, R.; Yasuhara, K.; Deguchi, S. Effect of Molecular Distortion on the Optical Properties of Carotenoid-Based Nanoparticles. *J. Phys. Chem. C* **2022**, *126*, 2607–2613. [CrossRef]

104. Anarjan, N.; Tan, C.P.; Nehdi, I.A.; Ling, T.C. Colloidal astaxanthin: Preparation, characterisation and bioavailability evaluation. *Food Chem.* **2012**, *135*, 1303–1309. [CrossRef] [PubMed]

105. McClements, D.J. Crystals and crystallization in oil-in-water emulsions: Implications for emulsion-based delivery systems. *Adv. Colloid Interface Sci.* **2012**, *174*, 1–30. [CrossRef] [PubMed]

106. Chauhan, I.; Yasir, M.; Verma, M.; Singh, A.P. Nanostructured lipid carriers: A groundbreaking approach for transdermal drug delivery. *Adv. Pharm. Bull.* **2020**, *10*, 150. [CrossRef] [PubMed]

107. Doktorovova, S.; Shegokar, R.; Souto, E.B. Role of excipients in formulation development and biocompatibility of lipid nanoparticles (SLNs/NLCs). In *Nanostructures for Novel Therapy*; Elsevier: Amsterdam, The Netherlands, 2017; pp. 811–843.

108. Ribeiro, A.P.B.; Masuchi, M.H.; Miyasaki, E.K.; Domingues, M.A.F.; Stroppa, V.L.Z.; de Oliveira, G.M.; Kieckbusch, T.G. Crystallization modifiers in lipid systems. *J. Food Sci. Technol.* **2015**, *52*, 3925–3946. [CrossRef]
109. Weiss, J.; Decker, E.A.; McClements, D.J.; Kristbergsson, K.; Helgason, T.; Awad, T. Solid lipid nanoparticles as delivery systems for bioactive food components. *Food Biophys.* **2008**, *3*, 146–154. [CrossRef]
110. Gordillo-Galeano, A.; Mora-Huertas, C.E. Solid lipid nanoparticles and nanostructured lipid carriers: A review emphasizing on particle structure and drug release. *Eur. J. Pharm. Biopharm.* **2018**, *133*, 285–308. [CrossRef] [PubMed]
111. Azizi, M.; Li, Y.; Kaul, N.; Abbaspourrad, A. Study of the physicochemical properties of fish oil solid lipid nanoparticle in the presence of palmitic acid and quercetin. *J. Agric. Food Chem.* **2019**, *67*, 671–679. [CrossRef] [PubMed]
112. Helgason, T.; Awad, T.S.; Kristbergsson, K.; Decker, E.A.; McClements, D.J.; Weiss, J. Impact of surfactant properties on oxidative stability of β-carotene encapsulated within solid lipid nanoparticles. *J. Agric. Food Chem.* **2009**, *57*, 8033–8040. [CrossRef]
113. Gomes, G.V.d.L.; Borrin, T.R.; Cardoso, L.P.; Souto, E.; Pinho, S.C.d. Characterization and shelf life of β-carotene loaded solid lipid microparticles produced with stearic acid and sunflower oil. *Braz Arch Biol Technol.* **2013**, *56*, 663–671. [CrossRef]
114. Chen, Y.; He, N.; Yang, T.; Cai, S.; Zhang, Y.; Lin, J.; Huang, M.; Chen, W.; Zhang, Y.; Hong, Z. Fucoxanthin Loaded in Palm Stearin-and Cholesterol-Based Solid Lipid Nanoparticle-Microcapsules, with Improved Stability and Bioavailability In Vivo. *Mar. Drugs* **2022**, *20*, 237. [CrossRef]
115. Tamjidi, F.; Shahedi, M.; Varshosaz, J.; Nasirpour, A. Design and characterization of astaxanthin-loaded nanostructured lipid carriers. *Innov. Food Sci. Emerg. Technol.* **2014**, *26*, 366–374. [CrossRef]
116. Osanlou, R.; Emtyazjoo, M.; Banaei, A.; Hesarinejad, M.A.; Ashrafi, F. Preparation of solid lipid nanoparticles and nanostructured lipid carriers containing zeaxanthin and evaluation of physicochemical properties. *Colloids. Surf. A. Physicochem. Eng. Asp.* **2022**, *641*, 128588. [CrossRef]
117. Xia, Z.; McClements, D.J.; Xiao, H. Influence of physical state of β-carotene (crystallized versus solubilized) on bioaccessibility. *J. Agric. Food Chem.* **2015**, *63*, 990–997. [CrossRef] [PubMed]
118. Zhang, Y.; Yang, Y.; Mao, Y.; Zhao, Y.; Li, X.; Hu, J.; Li, Y. Effects of mono-and di-glycerides/phospholipids (MDG/PL) on the bioaccessibility of lipophilic nutrients in a protein-based emulsion system. *Food Funct.* **2022**, *13*, 8168–8178. [CrossRef] [PubMed]
119. Tang, B.; Cheng, G.; Gu, J.-C.; Xu, C.-H. Development of solid self-emulsifying drug delivery systems: Preparation techniques and dosage forms. *Drug Discov. Today* **2008**, *13*, 606–612. [CrossRef]
120. Kim, M.-S.; Ha, E.-S.; Choo, G.-H.; Baek, I.-H. Preparation and in vivo evaluation of a dutasteride-loaded solid-supersaturatable self-microemulsifying drug delivery system. *Int. J. Mol. Sci.* **2015**, *16*, 10821–10833. [CrossRef]
121. Dokania, S.; Joshi, A.K. Self-microemulsifying drug delivery system (SMEDDS)–challenges and road ahead. *Drug Deliv.* **2015**, *22*, 675–690. [CrossRef]
122. Quan, G.; Niu, B.; Singh, V.; Zhou, Y.; Wu, C.-Y.; Pan, X.; Wu, C. Supersaturable solid self-microemulsifying drug delivery system: Precipitation inhibition and bioavailability enhancement. *Int. J. Nanomed.* **2017**, *12*, 8801. [CrossRef]
123. Faisal, W.; Ruane-O'Hora, T.; O'Driscoll, C.M.; Griffin, B.T. A novel lipid-based solid dispersion for enhancing oral bioavailability of Lycopene–In vivo evaluation using a pig model. *Int. J. Pharm.* **2013**, *453*, 307–314. [CrossRef]
124. Aung, W.T.; Khine, H.E.E.; Chaotham, C.; Boonkanokwong, V. Production, physicochemical investigations, antioxidant effect, and cellular uptake in Caco-2 cells of the supersaturable astaxanthin self-microemulsifying tablets. *Eur. J. Pharm. Sci.* **2022**, *176*, 106263. [CrossRef]
125. Li, T.; Cipolla, D.; Rades, T.; Boyd, B.J. Drug nanocrystallisation within liposomes. *J. Control. Release* **2018**, *288*, 96–110. [CrossRef]
126. Pan, L.; Wang, H.; Gu, K. Nanoliposomes as vehicles for astaxanthin: Characterization, in vitro release evaluation and structure. *Molecules* **2018**, *23*, 2822. [CrossRef] [PubMed]

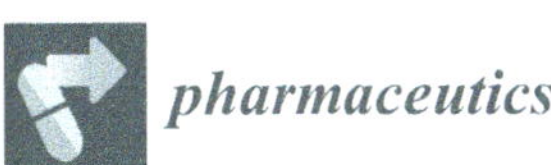

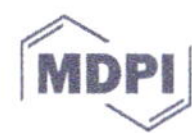

Article

Metformin-NSAIDs Molecular Salts: A Path towards Enhanced Oral Bioavailability and Stability

Francisco Javier Acebedo-Martínez [1], Alicia Domínguez-Martín [2], Carolina Alarcón-Payer [3], Carolina Garcés-Bastida [1], Cristóbal Verdugo-Escamilla [1], Jaime Gómez-Morales [1] and Duane Choquesillo-Lazarte [1,*]

[1] Laboratorio de Estudios Cristalográficos, IACT, CSIC-Universidad de Granada, Avda. de las Palmeras 4, 18100 Armilla, Spain
[2] Department of Inorganic Chemistry, Faculty of Pharmacy, University of Granada, 18071 Granada, Spain
[3] Servicio de Farmacia, Hospital Universitario Virgen de las Nieves, 18014 Granada, Spain
* Correspondence: duane.choquesillo@csic.es

Abstract: According to the World Health Organization, more than 422 million people worldwide have diabetes. The most common oral treatment for type 2 diabetes is the drug metformin (MTF), which is usually formulated as a hydrochloride to achieve higher water solubility. However, this drug is also highly hygroscopic, thus showing stability problems. Another kind of worldwide prescribed drug is the non-steroidal anti-inflammatory drug (NSAID). These latter, on the contrary, show a low solubility profile; therefore, they must be administered at high doses, which increases the probability of secondary effects. In this work, novel drug-drug pharmaceutical solids combining MTF-NSAIDs have been synthesized in solution or by mechanochemical methods. The aim of this concomitant treatment is to improve the physicochemical properties of the parent active pharmaceutical ingredients. After a careful solid-state characterization along with solubility and stability studies, it can be concluded that the new molecular salt formulations enhance not only the stability of MTF but also the solubility of NSAIDs, thus giving promising results regarding the development of these novel pharmaceutical multicomponent solids.

Keywords: metformin; NSAIDs; molecular salts; crystal engineering; mechanochemistry

Citation: Acebedo-Martínez, F.J.;
Domínguez-Martín, A.;
Alarcón-Payer, C.; Garcés-Bastida, C.;
Verdugo-Escamilla, C.; Gómez-Morales,
J.; Choquesillo-Lazarte, D.
Metformin-NSAIDs Molecular Salts:
A Path towards Enhanced Oral
Bioavailability and Stability.
Pharmaceutics **2023**, *15*, 449.
https://doi.org/10.3390/
pharmaceutics15020449

Academic Editor: Hisham Al-Obaidi

Received: 29 December 2022
Revised: 24 January 2023
Accepted: 26 January 2023
Published: 29 January 2023

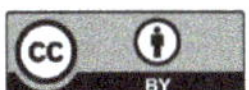

1. Introduction

According to the World Health Organization (WHO), diabetes is defined as a "chronic, metabolic disease characterized by elevated levels of blood glucose" [1]. WHO estimates as 422 million the number of worldwide adult patients diagnosed with diabetes, and this number rises to 537 million according to the International Diabetes Federation [2]. In 2045, the number of patients with diabetes is believed to reach 784 million, therefore being diabetes a real challenge for healthcare systems [1,2]. There are two types of diabetes. Type 1 diabetes, once so-called juvenile diabetes, occurs when the pancreas does not produce insulin, whereas type 2 diabetes occurs when the body becomes resistant to insulin, and it most often develops in adults. Nonetheless, the prevalence of overweight individuals and obesity in the younger age populations, along with insufficient physical activity, is directly related to the increasing occurrence of type 2 diabetes in younger populations, too [1,3].

Metformin (MTF) is a biguanide antihyperglycemic agent (Scheme 1) used as a first-line pharmacological treatment in the management of type 2 diabetes due to its efficacy, safety profile, and low cost for patients [4,5]. MTF exerts its antihyperglycemic action by increasing insulin sensitivity in peripheral tissues and reducing hepatic gluconeogenesis [6]. It is most commonly prescribed alone as metformin hydrochloride (MTF·HCl), i.e., chemically defined as a salt, in order to increase solubility and stability [7–9]. Although MTF·HCl solubility is outstanding [10], the low gastrointestinal permeability of MTF [11] eventually leads to gastrointestinal disorders in about 20–30% of chronic patients due to accumulation in the enterocytes within the small intestine [12,13]. Regarding the molecular stability of metformin, the instability profile and degradation products are detailed in its official Pharmacopeia monograph [14]. In addition, several stability assessments on aqueous media agree on metformin's instability in alkaline solutions and its being less sensitive to oxidants [15,16]. Unfortunately, glycemic control with MTF in type 2 diabetes is still a challenge that concerns physicians due to its complexity [17]. Hence, its prescription, along with other antidiabetic drugs, is not rare in clinics.

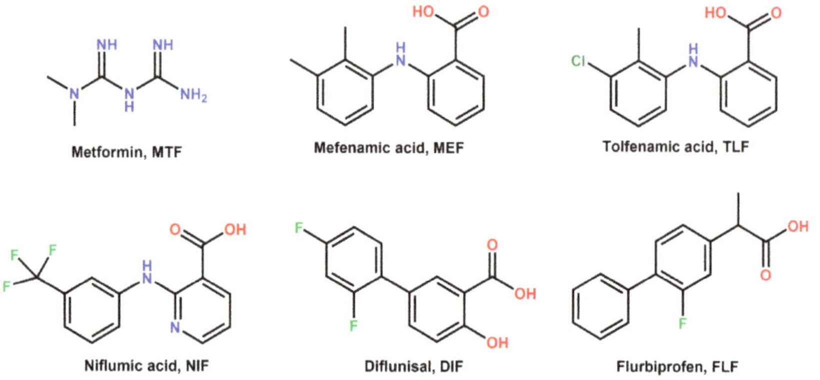

Scheme 1. Chemical formula of metformin (MTF), mefenamic acid (MEF), tolfenamic acid (TLF), niflumic acid (NIF), diflunisal (DIF), and flurbiprofen (FLP).

Non-steroidal anti-inflammatory drugs (NSAIDs) work to relieve pain, reduce inflammation, and bring down fever [18], thus being one of the most commonly prescribed medications worldwide. Despite their chemical diversity, they are generally poorly soluble [18], which is an important drawback of this kind of drug. This fact requires an increase in their dosage, increasing the probability of side effects and drug interactions. Therefore, enhancing the solubility of NSAIDs is also quite an active research area within the pharmaceutical industry.

Diabetic neuropathy is a serious diabetes complication in which overall peripheral nerves are affected, whose symptoms include pain and numbness in extremities [19]. Thereby the concomitant administration of MTF and NSAIDs is very frequent [20], even if NSAIDs are not considered especially effective at treating neuropathic pain unless there is inflammation [19]. Despite the latter, their massive use is a reality in clinics, most likely due to: (i) the lack of non-opioid alternatives in the treatment of mild-moderate pain, (ii) the 'over the counter' (OTC) character of several NSAIDs, and (iii) their safety profile. Even if they are generally regarded as safe, a rare, although serious, condition known as lactic acidosis has been reported for long-term MTF treatments connected to acute renal failure [21,22]. On the other hand, NSAIDs are known for their nephrotoxicity [23]. Therefore, patients with concomitant and chronic treatments of MTF and NSAIDs are more susceptible to developing renal impairment [24].

In this work, crystal engineering tools have been used to yield drug–drug multicomponent pharmaceutical solids. This novel approach is rather interesting for the pharmaceutical industry since it allows for the improvement of the physicochemical properties of parent active pharmaceutical ingredients (APIs) without modifying their chemical structure, thus being a relatively inexpensive method compared to the development of a complete drug pipeline [25]. The proposed novel formulations involve the antidiabetic drug metformin (MTF) and five different NSAIDs, i.e., Niflumic acid (NIF), Diflunisal (DIF), Mefenamic acid (MEF), Tolfenamic acid (TLF), and Flurbiprofen (FLF) (Scheme 1).

The aim of the study is to explore novel treatment alternatives that might increase the oral bioavailability of the aforementioned drugs via the formation of multidrug salts, as well as reduce the side effects associated with this combined therapy. To this purpose, five

(MTF)(NSAIDs) salts have been synthesized. Structure-physicochemical properties relationships of the new multicomponent pharmaceutical solids have been assessed thanks to a comprehensive solid-state analysis of the crystallographic structures. Moreover, solubility and stability have been evaluated in the new formulations and compared to the isolated parent APIs, showing promising results.

2. Materials and Methods

2.1. Materials

All APIs and solvents used in this work were purchased from commercial sources and used as received. Metfomin·HCl, tolfenamic acid, niflumic acid, and flurbiprofen were obtained from TCI Europe (Zwijndrecht, Belgium). Diflunisal and mefenamic acid were obtained from Sigma-Aldrich (St. Louis, CA, USA). Ethyl acetate HPLC grade and absolute ethanol were obtained from labkem (Barcelona, Spain).

2.2. Salt Syntheses

2.2.1. Metformin Hydrochloride Neutralization

To obtain the MTF base, MTF·HCl was neutralized by stirring 10 mmol of MTF·HCl (1.656 g) and 10 mmol of NaOH (0.4 g) in 60 mL of isopropanol at room temperature, using a magnetic stirrer and a sealed glass beaker to avoid evaporation. After 24 h, the solution was filtered using 0.22 μm syringe filters to remove the NaCl (insoluble in isopropanol). The solvent of the clear filtered obtained (containing the MTF base) was removed using a rotatory evaporator set at 50 °C and 30 rpm. The remaining powder was dried and characterized by powder X-ray diffraction (PXRD) to confirm the purity of the MTF base obtained.

2.2.2. Mechanochemical Synthesis

The mechanochemical synthesis of MTF salts was conducted using Liquid-Assisted Grinding (LAG) in a Retsh MM2000 ball mill (Retsch, Haan, Germany), operating at a 25-Hz frequency, using stainless steel jars along with stainless steel balls 7 mm in diameter.

MTF–MEF was obtained by LAG of a mixture of MTF (0.5 mmol, 64.58 mg) and MEF (0.5 mmol, 120.64 mg) in a 1:1 stoichiometric ratio with 100 μL of ultrapure water as a liquid additive.

MTF–FLP and MTF–TLF were obtained using LAG of a mixture of MTF (0.5 mmol, 64.58 mg) and the respective coformer (130.85 mg of TLF, 122.13 mg of FLP) in a 1:1 stoichiometric ratio, along with 100 μL of ethanol as a liquid additive.

MTF–DIF and MTF–NIF hydrates were obtained using LAG of a mixture of MTF (0.5 mmol, 64.58 mg) and the respective coformer (125.10 mg of DIF, 141.11 mg of NIF) in a 1:1 stoichiometric ratio, along with 100 μL of ultrapure water as a liquid additive.

To obtain MTF–DIF and MTF–NIF as anhydrated salts, the product of the mechanochemical synthesis was heated at 100 °C for 2 h.

All reaction syntheses lasted for 30 min and were repeated to ensure reproducibility. Bulk materials were further evaluated using PXRD to determine the salt formation.

2.2.3. Preparation of Single Crystals

Single crystals of MTF–based salts were obtained by dissolving the product of the LAGs in ethanol (for MTF–NIF·2H$_2$O, MTF–MEF, MTF–FLP, and MTF–TLF) and ethyl acetate (for MTF–NIF). MTF–DIF single crystals were obtained using a hydrothermal reaction by placing a mixture of 0.2 mmol of MTF (25.8 mg) and 0.2 mmol of DIF (50.4 mg) in a hydrothermal reactor along with 3 mL of distilled water. The reactor was sealed and heated at 110 °C for 24 h. After cooling down to room temperature, the reactor was opened, and single crystals were separated from the solution for further characterization.

2.3. X-ray Diffraction Analysis

Single-crystal X-ray diffraction (SCXRD) data were acquired at room temperature on a Bruker D8 Venture diffractometer (Bruker-AXS, Karlsruhe, Germany) using CuKα radiation ($\lambda = 1.54178$ Å). The data were processed with the APEX4 suite [26]. The structures were solved with intrinsic phasing (SHELXT) [27] and refined with full-matrix least squares on F^2 [28] using Olex2 as a graphical interface [29]. The non-hydrogen atoms were refined anisotropically. For all structures, hydrogen atoms were located in difference Fourier maps and included as fixed contributions riding on attached atoms with isotropic thermal displacement parameters 1.2 or 1.5 times those of the respective atom. Mercury [30], Platon [31], and Olex2 [29] were used for the analysis and visualization of the structures and also for graphic material preparation. All deposited CIF files are in the Cambridge Structural Database (CSD) under the CCDC numbers 2232928–2232933. Copies of the data can be obtained free of charge at https://www.ccdc.cam.ac.uk/structures/ (accessed on 29 December 2022).

Powder X-ray diffraction (PXRD) analysis was performed at room temperature on a Bruker D8 Advance Vαrio diffractometer (Bruker-AXS, Karlsruhe, Germany) diffractometer equipped with a LYNXEYE detector and CuKα$_1$ radiation (1.5406 Å). The diffractograms were collected over an angular range of 5–40° (2θ) with a step size of 0.02° (2θ) and a constant counting time of 5 s per step.

2.4. Differential Scanning Calorimetry

A differential scanning calorimetry (DSC) study was performed with a Mettler-Toledo SC-822e calorimeter (Mettler Toledo, Columbus, OH, USA). Experimental conditions: aluminum crucibles of 40 μL volume, an atmosphere of dry nitrogen with 50 mL/min flow rate, and heating rates of 1 °C/min and 10 °C/min. The calorimeter was calibrated with indium of 99.99% purity (m.p.: 156.4 °C; DH: 28.14 J/g).

2.5. Stability Studies

Stability in an aqueous solution was evaluated through slurry experiments. An excess of powder samples of each phase was added to 1 mL of buffer phosphate (pH 6.8) and stirred for 24 h in sealed vials. The solids were collected, filtered, dried, and analyzed with PXRD.

Stability at accelerated aging conditions was also studied: 200 mg of solid was placed in watch glasses and left at 40 °C in 75% relative humidity using a Memmert HPP110 climate chamber (Memmert, Schwabach, Germany). Under the above-accelerated aging conditions, the stability of the solid forms was periodically monitored using PXRD for two months.

2.6. Solubility Studies

Samples for the solubility studies were prepared following the shake-flask method [32]. Saturated solutions were obtained by stirring an excess amount of APIs in 10 mL of pH 6.8 phosphate buffer at 25 °C until the thermodynamic equilibrium was reached after 24 h. Thermodynamic equilibrium was tested using UV spectroscopy by following the global solubility of the molecular salt over time until the plateau region was reached (3 h) and sustained more than 24 h. The solutions were then centrifuged, filtered through 0.22 μm polyether sulfone (PES) filters, and directly measured using high-performance liquid chromatography (HPLC). Appropriate dilutions were made to obtain measurable absorbance values. The absorbance measurements were thereafter used to quantify the MTF dissolved in each sample. The remaining solids were analyzed using PXRD to identify the crystalline phases and, thus, to check the stability of the initial crystalline phase.

HPLC experiments were performed with an Agilent 1200 HPLC system (Agilent Technologies, Santa Clara, CA, USA) equipped with a solvent degasser, pump, auto-sampler, and diode array detector. A Scharlau (Barcelona, Spain) 100 C18 chromatographic column (3 μm, 150 × 4.6 mm) was the thermostat at 25 °C and used for compound separation, using an isocratic elution method. The mobile phase was composed of a mixture of 10% acetonitrile (0.1% Formic acid, v/v) and 90% water (0.1% Formic acid, v/v). The flow rate was 1 mL/min, and the injection volume was 10 µL. The absorbance was measured at 233 nm, i.e., the maximum absorbance for metformin. Data acquisition and analysis were performed using the software ChemStation (Agilent Technologies, Santa Clara, CA, USA). The retention time for MTF was 1 min 54 s, and the concentration for the calibration curve was determined from the area under the MTF peak. The conditions are summarized in Supplementary Table S1.

3. Results and Discussion

3.1. Salt Synthesis

Mechanochemistry, especially liquid-assisted grinding (LAG), has been widely used in the pharmaceutical industry for the synthesis of new multicomponent materials. This methodology is well known to be efficient, quick, and reproducible, requiring a minimum amount of organic solvents compared with other traditional techniques [33].

In this work, LAG reactions were performed using a 1:1 stoichiometric mixture of metformin base, previously neutralized, and the corresponding NSAIDs, along with ultrapure water or ethanol as an additive solvent. After 30 min of reaction, the powder obtained in each reaction was characterized using PXRD and compared with the corresponding parent APIs to evaluate the formation of the new salts. PXRD patterns demonstrated the formation of five new phases after LAG reactions and their purity (Figures 1 and S1).

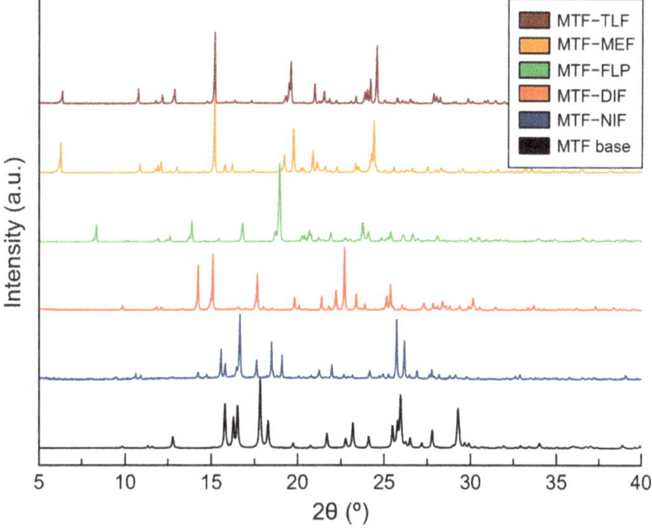

Figure 1. PXRD patterns of MTF base and the novel salts obtained by mechanochemical synthesis.

To obtain more information about the crystalline structure of the new phases, the polycrystalline products of the LAGs were used for recrystallization by dissolving them in ethanol and ethyl acetate. After slow solvent evaporation at room temperature, suitable crystals for single-crystal X-ray diffraction (SCXRD) were obtained.

From these experiments, MTF–TLF, MTF–MEF, MTF–FLP, and MTF–NIF structures were obtained. The structural information allowed the simulation of a calculated PXRD for each salt (Figure S1), which confirmed the phase purity of the bulk products obtained from LAG except for MTF–NIF, whose calculated powder pattern did not match the product obtained from the LAG reaction, thus indicating the formation of an intermediate phase or a hydrate phase. For that reason, the product of the LAG of MTF and NIF was heated at 100 °C for 2 h. After the thermal treatment, the PXRD pattern was in good agreement with the calculated powder pattern for MTF–NIF anhydrate salt. To confirm the formation of a hydrated phase during the LAG recrystallization, single crystals of MTF–NIF·2H$_2$O were obtained and analyzed, which allowed the use of the calculated PXRD pattern to compare with the initial mechanochemical reaction. As expected, however, the PXRD patterns of MTF–NIF·2H$_2$O and the product obtained from LAG synthesis did not match since they are different hydrated forms (Figure S2).

Similar results were obtained for MTF–DIF. Although good-quality single crystals were obtained from hydrothermal reactions, the bulk material obtained from LAG did not match the PXRD pattern of the anhydride phase. Following the previous methodology, the product of the LAG was heated at 100 °C for 2 h. After the treatment, the PXRD patterns matched perfectly. For MTF–DIF, no crystalline structure of a hydrate form was found.

3.2. Salt Screening

The Cambridge Structural Database (CSD version 5.43, update 4 from November 2022) was searched for MTF complexes resulting in 59 hits. After excluding entries corresponding to the MTF base molecule and its inorganic salts (4) as well as MTF metal complexes (29), the remaining dataset contained 26 molecular salts (44%). From the remaining molecular salts, 13 entries corresponded to MTF–drug salts, mainly antidiabetic drugs [34–38]. Only three salt structures containing MTF and an NSAID as counterion have been reported: MTF–diclofenac [39], MTF–salicylate [40], and MTF–aspirin [41] salts. The high number of observed molecular salts agrees with the strong basic nature of MTF. Table 1 evidences a significant difference in pK_a values between the ionizable groups of MTF and the selected NSAIDs. Thereby, proton transfer is expected from the carboxylic group present in NSAIDs to an amine moiety in MTF, according to the well-known pK_a rule widely used in the pharmaceutical industry [42–44]. Indeed, crystal structures of the multi-component drug–drug materials reported in this work confirm the molecular salt nature of these solids, which is consistent with other multicomponent pharmaceutical solids involving MTF published very recently [41,45,46].

Table 1. Molecules used to make salts with MTF and their corresponding pK_a values.

APIs	Reported pK_a Values	References	Calculated pK_a Values *	Calculated MTF-NSAID ΔpK_a
Metformin	12.4	[47]	12.30	-
Mefenamic Acid	3.93	[48]	3.89	8.41
Tolfenamic Acid	4.3	[49]	3.88	8.42
Niflumic acid	1.88	[50]	1.88	10.42
Diflunisal	2.69	[50]	2.69	9.61
Flurbiprofen	4.2	[51]	4.42	7.88

* Estimated using the pK_a plugin in MarvinSketch software [52].

3.3. Crystal Structure Analysis of Molecular Salts

Single crystals of molecular salts suitable for structural purposes were obtained, and their structures were determined using SCXRD. Crystallographic data for these salts are summarized in Table 2. Asymmetric units of the salts are represented in Figure S3, and hydrogen bond information is presented in Table S2. SCXRD data confirmed the proton transfer from the acid groups of NSAIDs to the basic nitrogen site of metformin. This finding was also evidenced in the experimental electron density map and confirmed by the analysis of the C–O bond distances of the carboxylate group of NSAIDs, with ΔD$_{C-O}$ values being similar to those observed in salts, in the range 0.008–0.024 Å [53]. Due to the protonation of MTF, the resulting MTF$^+$ cation is able to participate in hetero-synthons with the NSAID anion through guanidinium···carboxylate synthons, engaged through the $R_2^2(8)$ ring motif [54,55].

Table 2. Crystallographic data and structure refinement details of MTF—NSAIDs molecular salts.

Compound Name	MFT–MEF	MFT–TLF	MFT–NIF	MFT–NIF·2H$_2$O	MTF–DIF	MFT–FLP
Formula	C$_{19}$H$_{26}$N$_6$O$_2$	C$_{18}$H$_{23}$ClN$_6$O$_2$	C$_{17}$H$_{20}$F$_3$N$_7$O$_2$	C$_{17}$H$_{24}$F$_3$N$_7$O$_4$	C$_{17}$H$_{19}$F$_2$N$_5$O3	C$_{19}$H$_{24}$FN$_5$O$_2$
Formula weight	370.46	390.87	411.40	447.43	379.37	373.43
Crystal system	Monoclinic	Monoclinic	Monoclinic	Monoclinic	Monoclinic	Triclinic
Space group	P2$_1$/c	P2$_1$/c	P2$_1$/n	P2$_1$/c	C2/c	P-1
a/Å	15.5701(19)	15.5584(15)	6.2011(16)	19.9296(15)	36.998(2)	8.7587(5)
b/Å	8.7141(11)	8.7072(8)	32.216(8)	7.9245(6)	6.7220(5)	10.5391(7)
c/Å	16.239(2)	16.3668(16)	9.846(3)	14.6836(11)	15.0427(9)	10.5990(6)
α/°	90	90	90	90	90	90.265(2)
β/°	116.408(4)	117.919(4)	101.051(13)	109.362(4)	104.981(3)	96.217(2)
γ/°	90	90	90	90	90	94.624(2)
V/Å^3	1973.4(4)	1959.2(3)	1930.6(8)	2187.9(3)	3614.0(4)	969.37(10)
Z	4	4	4	4	8	2
D$_c$/g cm^{-3}	1.247	1.325	1.415	1.358	1.394	1.279
F(000)	792	824	856	936	1584	398
Reflections collected	20,802	19,113	19,888	17,437	18,152	14,188
Unique reflections	3509	3452	3396	3853	3155	3366
Data/restraints/parameters	3509/0/251	3452/0/248	3396/0/264	3853/0/288	3155/5/258	3366/0/248
Goodness-of-fit on F^2	1.053	1.048	1.036	1.026	1.037	1.068
R1 (I > 2σ(I))	0.0398	0.0477	0.0640	0.0633	0.0380	0.0551
wR2 (I > 2σ(I))	0.1153	0.1315	0.1758	0.1673	0.1044	0.1622

3.3.1. MTF–MEF and MTF–TLF Salts

Molecular salts of MTF and the fenamic acids reported in this study (MEF and TLF) are isostructural (have the same crystal structure) and, in addition, isomorphous (have the same unit-cell dimensions and spacegroup [56]). The unit-cell parameters of two crystal structures were used to calculate the unit-cell similarity index Π (Equation (1)) [57]. A Π value of 0.003 confirms the isomorphous nature of the MTF–fenamate pairs. Moreover, PXRD similarity index scores for each pair and the RMSDs (root-mean-square deviations) were calculated from the packing similarity tool in Mercury [30] (overlay with 20 molecules and allowing molecular differences). The results obtained from these calculations showed that 20 out of 20 molecules were matched in the pairs of fenamate salts (PXRD similarity: 0.986; RMSD (Å): 0.131), suggesting that these molecular salts have identical intermolecular interactions and therefore affording the same crystal packing.

$$\Pi = \frac{(a + b + c)}{(a' + b' + c')} - 1 \tag{1}$$

These molecular salts crystallize in the monoclinic P2$_1$/c space group, with one monoprotonated MTF$^+$ cation and one fenamate (MEF or TLF) anion in the asymmetric unit as ionic pair. In the molecular salt, the ions are associated through the $R_2^2(8)$ ring motif built by the COO$^-$ group and the terminal amines moiety of the MTF$^+$ cation (Figure 2). Ionic pairs are aligned in a 1D-chain along [010] direction by the N–H···O H-bond (N2–H2D···O1) formed between the NH$_2$ group in MTF$^+$ cations and the COO$^-$ group of fenamate anions. Along [001] direction, adjacent chains are held together through the $R_4^2(8)$ homo dimeric motif between two MTF$^+$ fenamate pairs related by an inversion center, generating a ribbon structure. A layered 2D structure is further generated with π,π-stacking interactions between the substituted rings of fenamate ions. The supramolecular structure is then obtained by stacking these layers with H-bonds involving amine groups of MTF$^+$ and carboxylate groups of fenamates (Figure 2c).

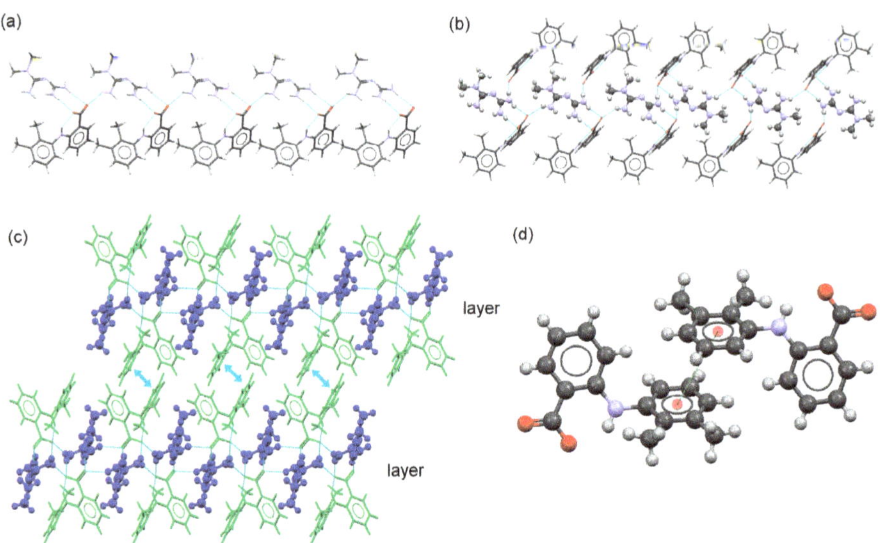

Figure 2. (**a**) Fragment of 1D-chain structure in the crystal structure of MTF–MEF. (**b**) Detailed view of the ribbon structure in the molecular salt MTF–MEF. MTF$^+$ cations are represented as balls and sticks. (**c**) Detailed view of the packing arrangement of MTF cations (blue) and MEF anions (green) in the crystal structure of MTF–MEF. MTF$^+$ cations are represented as balls and sticks. (**d**) A pair of stacked MEF–MEF anions.

3.3.2. MTF–NIF Salts and MTF–NIF·2H$_2$O Hydrate Salt

MTF–NIF salt crystallizes in the monoclinic system spacegroup P2$_1$/n. The asymmetric unit of this crystal phase contains one MTF$^+$ cation and a niflumate anion. The ion pair is associated with a charge-assisted hydrogen bond involving the guanidium moiety of MTF and the carboxylate group of NIF. As in the previously described salt structures containing MEF and TLF, adjacent ion pairs are H-bonded to build a 1D chain (along the a-axis). π,π-stacking interactions between each one of the rings of NIF reinforce the chains. A 2D layered structure is then generated through H-bonds between amine groups of MTF cations and carboxylate groups of NIF anions. Finally, the supramolecular structure is obtained by stacking these layers (along the b-axis) facing –CF$_3$ groups of NIF (Figure 3).

MTF–NIF·2H$_2$O crystallized in the monoclinic system spacegroup P2$_1$/c. The asymmetric unit of this crystal phase contains one MTF$^+$ cation, a niflumic anion, and two water molecules, resulting in a salt hydrate. In the asymmetric unit, the ions are connected by charge-assisted hydrogen bonds between the guanidinium moiety of MTF and a carboxylate group of NIF. Unlike the previously described structures, this interaction involves only one oxygen atom from the carboxylate group of NIF ($R_2^1(6)$ graph set). Water molecules and ion pars are connected by H-bonding interactions to build a ribbon structure that extends along the b-axis, locating the –CF$_3$ groups in the periphery. Additional H-bonding interactions involving the terminal amino group of the MTF$^+$ cation and water molecules connect ribbons to build a 2D layered structure that extends parallel to the bc- plane of the crystal. Finally, the supramolecular 3D structure is generated by stacking these layers along the a-axis facing the -CF$_3$ containing rings of NIF anions (Figure 4).

A possible explanation for the transformation of the anhydrate salt into the hydrate salt form can be obtained from the study of the predicted crystal morphology of MTF–NIF (Figure 5). BFDH morphology of the anhydrate MTF–NIF salt was calculated by using the Bravais–Friedel–Donnay–Harker (BFDH) method included in the latest release of the visualization software package Mercury [30]. In the case of MTF–NIF, the faces {−110}, {−1–10}, {1 1 0} and {1 −1 0} (corresponding to 14.4 % of the total surface) and the faces

{1 −1 −1}, {1 1 −1}, {−1 −1 1} and {−1 1 1} (corresponding to 32 % of the total surface) expose amino groups of MTF and carboxylate groups of NIF to the surface and coincide with the crystal structure region where the ion pairs form the tape-like structures. Therefore, it seems reasonable that water molecules can access and form additional H-bonds with the groups involved resulting in the hydrated structure as reported herein.

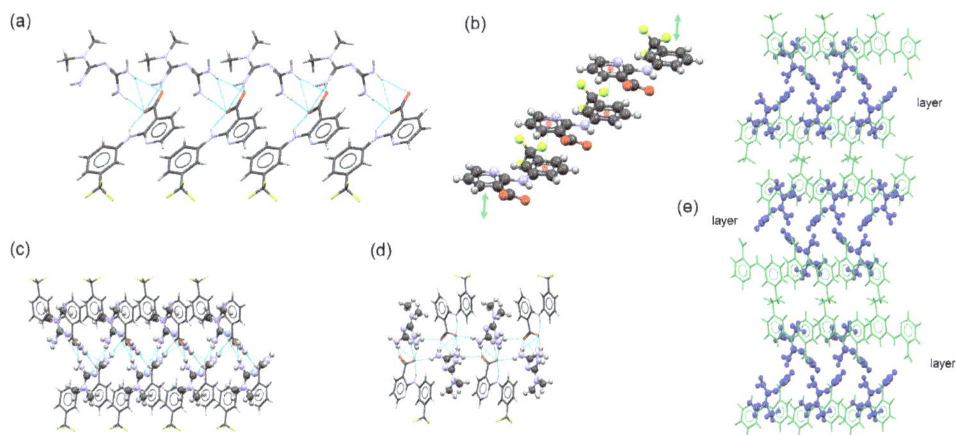

Figure 3. (**a**) Fragment of 1D-chain structure in the crystal structure of MTF–NIF. (**b**) Detailed view of multi-stacking π,π-interaction between NIF anions. (**c**) Detailed view of the ribbon structure in the molecular salt MTF–NIF. MTF$^+$ cations are represented as balls and sticks. (**d**) Fragment of the 2D-layered structure in the molecular salt MTF–NIF. (**e**) Packing arrangement of MTF cations (blue) and NIF anions (green) in the crystal structure of MTF–NIF.

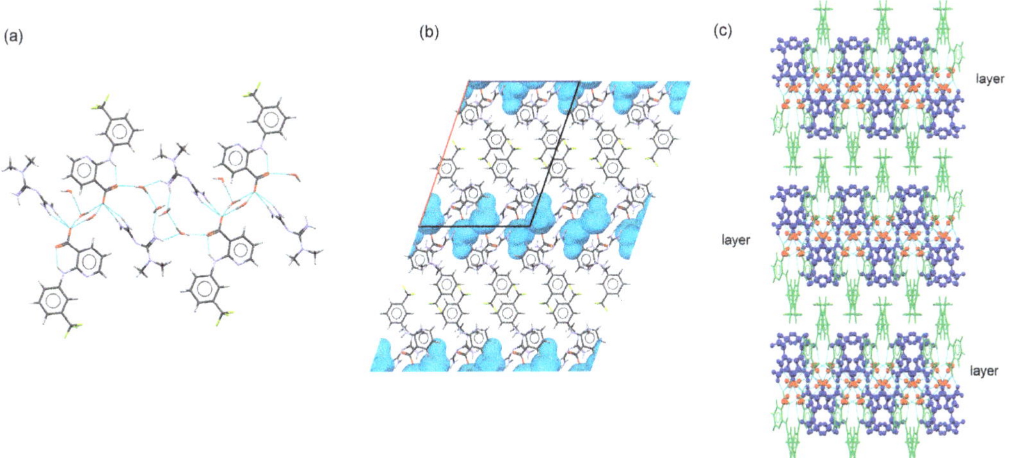

Figure 4. (**a**) Fragment of ribbon structure in the crystal structure of MTF–NIF·2H$_2$O. (**b**) Detailed view voids where water molecules are located in MTF–NIF·2H$_2$O. (**c**) Packing arrangement of MTF cations (blue), water molecules (red), and NIF anions (green) in the crystal structure of MTF–NIF·2H$_2$O. MTF cations are represented as balls and sticks.

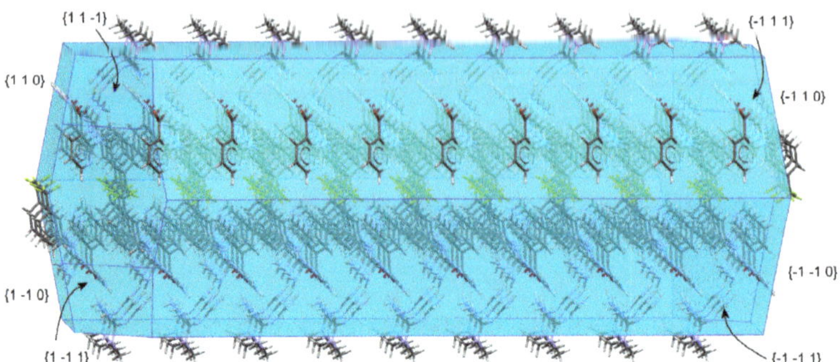

Figure 5. BFDH−predicted morphology of MTF–NIF salt.

3.3.3. MTF–DIF Salt

MTF–DIF crystallized in the monoclinic system spacegroup C2/c, with one MTF$^+$ cation and one DIF anion in the asymmetric unit. A trimer was formed by MTF and two DIF ions through guanidinium···carboxylate, N4–H4E···O2 (3.01 Å) and N5–H5B···O1 (2.96 Å) ($R_2^2(8)$ graph set), and N2–H2A···O2 (2.92 Å) hydrogen bonds (Figure 6). The trimers are then linked to build a ribbon structure through N5–H5A···O2 (3.05 Å) hydrogen bonds along the b-axis (Figure 6b). Additional H-bond involving amine groups of MTF$^+$ and carboxylate groups of DIF generate a 2D layered structure running parallel to the bc-plane of the crystal. C-H···F contacts participate in the cohesion of these structures. The supramolecular structure is finally built with stacks of layers facing 2,4-difluorophenyl rings of DIF (Figure 6).

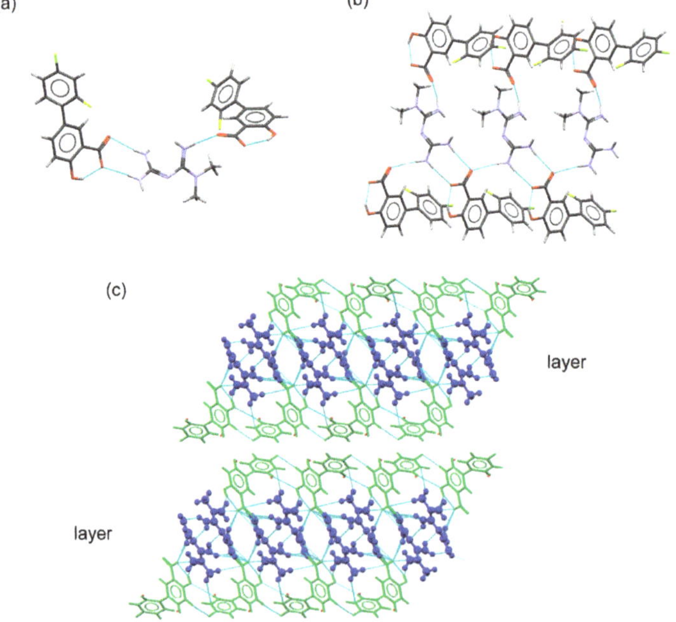

Figure 6. (**a**) Trimer structure generated by H-bonding interactions in the MTF–DIF salt. (**b**)Fragment of the ribbon structure generated using connecting trimers with H-bonding interactions. (**c**) Detailed view of the packing arrangement of MTF cations (blue) and DIF anions (green) in the crystal structure of MTF–DIF. MTF cations are represented as balls and sticks.

3.3.4. MTF–FLP Salt

This molecular salt crystallizes in the triclinic system space group P-1, with one monoprotonated MTF$^+$ cation and one FLP anion in the asymmetric unit as ionic pair. Both ions are associated with a charge-assisted H-bond through the guanidinium moiety of MTF$^+$ and the carboxylate group of FLP anion ($R_2^2(8)$ graph set). Adjacent pairs are further connected by H-bonds ($R_4^2(8)$ graph set) to build a ribbon structure that extends along the c-axis, locating the FLP ions outside. 2D-layered structures are then generated by connecting ribbons involving non-terminal amine groups of MTF$^+$ and carboxylate groups. The 3D supramolecular architecture is built through π,π-stacking interactions between the non-substituted aromatic ring of FLP anions that connect adjacent layers (Figure 7).

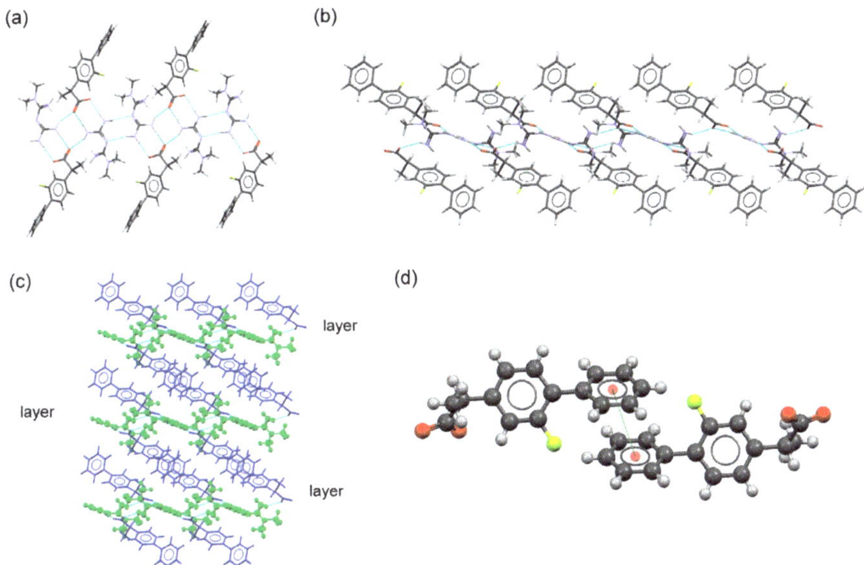

Figure 7. (**a**) Fragment of ribbon structure in the crystal structure of MTF–FLP. (**b**) Fragment of the 2D-layered structure in the molecular salt MTF–FLP. (**c**) Packing arrangement of MTF cations (blue) and NIF anions (green) in the crystal structure of MTF–DIF. (**d**) A pair of stacked FLP–FLP anions.

3.4. Thermal Analysis

Differential scanning calorimetry (DSC) was used to evaluate the thermal stability and determine the melting point of the new phases. Figure 8 shows the DSC traces and the endothermic events occurring during the experiments, which correspond to the melting point of the salts. The existence of one single and well-defined endothermic event confirms the purity of the phases, which is in good agreement with the results obtained using PXRD. In addition, the presence of only one endothermic event demonstrates the stability of the phase under the melting point. Over the transition state, other endothermic events are observed, ascribed to the degradation of the samples.

With the exception of MTF–FLP, all the molecular salts show a melting point in a range between the melting point of the MTF base (117 °C) and the corresponding NSAID coformer (MEF 230 °C, DIF 210–211 °C, TLF 207 °C, NIF 204 °C), increasing the thermal stability of the MTF base in all cases, although still under the melting point of the commercially available MTF·HCl (231.5 °C) [46]. This behavior has already been described by other researchers, demonstrating the ability of multicomponent materials to modulate the thermal behavior of APIs [58]. Interestingly, the melting point of MTF–FLP is 200 °C, while the melting point of the components goes from 110 to 117 °C, increasing the thermal stability and the melting point of both APIs by more than 80 °C.

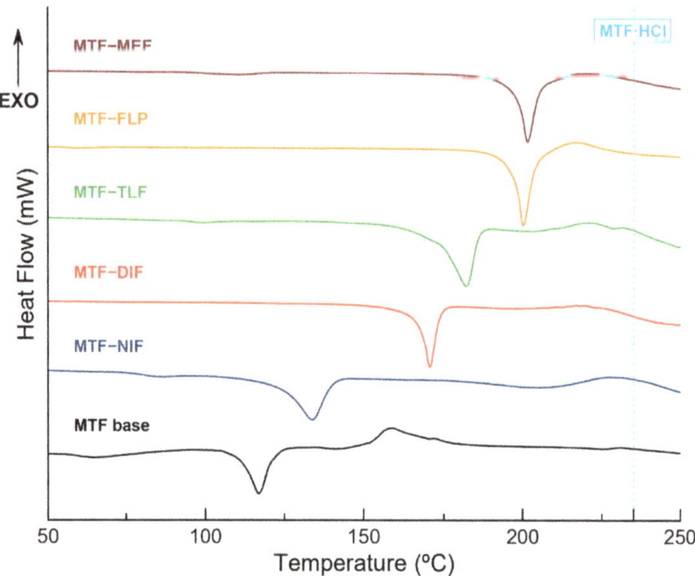

Figure 8. DSC traces of the pure molecular salts and MTF base. Blue-dotted line corresponds to the melting point of MTF·HCl.

3.5. Stability Studies

The thermodynamic stability of molecular salts was studied by conducting aqueous slurry experiments at 25 °C. After 24 h, the suspensions were filtered, air-dried at room temperature, and characterized using PXRD (Figure S4). No observable changes in color or texture were observed for the samples. Despite MTF–NIF and MTF–DIF displaying a phase transition indicating low stability in solution, MTF–TLF, MTF–MEF, and MTF–FLP remained stable upon slurrying, as the crystallinity and the initial crystal structures remained intact. SCXRD and further PXRD confirmed the formation of the dihydrate salt of MTF–NIF, but it was impossible to determine the final phase of MTF–DIF. Interestingly, this unknown phase agrees with the phase obtained directly from the LAG reaction using water as a liquid additive (Figure S5), suggesting the formation of a hydrate form of MTF–DIF salt.

The molecular salts were also stored under accelerated aging conditions (40 °C and 75% RH). Under these conditions, all the samples remained stable after four months, with the exception of MTF–NIF (Figure S6), which presented a partial phase transition on the third day, with a final conversion at one week. This new phase matched neither the already determined dihydrate salt form nor the product of the LAG in water, suggesting the formation of different grades of hydrate salt for the MTF–NIF system.

3.6. Solubility Studies

Solubility and oral bioavailability are closely related. Therefore, solubility enhancement is one of the most common approaches to increasing the bioavailability of poorly soluble drugs [59–61].

In this work, HPLC was used to determine the solubility of the proposed MTF molecular salts. The solubility improvement of NSAID coformers was also assessed through data normalization, using the corresponding stoichiometry and molecular weight of MTF-NSAID salts and isolated components. It should be noted that this procedure can only be applied to stable phases in which the stoichiometry MTF:NSAID is maintained.

Low stability was observed for MTF–NIF, and MTF–DIF in the stability test performed in aqueous media. A phase transformation for MTF–NIF was confirmed through the obtention of MTF–NIF·$2H_2O$ single crystals. For this reason, the solubility of MTF–NIF could not be determined at the reported experimental conditions. Instead, the solubility corresponding to the MTF–NIF salt hydrate was obtained. On the other hand, the phase transformation for MTF–DIF could not be determined, thus, making MTF–DIF unsuitable for solubility studies.

Table 3 shows a notorious increase in the solubility of NSAIDs when compared with the reported isolated APIs: MTF–TLF increased solubility 111 times, MTF–MEF 208 times, MTF–NIF·2H$_2$O 574 times, and finally MTF–FLP 1110 times, while exhibiting good stability. Furthermore, an interesting modulation of MTF solubility is also observed in the novel multicomponent molecular salts when compared with the solubility of MTF·HCl (ranging from 250 mg/mL [46,62,63]). In all reported MTF–NSAID salts, the solubility is reduced more than 50 times, with MTF–TLF decreasing the solubility of MTF by 90 times. Bearing in mind that clinical side effects of metformin were mainly caused by the gastrointestinal accumulation of MTF·HCl due to its extreme solubility [12], the obtention of a less soluble phase might reduce such side effects.

The remaining solids were finally analyzed using PXRD to identify the crystalline phases, thus confirming the stability of the initial phases and the congruent solubility of these new salts.

The remarkable solubility values obtained for the novel MTF–NSAID salts are consistent with the formation of molecular salts [7], as already expected from their pK_a values. Furthermore, it is well known that the physicochemical properties of solids, such as solubility, are also strongly dependent on their intimate crystal structure. Herein, the layered arrangement exhibited by the APIs and the presence of charge-assisted hydrogen bonds in the crystal structure [64,65] are eventually responsible for the new solubility properties.

Table 3. HPLC solubilities of the pure salts compared with their corresponding components.

Compound	MTF Solubility in the Salts [mg/mL]	NSAID Solubility in the Salts [mg/mL]	Solubility Enhancement over MTF·HCl/NSAID	NSAID Solubility [mg/mL]	Ref.
MTF–NIF·2H$_2$O	5.290	11.493	0.0212x/574x	<0.02	[66]
MTF–FLP	4.775	5.552	0.0191x/1110x	<0.005	[67]
MTF–MEF	3.185	5.950	0.0127x/119x	<0.05	[68,69]
MTF–TLF	2.740	10.397	0.0110x/208x	<0.05	[68]

4. Conclusions

The novel multicomponent MTF–NSAID solids succeeded in overcoming two of the main problems that these APIs have when administered separately. On the one hand, MTF stability has been improved while achieving an outstanding solubility profile. For instance, the reported MTF–NSAID solids are more soluble than MTF base but less soluble than MTF·HCl salt, thus potentially reducing improper intestinal accumulation, which is one of the most common side effects associated with the current MTF·HCl chronic treatment. On the other hand, MTF–NSAID molecular salts, thanks to the salification strategy, are able to significantly enhance the solubility of NSAIDs, thus reducing the dosage and the undesired gastrointestinal dose-dependent side effects of these drugs.

Interestingly, structure-properties relationships could be gathered from the thorough study of the intimate crystal structure of the new multicomponent MTF–NSAIDs molecular salts. The disruption of the robust NSAID–NSAID dimers present in the crystal structure of isolated NSAIDs is key for understanding their enhancement in solubility. Moreover, the new layered NSAID–MTF–NSAID structure in the novel multicomponent materials protects MTF from water, explaining the higher stability and the new solubility profile.

Considering all the above, the novel drug–drug molecular salts are worthy of further investigation. Our results confirm improved physicochemical properties thanks to the novel formulation, among which a better solubility profile should be remarked. Improving solubility should not be underestimated since a poor solubility profile is currently the most important limitation of oral biopharmaceutics in the pharmaceutical industry. Likewise, optimized solubility opens the door to dosage reduction and consequently might reduce those side effects associated with MTF–NSAID treatments.

Supplementary Materials: The following supporting information can be downloaded at: https://www.mdpi.com/article/10.3390/pharmaceutics15020449/s1, Figure S1: PXRD patterns of the molecular salts obtained using LAG, compared with their respective components; Figure S2: PXRD pattern of MTF–NIFH2O, compared with the product of the LAG in water; Figure S3: ORTEP representation showing the asymmetric unit of MTF—MEF (a), MTF—TLF (b), MTF—NIF (c), MTF—NIF·2H2O (d), MTF—DIF (e), and MTF—FLP (f) with an atom numbering scheme (thermal ellipsoids are plotted with a 50% probability level); Figure S4: PXRD patterns of the reported molecular salts after aqueous slurrying for 24 h; Figure S5: PXRD pattern of LAG of the mixture of MTF and DIF using water as liquid additive compared with the product after the slurry of MTF—DIF in aqueous media; Figure S6: PXRD patterns of reported molecular salts under accelerated aging conditions for 4 months; Figure S7: Calibration curve of MTF·HCl determined from HPLC data; Table S1: HPLC method parameters; Table S2: Hydrogen bonds for MTF—NSAIDs molecular salts [Å and deg.]; Table S3: π,π-stacking interactions analysis of compounds MTF—MEF, MTF—TLP, and MTF—FLP.

Author Contributions: Conceptualization and methodology, D.C.-L.; formal analysis and investigation, C.A.-P., F.J.A.-M., J.G.-M., C.V.-E., A.D.-M. and C.G.-B.; funding acquisition, A.D.-M., J.G.-M. and D.C.-L.; supervision, D.C.-L.; writing—original draft preparation, D.C.-L., A.D.-M. and F.J.A.-M.; writing—review and editing, D.C.-L. and A.D.-M. All authors have read and agreed to the published version of the manuscript.

Funding: This research was funded by Project B-FQM-478-UGR20 (FEDER-Universidad de Granada, Spain).

Institutional Review Board Statement: Not applicable.

Informed Consent Statement: Not applicable.

Data Availability Statement: The Crystallographic Information File with the structural data of the new phase can be obtained from the CCDC and requested with the references 2232928-2232933 at https://www.ccdc.cam.ac.uk/structures/ (accessed on 29 December 2022).

Acknowledgments: F.J.A.-M. wants to acknowledge an FPI grant (Ref. PRE2019-088832). C.V.-E. acknowledges Project PTA2020-019483-I funded by the Spanish Agencia Estatal de Investigación of the Ministerio de Ciencia e Innovación.

Conflicts of Interest: The authors declare no conflict of interest.

References

1. World Health Organization (WHO) Diabetes. Available online: https://www.who.int/health-topics/diabetes#tab=tab_1 (accessed on 21 November 2022).
2. International Diabetes Federation Diabetes. Available online: https://idf.org/ (accessed on 21 November 2022).
3. Centers for Disease Control and Prevention. Type 2 Diabetes. Available online: https://www.cdc.gov/diabetes/basics/type2.html (accessed on 21 November 2022).
4. U.S. Food and Drug Administration. *(FDA) Approved Drug Products: Metformin*; FDA: Silver Spring, MD, USA, 2018.
5. Viollet, B.; Guigas, B.; Sanz Garcia, N.; Leclerc, J.; Foretz, M.; Andreelli, F. Cellular and Molecular Mechanisms of Metformin: An Overview. *Clin. Sci.* **2012**, *122*, 253. [CrossRef] [PubMed]
6. Rena, G.; Hardie, D.G.; Pearson, E.R. The Mechanisms of Action of Metformin. *Diabetologia* **2017**, *60*, 1577. [CrossRef] [PubMed]
7. Serajuddin, A.T.M. Salt Formation to Improve Drug Solubility. *Adv. Drug Deliv. Rev.* **2007**, *59*, 603–616. [CrossRef] [PubMed]
8. Sun, X.; Du, S.; Sun, Y.; Li, H.; Yu, C.P.; Guo, J.; Wang, Y.; Yu, S.; Cheng, Y.; Xue, F. Solubility Measurement and Data Correlation of Metformin Hydrochloride in Four Aqueous Binary Solvents and Three Pure Solvents from 283.15 to 323.15 K. *J. Chem. Eng. Data* **2021**, *66*, 3282–3292. [CrossRef]
9. Klepser, T.B.; Kelly, M.W. Metformin Hydrochloride: An Antihyperglycemic Agent. *Am. J. Health Syst. Pharm.* **1997**, *54*, 893–903. [CrossRef] [PubMed]
10. Bretnall, A.A.; Clarke, G.S. *Analytical Profiles of Drug Substances and Excipients*; Brittain, H., Ed.; Academic Press: Millbrae, CA, USA, 1998; Volume 25.
11. Nicklin, P.; Keates, A.C.; Page, T.; Bailey, C.J. Transfer of Metformin across Monolayers of Human Intestinal Caco-2 Cells and across Rat Intestine. *Int. J. Pharm.* **1996**, *128*, 155–162. [CrossRef]
12. McCreight, L.J.; Bailey, C.J.; Pearson, E.R. Metformin and the Gastrointestinal Tract. *Diabetologia* **2016**, *59*, 426–435. [CrossRef] [PubMed]

13. Wilcock, C.; Bailey, C.J. Accumulation of Metformin by Tissues of the Normal and Diabetic Mouse. *Xenobiotica* **1994**, *24*, 49–57. [CrossRef] [PubMed]
14. Council of Europe (Ed.) *European Pharmacopeia*, 9th ed.; Council of Europe: Strasbourg, France, 2016.
15. Hamdan, I.I.; Jaber, A.K.B.; Abushoffa, A.M. Development and Validation of a Stability Indicating Capillary Electrophoresis Method for the Determination of Metformin Hydrochloride in Tablets. *J. Pharm. Biomed. Anal.* **2010**, *53*, 1254–1257. [CrossRef] [PubMed]
16. Gumieniczek, A.; Berecka-Rycerz, A.; Mroczek, T.; Wojtanowski, K. Determination of Chemical Stability of Two Oral Antidiabetics, Metformin and Repaglinide in the Solid State and Solutions Using LC-UV, LC-MS, and FT-IR Methods. *Molecules* **2019**, *24*, 4430. [CrossRef] [PubMed]
17. Inzucchi, S.E.; Bergenstal, R.M.; Buse, J.B.; Diamant, M.; Ferrannini, E.; Nauck, M.; Peters, A.L.; Tsapas, A.; Wender, R.; Matthews, D.R. Management of Hyperglycaemia in Type 2 Diabetes: A Patient-Centered Approach. Position Statement of the American Diabetes Association (ADA) and the European Association for the Study of Diabetes (EASD). *Diabetologia* **2012**, *55*, 1577–1596. [CrossRef] [PubMed]
18. NHS Non-Steroidal Anti-Inflammmatory Drugs. Available online: https://www.southtees.nhs.uk/resources/information-for-adult-patients-prescribed-non-steroidal-antiinflammatory-drugs-for-pain/ (accessed on 29 December 2022).
19. Schreiber, A.K.; Nones, C.F.; Reis, R.C.; Chichorro, J.G.; Cunha, J.M. Diabetic Neuropathic Pain: Physiopathology and Treatment. *World J. Diabetes* **2015**, *6*, 432. [CrossRef] [PubMed]
20. Moore, R.A.; Chi, C.C.; Wiffen, P.J.; Derry, S.; Rice, A.S.C. Oral Nonsteroidal Anti-Inflammatory Drugs for Neuropathic Pain. *Cochrane Database Syst. Rev.* **2015**, *10*, CD010902. [CrossRef] [PubMed]
21. Assan, R.; Heuclin, C.; Ganeval, D.; Bismuth, C.; George, J.; Girard, J.R. Metformin-Induced Lactic Acidosis in the Presence of Acute Renal Failure. *Diabetologia* **1977**, *13*, 211–217. [CrossRef] [PubMed]
22. Vecchio, S.; Giampreti, A.; Petrolini, V.M.; Lonati, D.; Protti, A.; Papa, P.; Rognoni, C.; Valli, A.; Rocchi, L.; Rolandi, L.; et al. Metformin Accumulation: Lactic Acidosis and High Plasmatic Metformin Levels in a Retrospective Case Series of 66 Patients on Chronic Therapy. *Clin. Toxicol.* **2014**, *52*, 129–135. [CrossRef] [PubMed]
23. Whelton, A. Nephrotoxicity of Nonsteroidal Anti-Inflammatory Drugs: Physiologic Foundations and Clinical Implications. *Am. J. Med.* **1999**, *106*, 13S–24S. [CrossRef] [PubMed]
24. Chan, N.N.; Fauvel, N.J.; Feher, M.D. Non-Steroidal Anti-Inflammatory Drugs and Metformin: A Cause for Concern? *Lancet* **1998**, *352*, 201. [CrossRef] [PubMed]
25. Berry, D.J.; Steed, J.W. Pharmaceutical Cocrystals, Salts and Multicomponent Systems; Intermolecular Interactions and Property Based Design. *Adv. Drug Deliv. Rev.* **2017**, *117*, 3–24. [CrossRef] [PubMed]
26. Bruker APEX4. In *APEX4 V2022.1*; Bruker-AXS: Madison, WI, USA, 2022.
27. Sheldrick, G.M. SHELXT—Integrated Space-Group and Crystal-Structure Determination. *Acta Cryst. A* **2015**, *71*, 3–8. [CrossRef]
28. Sheldrick, G.M. Crystal Structure Refinement with SHELXL. *Acta Cryst. C Struct. Chem.* **2015**, *71*, 3–8. [CrossRef] [PubMed]
29. Dolomanov, O.V.; Bourhis, L.J.; Gildea, R.J.; Howard, J.A.K.; Puschmann, H. OLEX2: A Complete Structure Solution, Refinement and Analysis Program. *J. Appl. Cryst.* **2009**, *42*, 339–341. [CrossRef]
30. MacRae, C.F.; Sovago, I.; Cottrell, S.J.; Galek, P.T.A.; McCabe, P.; Pidcock, E.; Platings, M.; Shields, G.P.; Stevens, J.S.; Towler, M.; et al. Mercury 4.0: From Visualization to Analysis, Design and Prediction. *J. Appl. Cryst.* **2020**, *53*, 226–235. [CrossRef] [PubMed]
31. Spek, A.L. Structure Validation in Chemical Crystallography. *Acta Cryst. D Biol. Cryst.* **2009**, *65*, 148–155. [CrossRef] [PubMed]
32. Glomme, A.; März, J.; Dressman, J.B. Comparison of a Miniaturized Shake-Flask Solubility Method with Automated Potentiometric Acid/Base Titrations and Calculated Solubilities. *J. Pharm. Sci.* **2005**, *94*, 1–16. [CrossRef] [PubMed]
33. Braga, D.; Maini, L.; Grepioni, F. Mechanochemical Preparation of Co-Crystals. *Chem. Soc. Rev.* **2013**, *42*, 7638–7648. [CrossRef] [PubMed]
34. Jia, L.; Wu, S.; Gong, J. A Tolbutamide Metformin Salt Based on Antidiabetic Drug Combinations: Synthesis, Crystal Structure Analysis and Pharmaceutical Properties. *Acta Cryst. C Struct. Chem* **2019**, *75*, 1250–1258. [CrossRef] [PubMed]
35. Bian, X.; Jiang, L.; Gan, Z.; Guan, X.; Zhang, L.; Cai, L.; Hu, X. A Glimepiride-Metformin Multidrug Crystal: Synthesis, Crystal Structure Analysis, and Physicochemical Properties. *Molecules* **2019**, *24*, 3786. [CrossRef] [PubMed]
36. Bian, X.; Jiang, L.; Zhou, J.; Guan, X.; Wang, J.; Xiang, P.; Pan, J.; Hu, X. Improving Dissolution and Cytotoxicity by Forming Multidrug Crystals. *Molecules* **2020**, *25*, 1343. [CrossRef] [PubMed]
37. Putra, O.D.; Furuishi, T.; Yonemochi, E.; Terada, K.; Uekusa, H. Drug-Drug Multicomponent Crystals as an Effective Technique to Overcome Weaknesses in Parent Drugs. *Cryst. Growth Des.* **2016**, *16*, 3577–3581. [CrossRef]
38. Sun, J.; Jia, L.; Wang, M.; Liu, Y.; Li, M.; Han, D.; Gong, J. Novel Drug-Drug Multicomponent Crystals of Epalrestat-Metformin: Improved Solubility and Photostability of Epalrestat and Reduced Hygroscopicity of Metformin. *Cryst. Growth Des.* **2022**, *22*, 1005–1016. [CrossRef]
39. Feng, W.Q.; Wang, L.Y.; Gao, J.; Zhao, M.Y.; Li, Y.T.; Wu, Z.Y.; Yan, C.W. Solid State and Solubility Study of a Potential Anticancer Drug-Drug Molecular Salt of Diclofenac and Metformin. *J. Mol. Struct.* **2021**, *1234*, 130166. [CrossRef]
40. Pérez-Fernández, R.; Fresno, N.; Goya, P.; Elguero, J.; Menéndez-Taboada, L.; García-Granda, S.; Marco, C. Structure and Thermodynamical Properties of Metformin Salicylate. *Cryst. Growth Des.* **2013**, *13*, 1780–1785. [CrossRef]
41. Zhou, W.-X.; Zhao, H.-W.; Chen, H.-H.; Zhang, Z.-Y.; Chen, D.-Y. Characterization of Drug–Drug Salt Forms of Metformin and Aspirin with Improved Physicochemical Properties. *CrystEngComm* **2019**, *21*, 3770–3773. [CrossRef]

42. Johnson, S.L.; Rumon, K.A. Infrared Spectra of Solid 1:1 Pyridine-Benzoic Acid Complexes; the Nature of the Hydrogen Bond as a Function of the Acid-Base Levels in the Complex. *J. Phys. Chem.* **1965**, *69*, 74–86. [CrossRef]

43. Tong, W.Q.; Whitesell, G. In Situ Salt Screening-A Useful Technique for Discovery Support and Preformulation Studies. *Pharm. Dev. Technol.* **1998**, *3*, 215–223. [CrossRef] [PubMed]

44. Cruz-Cabeza, A.J. Acid-Base Crystalline Complexes and the PKa Rule. *CrystEngComm* **2012**, *14*, 6362–6365. [CrossRef]

45. Verdugo-Escamilla, C.; Alarcón-Payer, C.; Acebedo-Martínez, F.J.; Domínguez-Martín, A.; Choquesillo-Lazarte, D. New Metformin-Citric Acid Pharmaceutical Molecular Salt: Improving Metformin Physicochemical Properties. *Crystals* **2022**, *12*, 1748. [CrossRef]

46. Diniz, L.F.; Carvalho, P.S.; Gonçalves, J.E.; Diniz, R.; Fernandes, C. Solid-State Landscape and Biopharmaceutical Implications of Novel Metformin-Based Salts. *New J. Chem.* **2022**, *46*, 13725–13737. [CrossRef]

47. Jones, O.A.H.; Voulvoulis, N.; Lester, J.N. Aquatic Environmental Assessment of the Top 25 English Prescription Pharmaceuticals. *Water Res.* **2002**, *36*, 5013–5022. [CrossRef] [PubMed]

48. Avdeef, A. Solubility of Sparingly-Soluble Ionizable Drugs. *Adv. Drug Deliv. Rev.* **2007**, *59*, 568–590. [CrossRef] [PubMed]

49. Pentikäinen, P.J.; Tokola, O.; Alhava, E.; Penttilä, A. Pharmacokinetics of Tolfenamic Acid: Disposition in Bile, Blood and Urine after Intravenous Administration to Man. *Eur. J. Clin. Pharmacol.* **1984**, *27*, 349–354. [CrossRef] [PubMed]

50. Wishart, D.S.; Feunang, Y.D.; Guo, A.C.; Lo, E.J.; Marcu, A.; Grant, J.R.; Sajed, T.; Johnson, D.; Li, C.; Sayeeda, Z.; et al. DrugBank 5.0: A Major Update to the DrugBank Database for 2018. *Nucleic Acids Res.* **2018**, *46*, D1074–D1082. [CrossRef] [PubMed]

51. Somasundaram, S.; Rafi, S.; Hayllar, J.; Sigthorsson, G.; Jacob, M.; Price, A.B.; Macpherson, A.; Mahmod, T.; Scott, D.; Wrigglesworth, J.M.; et al. Mitochondrial Damage: A Possible Mechanism of the "topical" Phase of NSAID Induced Injury to the Rat Intestine. *Gut* **1997**, *41*, 344–353. [CrossRef] [PubMed]

52. ChemAxon MarvinSketch 2020. Available online: https://chemaxon.com/marvin (accessed on 29 December 2022).

53. Childs, S.L.; Stahly, G.P.; Park, A. The Salt-Cocrystal Continuum: The Influence of Crystal Structure on Ionization State. *Mol. Pharm.* **2007**, *4*, 323–338. [CrossRef]

54. Etter, M.C.; MacDonald, J.C.; Bernstein, J. Graph-Set Analysis of Hydrogen-Bond Patterns in Organic Crystals. *Acta Cryst. B* **1990**, *46*, 256–262. [CrossRef]

55. Etter, M.C. Encoding and Decoding Hydrogen-Bond Patterns of Organic Compounds. *Acc. Chem. Res.* **1990**, *23*, 120–126. [CrossRef]

56. Kálmán, A.; Párkányi, L.; Argay, G. Classification of the Isostructurality of Organic Molecules in the Crystalline State. *Acta Cryst. Sect. B* **1993**, *49*, 1039–1049. [CrossRef]

57. Oliveira, M.A.; Peterson, M.L.; Klein, D. Continuously Substituted Solid Solutions of Organic Co-Crystals. *Cryst. Growth Des.* **2008**, *8*, 4487–4493. [CrossRef]

58. Perlovich, G. Melting Points of One- and Two-Component Molecular Crystals as Effective Characteristics for Rational Design of Pharmaceutical Systems. *Acta Cryst. B Struct. Sci. Cryst. Eng. Mater.* **2020**, *76*, 696–706. [CrossRef]

59. Sathisaran, I.; Dalvi, S.V. Engineering Cocrystals of Poorlywater-Soluble Drugs to Enhance Dissolution in Aqueous Medium. *Pharmaceutics* **2018**, *10*, 108. [CrossRef]

60. Varshosaz, J.; Ghassami, E.; Ahmadipour, S. Crystal Engineering for Enhanced Solubility and Bioavailability of Poorly Soluble Drugs. *Curr. Pharm. Des.* **2018**, *24*, 2473–2496. [CrossRef] [PubMed]

61. Patel, J.N.; Rathod, D.M.; Patel, N.A.; Modasiya, M.K. Techniques to Improve the Solubility of Poorly Soluble Drugs. *Int. J. Pharm. Life Sci.* **2012**, *3*, 1459–1469.

62. Cheng, C.L.; Yu, L.X.; Lee, H.L.; Yang, C.Y.; Lue, C.S.; Chou, C.H. Biowaiver Extension Potential to BCS Class III High Solubility-Low Permeability Drugs: Bridging Evidence for Metformin Immediate-Release Tablet. *Eur. J. Pharm. Sci.* **2004**, *22*, 297–304. [CrossRef] [PubMed]

63. Kim, D.W.; Park, J.B. Development and Pharmaceutical Approach for Sustained-Released Metformin Succinate Tablets. *J. Drug Deliv. Sci. Technol.* **2015**, *30*, 90–99. [CrossRef]

64. Gould, P.L. Salt Selection for Basic Drugs. *Int. J. Pharm.* **1986**, *33*, 201–217. [CrossRef]

65. Putra, O.D.; Umeda, D.; Fujita, E.; Haraguchi, T.; Uchida, T.; Yonemochi, E.; Uekusa, H. Solubility Improvement of Benexate through Salt Formation Using Artificial Sweetener. *Pharmaceutics* **2018**, *10*, 64. [CrossRef]

66. Kim, S.; Chen, J.; Cheng, T.; Gindulyte, A.; He, J.; He, S.; Li, Q.; Shoemaker, B.A.; Thiessen, P.A.; Yu, B.; et al. PubChem in 2021: New Data Content and Improved Web Interfaces. *Nucleic Acids Res.* **2021**, *49*, D1388–D1395. [CrossRef]

67. Oh, D.H.; Park, Y.J.; Kang, J.H.; Yong, C.S.; Choi, H.G. Physicochemical Characterization and in Vivo Evaluation of Flurbiprofen-Loaded Solid Dispersion without Crystalline Change. *Drug Deliv.* **2011**, *18*, 46–53. [CrossRef]

68. Avdeef, A.; Bendels, S.; Tsinman, O.; Tsinman, K.; Kansy, M. Solubility-Excipient Classification Gradient Maps. *Pharm. Res.* **2007**, *24*, 530–545. [CrossRef]

69. Gao, L.; Zheng, W.Y.; Yang, W.L.; Zhang, X.R. Drug-Drug Salt Forms of Vortioxetine with Mefenamic Acid and Tolfenamic Acid. *J. Mol. Struct.* **2022**, *1268*, 133725. [CrossRef]

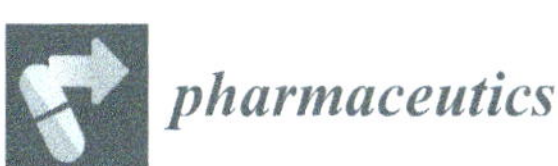 *pharmaceutics*

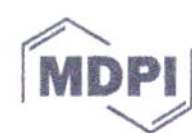

Article

The Formulation of Curcumin: 2-Hydroxypropyl-β-cyclodextrin Complex with Smart Hydrogel for Prolonged Release of Curcumin

Ljubiša Nikolić [1,*], Maja Urošević [1], Vesna Nikolić [1], Ivana Gajić [1], Ana Dinić [1], Vojkan Miljković [1], Srđan Rakić [2], Sanja Đokić [3], Jelena Kesić [3], Snežana Ilić-Stojanović [1] and Goran Nikolić [1]

[1] Faculty of Technology, University of Niš, Bulevar Oslobodjenja 124, 16000 Leskovac, Serbia
[2] Department of Physics, Faculty of Sciences, University of Novi Sad, Trg Dositeja Obradovica 4, 21000 Novi Sad, Serbia
[3] Department of Chemistry, Biochemistry and Environmental Protection, Faculty of Sciences, University of Novi Sad, Trg Dositeja Obradovića 3, 21000 Novi Sad, Serbia
* Correspondence: nljubisa@tf.ni.ac.rs

Abstract: Curcumin comes from the plant species *Curcuma longa* and shows numerous pharmacological activities. There are numerous curcumin formulations with gels or cyclodextrins in order to increase its solubility and bioavailability. This paper presents the formulation of complex of curcumin with 2-hydroxypropyl-β-cyclodextrin in a thermosensitive hydrogel, based on N-isopropylmethacrylamide and N-isopropylacrylamide with ethylene glycol dimethacrylate as a crosslinker. The product was characterized by chemical methods and also by FTIR, HPLC, DSC, SEM, XRD. The results show that synthesis was successfully done. With an increase in the quantity of crosslinker in the hydrogels, the starting release and the release rate of curcumin from the formulation of the complex with hydrogels decreases. The release rate of curcumin from the gel complex formulation is constant over time. It is possible to design a formulation that will release curcumin for more than 60 days. In order to determine the mechanism and kinetics of curcumin release, various mathematical models were applied by using the DDSolver package for Microsoft Excel application. The Korsmeyer-Peppas model best describes the release of curcumin from the gel formulation of the complex, while the values for the diffusion exponent (0.063–0.074) shows that mechanism of the release rate is based on diffusion.

Keywords: curcumin; 2-hydroxypropyl-β-cyclodextrin; complex; N-isopropylmethacrylamide; N-isopropylacrylamide; smart hydrogel

1. Introduction

Curcumin ((1E,6E)-1,7-bis(4-hydroksy-3-methoxyphenyl)-1,6-heptadiene-3,5-dione), Figure 1, is a natural polyphenol isolated from the rhizome of the plant species *Curcuma longa* which shows numerous pharmacological activities by the modulation of physiological and biochemical processes. Research shows that curcumin possesses hypoglycemic [1], antimicrobial [2], hepatoprotective [3], anti-inflammatory [4], antioxidant [5], anticancer [6], antiviral [7] and many other effects. Various animal studies and clinical trials have shown that curcumin is safe to apply at high doses because it does not affect liver and kidney function. However, due to poor water solubility and low bioavailability, it is classified as a drug of group IV by the biopharmaceutical classification system, and its therapeutic application is limited [8–11]. In order to improve the physicochemical properties, different systems for curcumin delivery were used: cyclodextrins for the formation of inclusion complexes [12–15], micelles [16], liposomes [17,18], nanoemulsions [19], hydrogels [20], polymers formed by cross-linking of cyclodextrin [21–23], polymer nanofibers [24–26], complexes with cyclodextrin incorporated into polymers [27–29] and

Citation: Nikolić, L.; Urošević, M.; Nikolić, V.; Gajić, I.; Dinić, A.; Miljković, V.; Rakić, S.; Đokić, S.; Kesić, J.; Ilić-Stojanović, S.; et al. The Formulation of Curcumin: 2-Hydroxypropyl-β-cyclodextrin Complex with Smart Hydrogel for Prolonged Release of Curcumin. *Pharmaceutics* **2023**, *15*, 382. https://doi.org/10.3390/pharmaceutics15020382

Academic Editor: Hisham Al-Obaidi

Received: 15 December 2022
Revised: 16 January 2023
Accepted: 18 January 2023
Published: 22 January 2023

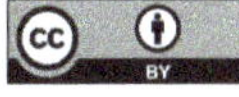

other nanoparticles [2,30]. In the study of Purpura et al., the bioavailability of formulation of curcumin with β-cyclodextrin was examined. The results of the study show that the formulation of β-cyclodextrin with curcumin significantly improves the absorption of curcumin in healthy people [31]. In the experiment of Jafer et al., with the aim of improving the delivery of curcumin in the treatment of cancer cells, an inclusion complex of β-cyclodextrin with curcumin was prepared. The obtained results show that the complex of β-cyclodextrin with curcumin improved the delivery and antiproliferative effect to the MCF-7 breast cancer cells [14]. The inclusion complex of curcumin with β-cyclodextrin obtained by coprecipitation method increased the water solubility of curcumin from 0.00122 to 0.721 mg/cm^3. The release of the inclusion complex from nanocomposite and conventional poly(N-isopropylacrylamide/sodium alginate) hydrogels crosslinked with N,N$'$methylenebis(acrylamide) (BIS), respectively, was tested under simulated gastrointestinal conditions. At pH = 1.2, hydrogels showed the lowest release and swelling ratio, but at pH = 6.8 the highest release to swelling ratios of curcumin were achieved [28]. A thermosensitive hydrogel was synthesized, poly(D,L-lactide-co-glycolide)-poly(ethyleneglycol)-poly(D,L-lactide-co-glycolide), as a carrier for the delivery of doxorubicin in combination with an inclusion complex of curcumin with β-cyclodextrin for the treatment of cancer cells. Combined therapy based on doxorubicin and inclusion complex of curcumin with β-cyclodextrin showed greater antitumor activity than monotherapy in vitro [29]. Zhang et al., synthesized in situ forming hydrogels based on polyvinyl pyrrolidone, encapsulated with a solid dispersion of curcumin for the healing of vaginal wounds and the treatment of vaginal bacterial infections. After local application for treatment of the vaginal infection caused by *Escherichia coli* and *Staphylococcus aureus*, high efficiency in therapeutic treatment has been confirmed, along with inflammation reduction and improved healing of vaginal wounds [32]. Shefa et al. have synthesized a biocompatible and biodegradable hydrogel system for the delivery of curcumin based on polyvinyl alcohol and oxidized cellulose nanofibers, in order to improve the wound healing process [33]. Thermosensitive β-glycerophosphate/chitosan hydrogels, with an encapsulated complex of curcumin:β-cyclodextrin for the treatment of skin wound infections, were synthesized in work of Zao et al. The ability of wound healing using the above mentioned hydrogel was tested on induced superficial wounds in rats. By analyzing the results, it was observed that the wounds treated with hydrogel containing the complex of curcumin:β-cyclodextrin showed a faster healing rate compared to wounds that were covered only with gauze [34]. A drug delivery system based on poly(N-isopropylacrylamide), p(NiPAm), hydrogel and a suitable solvent for improvement of solubility and local release of curcumin was also synthesized in the experimental work of Ayar et al. Curcumin was incorporated in p(NiPAm) hydrogel during swelling by using methanol or polyethylene glycol of low molecular weight (PEG200). The obtained results show that PEG200 increases curcumin solubility more than methanol, and shows a superior effect on the cumulative quantitative of curcumin released over 7 days (33.163 $\pm$ 0.319 mg/cm^3) compared to methanol (8.765 $\pm$ 0.544 mg/cm^3). P(NiPAm) hydrogel combined with PEG200 did not show any cytotoxicity, and can be used as an effective sustained release system for curcumin [35].

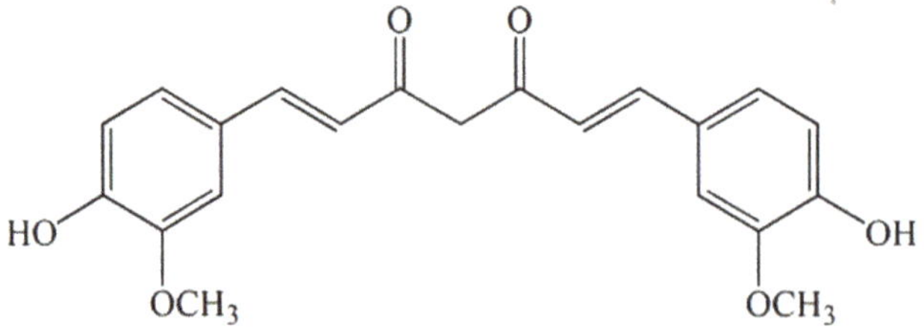

Figure 1. Chemical structure of curcumin.

In recent years, highly advanced curcumin delivery systems have been developed such as nanoparticles, ultrasound microbubbles, exosomes, biopolymer nanoparticles [36], nanogels, nanosuspensions, nanoemulsions and dendrimer [37]. The goal for creating such formulations was to improve the stability and solubility of curcumin.

The polymer hydrogels based on N- isopropylmethacrylamide (NiPMAm) and/or N-isopropylacrylamide (NiPAm) are well known because of their good property to respond to temperature changes by changing the degree of swelling [38,39]. To create a three-dimensional network of these gels, ethylene glycol dimethacrylate (EGDM) is often used as a networker. If in their structure they contain a copolymerized organic acid (acrylic acid, methacrylic acid, etc.), the degree of swelling of these gels will also change with the change in the pH value of the environment [40]. That is why these gels are called smart hydrogels, because they react by changing the degree of swelling with the change of the conditional parameters in which they are found. Namely, if the temperature of these swollen hydrogels is increased, their degree of swelling decreases and they squeeze out liquid and vice versa, but if their pH value is lowered the degree of swelling increases and vice versa. These kinds of gels have been used as matrix systems for medicinal substances [41]. In Figure 2, chemical structures of N-isopropylmethacrylamide, N- isopropylacrylamide and ethylene glycol dimethacrylate are shown.

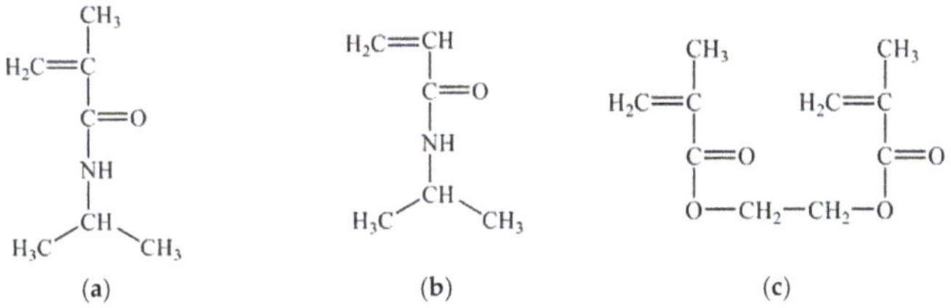

Figure 2. Chemical structure: (**a**) N-isopropylmethacrylamide, (**b**) N-isopropylacrylamide and (**c**) ethylene glycol dimethacrylate.

The topic of this paper is the development of a new matrix system based on a smart polymer carrier crosslinked with poly(N-isopropylmethacrylamide-co-N-isopropylacrylamide), with an incorporated inclusion complex of curcumin: 2-hydroxypropyl-β-cyclodextrin, with the aim of increasing the solubility of curcumin. With this system, targeted delivery and sustained release of curcumin can be performed. In Figure 3, part of a cyclic structure of a seven-membered ring molecule of 2-hydroxypropyl-β-cyclodextrin is shown.

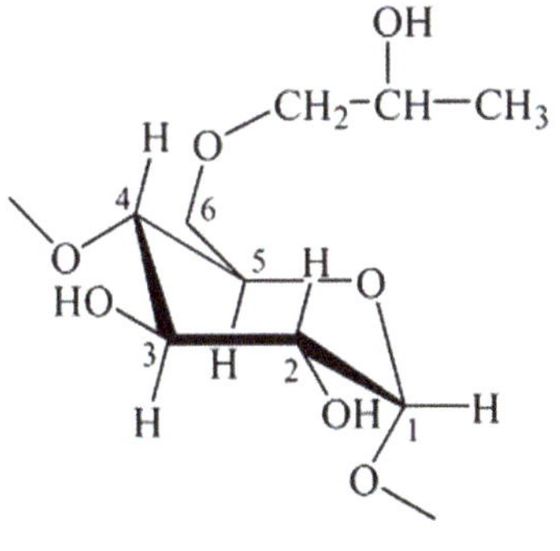

Figure 3. Chemical structure of a seven-membered ring molecule part of 2-hydroxypropyl-β-cyclodextrin.

2. Materials and Methods

2.1. Reagents

N-isopropylmethacrylamide (NiPMAm) 97%, N-isopropylacrylamide (NiPAm) 99%, 2,2′-azobis(2-methylpropionitrile) (AIBN) 98% (Acros Organics, New Jersey, NJ, USA); ethylene glycol dimethacrylate (EGDM) 97% (Fluka Chemical Corp, Buchs, Switzerland);

curcumin (CU) 97%, 2-hydroxypropyl-β-cyclodextrin (2-HP-β-CD) 97% (Tokyo Chemical Industry Co., Ltd., Tokyo, Japan); Tween 20 (Alfa Aesar, ThermoFisher, Kandel, Germany), potassium bromide (KBr) 99%, ethanol (Et) 99.5%, methanol for HPLC (Me) ≥99.9% (Merck KGaA, Darmstadt, Germany); Hanks' buffered solution pH 7.4 GmbH (PAA Laboratories, Pasching, Austria). All reagents were used with no further purification.

2.2. Synthesis of Hydrogels

Hydrogels samples were synthesized according to the procedure described previously [39]. In short, hydrogels poly(N-isopropylmethacrylamide-*co*-N-isopropylacrylamide), p(NiPMAm/NiPAm), in the molar ratio 10/90 were synthesized by radical polymerization of monomers NiPMAm and NiPAm, with EGDM as a crosslinker in 2 and 3 mol% relative to the total amount of monomer. Obtained gels were marked 10/90/2 and 10/90/3, respectively. Ethanol was used as a solvent and 30 mg of AIBN for initiation of the polymerization reaction. After dissolving the reactants, the homogenized reaction mixtures were injected into glass ampoules which were then heat sealed. The polymerization reaction was performed in the mode: 0.5 h at 70 °C, 2 h at 80 °C and 0.5 h at 85 °C. After polymerization and cooling of the samples at room temperature, copolymerized p(NiPMAm/NiPAm) hydrogels were obtained in the form of long cylinders and cut into discs of thickness 5 mm. Hydrogels prepared in this way were extracted with methanol during 168 h in order to remove unreacted reactants, then washed off with water for 24 h to remove methanol and after that, dried at 40 °C to constant weight.

2.3. Lyophilization of Gels

Lyophilization p(NiPMAm/NiPAm) of hydrogels swollen up to the equilibrium was performed on the apparatus LH Leybold Heraeus, Lyovac GT2 (Labexchange, Frekendorf, Switzerland). The synthesized hydrogels are firstly frozen at a temperature of −40 °C during 24 h. In first subphase of drying, the volume of solution was reduced by sublimation at −30 °C and pressure of 5 Pa during 12 h. In the second subphase of drying, i.e., isothermal desorption, the hydrogels were heated up to 20 °C during 6 h at the pressure of 5 Pa, with removal of steam. Lyophilized samples of hydrogels were packed under vacuum condition and stored in a refrigerator at 5 °C.

2.4. Obtaining of the Complex

Curcumin (368.38 mg) was dissolved in 200 cm^3 of absolute ethanol and added to the solution of 2-hydroxypropyl-β-cyclodextrin obtained by dissolution of 1541.54 mg 2-hydroxypropyl-β-cyclodextrin in 100 cm^3 of distilled water. The mixture obtained like this was equilibrated by mixing on a magnetic stirrer at room temperature during 96 h, protected from light. The resulting solution was concentrated on a vacuum evaporator at 40 °C to the minimum volume, and then dried in a desiccator over a dehydrating agent at room temperature to constant mass. The molar ratio of curcumin and 2-hydroxypropyl-β-cyclodextrin in inclusion complex was 1:1.

2.5. Phase Solubility

Phase solubility study was performed according to method described by Higuchi & Connors [42]. Surplus of curcumin (each 10 mg) was added in 2.5 cm^3 water solution of 2-hydroxypropyl-β-cyclodextrin of concentration 0–10 mmol/dm^3. The samples were stirred at room temperature during 24 h, and then filtered through a membrane filter with a pore diameter 0.45 μm (Econofilters, Agilent Technologies, Waldborn, Germany). The quantity of dissolved curcumin was determined by application of UV/V method on the basis of constructed calibration curves of absorbance dependence on concentration. Measurements were performed by spectrophotometer Cary-100 Conc (Varian PTY LTD, Springvale, Australia) at wavelength 429 nm, in quartz cuvettes ($1 \times 1 \times 4.5$ cm) at room temperature. Distilled water was used as a blank solution. The presence of 2-hydroxypropyl-β-cyclodextrin does not affect the absorbance of curcumin at 429 nm, because its absorption at that wavelength is equal to 0. The constant of stability ($K_{1:1}$) of inclusion complex was calculated based on the phase solubility diagram according to Equation (1):

$$K_{1:1} = \frac{slope}{S_0(1 - slope)}, \tag{1}$$

where S_0 is solubility of curcumin at 25 °C in the absence of cyclodextrin (intercept) and slope represents the value from the phase solubility graph.

2.6. Incorporation of Complex of Curcumin: 2-Hydroxypropyl-β-cyclodextrin into p(NiPMAm/NiPAm) Gels

Matrix systems with a curcumin: 2-hydroxypropyl-β-cyclodextrin complex and p(NiPMAm/NiPAm) hydrogels were obtained by swelling the hydrogels to equilibrium in ethanol in which the inclusion complex of curcumin: 2-hydroxypropyl-β-cyclodextrin in concentration of 1.23 mg/cm^3 was dissolved, at a temperature of 25 °C. Weighed samples of xerogels p(NiPMAm/NiPAm), 50 mg, were covered with a solution of curcumin inclusion complex (5 cm^3) and left to swell at room temperature, protected from light. After reaching equilibrium, swollen p(NiPMAm/NiPAm) the hydrogels were separated from the remaining solution by decantation, washed with distilled water in order to remove the unincorporated amount of the inclusion complex of curcumin: 2-hydroxypropyl-β-cyclodextrin, and after that extra water was removed from the surface of the matrix gels. The quantity of incorporated curcumin in p(NiPMAm/NiPAm) was determined based on the difference in the quantities of curcumin in the initial solution of the inclusion complex curcumin: 2-hydroxypropyl-β-cyclodextrin, and the supernatant after equilibrium was reached by using the HPLC method. The efficiency of incorporation of curcumin in hydrogel, η, was calculated according to Equation (2):

$$\eta(\%) = \frac{L_g}{L_u} \cdot 100, \tag{2}$$

where L_g is mass of curcumin incorporated in p(NiPMAm/NiPAm) hydrogel, mg/g$_{xerogel}$, and L_u initial mass of curcumin entered by the solution of the curcumin: 2-hydroxypropyl-β-cyclodextrin inclusion complex for swelling and incorporating into xerogel, mg/g$_{xerogel}$.

The schematic view of obtaining the formulation of curcumin: 2-hydroxypropyl-β-cyclodextrin complex with p(NiPMAm/NiPAm) hydrogel is shown in Figure 4.

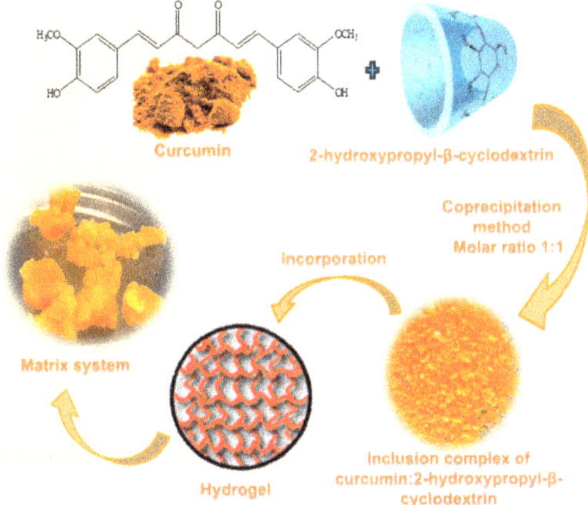

Figure 4. The schematic view of obtaining the formulation of curcumin: 2-hydroxypropyl-β-cyclodextrin complex with p(NiPMAm/NiPAm) hydrogel.

2.7. The Release of Curcumin from Matrix System

In vitro study of the release of curcumin from swollen p(NiPMAm/NiPAm) hydrogels with incorporated inclusion complex of curcumin: 2-hydroxypropyl-β-cyclodextrin was carried out in a medium that simulates physiological conditions. Each sample was covered with 10 cm^3 of solution (9 cm^3 Hank's BSS buffer with pH value 7.4 and 1 cm^3 of Tween 20 solution concentration of 1.52 mg/cm^3). The samples were thermostated in a water bath at 37 °C with stirring on a magnetic stirrer (Hanna Instruments, Magnetic stirrer HI 190M) during 48 h. The amount of curcumin released was monitored by sampling 200 μL of solution over time, which were then filled up with methanol up to 1 cm^3, filtered on a cellulose membrane filter with a pore diameter 0.45 μm and analyzed by HPLC method. The kinetics of the curcumin release from the matrix system was evaluated by different mathematical models (Higuchi, Korsmeyer–Peppas, Baker–Lonsdale) with DDSolver package for Microsoft Excel applications.

2.8. Determination of the Concentration of Some Compounds by Using High Pressure Liquid Chromatography (HPLC)

The content of residual reactant (monomers and crosslinkers) in samples of synthesized p(NiPMAm/NiPAm) hydrogels was calculated by HPLC method. The analysis was performed by using the apparatus HPLC Agilent 1100 Series (Waldborn, D) equipped with diode-array detector, DAD 1200 Series. Conditions for chromatography performance: column Zorbax Eclipse XDB-C18 (4.6 × 250 mm, 5 μm) (Agilent Technologies, Inc., Santa Clara, CA, USA); temperature 25 °C; injected volume of samples 10 μL; detection wavelength 210 nm; mobile phase consists of methanol/redistilled water 70/30, v/v; mobile phase flow was 0.5 cm^3/min. The results obtained were processed by software Agilent Chemstation. On the basis of constructed calibration curves for the linear dependence, the equations were obtained for determining the content of NiPMAm, NiPAm and EGDM in methanol extracts obtained by the processing of synthesized p(NiPMAm/NiPAm) hydrogels.

The dependence of the peak area on the concentration of NiPMAm is linear in range of 0.005–0.250 mg/cm^3. For the straight part of the calibration curve of NiPMAm the Equation (3) applies with a linear correlation coefficient R^2 = 0.995.

$$c = \frac{A - 572.14}{97110.1}, \tag{3}$$

Dependence of peak area on concentration of NiPAm is linear in range of 0.005–0.250 mg/cm^3 and in the straight part of the calibration curve the Equation (4) applies, R^2 = 0.997.

$$c = \frac{A - 594.72}{137938.4}, \tag{4}$$

Dependence of peak area on concentration of EGDM is linear in range 0.005–0.250 mg/cm^3. For the straight part of the calibration curve of EGDM the Equation (5) applies, R^2 = 0.998.

$$c = \frac{A - 911.18}{171,931}, \tag{5}$$

In Equations (2)–(4), A is pick area (mAU·s), and c is concentration of reactants (mg/cm^3) NiPMAm, NiPAm either EGDM.

Determination of the quantity of curcumin that was not incorporated into the hydrogels, as well as monitoring of curcumin release from the hydrogels, was performed by using liquid chromatography HPLC method at these conditions: column Zorbax Eclipse XDB-CN 250 × 4.6 mm, 5 μm (Agilent Technologies, Inc., Santa Clara, CA, USA); eluent was methanol: mobile phase flow was 1 cm^3/min; volume of injected samples 20 μL; column temperature 40 °C; detection wavelength 425 nm. For the straight line part of the curcumin calibration curve in range 0.53–106 µg/cm^3, Equation (6) applies with a linear correlation coefficient R^2 = 0.999.

$$c = \frac{A + 158.26}{184.15},$$

(6)

where A is pickk area (mAU·s), and c is concentration of curcumin (µg/cm^3).

2.9. Swelling of Hydrogels

Swelling of synthesized p(NiPMAm/NiPAm) xerogels was monitored gravimetrically. A known quantity of p(NiPMAm/NiPAm) xerogels was immersed in a water solution of a certain pH value and temperature, and then the mass of the sample was measured at certain time intervals until equilibrium was reached, i.e., until constant mass of hydrogels was reached. Aqueous mediums for swelling were prepared by adjusting the pH value by addition of 0.1 M solution of sodium hydroxide (Centrohem, Beograd, Serbia) or 0.1 M solution of hydrochloric acid (Zorka, Šabac, Serbia) while observing the value on pH meter (HI9318-HI9219, Hanna, P). The thermosensitivity of hydrogels was tested in the temperature range of 25 to 80 °C in a water bath. The degree of swelling, α, was calculated according to Equation (7).

$$\alpha = \frac{m - m_0}{m_0},$$

(7)

where m_0—is mass of dry gel, m—mass of swollen gel in a point of time t.

To analyze the type of solvent diffusion process inside hydrogels, Equation (8) applies, which stands for condition ($Mt/Me \leq 0.6$) [43,44]:

$$F = \frac{M_t}{M_e} = k \cdot t^n,$$

(8)

where F—is the fractional sorption, M_t—mass of the absorbed solvent in a point of time, M_e—mass of the absorbed solvent in equilibrium, k—a constant that is characteristic for a certain type of polymer network (min$^{1/n}$) and n—diffusion exponent. By logarithmizing Equation (8) comes a linear Equation (9) that can be applied to calculate the constant k and an exponent n.

$$\ln \frac{M_t}{M_e} = \ln k + n \cdot \ln t,$$

(9)

The value of diffusion exponent n determines the mechanism of fluid diffusion. For value $n = 0.5$ the fluid diffusion mechanism corresponds to Fick's law of diffusion (case I), where the rate of solvent transport into the gel is lower than the rate of relaxation of polymer chains. When the value for diffusion exponent is lower than 0.5, the penetration of solvent is much slower than the polymer chains relaxation. The solvent transportation mechanism is a part of Fick's diffusion and is called "less to Fick's" diffusion. Anomalous diffusion mechanism (non-Fick's diffusion) occurs with $0.5 < n < 1$, and then the hydrogels swelling is under control by both solvent diffusion in matrix and polymer chains relaxation. The diffusion process is a lot faster when the diffusion exponent has value 1 in comparison to the polymer system chains relaxation (case II), while when $n > 1$ the polymer chains relaxation is under control of gels swelling (case III, Super case II). The diffusion coefficient of solvent molecules in hydrogel (D) is most often determined by applying the Equation (10) which takes into account only the initial stage of swelling (60% of swelling) during which the thickness of the polymer remains approximately constant [45,46]:

$$\frac{M_t}{M_e} = 4 \cdot \left(\frac{Dt}{\pi l^2} \right)^{1/2},$$

(10)

where D stands for diffusion coefficient (cm^2/min), and l for the thickness of the dry hydrogel, xerogel (cm). By logarithmization of Equation (10), linear dependence comes between $\ln(M_t/M_e)$ and $\ln t$ (Equation (11)) from the section of which the diffusion coefficient D is calculated,

$$\ln \frac{M_t}{M_e} = \left(\frac{4D^{1/2}}{\pi^{1/2}l} \right) + \frac{1}{2} \ln t, \tag{11}$$

2.10. Fourier Transform Infrared Spectroscopy (FTIR)

The FTIR spectra of monomers, synthesized p(NiPMAm/NiPAm) xerogels, curcumin, 2-hydroxypropyl-β-cyclodextrin, inclusion complex of curcumin: 2-hydroxypropyl-β-cyclodextrin, xerogels with incorporated complex of curcumin: 2-hydroxypropyl-β-cyclodextrin, were recorded by the thin transparent tablets technique with potassium bromide of spectroscopic purity, by vacuuming and pressing under a pressure of approximately 200 MPa. The preparation of tablets was measured by 150 mg of potassium bromide and 0.7 mg each sample which were pulverized on an amalgamator (WIG-L-Bug, Dentsply RINN, a Division of Dentsply International Inc., York, PA, USA). Crosslinker EGDM was recorded in the form of a thin film between two plates of zinc selenide (ZnSe). The recording was performed on FTIR spectrophotometer BOMEM MB-100 (Hartmann & Braun, Baptiste, Quebec, QC, Canada) in the wavenumber range of 4000 to 400 cm^{-1}. Spectra were processed by application Win-Bomem Easy software.

2.11. Scanning Electron Microscopy (SEM)

The morphology of curcumin, complex of curcumin: 2-hydroxypropyl-β-cyclodextrin, lyophilized p(NiPMAm/NiPAm) hydrogels and p(NiPMAm/NiPAm) hydrogels with incorporated complex of curcumin: 2-hydroxypropyl-β-cyclodextrin was examined by scanning electron microscopy. Before analysis, the pulverized sample was coated with gold/palladium alloy (15/85) by using a sprayer JEOL Fine Coat JFC 1100E Ion Sputter (JEOL Ltd., Tokyo, Japan) and recorded on apparatus JEOL Scaning Electron Microscope JSM-5300 (JEOL Ltd., Tokyo, Japan).

2.12. Differential Scanning Calorimetry (DSC)

For testing the thermal properties of curcumin, 2-hydroxypropyl-β-cyclodextrin, inclusion complex of curcumin: 2-hydroxypropyl-β-cyclodextrin, empty p(NiPMAm/NiPAm) hydrogels and hydrogels with incorporated complex of curcumin: 2-hydroxypropyl-β-cyclodextrin differential scanning calorimetry method was applied. The sample (about 3 mg) was placed in a vessel and heated in one cycle from room temperature up to 250 °C heating dynamics 10 °C/min in a nitrogen atmosphere. This testing was performed by using apparatus differential scanning calorimeter TA Instruments Q20 (TA Instruments, New Castle, DE, USA).

2.13. X-ray Diffraction (XRD)

XRD spectra of curcumin, 2-hydroxypropyl-β-cyclodextrin, inclusion complex of curcumin: 2-hydroxypropyl-β-cyclodextrin, empty p(NiPMAm/NiPAm) hydrogels and hydrogels with incorporated complex of curcumin: 2-hydroxypropyl-β-cyclodextrin were recorded at these conditions: samples were marked by monochrome CuKα radiation and analyzed at an angle 2θ between 5 and 75° with a sequence of 0.05° and recording time τ = 5 s. During recording, voltage and current used were 40 kV and 20 mA, respectively. All tested samples were recorded by a powder diffractometer Rigaku MiniFlex 600 (Rigaku, Tokyo, Japan).

2.14. Nuclear Magnetic Resonance (^{1}H-NMR)

^{1}H-NMR spectra of 2-hydroxypropyl-β-cyclodextrin and of curcumin: 2-hydroxypropyl-β-cyclodextrin inclusion complex were recorded on Bruker Avance III NMR, 400 MHz (BRUKER AXS GmbH, Karlsruche, Deutschland) apparatus in a glass cuvette with a diameter of 5 mm at room temperature by the pulse method, with multiple repetition of pulses.

The samples were dissolved in deuterated water (D$_2$O) and the solutions were treated in an ultrasonic bath for 25 min before recording.

3. Results

3.1. Phase Solubility

Phase solubility analysis was performed in order to determine and compare the solvation and complexation power of 2-hydroxypropyl-β-cyclodextrin to curcumin. From Figure 5 it can be seen that phase solubility diagram is of "A$_L$" type [42]. This indicates that the molar ratio between host and guest molecule in the inclusion complex is 1:1, and that the solubility of curcumin is increasing linearly with the increase of 2-hydroxypropyl-β-cyclodextrin concentration. By linear fitting, using the data from Figure 5 the following is obtained: slope = 9.953 × 10^{-4}, intercept = 8.571 × 10^{-6} mol/dm^3. By using the data from Figure 5 for slope and intercept and Equation (1), the value of the stability constant of the curcumin and 2-hydroxypropyl-β-cyclodextrin complex was calculated: K$_{1:1}$ = 116.23, and solubilization efficiency (ratio of curcumin solubility in water solution in presence of highest tested concentration of 2-hydroxypropyl-β-cyclodextrin, 10 mmol/dm^3, and solubility of pure curcumin itself in water) was 1237.18.

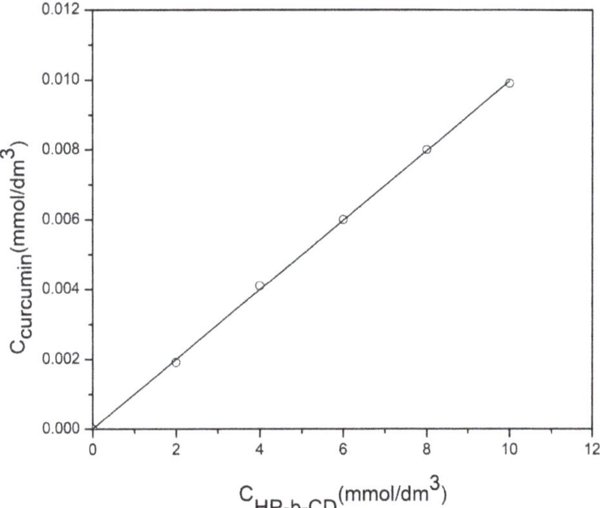

Figure 5. Phase solubility diagram of curcumin in the presence of 2-hydroxypropyl-β-cyclodextrin in water solution at 25 °C.

3.2. The Swelling

Dependence of the degree of swelling on time of p(NiPMAm/NiPAm) of lyophilized hydrogels (10/90/2 i 10/90/3) in solution with pH = 7.4 on different temperatures (25 and 37 °C) is shown in Figure 6a,b, one after the other. From these experiments, the equilibrium values of the degree of swelling for the corresponding gels and temperatures was determined. The dependence of the degree of swelling on temperature is shown in Figure 7, and it can be seen that degree of swelling decreases when temperature increases. There is a phase transition—the lower critical temperature of solution (LCST), at a temperature of approximately 37 °C for this hydrogel composition—when hydrogel transforms from hydrophilic to hydrophobic form. At temperatures above the temperature of phase transition, the breakup of hydrogen bonds with water molecules occurs, the hydrophobic interactions become dominant and the polymer network contracts [47].

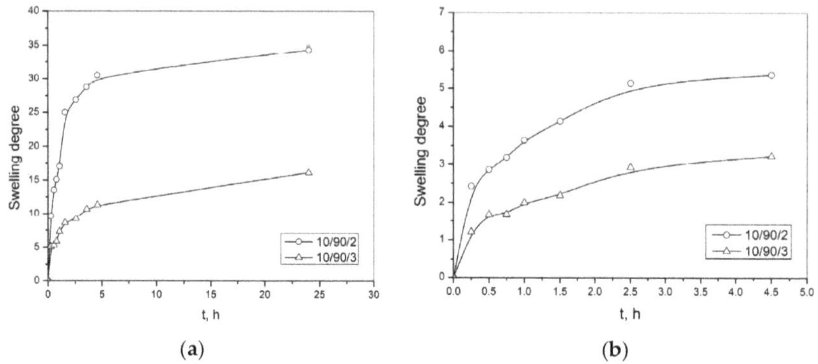

Figure 6. Dependence of the degree of swelling on time of p(NiPMAm/NiPAm) hydrogels in the solution which pH value is 7.4 at the temperature: (a) 25 °C and (b) 37 °C.

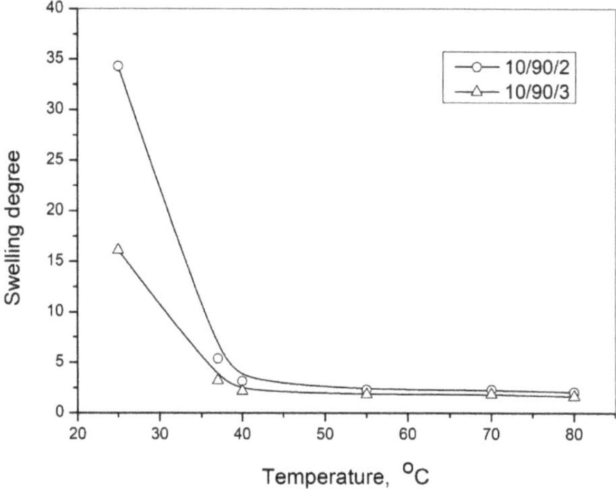

Figure 7. Dependence of the degree of swelling on temperature in the solution in which pH value is 7.4.

That is why this type of hydrogel has a higher degree of swelling at lower temperatures, and this property can be used to enter a larger amount of active substance into the hydrogel structure at lower temperatures. On the contrary, when the temperature increases, these hydrogels have a lower swelling degree. This means that they show a tendency to squeeze some of the liquid out of their structure. Therefore, the concept of this work was to conduct the experiment on the release of curcumin from the hydrogel complex formulation at a temperature of 37 °C, when equilibrium is established in the structure throughout the time of swelling.

In Table 1 the values are shown for kinetic parameters: the constants that are characteristic for certain types of polymer network, diffusion exponents and diffusion coefficients for swelling of p(NiPMAm/NiPAm) hydrogels at 25 and 37 °C with pH 7.4, obtained by the application of Equations (9) and (11).

The transport of solution into the polymeric matrix of p(NiPMAm/NiPAm) hydrogels at a temperature 25 °C and pH 7.4 presents the anomalous type of diffusion (non-Fick's diffusion), where the value of the diffusion exponent has to be in the range of $0.5 < n < 1$. For the tested samples it is in the range 0.60–0.82. At a temperature of 37 °C and pH = 7.4, the swelling process of p(NiPMAm/NiPAm) hydrogels 10/90/2 is determined by the diffusion of the aqueous solution ("less to Fick's" diffusion, $n = 0.49 \approx 0.5$), while for the hydrogel sample, 10/90/3 solvent diffusion into the matrix and the polymer chain relaxation controls the swelling because of the diffusion exponent value 0.63.

Table 1. Kinetic parameters of swelling of p(NiPMAm/NiPAm) hydrogels at pH 7.4.

Temperature, °C	Sample	n	k, min$^{1/n}$	D, cm^2/min
25	10/90/2	0.82	0.092	$1.65 \cdot 10^{-5}$
	10/90/3	0.60	0.127	$3.17 \cdot 10^{-5}$
37	10/90/2	0.49	0.231	$1.05 \cdot 10^{-4}$
	10/90/3	0.63	0.164	$5.26 \cdot 10^{-5}$

n-diffusion exponent; k-the constant characteristic for certain types of polymer network (min$^{1/n}$); D-diffusion coefficient (cm^2/min).

3.3. Residual Monomers Analysis

By using the HPLC method, the content of unreacted reactants in p(NiPMAm/NiPAm) hydrogels synthesis process was determined, using calibration curves for monomers (NiPMAm and NiPAm) and crosslinker (EGDM). At selected conditions for chromatographic analysis the retention time (R_t) for monomer NiPMAm was 6.693 min, NiPAm 6.176 min and crosslinker EGDM 12.812 min. Residual quantities of monomers in copolymer samples of p(NiPMAm/NiPAm) in relation to their initial quantity in the reaction mixture are shown in Table 2.

Table 2. The content of residual monomers in synthesized p(NiPMAm/NiPAm) hydrogels.

Sample	The Content of Residual Monomers in Sample, %		
	NiPMAm	NiPAm	EGDM
10/90/2	0.11	0.28	0.07
10/90/3	0.13	0.30	0.08

Since the toxicity of the residual monomers is limited by their content in the copolymer, and that in the synthesized samples their content is acceptable (<0.3%), synthesized p(NiPMAm/NiPAm) hydrogels can be considered as safe for use as carriers for bioactive substances.

The procedure with variable temperature used for the synthesis of these hydrogels, which was developed through research in the previous period, enables such a low content of residual monomers. This is the minimum amount of residual monomers achieved by the synthesis. Hydrogels can even get rid of these low amounts of residual monomers by extraction with methanol and then washing with water. In this way, a hydrogel without residual monomers will be obtained, which is the most favorable for the production of pharmaceutical formulations.

3.4. FTIR Spectroscopy Analysis

Structural analyses of the starting monomers NiPMAm, NiPAm, crosslinker EGDM and synthesized 2 mol% EGDM p(NiPMAm/NiPAm) xerogel were carried out by using the FTIR method (Figure 8). In addition, the structure of the inclusion complex of curcumin: 2-hydroxypropyl-β-cyclodextrin, as well as the matrix system, p(NiPMAm/NiPAm) gel in which was incorporated curcumin: 2-hydroxypropyl-β-cyclodextrin inclusion complex were examined by using this method. In Figure 8, FTIR spectra of NiPMAm monomers, comonomers NiPAm, crosslinker EGDM and synthesized p(NiPMAm/NiPAm) xerogel containing 2 mol% of EGDM are shown.

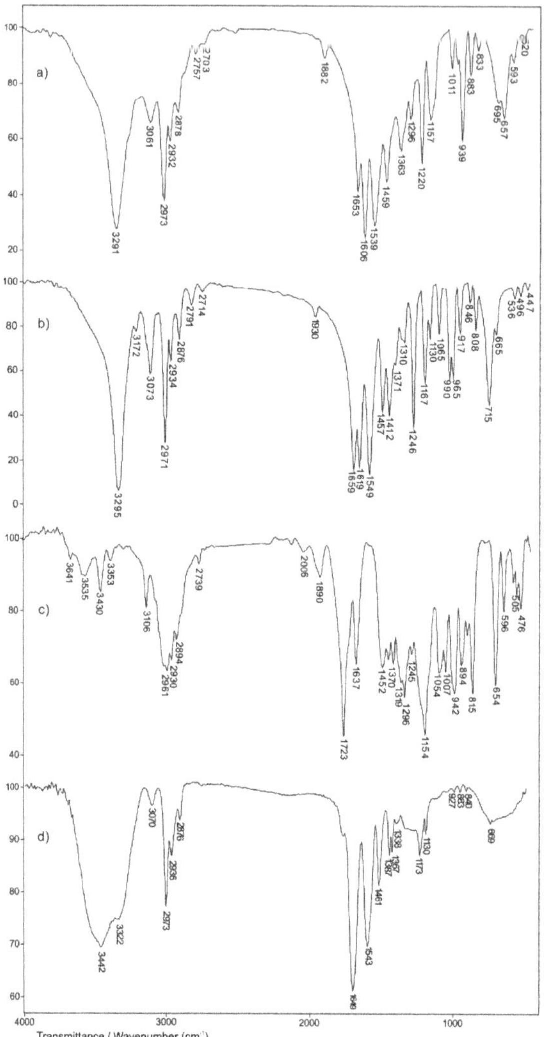

Figure 8. FTIR spectra: (**a**) NiPMAm monomer, (**b**) NiPAm monomer, (**c**) crosslinker EGDM and (**d**) synthesized p(NiPMAm/NiPAm) copolymer with 2 mol% of EGDM.

In the FTIR spectrum of NiPMAm monomer (Figure 8a), the absorption band 3291 cm^{-1} is a result of valence N-H vibrations, ν(N-H). Asymmetric valence vibrations of C-H bond of the vinyl group, νas(=C-H), give an absorption band with a maximum at 3061 cm^{-1}. The absorption bands at 2973 and 2878 cm^{-1} are from asymmetric and symmetric valence of the methyl group in the NiPMAm monomer structure, respectively. The proof for the presence of the amide group in the monomer structure are absorption bands with maximums at 1653 cm^{-1} (Amide band I) and 1539 cm^{-1} (Amide band II). It can be assumed that amide band I is from the valence vibrations of the keto group, while Amide band II arises by coupling of N-H deformation vibrations and valence C-N vibrations. The valence vibrations of C=C bond in FTIR spectrum of NiPMAm monomer (Figure 8a) give an absorption band with a maximum at 1606 cm^{-1}. The absorption band of asymmetric deformative C-H vibration in the plane of CH$_3$-C group in the monomer spectrum is present at 1459 cm^{-1}. The valence vibrations of C-H bond of isopropyl group give an absorption band with a maximum at 1363 cm^{-1}. The presence of the isopropyl group in the monomer structure is also confirmed by the presence of an absorption band at 1157 and 1011 cm^{-1}.

In FTIR spectrum of NiPAm comonomers in the wavelength range of 3000 cm^{-1} (Figure 8b), two absorption bands with different intensity can be observed. The high intensity absorption band with a maximum at 3295 cm^{-1} is attributed to valence vibrations of the secondary amino group, ν(N-H) which is in agreement with the research of other authors [48], while the absorption band at 3073 cm^{-1}, is a result of asymmetric vibrations of vinyl group, ν_{as}(=C-H). In FTIR spectrum of NiPAm comonomer (Figure 8b), absorption bands with a maximum at 2971 cm^{-1} and 2876 cm^{-1} come from asymmetric and symmetric valence vibrations of C-H bond from the methyl group, respectively. The absorption band of medium intensity with a maximum at 2934 cm^{-1} comes from asymmetric valence vibrations, ν_{as}(C-H), of C-H bonds in isopropyl group of NiPAm. The Amide bands I, II and III with a maximum at 1659 cm^{-1}, 1549 cm^{-1}, 1310 cm^{-1}, respectively, confirm the presence of an amide group in the molecule of NIPAM [49]. The valence vibrations of C=C bond in FTIR spectrum of NiPAm monomer (Figure 8b) provides an absorption band with a maximum at 1619 cm^{-1}. The absorption band of medium intensity at 1371 cm^{-1}, relates to deformation vibrations in the plane δ(C-H), of C-H bond in isopropyl group of NiPAm. The high intensity band with a maximum at 1167 cm^{-1} in the comonomer spectrum also confirms the presence of the isopropyl group in the structure of NiPAm. The appearance of absorption bands which come from deformation vibrations in the plane δ(=C-H), at 1412 cm^{-1} and deformation vibrations out of the plane γ(=C-H), at 990 and 917 cm^{-1} confirms the presence of the vinyl group in the structure of the comonomer [49].

In the FTIR spectrum of crosslinker EGDM (Figure 8c), there are absorption bands characteristic for ester and vinyl functional groups present in the molecule. Sharp absorption bands of high intensity with a maximum at 1723 cm^{-1} in FTIR spectrum of EGDM, comes from valence vibrations of the carbonyl group that is conjugated by a double bond, which is why the medium intensity band that corresponds to the valence vibrations of the C=C bond is noticeable at 1637 cm^{-1}. The valence vibrations of C-O bond give an absorption band with a maximum of absorption at 1154 cm^{-1}. In the FTIR spectrum of crosslinker EGDM, absorption bands with a maximum at 2894 cm^{-1} from ν_s(CH$_3$), at 2961 cm^{-1} from ν_{as}(CH$_3$), at 2930 cm^{-1} from ν_{as}(CH$_2$) and at 3106 cm^{-1} from the vinyl group ν_{as}(=CH) are present, which is in accordance with the literature data [39].

By comparing the FTIR spectrum of p(NiPMAm/NiPAm) copolymer with 2 mol% of EGDM (Figure 8d) to the spectrum of NiPMAm monomer (Figure 8a) and NiPAm (Figure 8b), there is a clear difference that indicates the difference in structure between the synthesized polymer and the initial reactants. The shift and absence of some absorption bands from the characteristic functional groups of monomers was observed, which indicates the creation of a new structure. A broad absorption band of high intensity from valence vibrations of the N-H bond in the FTIR spectrum of copolymer at 3442 cm^{-1} is shifted to higher wavenumbers compared to the same band in the FTIR spectrum of monomer NiPMAm (Figure 8a) and comonomer NiPAm (Figure 8b). The displacement of the centroid of this band indicates the involvement of the amino group in the formation of the hydrogen bond. This fact is supported by displacement of amide band II compared to its placement in the FTIR spectrum of the monomer. An absorption band of the copolymer related to valence vibrations of the C=O group (amide band I) appears at 1649 cm^{-1} and shifted to lower wavenumbers compared to the absorption band in the FTIR spectra of NiPMAm and NiPAm by 4 and 10 units, respectively. The absorption bands at 1387 and 1367 cm^{-1} confirm the presence of an isopropyl group in the structure of the copolymer p(NiPMAm/NiPAm) and indicate that this group, that is present in monomers, was not involved in the polymerization process. The absence of an absorption band in the valence vibrations of the C=C bond, and which for monomers appears around wave numbers in the range of 1600–1640 cm^{-1}, clearly indicates that the polymerization reaction of the NiPMAm and NiPAm monomers happened by the breaking of double bonds.

In the FTIR spectrum of curcumin (Figure 9a), a broad absorption band appears at 3421 cm^{-1} as a result of the valence vibrations of the free phenolic OH group. In the wavenumber range of 2800–3000 cm^{-1} in the FTIR spectrum of curcumin, two characteristic absorption bands appear with a maximum at 2967 and 2841 cm^{-1} that come from the asymmetric valence vibrations of the methyl group and the valence vibrations of the methoxy group, respectively [50–52]. The presence of an aromatic structure is confirmed by the absorption bands of valence vibrations of the C=C group which appears in the wavenumber range of 1600–1450 cm^{-1}, and in the FTIR spectrum of curcumin are present with a maximum at 1627, 1590, 1512 and 1459 cm^{-1}. In accordance with literature data, the absorption band with a maximum at 1627 cm^{-1} can be related to valence vibrations of the carbonyl group [53]. The absorption band with a maximum at 1209 cm^{-1} comes from valence vibrations of the C-O phenolic group, while the absorption band that comes from the C-O-C bond in the FTIR spectrum of curcumin appears at 1031 cm^{-1} [54]. In the wavenumber range 730–860 cm^{-1} absorption bands are present which come from deformative vibrations out of the C-H plane of the aromatic ring.

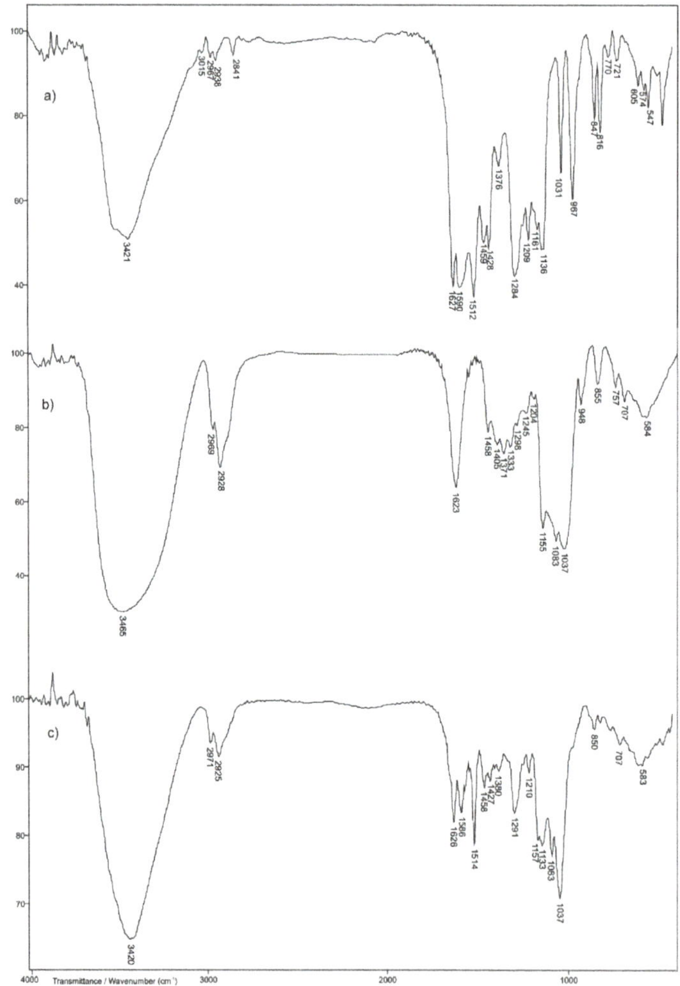

Figure 9. The FTIR spectra: (**a**) curcumin, (**b**) 2-hydroxypropyl-β-cyclodextrin, (**c**) curcumin: 2-hydroxypropyl-β-cyclodextrin inclusion complex.

The broad absorption band, with a maximum of absorption at 3465 cm^{-1} in the FTIR spectrum of 2-hydroxypropyl-β-cyclodextrin (Figure 9b), is a result of valence vibrations of the hydroxyl group from 2-hydroxypropyl-β-cyclodextrin. The absorption bands coming from valence vibrations of C-H bound are appearing in the FTIR spectrum with a maximum at 2928 and 2969 cm^{-1} [55]. In the FTIR spectrum of 2-hydroxypropyl-β-cyclodextrin, the absorption band with a maximum at 1623 cm^{-1} comes from O-H deformative vibration in the plane [56]. The asymmetric and symmetric C–H deformative vibrations in the plane give absorption bands at 1458 and 1371 cm^{-1} in the FTIR spectrum of 2-hydroxypropyl-β-cyclodextrin, respectively. The absorption band at 1155 cm^{-1} indicates the valence vibrations of the C–C group, while absorption bands with maximums at 1083 and 1037 cm^{-1} confirm the presence of valence vibrations of the C–O bond at ether and hydroxyl groups of 2-hydroxypropyl-β-cyclodextrin. In the range of 1000–700 cm^{-1} valence and deformation vibration bands of glucopyranose units appear [57].

By comparative analysis of FTIR spectra of curcumin and 2-hydroxypropyl-β-cyclodextrin with the FTIR spectrum of curcumin: 2-hydroxypropyl-β-cyclodextrin complex (Figure 9c), changes in appearance of FTIR spectra of complex compared to the FTIR spectra of pure substances are noticed. The broad absorption band with the maximum of absorption at 3420 cm^{-1} in the FTIR spectrum of curcumin: 2-hydroxypropyl-β-cyclodextrin complex (Slika 9c) is shifted to lower wavenumbers by 45 units compared to the position of the same absorption band in the FTIR spectrum of 2-hydroxypropyl-β-cyclodextrin (Slika 9b). In the FTIR spectrum of complex of curcumin: 2-hydroxypropyl-β-cyclodextrin the absence of two characteristic absorption bands with maximums of absorptions at 2967 and 2841 cm^{-1} that come from asymmetric and symmetric vibrations of methyl group and valence vibrations of methoxy group of curcumin (Figure 9a), respectively, is noticed. The absorption bands that come from C-H valence vibrations with the maximums at 2928 and 2969 cm^{-1} in the FTIR spectrum of 2-hydroxypropyl-β-cyclodextrin are shifted by 3 units to lower i.e., by 2 units to higher wavelength numbers in the FTIR spectrum of curcumin: 2-hydroxypropyl-β-cyclodextrin (Figure 9c) and appear at 2925 cm^{-1} and 2971 cm^{-1}, respectively. These changes may indicate the interaction of these groups from 2-hydroxypropyl-β-cyclodextrin with appropriate groups from the molecule of curcumin. The absorption band which comes from C-O-C bond in the FTIR spectrum of curcumin and appears at 1031 cm^{-1} is not present in the FTIR spectrum of curcumin: 2-hydroxypropyl-β-cyclodextrin complex (Figure 9c). The absorption band of C–O valence vibrations from 2-hydroxypropyl-β-cyclodextrin in the FTIR spectrum of complex is shifted by 2 units to higher wavelength numbers. The absence and shift of some absorption bands in the FTIR spectrum of curcumin: 2-hydroxypropyl-β-cyclodextrin complex indicate the incorporation of curcumin in holes of cyclodextrin, which is in accordance with literature data [58].

By incorporation of curcumin into p(NiPMAm/NiPAm) hydrogels, it is expected that the establishment of intermolecular interactions of the type hydrogen bondage between phenolic OH groups of curcumin as a proton-donor, with oxygen from the C=O group as a proton-acceptor of side chains of p(NiPMAm/NiPAm) copolymer occur. In addition, the C=O group of curcumin can form hydrogen bonds with NH proton donor groups of side chains of p(NiPMAm/NiPAm) hydrogels.

In the FTIR spectrum of p(NiPMAm/NiPAm), hydrogels containing 2 mol% of crosslinker with incorporated curcumin: 2-hydroxypropyl-β-cyclodextrin inclusion complex (Figure 10b), at the wavelength number range of 3500–3200 cm^{-1} broad absorption band with the maximum at 3430 cm^{-1} that comes from valence vibrations of N-H bond of hydrogels and valence vibrations of the phenolic OH group of curcumin, can be noticed. The maximum of this band is shifted by 12 units to lower wavelength numbers compared to the position of the same absorption band in the FTIR spectrum of empty hydrogel (Figure 10a), and by 9 units to higher wavelength numbers compared to the position of the absorption band in the FTIR spectrum of curcumin (Figure 9a). This indicates that the mentioned groups are involved in the formation of hydrogen bonds between curcumin molecules and the hydrogel. The amide absorption band I, ν(C=O), appears at 1653 cm^{-1}, while the amide absorption band II, δ(N-H), appears at 1549 cm^{-1}, and their maximums are shifted by 4, that is, 6 units to higher wavelength numbers, compared to the spectrum of hydrogel only (Figure 10a). The maximum of absorption that comes from valence vibrations of C=O in the FTIR spectrum of hydrogels with incorporated curcumin (Figure 10b) is shifted by 26 units to higher wavelength numbers, compared to the position of the same absorption band in the FTIR spectrum of curcumin (Figure 9a). The shiftment of the maximum of amide absorption bands and the decrease in their intensity compared to hydrogel only, indicates the involvement of C=O and –NH groups in the formation of hydrogen bonds. The absorption band that comes from valence vibrations of the C-O-C bond is present with a maximum at 1034 cm^{-1} and is shifted to higher wavelength numbers by 3 units, compared to the position of the same band in the FTIR spectrum of curcumin. The results of FTIR analysis show that the change in intensity and the shift of the characteristic absorption bands of curcumin and hydrogel to lower or higher values of wavelength numbers happened, which indicates the incorporation of curcumin into the hydrogel structure.

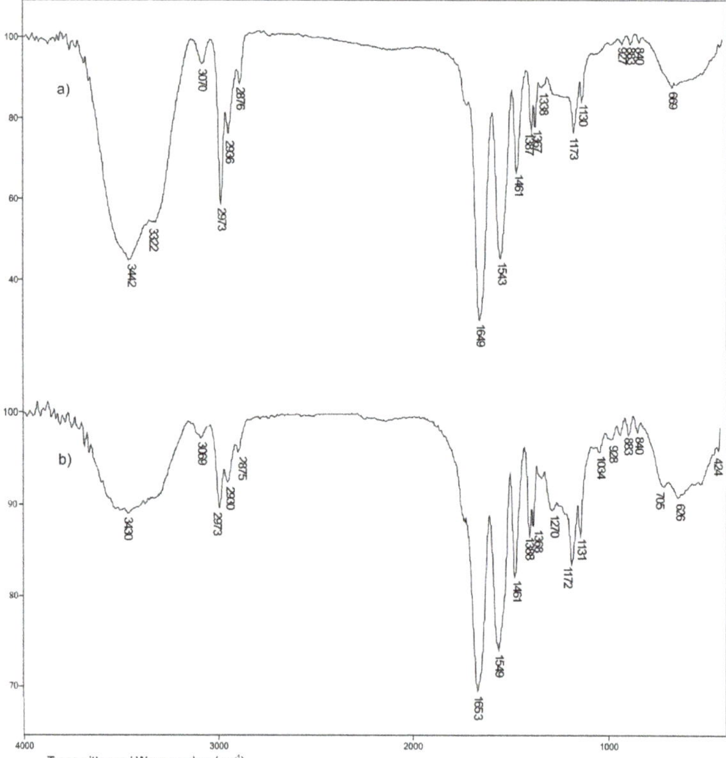

Figure 10. The FTIR spectra: (**a**) copolymer p(NiPMAm/NiPAm), sample 10/90/2 and (**b**) matrix system of p(NiPMAm/NiPAm) with incorporated inclusion complex of curcumin: 2-hydroxypropyl-β-cyclodextrin.

Shifts of the corresponding absorption maxima by several units of cm^{-1} indicate the formation of weak hydrogen bonds, which is favorable from the aspect of formulation development. This indicates that these weak hydrogen bonds will possibly slow down the diffusion of curcumin molecules from the hydrogel structure, and enable the release of curcumin from the formulation for a longer period of time.

3.5. Scanning Electron Microscopy (SEM)

The morphology of curcumin, curcumin: 2-hydroxypropyl-β-cyclodextrin complex, synthesized p(NiPMAm/NiPAm) hydrogel containing 2 mol% crosslinker and p(NiPMAm/NiPAm) hydrogel with incorporated complex of curcumin: 2-hydroxypropyl-β-cyclodextrin, was examined by SEM method. Hydrogel samples were swollen to equilibrium and then lyophilized in order to better understand their morphology. Obtained SEM micrographs are shown in Figure 11.

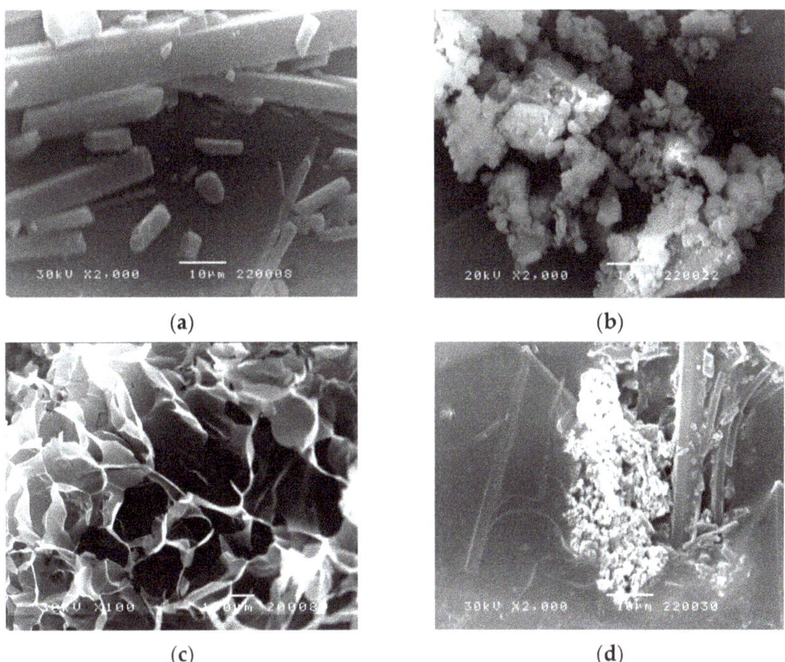

Figure 11. Scanning electron microscopy micrographs (SEM): (**a**) curcumin, (**b**) curcumin: 2-hydroxypropyl-β-cyclodextrin complex, (**c**) p(NiPMAm/NiPAm) hydrogel containing 2 mol% EGDM, (**d**) p(NiPMAm/NiPAm) hydrogel containing 2 mol% of crosslinker with incorporated curcumin: 2-hydroxypropyl-β-cyclodextrin complex.

In Figure 11a curcumin crystals are clearly visible, while in Figure 11b crystal structure of curcumin: 2-hydroxypropyl-β-cyclodextrin complex cannot be seen. By analyzing the SEM micrographs, a clear difference between the look of the surface structure of the empty hydrogel (Figure 11c) and hydrogel with incorporated curcumin: 2-hydroxypropyl-β-cyclodextrin complex can be observed (Figure 11d). The structure of p(NiPMAm/NiPAm) hydrogel containing 2 mol% EGDM is porous, with a pore diameter in the range of 100 to 300 μm (Figure 11c). In micrography 7d, the presence of curcumin: 2-hydroxypropyl-β-cyclodextrin complex in holes of hydrogel can be seen, whose structure matches the structure of curcumin: 2-hydroxypropyl-β-cyclodextrin complex (Figure 11b). This indicates a successful incorporation of curcumin: 2-hydroxypropyl-β-cyclodextrin inclusion complex into holes of the synthesized p(NiPMAm/NiPAm) gel, and is in accordance with the result obtained by FTIR analysis.

3.6. Differential Scanning Calorimetry (DSC)

In Figure 12 are shown DSC curves of curcumin, 2-hydroxypropyl-β-cyclodextrin, curcumin: 2-hydroxypropyl-β-cyclodextrin complex, p(NiPMAm/NiPAm) 10/90/2 hydrogel and p(NiPMAm/NiPAm) 10/90/2 hydrogel with incorporated curcumin: 2-

hydroxypropyl-β-cyclodextrin complex. In the DSC curve that comes from curcumin (curve 1 in Figure 12) can be seen the endothermic melting peak of curcumin at 188 °C and the peak area correspond to the curcumin melting enthalpy of 171.5 J/g. Considering that curcumin complexation occurred in the presence of 2-hydroxypropyl-β-cyclodextrin, the curcumin molecules in the complex and in the gel complex formulation cannot form curcumin crystals that would give an endothermic melting peak. Nevertheless, in the endothermic peak of the complex, a weak peak is observed at 186 °C, which may indicate that the curcumin molecules have not completely entered the holes of 2-hydroxypropyl-β-cyclodextrin (curve 3 in Figure 12). In the formulation of the complex with gel (curve 2 in Figure 12), the endothermic peak from the melting of curcumin can no longer be observed. This indicates that the supramolecular structures of the complexes are now already distributed in the gel, and that a constant release rate of curcumin could be expected from this formulation of the curcumin complex in the gel.

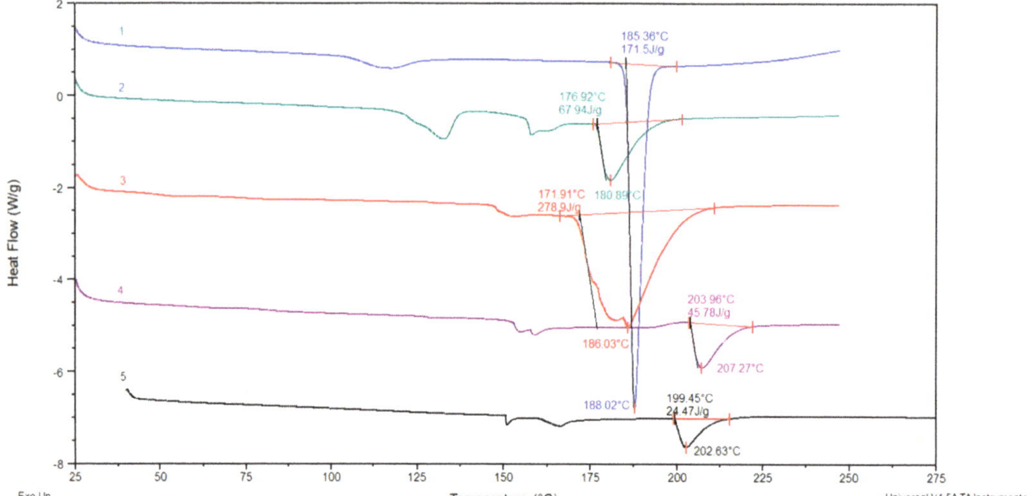

Figure 12. DSC curves: 1. curcumin, 2. p(NiPMAm/NiPAm) 10/90/2 hydrogel containing curcumin: 2-hydroxypropyl-β-cyclodextrin complex, 3. curcumin: 2-hydroxypropyl-β-cyclodextrin complex, 4. p(NiPMAm/NiPAm)10/90/2 hydrogel, 5. 2-hydroxypropyl-β-cyclodextrin.

3.7. X-ray Diffraction (XRD)

The XRD spectra of curcumin, 2-hydroxypropyl-β-cyclodextrin, curcumin: 2-hydroxypropyl-β-cyclodextrin complex, synthesized p(NiPMAm/NiPAm) hydrogel containing 2 mol% EGDM and p(NiPMAm/NiPAm) hydrogel with incorporated curcumin: 2-hydroxypropyl-β-cyclodextrin complex are shown in Figure 13.

In the X-ray diffractogram of curcumin (Figure 13a), sharp peaks are present at the values of diffraction angle 2 θ: 7.6; 8.7; 16; 17.5; 21 and 42.55° that indicates that pure curcumin is in crystalline form, which is in agreement with the literature data [22]. Two broad peaks without high maximums that appear in the range of 2 θ = 5–15° and 2 θ = 15–22.5° in diffractogram of 2-hydroxypropyl-β-cyclodextrin (Figure 13b) indicate its amorphous structure [59]. By comparative analysis of diffractograms in Figure 13, it can be observed that in the diffractogram of the inclusion complex of curcumin: 2-hydroxypropyl-β-cyclodextrin (Figure 13c), there are no sharp peaks present in the diffractogram of pure crystalline curcumin. The appearance of new peaks in the diffractogram of the inclusion complex clearly indicates the formation of a new supramolecular structure. Sharp peaks at the values of the diffraction angle 2 θ: 7, 13.5, 16, 19 and 27° in diffractogram of the curcumin: 2-hydroxypropyl-β-cyclodextrin complex indicate that the curcumin molecule did not completely enter into the hole of the 2-hydroxypropyl-β-cyclodextrin from inclusion complex. This is understandable, since one molecule of curcumin requires two molecules of 2-hydroxypropyl-β-cyclodextrin to be completely included in the cavities of 2-hydroxypropyl-β-cyclodextrin [24]. However, that was not necessary in this case because the further homogenization was carried over by the gel. By comparative analysis of the diffractogram of the empty hydrogel and the hydrogel with incorporated complex of curcumin: 2-hydroxypropyl-β-cyclodextrin (Figure 13d and e, respectively), great similarity was observed considering the shape and position of the peaks that appear as broad in the range of 2 θ = 5–10 and 2 θ = 15–32.5, and they correspond to the peaks that appear in the diffractogram of the empty hydrogel. This indicates that the structure of the hydrogel after incorporation of the inclusion complex did not significantly change, and that the complex of curcumin: 2-hydroxypropyl-β-cyclodextrin was relatively uniformly distributed into the gel.

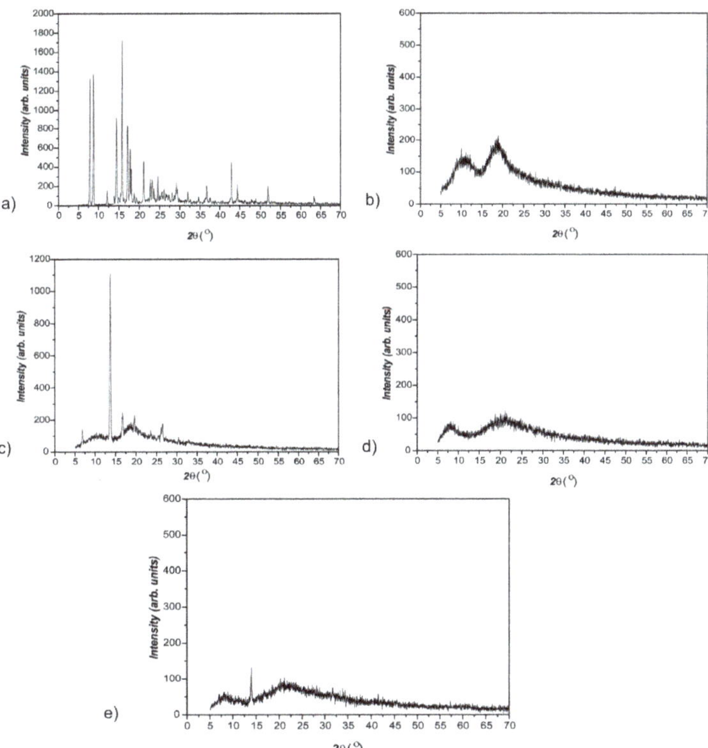

Figure 13. The XRD diffractograms: (**a**) curcumin, (**b**) 2-hydroxypropyl-β-cyclodextrin, (**c**) inclusion complex of curcumin: 2-hydroxypropyl-β-cyclodextrin, (**d**) p(NiPMAm/NiPAm) hydrogel containing 2 mol% of crosslinker, and (**e**) p(NiPMAm/NiPAm) hydrogel with incorporated curcumin: 2-hydroxypropyl-β-cyclodextrin complex.

3.8. Nuclear Magnetic Resonance (^{1}H-NMR)

In Figure 14 are shown ^{1}H-NMR spectra of 2-hydroxypropyl-β-cyclodextrin and the complex of curcumin: 2-hydroxypropyl-β-cyclodextrin. In Table 3 are shown values for chemical shifts of 2-hydroxypropyl-β-cyclodextrin and the complex of curcumin: 2-hydroxypropyl-β-cyclodextrin, and the change in chemical shifts of protons which originate from 2-hydroxypropyl-β-cyclodextrin in the complex. Considering that the solubility of curcumin in water is very weak, the analysis is aimed at monitoring the chemical shifts of protons from 2-hydroxypropyl-β-cyclodextrin. The changes in chemical shifts of protons

Δδ which are shown in Table 3, indicate the formation of weak hydrogen bonds in which protons from 2-hydroxypropyl-β-cyclodextrin are involved which indicates the possible inclusion and creation of the inclusion complex.

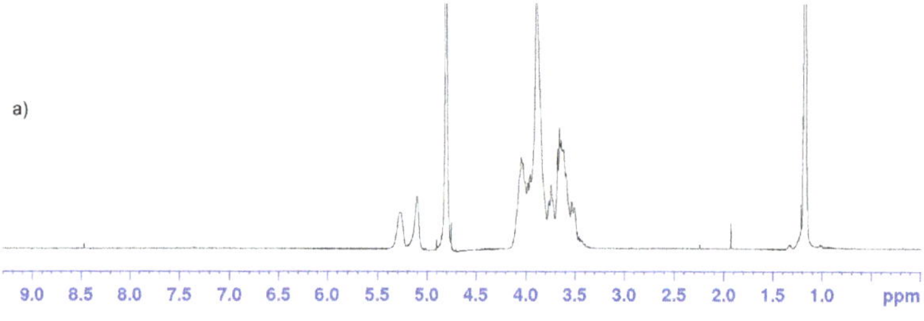

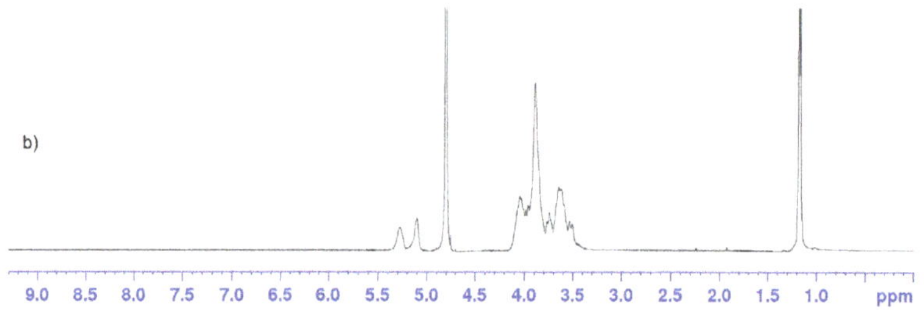

Figure 14. ^{1}H-NMR spectrum: (**a**) complex of curcumin: 2-hydroxypropyl-β-cyclodextrin and (**b**) 2-hydroxypropyl-β-cyclodextrin.

Table 3. Chemical shifts values δ for 2-hydroxypropyl-β-cyclodextrin (2-HP-β-CD) and for complex of curcumin: 2-hydroxypropyl-β-cyclodextrin (Complex) and changes in chemical shifts Δδ for protons originate from 2-hydroxypropyl-β-cyclodextrin in complex.

Type of Proton	Chemical Shifts Values δ		Δδ
	2-HP-β-CD	**Complex**	
CH$_3$	1.1692	1.1678	+0.0014
H-C$_1$	5.1005	5.0993	+0.0012
H-C$_2$	5.2732	5.2743	−0.0011

3.9. The Loading Efficiency of Curcumin into the p(NiPMAm/NiPAm) Hydrogel

By knowing that curcumin does not dissolve in aqueous media, the incorporation of curcumin into the hydrogel was accomplished by incorporating the curcumin: 2-hydroxypropyl-β-cyclodextrin complex into samples of hydrogels. The efficiency of curcumin incorporation, η, was calculated according to Equation (2), in terms of the total starting mass of curcumin available in the complex. The data are shown in Table 4.

Table 4. The efficiency of curcumin incorporation (η) into p(NiPMAm/NiPAm) xerogels.

Sample	η of Curcumin (%)
10/90/2	78.35
10/90/3	67.58

The efficiency of curcumin incorporation into the inclusion complex of p(NiPMAm/NiPAm) 10/90/2 xerogel is greater than for 10/90/3, that is in agreement with the results for the swelling for synthesized gels. These values are satisfying considering that the water solubility of curcumin is very low. By complexation with 2-hydroxypropyl-β-cyclodextrin, its water solubility is increased 1237 times, and this provides easier incorporation into synthesized hydrogels as well as a release in physiological mediums.

3.10. In Vitro Release of Curcumin from p(NiPMAm/NiPAm) Gels

The release of curcumin from p(NiPMAm/NiPAm) gels containing 2 and 3 mol% of EGDM was monitored under in vitro conditions at temperature 37 °C and pH 7.4, that simulate the body temperature and pH conditions as in the small intestine, by applying the HPLC method (Figure 15). The release of curcumin from the gels was monitored during 48 h.

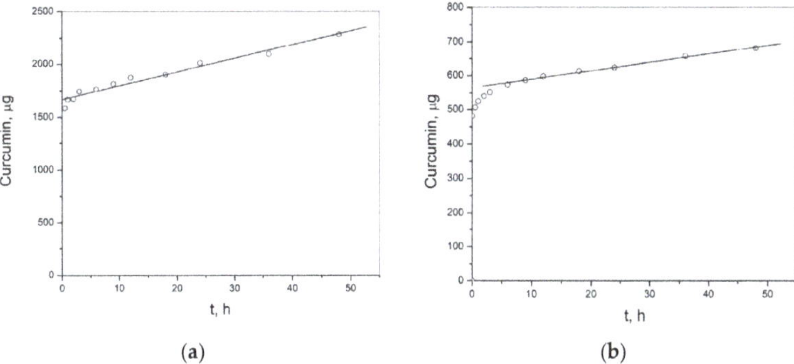

Figure 15. Profile of curcumin release from p(NiPMAm/NiPAm) hydrogels: (**a**) sample 10/90/2 and (**b**) sample 10/90/3.

The release rate of curcumin from p(NiPMAm/NiPAm) hydrogels containing 2 mol% of EGDM is 13.13 μg/h, and for hydrogels containing 3 mol% of EGDM it is 2.51 μg/h, which provides a prolonged release of curcumin during 366.5 h (15.27 days) and 1653.6 h (68.9 days), respectively. In Figure 15a it can be seen that there is also an initial release of curcumin in an amount of approximately 1600 μg from the formulation of sample 10/90/2, and approximately 500 μg from the formulation of sample 10/90/3 (Figure 15b). The results obtained indicate the possibility that thermosensitive p(NiPMAm/NiPAm) hydrogels could find application in the development of formulations with the prolonged release of curcumin. These results shows that there is a possibility of tailoring the formulation in terms of the amount of curcumin that should be incorporated into the gel through the complex, for tailoring the time and rate of curcumin release from this formulation as well as the intensity of the initial release; for example, by changing the crosslinker concentration. The amount of crosslinker for synthesis of gel will determine the density of the nodes in the network and the length of the branches in the gel network, that will affect the diffusion of curcumin molecules through the mass of gel. In a polymer network created with a higher concentration of crosslinker, the branches will be shorter and the concentration of nodes will be higher, and like this the diffusion of curcumin molecules will slow down. Analysis of the release mechanism of curcumin from the formulation of the complex in gel can be helpful for this purpose.

With the aim to further study the curcumin release mechanism from p(NiPMAm/NiPAm), hydrogels with the incorporated inclusion complex of curcumin: 2-hydroxypropyl-β-cyclodextrin, the experimental data obtained in this work are fitted by appropriate mathematical models: Higuchi, Korsmeyer–Peppes and Baker–Lonsdale, and the obtained parameters are shown in Table 5.

Table 5. The kinetic of curcumin release from p(NiPMAm/NiPAm) hydrogels.

Kinetic Model	Parameter	Sample 10/90/2	Sample 10/90/3
Higuchi $F = k_H \cdot t^{1/2}$	k_H R^2 AIC	9.218 −0.918 97.98	3.350 −1.147 74.811
Korsmeyer–Peppas $F = k_{KP} \cdot t^n$	k_{KP} n R^2 AIC	33.247 0.074 0.984 41.036	12.499 0.063 0.996 −2.927
Baker–Lonsdale $3/2[1-(1-F/100)^{2/3}]-F/100 = k_{BL} \cdot t$	k_{BL} R^2 AIC	0.002 −0.636 96.078	0 −1.054 74.27

k_H: the constant of release at Higuchi model; R^2: coefficient of determination; AIC: Akaik's information criterion; F: the fraction of released drug in function of time t; k_{KP}: the constant of release at Korsmeyer-Peppes model that takes into account structural and geometrical characteristics of dosage form; n: the exponent of release/diffusion; k_{BL}: combined constant of release at Baker-Lonsdale model; [60–62].

The highest coefficient of determination (R^2) and the lowest AIC indicate that Korsmeyer-Peppes's model best describes the release of curcumin from the formulation of p(NiPMAm/NiPAm) hydrogels containing curcumin: 2-hydroxypropyl-β-cyclodextrin complex. The value for the diffusion exponent of the hydrogel sample p(NiPMAm/NiPAm) containing 2 mol% EGDM is 0.074, but 0.063 for the sample of p(NiPMAm/NiPAm) hydrogel containing 3 mol% of EGDM, and that shows that the release mechanism of curcumin, is based on diffusion from the polymer matrix of the gels. This definitely confirms the conclusion that the right choice on the crosslinker concentration to be used for the synthesis process of p(NiPMAm/NiPAm) hydrogels can have an influence on the release rate of curcumin from the gel formulation with curcumin: 2-hydroxypropyl-β-cyclodextrin complex. The form of curcumin: 2-hydroxypropyl-β-cyclodextrin complex was applied to provide a larger amount of curcumin into the gel.

If the overall results are considered, it can be concluded that a system for the sustained release of curcumin from a formulation base on hydrogel has been developed. This was achieved primarily by increasing solubility by including curcumin to 2-hydroxypropyl-β-cyclodextrin, which enabled the required amount of curcumin to enter into the hydrogel. Incorporation of pure curcumin into the hydrogel would create curcumin agglomerates in the formulation, while the cyclodextrin complex enabled individual curcumin molecules to diffuse through the gel. By that, the entire formulation significantly contributed to increasing the solubility of curcumin.

4. Conclusions

In this work, the synthesis and characterization of p(NiPMAm/NiPAm) hydrogels with two different concentrations of crosslinker was done. The results show that less than 0.3% of residual monomers is present in synthesized hydrogels. The FTIR analysis of reactants at the beginning of the synthesis, synthesized hydrogels, curcumin: 2-hydroxypropyl-β-cyclodextrin complex and the formulation of hydrogel with complex of curcumin: 2-hydroxypropyl-β-cyclodextrin showed that the complexation and formulation of complexes with the gel were done by the help of hydrogen bonds formation. The water swelling process is controlled by the mechanisms called "non-Fick's diffusion" and "less to Fick's diffusion". The phase solubility of curcumin in solution of 2-hydroxypropyl-β-cyclodextrin showed increased solubility by 1237 times. The SEM analysis showed the loss of the crystal structure of curcumin in the complex and in the formulation of the complex with gel, which was additionally confirmed by DSC and XRD analyses. Since the water solubility of curcumin is low (3 mg/dm^3), the complexation with 2-hydroxypropyl-β-cyclodextrinthe made incorporation of curcumin into hydrogels easier by increasing the solubility. The monitoring of the curcumin release profile from the formulation of curcumin: 2-hydroxypropyl-β-cyclodextrin complex with p(NiPMAm/NiPAm) hydrogels, shows the starting release of curcumin from the formulation that slows with the increasement of crosslinker in the composition of the reaction mixture for hydrogel synthesis. In addition, with an increase in the concentration of the crosslinker, the release rate of curcumin from the formulation also decreases, which gives the possibility of tailoring the release rate from the formulation. The release rate of curcumin from the formulation of the complex with gel is constant in the function of time, and is dependent on the amount of curcumin in the formulation and the release rate. This is a formulation from which the curcumin will be released over a longer period of time can be designed, more than over 60 days. The kinetic analysis of data for curcumin release from the formulation of curcumin-gel complex showed that the mechanism of curcumin release is based on diffusion from the polymer matrix of the gels.

5. Patents

Patent Application RS2022P0287, Urošević, M.; Nikolić, Lj.; Gajić, I.; Nikolić, V.; Dinić, A.; Ilić-Stojanović, S.; Miljković, V.; Nikolić, G.; Cakić, S. Formulation of the matrix system with curcumine, Priority 17 Mart 2022, the Intellectual Property Office of the Republic of Serbia.

Author Contributions: Conceptualization, L.N., M.U., V.N., I.G. and A.D.; methodology, L.N., M.U., V.N., I.G., A.D., V.M., S.R., S.Đ., J.K., S.I.-S. and G.N.; formal analysis, L.N., M.U., V.N., I.G., A.D., V.M., S.R., S.Đ., J.K., S.I.-S. and G.N.; investigation, L.N., M.U., V.N., I.G., A.D., V.M., S.R., S.Đ., J.K., S.I.-S. and G.N.; writing—original draft preparation, L.N., M.U., V.N., I.G. and A.D.; writing—review and editing, L.N., M.U., V.N., I.G. and A.D. All authors have read and agreed to the published version of the manuscript.

Funding: This research received no external funding.

Institutional Review Board Statement: Not applicable.

Informed Consent Statement: Not applicable.

Data Availability Statement: Not applicable.

Acknowledgments: The authors wish to thank Republic of Serbia—Ministry of Education, Science and Technological Development Program, for financing scientific research work, number 451-03-68/2022-14/200133, University of Niš, Faculty of Technology.

Conflicts of Interest: The authors declare no conflict of interest.

References

1. Xia, Z.H.; Chen, W.B.; Shi, L.; Jiang, X.; Li, K.; Wang, Y.X.; Liu, Y.Q. The underlying mechanisms of curcumin inhibition of hyperglycemia and hyperlipidemia in rats fed a high-fat diet combined with STZ treatment. *Molecules* **2020**, *25*, 271. [CrossRef] [PubMed]
2. Trigo-Gutierrez, J.K.; Vega-Chacón, Y.; Soares, A.B.; Mima, E.G.D.O. Antimicrobial activity of curcumin in nanoformulations: A comprehensive review. *Int. J. Mol. Sci.* **2021**, *22*, 7130. [CrossRef] [PubMed]
3. Kheiripour, N.; Plarak, A.; Heshmati, A.; Asl, S.S.; Mehri, F.; Ebadollahi-Natanzi, A.; Ranjbar, A.; Hosseini, A. Evaluation of the hepatoprotective effects of curcumin and nanocurcumin against paraquat-induced liver injury in rats: Modulation of oxidative stress and Nrf2 pathway. *J. Biochem. Mol. Toxicol.* **2021**, *35*, e22739. [CrossRef] [PubMed]
4. González-Ortega, L.A.; Acosta-Osorio, A.A.; Grube-Pagola, P.; Palmeros-Exsome, C.; Cano-Sarmiento, C.; García-Varela, R.; García, H.S. Anti-inflammatory activity of curcumin in gel carriers on mice with atrial edema. *J. Oleo Sci.* **2020**, *69*, 123–131. [CrossRef]
5. Belhan, S.; Yıldırım, S.; Huyut, Z.; Özdek, U.; Oto, G.; Algül, S. Effects of curcumin on sperm quality, lipid profile, antioxidant activity and histopathological changes in streptozotocin-induced diabetes in rats. *Andrologia* **2020**, *52*, e13584. [CrossRef]
6. Mirzaei, H.; Bagheri, H.; Ghasemi, F.; Khoi, J.M.; Pourhanifeh, M.H.; Heyden, Y.V.; Mortezapour, E.; Nikdasti, A.; Jeandet, P.; Khan, H.; et al. Anti-cancer activity of curcumin on multiple myeloma. *Anti Cancer Agents Med. Chem.* **2021**, *21*, 575–586. [CrossRef]
7. Loutfy, S.A.; Elberry, M.H.; Farroh, K.Y.; Mohamed, H.T.; Mohamed, A.A.; Mohamed, E.B.; Faraag, A.H.I.; Mousa, S.A. Antiviral Activity of Chitosan Nanoparticles Encapsulating Curcumin Against Hepatitis C Virus Genotype 4a in Human Hepatoma Cell Lines. *Int. J. Nanomed.* **2022**, *17*, 2891–2892. [CrossRef]

8.	Mai, N.N.S.; Nakai, R.; Kawano, Y.; Hanawa, T. Enhancing the solubility of curcumin using a solid dispersion system with hydroxypropyl-β-cyclodextrin prepared by grinding, freeze-drying, and common solvent evaporation methods. *Pharmacy* **2020**, *8*, 203. [CrossRef]

9.	Witika, B.A.; Makoni, P.A.; Matafwall, S.K.; Mweetwa, L.L.; Shandele, G.C.; Walker, R.B. Enhancement of biological and pharmacological properties of an encapsulated polyphenol: Curcumin. *Molecules* **2021**, *26*, 4244. [CrossRef]

10.	Rahmani, A.H.; Alsahli, M.A.; Aly, S.M.; Khan, M.A.; Aldebasi, Y.H. Role of curcumin in disease prevention and treatment. *Adv. Biomed. Res.* **2018**, *7*, 1–9. [CrossRef]

11.	Khosropanah, M.H.; Dinarvand, A.; Nezhadhosseini, A.; Haghighi, A.; Hashemi, S.; Nirouzad, F.; Dehghani, H. Analysis of the antiproliferative effects of curcumin and nanocurcumin in MDA-MB231 as a breast cancer cell line. *Iran J. Pharm. Res.* **2016**, *15*, 231.

12.	Arya, P.; Raghav, N. In-vitro studies of Curcumin-β-cyclodextrin inclusion complex as sustained release system. *J. Mol. Struct.* **2021**, *1228*, 129774. [CrossRef]

13.	Mangolim, C.S.; Moriwaki, C.; Nogueira, A.C.; Sato, F.; Baesso, M.L.; Neto, A.M.; Matioli, G. Curcumin–β-cyclodextrin inclusion complex: Stability, solubility, characterisation by FT-IR, FT-Raman, X-ray diffraction and photoacoustic spectroscopy, and food application. *Food Chem.* **2014**, *153*, 361–370. [CrossRef]

14.	Jáfar, M.H.; Kamal, N.N.S.N.M.; Hui, B.Y.; Kamaruzzaman, M.F.; Zain, N.N.M.; Yahaya, N.; Raoov, M. Inclusion of Curcumin in β-cyclodextrins as Potential Drug Delivery System: Preparation, Characterization and Its Preliminary Cytotoxicity Approaches. *Sains Malays* **2018**, *47*, 977–989. [CrossRef]

15.	Jantarat, C.; Sirathanarun, P.; Ratanapongsai, S.; Watcharakan, P.; Sunyapong, S.; Wadu, A. Curcumin-Hydroxypropyl-β-Cyclodextrin Inclusion Complex Preparation Methods: Effect of Common Solvent Evaporation, Freeze Drying, and pH Shift on Solubility and Stability of Curcumin. *Trop. J. Pharm. Res.* **2014**, *13*, 1215. [CrossRef]

16.	Rashidzadeh, H.; Rezaei, S.J.T.; Zamani, S.; Sarijloo, E.; Ramazani, A. pH-sensitive curcumin conjugated micelles for tumor triggered drug delivery. *J. Biomater. Sci.* **2021**, *32*, 320–336. [CrossRef]

17.	Odeh, F.; Nsairat, H.; Alshaer, W.; Alsotari, S.; Buqaien, R.; Ismail, S.; Awidi, A.; Bawab, A.A. Remote loading of curcumin-in-modified β-cyclodextrins into liposomes using a transmembrane pH gradient. *RSC Adv.* **2019**, *9*, 37148–37161. [CrossRef]

18.	Tai, K.; Rappolt, M.; Mao, L.; Gao, Y.; Li, X.; Yuan, F. The stabilization and release performances of curcumin-loaded liposomes coated by high and low molecular weight chitosan. *Food Hydrocoll.* **2020**, *99*, 105355. [CrossRef]

19.	Md Saari, N.H.; Chua, L.S.; Hasham, R.; Yuliati, L. Curcumin-loaded nanoemulsion for better cellular permeation. *Sci. Pharm.* **2020**, *88*, 44. [CrossRef]

20.	Wei, Z.; Lin, Q.; Yang, J.; Long, S.; Zhang, G.; Wang, X. Fabrication of novel dual thermo-and pH-sensitive poly (N-isopropylacrylamide-N-methylolacrylamide-acrylic acid) electrospun ultrafine fibres for controlled drug release. *Mater. Sci. Eng. C* **2020**, *115*, 111050. [CrossRef]

21.	Karpkird, T.; Khunsakorn, R.; Noptheeranuphap, C.; Midpanon, S. Inclusion complexes and photostability of UV filters and curcumin with beta-cyclodextrin polymers: Effect on cross-linkers. *J. Incl. Phenom. Macrocycl. Chem.* **2018**, *91*, 37–45. [CrossRef]

22.	Chen, J.; Qin, X.; Zhong, S.; Chen, S.; Su, W.; Liu, Y. Characterization of Curcumin/Cyclodextrin Polymer Inclusion Complex and Investigation on Its Antioxidant and Antiproliferative Activities. *Molecules* **2018**, *23*, 1179. [CrossRef] [PubMed]

23.	Chen, J.; Li, J.; Fan, T.; Zhong, S.; Qin, X.; Li, R.; Gao, J.; Liang, Y. Protective effects of curcumin/cyclodextrin polymer inclusion complex against hydrogen peroxide-induced LO2 cells damage. *Food Sci. Nutr.* **2022**, *10*, 1649–1656. [CrossRef] [PubMed]

24.	Celebioglu, A.; Uyar, T. Fast-dissolving antioxidant curcumin/cyclodextrin inclusion complex electrospun nanofibrous webs. *Food Chem.* **2020**, *317*, 126397. [CrossRef] [PubMed]

25.	Aytac, Z.; Uyar, T. Core-shell nanofibers of curcumin/cyclodextrin inclusion complex andpolylactic acid: Enhanced water solubility and slow release of curcumin. *Int. J. Pharm.* **2017**, *518*, 177–184. [CrossRef]

26.	Rezaei, A.; Nasirpour, A. Evaluation of Release Kinetics and Mechanisms of Curcumin and Curcumin-β-Cyclodextrin Inclusion Complex Incorporated in Electrospun Almond Gum/PVA Nanofibers in Simulated Saliva and Simulated Gastrointestinal Conditions. *Bionanoscience* **2019**, *9*, 438–445. [CrossRef]

27.	Zhang, Y. Enhancing Antidepressant Effect of Poloxamer/Chitosan Thermosensitive Gel Containing Curcumin-Cyclodextrin Inclusion Complex. *Int. J. Polym. Sci.* **2018**, *2018*, 3041417. [CrossRef]

28.	Kasapoglu-Calik, M.; Ozdemir, M. Synthesis and controlled release of curcumin-β-cyclodextrin inclusion complex from nanocomposite poly(N-isopropylacrylamide/sodium alginate) hydrogels. *J. App. Polym. Sci.* **2019**, *136*, 47544. [CrossRef]

29.	Yang, Z.; Liu, J.; Lu, Y. Doxorubicin and CD CUR inclusion complex co loaded in thermosensitive hydrogel PLGA PEG PLGA localized administration for osteosarcoma. *Int. J. Oncol.* **2020**, *57*, 433–444. [CrossRef]

30.	Duse, L.; Agel, M.R.; Pinnapireddy, S.R.; Schäfer, J.; Selo, M.A.; Ehrhardt, C.; Bakowsky, U. Photodynamic therapy of ovarian carcinoma cells with curcumin-loaded biodegradable polymeric nanoparticles. *Pharmaceutics* **2019**, *11*, 282. [CrossRef]

31.	Purpura, M.; Lowery, R.P.; Wilson, J.M.; Mannan, H.; Münch, G.; Razmovski-Naumovski, V. Analysis of different innovative formulations of curcumin for improved relative oral bioavailability in human subjects. *Eur. J. Nutr.* **2018**, *57*, 929–938. [CrossRef]

32.	Zhang, M.; Zhuang, B.; Du, G.; Han, G.; Jin, Y. Curcumin solid dispersion-loaded in situ hydrogels for local treatment of injured vaginal bacterial infection and improvement of vaginal wound healing. *J. Pharm. Pharmacol.* **2019**, *71*, 1044–1054. [CrossRef]

33.	Shefa, A.A.; Sultana, T.; Park, M.K.; Lee, S.Y.; Gwon, J.; Lee, B. Curcumin incorporation into an oxidized cellulose nanofiber-polyvinyl alcohol hydrogel system promotes wound healing. *Mater. Des.* **2020**, *186*, 108313. [CrossRef]

34. Zhao, Y.; Liu, J.G.; Chen, W.M.; Yu, A.C. Efficacy of thermosensitive chitosan/β-glycerophosphate hydrogel loaded with β-cyclodextrin-curcumin for the treatment of cutaneous wound infection in rats. *Exp. Ther. Med.* **2018**, *14*, 1304–1313. [CrossRef]
35. Ayar, Z.; Shafieian, M.; Mahmoodi, N.; Sabzevari, O.; Hassannejad, Z. A rechargeable drug delivery system based on pNIPAM hydrogel for the local release of curcumin. *J. Appl. Polym. Sci.* **2021**, *138*, 51167. [CrossRef]
36. Zielinska, A.; Alves, H.; Marques, V.; Durazzo, A.; Lucarini, M.; Alves, T.; Morsink, M.; Willemen, N.; Eder, P.; Chaud, M.; et al. Properties, Extraction Methods, and Delivery Systems for Curcumin as a Natural Source of Beneficial Health Effects. *Medicina* **2020**, *56*, 336. [CrossRef]
37. Sun, M.; Su, X.; Ding, B.; He, X.; Liu, X.; Yu, A.; Lou, H.; Zhai, G. Advances in nanotechnology-based delivery systems for curcumin. *Nanomedicine* **2012**, *7*, 1. [CrossRef]
38. Ilić-Stojanović, S.; Nikolić, L.; Nikolić, V.; Ristić, I.; Budinski-Simendić, J.; Kapor, A.; Nikolić, G.M. The Structure Characterization of Thermosensitive Poly(N-isopropylacrylamide-co-2-hydroxypropyl methacrylate) Hydrogel. *Polym. Int.* **2014**, *63*, 973–981. [CrossRef]
39. Ilic-Stojanovic, S.; Urosevic, M.; Nikolic, L.; Petrovic, D.; Stanojevic, J.; Najman, S.; Nikolic, V. Intelligent Hydrogels Poly(N-Isopropylmethacrylamide): Synthesis, Structure Characterization, Swelling Properties and their Radiation Decomposition. *Polymers* **2020**, *12*, 1112. [CrossRef]
40. Zdravković, A.; Nikolić, L.; Ilić-Stojanović, S.; Nikolić, V.; Najman, S.; Mitić, Ž.; Ćirić, A.; Petrović, S. Removal of heavy metal ions from aqueous solutions by hydrogels based on N-isopropylacrylamide and acrylic acid. *Polym. Bull.* **2018**, *75*, 4797–4821. [CrossRef]
41. Ilić-Stojanović, S.; Nikolić, L.; Nikolić, V.; Petrović, S.; Najman, S.; Mitić, Ž.; Oro, V. Semi-crystalline copolymer hydrogels as smart drug carriers: In vitro thermo-responsive naproxen release. *Pharmaceutics* **2021**, *13*, 1–22. [CrossRef] [PubMed]
42. Higuchi, T.; Connors, K. Phase solubility techniques. *Adv. Anal. Chem. Instrum.* **1965**, *7*, 117–212.
43. Bajpai, S.K. Swelling–deswelling behavior of poly(acrylamide-co-maleic acid) hydrogels. *J. Appl. Polym. Sci.* **2001**, *80*, 2782–2789. [CrossRef]
44. Ritger, P.L.; Peppas, N.A. A simple equation for description of solute release II. Fickian and anomalous release from swellable devices. *J. Control. Release* **1987**, *5*, 37–42. [CrossRef]
45. Wang, J.; Wu, W.; Lin, Z. Kinetics and thermodynamics of the water sorption of 2-hydroxyethyl methacrylate/styrene copolymer hydrogels. *J. Appl. Polym. Sci.* **2008**, *109*, 3018–3023. [CrossRef]
46. Hansen, C.M. The significance of the surface condition in solutions to the diffusion equation: Explaining "anomalous" sigmoidal, Case II, and Super Case II absorption behavior. *Eur. Polym. J.* **2010**, *46*, 651–662. [CrossRef]
47. Heskins, M.; Guillet, J.E. Solution Properties of Poly(N-isopropylacrylamide). *J. Macromol. Sci. Pure Appl. Chem.* **1968**, *2*, 1441–1455. [CrossRef]
48. Rwei, S.P.; Anh, T.H.N.; Chiang, W.Y.; Way, T.F.; Hsu, Y.J. Synthesis and drug delivery application of thermo-and pH-sensitive hydrogels: Poly (β-CD-co-N-isopropylacrylamide-co-IAM). *Materials* **2016**, *9*, 1003. [CrossRef]
49. Tang, X.L.; Guo, S.M.; Liu, Z.D.; Tang, R.Z.; Pang, J.Y.; Chen, Y. Preparation of thermo-sensitive poly (N-isopropylacrylamide) film using KHz alternating current Dielectric barrier discharge. *Adv. Eng. Res.* **2018**, *120*, 598–602.
50. Kundu, S.; Nithiyanantham, U. In situ formation of curcumin stabilized shape-selective Ag nanostructures in aqueous solution and their pronounced SERS activity. *RSC Adv.* **2013**, *3*, 25278–25290. [CrossRef]
51. Safie, N.E.; Ludin, N.A.; Súait, M.S.; Hamid, N.H.; Sepeai, S.; Ibrahim, M.A.; Teridi, M.A.M. Preliminary study of natural pigments photochemical properties of curcuma longa l and lawsonia inermis l. as tio 2 photoelectrode sensitizer. *Malays. J. Anal. Sci.* **2015**, *19*, 1243–1249.
52. Ismail, E.H.; Sabry, D.Y.; Mahdy, H.; Khalil, M.M.H. Synthesis and Characterization of some Ternary Metal Complexes of Curcumin with 1, 10-phenanthroline and their Anticancer Applications. *J. Sci. Res.* **2014**, *6*, 509–519. [CrossRef]
53. Valand, N.N.; Patel, M.B.; Menon, S.K. Curcumin-p-sulfonatocalix [4] resorcinarene (p-SC [4]R) interaction: Thermo-physico chemistry, stability and biological evaluation. *RSC Adv.* **2015**, *5*, 8739–8752. [CrossRef]
54. Ali, M.S.; Pandit, V.; Jain, M.; Dhar, K.L. Mucoadhesive microparticulate drug delivery system of curcumin against Helicobacter pylori infection: Design, development and optimization. *J. Adv. Pharm. Technol. Res.* **2014**, *5*, 48–56. [CrossRef]
55. Mattos de Silva, M.R.; Santos, E.P.; Barros, R.C.S.A.; Garcia, S.; Albuquerque, M.G.; Oliveira, J.S.C.; Sader, M.S. The development of a new complexation technique of hydrocortisone acetate with 2-hydroxypropyl-β-cyclodextrin: Preparation and characterization. *J. Anal. Pharm. Res.* **2018**, *7*, 1–5. [CrossRef]
56. Wang, J.; Cao, Y.; Sun, B.; Wang, C. Physicochemical and release characterisation of garlic oil-β-cyclodextrin inclusion complexes. *Food Chem.* **2011**, *127*, 1680–1685. [CrossRef]
57. Nikolić, V.D.; Ilić-Stojanović, S.S.; Nikolić, L.B.; Cakić, M.D.; Zdravković, A.S.; Kapor, A.J.; Popsavin, M.M. Photostability of piroxicam in the inclusion complex with 2-hydroxypropyl-β-cyclodextrin. *Hem. Ind.* **2014**, *68*, 107–116. [CrossRef]
58. Rachmawati, H.; Edityaningrum, C.A.; Mauludin, R. Molecular inclusion complex of curcumin–β-cyclodextrin nanoparticle to enhance curcumin skin permeability from hydrophilic matrix gel. *AAPS Pharmscitech* **2013**, *14*, 1303–1312. [CrossRef]
59. Li, N.; Wang, N.; Wu, T.; Qiu, C.; Wang, X.; Jiang, S.; Wang, T. Preparation of curcumin-hydroxypropyl-β-cyclodextrin inclusion complex by cosolvency-lyophilization procedure to enhance oral bioavailability of the drug. *Drug Dev. Ind. Pharm.* **2018**, *44*, 1966–1974. [CrossRef]
60. Costa, P.; Lobo, J.M.S. Modeling and comparison of dissolution profiles. *Eur. J. Pharm. Sci.* **2001**, *13*, 123–133. [CrossRef]

61. Đorđević, S.; Isailović, T.; Cekić, N.; Vuleta, G.; Savić, S. Parenteralne nanoemulzije diazepama-fizičkohemijska karakterizacija i in vitro ispitivanje brzine oslobađanja. *Arh. Farm.* **2016**, *66*, 24–41
62. Zhang, Y.; Huo, M.; Zhou, J.; Zou, A.; Li, W.; Yao, C.; Xie, S. DDSolver: An add-in program for modeling and comparison of drug dissolution profiles. *AAPS J.* **2010**, *12*, 263–271. [CrossRef] [PubMed]

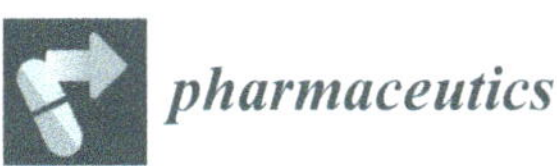 *pharmaceutics*

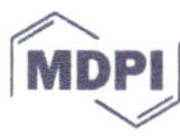

Article

The Solubility Studies and the Complexation Mechanism Investigations of Biologically Active Spiro[cyclopropane-1,3′-oxindoles] with β-Cyclodextrins

Anna A. Kravtsova [1,2], Anna A. Skuredina [1], Alexander S. Malyshev [2,3], Irina M. Le-Deygen [1,*], Elena V. Kudryashova [1] and Ekaterina M. Budynina [1]

[1] Department of Chemistry, Lomonosov Moscow State University, 119991 Moscow, Russia
[2] Faculty of Medicine, Lomonosov Moscow State University, 119991 Moscow, Russia
[3] Dukhov Research Institute of Automatics (VNIIA), 127030 Moscow, Russia
* Correspondence: i.m.deygen@gmail.com

Abstract: In this work, we first improved the aqueous solubility of biologically active spiro[cyclopropane-1,3′-oxindoles] (SCOs) via their complexation with different β-cyclodextrins (β-CDs) and proposed a possible mechanism of the complex formation. β-CDs significantly increased the water solubility of SCOs (up to fourfold). Moreover, the nature of the substituents in the β-CDs influenced the solubility of the guest molecule (MβCD > SBEβCD > HPβCD). Complexation preferably occurred via the inclusion of aromatic moieties of SCOs into the hydrophobic cavity of β-CDs by the numerous van der Waals contacts and formed stable supramolecular systems. The phase solubility technique and optical microscopy were used to determine the dissociation constants of the complexes ($K_c \sim 10^2 \ M^{-1}$) and reveal a significant decrease in the size of the formed crystals. FTIR-ATR microscopy, PXRD, and ^{1}H-^{1}H ROESY NMR measurements, as well as molecular modeling studies, were carried out to elucidate the host–guest interaction mechanism of the complexation. Additionally, in vitro experiments were carried out and revealed enhancements in the antibacterial activity of SCOs due to their complexation with β-CDs.

Keywords: β-cyclodextrins; cyclopropanes; spirooxindoles; inclusion complexes; solubility; antibacterial activity

Citation: Kravtsova, A.A.; Skuredina, A.A.; Malyshev, A.S.; Le-Deygen, I.M.; Kudryashova, E.V.; Budynina, E.M. The Solubility Studies and the Complexation Mechanism Investigations of Biologically Active Spiro[cyclopropane-1,3′-oxindoles] with β-Cyclodextrins. *Pharmaceutics* **2023**, *15*, 228. https://doi.org/10.3390/pharmaceutics15010228

Academic Editor: Hisham Al-Obaidi

Received: 6 December 2022
Revised: 5 January 2023
Accepted: 6 January 2023
Published: 9 January 2023

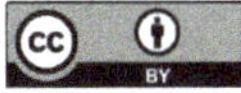

1. Introduction

Spirocyclic compounds have important applications in medicinal chemistry due to the tetrahedral nature of the spiro-linked carbon. Namely, spirooxindoles serve as privileged scaffolds in drug discovery [1]. Many spirooxindole derivatives were found to play fundamental roles in biological processes and exhibit important pharmacological activities [2]. Meanwhile, the spiro-fusion of the oxindole scaffold with a cyclopropane unit allows for the creation of perspective drug candidates due to the enhancement of conformational rigidity, as well as chemical and metabolic stability [3]. For example, CFI-400945, a potent Polo-like kinase 4 (PLK4) inhibitor, and RV-521, a viral fusion inhibitor, advanced into Phase II clinical trials for the treatment of human cancers and RSV infection, respectively (Figure 1) [4,5]. Additionally, several compounds bearing spirocyclopropaneoxindole (SCO) scaffolds are currently under active development: namely, anti-HIV agents [6], bromodomain-containing protein 4 inhibitors [7], progesterone receptor antagonists [8], thyroid hormone receptor-beta agonists [9], AMP-activated protein kinase activators [10], serotonergic agents [11], and non-receptor tyrosine kinase inhibitors [12].

In drug development, aqueous solubility is a critical factor in substrate selection; up to 77% of screened compounds were reported to have inadequate solubility for subsequent testing. Poor aqueous solubility may be responsible for the decrease in the pharmacological effect and may cause other biological problems [13]. Supramolecular hosts, such as cyclodextrins (CDs), are widely used to improve the aqueous solubility and other properties of drug-like molecules, e.g., stability and bioavailability [14].

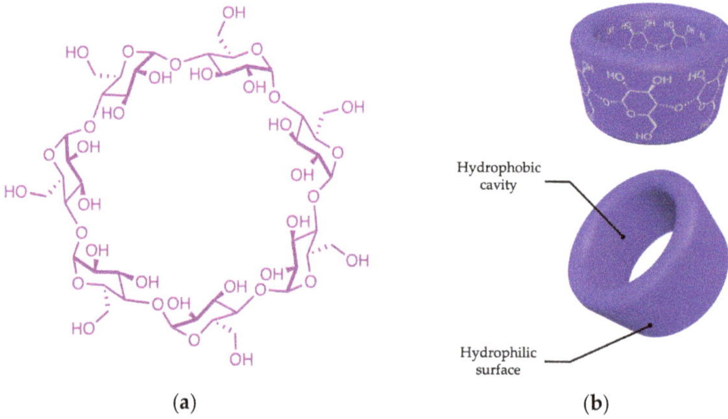

Figure 1. Examples of reported bioactive SCOs.

CDs are cyclic oligosaccharides containing five or more D-glucopyranose residues that are linked by $\alpha(1{\rightarrow}4)$-glycosidic bonds into a toroidal-shaped macrocycles (Figure 2). The external face of CDs is hydrophilic due to the presence of primary and secondary OH groups, whereas the internal cavity is relatively nonpolar [15]. These features of CD structures predispose them to encapsulate hydrophobic moieties, forming host-guest inclusion complexes and improving the guest molecule stability, solubility, and bioavailability [16].

Figure 2. Schematic representations of (**a**) general chemical structure and (**b**) 3D structure of β-CD.

The most common CDs, otherwise known as parent CDs, consist of six (α-CD), seven (β-CD), or eight (γ-CD) glucopyranose rings. The difference in the sizes of the inner cavity in the parent CDs steers them towards guest molecules with appropriate sizes and structures. For SCOs with aromatic fragments, β-CD is the most suitable host, as it has the most suitable cavity size for benzene ring entrapment [17,18]. Recently, CD derivatives with various substituents at the pyranose hydroxyl groups were used to increase the efficiency of complexation [19].

In this paper, we discuss an approach to improving the aqueous solubility of SCOs and, consequently, their biological activity via the formation of inclusive complexes with β-CDs. Therefore, 3′-Aryl-substituted SCOs **2** were synthesized as new model substrates to study the efficiency and the underlying mechanism of complexation with β-CDs.

2. Materials and Methods

2.1. Materials

The 2-hydroxypropyl β-cyclodextrin (HPβCD) and methyl β-cyclodextrin (MβCD) are both from Sigma-Aldrich (St. Louis, MO, USA). Sulfobutyl ether β-cyclodextrin sodium salt (SBEβCD) is from Zibo Qianhui Biotechnology Co. (Zibo, Shandong, China). Ethanol is from Reakhim (Moscow, Russia). Sodium phosphate buffer tablets for solution preparation were obtained from Pan-Eco (Russian Federation). *E. coli* ATCC 25922 is from the Russian collection of industrial microorganisms of the Kurchatov Institute, National Research Institute Centre.

2.2. Methods

2.2.1. Synthesis of Investigated Compounds

General Information

NMR spectra were acquired at room temperature; the chemical shifts δ were measured in ppm with respect to solvent (1H: CDCl$_3$, δ = 7.27 ppm; ^{13}C: CDCl$_3$, δ = 77.0 ppm). Splitting patterns are designated as s, singlet; d, doublet; t, triplet; m, multiplet; dd, double doublet. Coupling constants (*J*) are given in hertz. The structures of all compounds were elucidated with the aid of 1D NMR (1H, 13C) and 2D NMR (ROESY 1H−1H) spectroscopy. High-resolution mass spectra (HRMS) were performed using ESI and a TOF mass analyzer. Analytical thin-layer chromatography (TLC) was carried out with silica gel plates (silica gel 60, F254, supported on aluminum) and was visualized with a UV lamp (254 nm). Column chromatography was performed on silica gel 60 (230−400 mesh). NaH (60% dispersion in mineral oil) and trimethylsulfoxonium iodide are available commercially. Alkenes 1a–d and cyclopropanes 2a–d were prepared by Knoevenagel/Corey−Chaykovsky reactions [20,21], starting from the corresponding aldehydes, according to the published procedures [22]. Their spectra and physical data are consistent with earlier published data, except for the unreported compounds **1a,d** and **2a,d**. Their spectral and physical data are given in Supplementary Materials. All the reactions were carried out using freshly distilled and dry solvents.

General Procedure for the Synthesis of Alkenes 1

An aromatic aldehyde (1.1 equiv) was added to a solution of 1-methylindolin-2-one (1.0 equiv) in ethanol (1 M). The resulting solution was added dropwise to a solution of sodium hydroxide (2.0 equiv) in ethanol−water (1:2, 0.67 M) at 0 °C (ice bath). When the addition was completed, the reaction mixture was allowed to warm up to room temperature and was stirred for a specified time. Then, the reaction mixture was diluted with water and extracted with ethyl acetate. The organic layer was washed with water, dried with sodium sulfate, and concentrated under reduced pressure. Alkene 1 was purified by column chromatography on silica gel.

General Procedure for the Synthesis of Cyclopropanes 2

A suspension of sodium hydride (2.2 equiv) and trimethylsulfoxonium iodide (2.0 equiv) in DMF was stirred at room temperature for 30 min, then a solution of alkene 1 (1.0 equiv) in DMF was added dropwise. When addition was completed, the reaction mixture was stirred at room temperature for a specified time. Then, the reaction mixture was diluted with water and extracted with ethyl acetate. The organic layer was washed with water, dried with sodium sulfate, and concentrated under reduced pressure. The residue was washed with petroleum ether and dried.

2.3. Measurements

2.3.1. Solubility Studies

The samples solubility was studied by shake-flask method, as performed in [23]. Briefly, 5 mg of the sample was added to 5 mL of buffer solution in a glass vial. The solutions were intensely stirred at 25 °C for 6 h to achieve thermodynamic equilibrium. For dissolution rate studies, the aliquots were taken in the time range from 0.5 to 6 h. As sedimentation time significantly influences equilibrium solubility, all samples were stored without stirring for 18 h. Then, the concentration of dissolved sample was analyzed by UV spectroscopy. Physical mixture (PM) was performed by mixing 2a and CD powders. In the case of the kneading method (KM), the mixture was grinded until a homogeneous mass formed.

The phase solubility studies were conducted according to the well-known Higuchi and Connons method [24–26]. The K_c values of the complexes were calculated regarding the phase solubility diagram:

$$K_c = \frac{slope}{S_0(1 - slope)}$$

where S_0 is the solubility of **2**.

The experiments were carried out three times, and the values are presented with standard deviations.

2.3.2. UV Spectroscopy

The UV spectra were recorded by a Ultrospec 2100 pro instrument (Amersham Biosciences, Germany), within a wavelength range from 200 nm to 450 nm in a 1 mL quartz cell Hellma Analytics (Müllheim, Germany). The concentration of **2** was determined using the intensity at 265 nm.

2.3.3. FTIR Microscopy

The FTIR microscopy was performed by the Bruker LUMOS FTIR microscope (Bruker, Ettlingen, Germany). The FTIR spectra were recorded in 4000–800 cm^{-1} regions with 2 cm^{-1} spectral resolution in ATR mode. For each spectrum, 70-fold scanning and averaging were carried out. The background was recorded according to the measurement position. The spectra and images were analyzed by Opus 8.2.28 software.

2.3.4. Dynamic Light Scattering (DLS)

DLS was used to determine the size of the particles by a Zetasizer Nano S «Malvern» equipped with 4 mW He–Ne-laser 633 nm (Malvern Instruments, Malvern, UK). The experiments were performed three times for each sample at 25 °C, using the Correlator system K7032-09 Malvern (Worcestershire, UK) and the software Zetasizer Software (Malvern Instruments, Malvern, UK). The values are reported with standard deviations.

2.3.5. Powder X-ray Diffraction Analysis (PXRD)

PXRD patterns of **2** and their complexes with CDs (7–10 mg) were recorded using a Rigaku SmartLab (Rigaku Corporation, Tokyo, Japan), equipped with Cu-X-ray anode tube in the scanning range 1.5–80.0° with a step size of 5°/sec. X-rays were generated with 60 kV and 1.5 kW.

2.3.6. Minimum Inhibition Concentration (MIC)

The overnight culture was used for all in vitro experiments (the bacteria were grown in Luria Bertuni medium for 12 h). MIC was determined by agar well diffusion method [27]. Briefly, overnight bacteria (500 µL) were distributed over the solid agar surface (15 mL of Luria Bertuni medium) on Petri dishes. Four wells were incised in the medium by sterile plastic pipette tip (d = 10 mm). The 50 µL was put in the wells (three for the samples and one for negative control (sterile buffer)). The CD-SCO complexes were obtained by KM method (molar ratio 3: 1). In 20 min, the Petri dishes were placed into the incubator at

37 °C for 24 h. Then, the appeared inhibition zones were analyzed. The experiments were carried out three times. The MICs are reported with standard deviations.

2.3.7. System Preparation

Methyl-β-CD (MβCD) and ligands structures were constructed using the 3D-sketcher module in Maestro (Schrödinger, 2021) and then submitted to 10,000 steps of Polak–Ribiere conjugate gradient energy minimization by means of the Macromodel software (Schrödinger, 2021), using the OPLS3e force field [28] and GB/SA model as solvation treatment [29]. Docking studies were performed with the Glide program [30], using the centroid of MβCD to centre the grid box as docking space. Docking poses with RMS deviation <0.5 Å were discarded, and at most five docking poses were retrieved and subjected to a visual analysis. The best scoring pose of each stereoisomer was selected for further modeling (Table S1; Supplementary Materials).

2.3.8. Force-Field Parameterization

For MβCD and ligands, General Amber Force-Field 2 (GAFF2) parameterization [31,32] was chosen, and charges were assigned using the AM1-BCC method [33] with bond charge corrections. All parametrization procedures were made using the AnteChamber Python Parser Interface (ACPYPE) v. 2022.6.6 [34].

2.3.9. System Preparation and Simulation of Molecular Dynamics (MD)

Each system, consisting of MβCD molecule (168 atoms) and docked ligand (approx. 50 atoms), was immersed in the cell, with 1 nm distance between the solute and the cell, and filled with TIP3P water model [35]. The system energy was optimized using the gradient descent algorithm (1000 steps). For solvent equilibration, both temperature and pressure coupling with 5000 steps were performed. Classical MD simulations of 50 ns (25 ∗ 106 steps with a step length of 2 fs) trajectories for each system were performed (Figure S2; Supplementary Materials). For all simulation routines, including energy minimization and equilibration, the GROMACS [36] (v. 2021.3) program package was used as MD engine.

3. Results and Discussion

3.1. Synthesis of SCOs 2

Initially, we synthesized SCOs **2a–d** with various aryls at the three-membered ring via a two-step procedure starting from *N*-(*p*-methoxybenzyl)oxindole (*N*-PMB-oxindole) and the corresponding aromatic aldehydes (Figure 3). The synthetic sequence included Knoevenagel condensation and a Corey–Chaykovsky reaction [37,38]. This simple, cheap, and efficient method allows for a wide variation of substituents in the final SCOs by using various commercially available aldehydes and oxindoles. SCOs **2a–d** were obtained in good yields as diastereomeric mixtures.

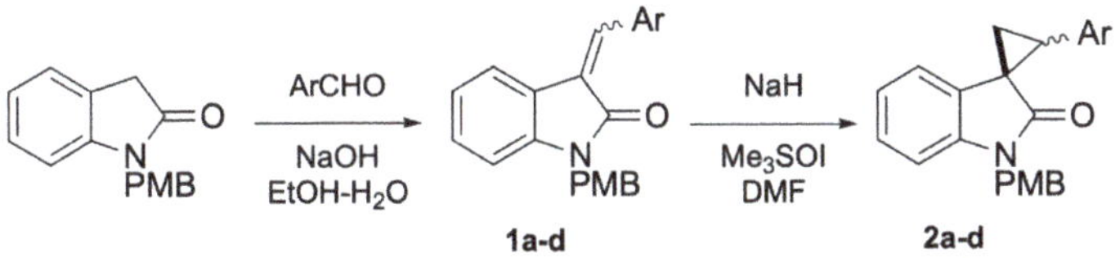

1a-d **2a-d**

2a: Ar = 2-ClC$_6$H$_4$, 92%, dr 71:29
2b: Ar = 4-NCC$_6$H$_4$, 83%, dr 58:42
2c: Ar = 4-*t*-BuC$_6$H$_4$, 82%, dr 70:30
2d: Ar = 3,4-(MeO)$_2$C$_6$H$_3$, 86%, dr 70:30

Figure 3. Synthesis of SCOs **2**.

3.2. Solubility of SCOs 2

As expected, SCOs **2a–d** are hydrophobic compounds due to the presence of three benzene rings in their molecules. Their intrinsic solubilities (*S*) were studied within two different aqueous media with the pH values of 7.4 (sodium phosphate buffer) and 2.0 (0.01 M HCl), simulating physiological conditions: blood plasma and stomach acid, respectively.

In the UV spectra of the resulting solutions, wide absorption bands with maxima at ca. 265 nm were detected in all cases.

We found that the increase in S strongly correlates with the increase in the polarity of aryl substituents in SCOs **2**: $S_{2c} < S_{2a} < S_{2d} < S_{2b}$ (Table 1). As the samples do not possess pH-sensitive groups, the changes in pH did not influence the S values in any noticeable way; thus, further experiments were conducted at neutral pH.

Table 1. Intrinsic solubilities (S) of SCOs **2**.

2	Ar	S [a], mg/mL
a	$2\text{-}ClC_6H_4$	0.18 ± 0.02
b	$4\text{-}NCC_6H_4$	0.84 ± 0.03
c	$4\text{-}t\text{-}BuC_6H_4$	0.11 ± 0.02
d	$3,4\text{-}(MeO)_2C_6H_3$	0.27 ± 0.03

[a] Suspensions of **2** (1 mg/mL) in sodium phosphate buffer (pH 7.4), shake-flask method.

Herein, we obtained SCOs with four substituents, with different position patterns and electronic effects. Although these groups seemed quite similar (primary as hydrophobic ones), some of them could participate in other interesting intermolecular interactions: -Cl participates in halogen bonding and hydrophobic interactions[39], and -CN can form intermolecular H-bonds by N as acceptor and, less often, hydrophobic contacts [40].

Thus, cyclopropanes **2a** and **2b** were chosen as model compounds in this study.

3.3. Preparation of SCO 2–β-CD Complexes

β-CD complexes with SCOs **2** were prepared using several techniques [41,42]. Among them, the physical mixture approach (PM) and the kneading method (KM) were found to be the most efficient and reliable for highly hydrophobic compounds. Additionally, these approaches can affect the size and morphology of the formed particles [41].

First, we tried obtaining the complexes of hydroxypropyl-β-CD (HPβCD) with SCOs **2** in a 3:1 molar ratio, assuming that all 3 aromatic units of **2** were participating in complexation. The HPβCD-**2a** complexes were employed as model compounds in our solubility study.

Visually, complexation led to a significant increase in S. Although the bulk of **2a** remained undissolved, the HPβCD-**2a** complexes prepared via both PM and KM afforded white suspensions (Figure S1). According to our optical microscopy study, the crystal size significantly decreased for HPβCD-**2a** vs. free **2a** (Figure 4). The sample of **2a** contained large particles with arbitrary shapes (Figure 4a), whereas in the samples of **HPβCD-2a** prepared via PM (Figure 4b) and KM (Figure 4c), noticeably smaller uniform particles could be found.

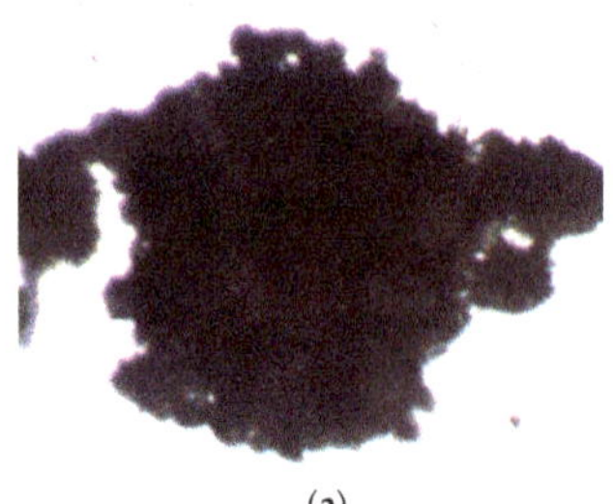
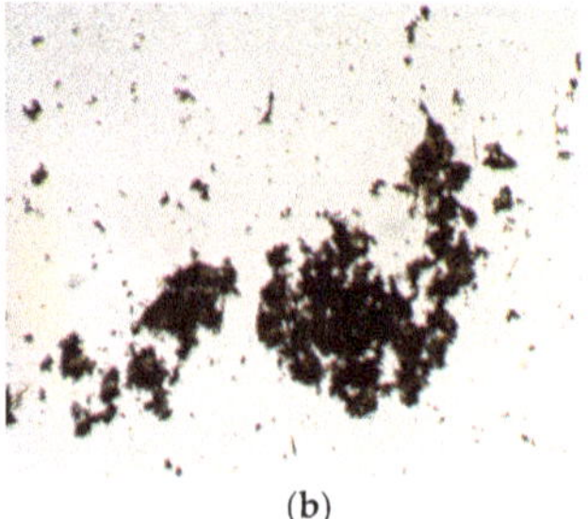
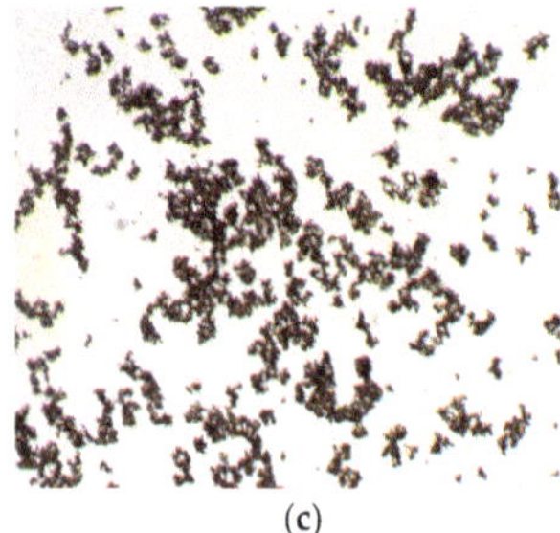

(a) (b) (c)

Figure 4. Influence of complexation with HPβCD on **2a** solubility (photomicrographs at ×10 magnification): suspensions of **2a** (a) and **HPβCD-2a** prepared by PM (b) and KM (c). $C_{2a} = 1$ mg/mL, $C_{HPβCD} = 12$ mg/mL, pH 7.4.

Next, the supernatants of these samples were analyzed via dynamic light scattering (DLS). Per this analysis, **2a** formed a homogenous solution with 1320 ± 32 nm particles (Figure 5, hydrodynamic diameter). The particles of the HPβCD-**2a** complex were significantly smaller: 490 ± 18 nm (PM) and 420 ± 20 nm (KM). This supports the increase in S upon complexation. The smaller size of particles provides a number of advantages: increased bioactivity, reduced side effects, and increased cell penetration.

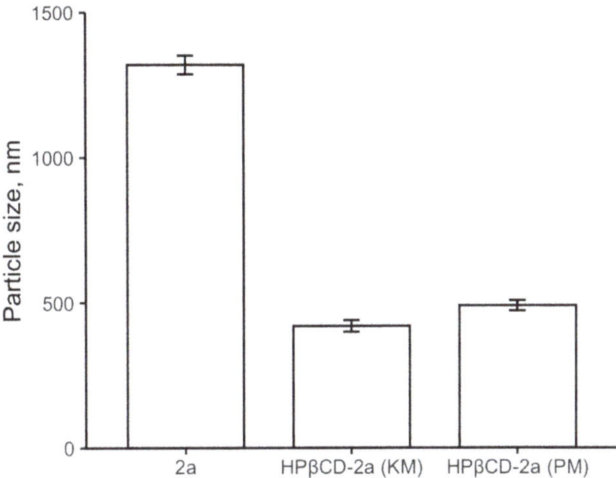

Figure 5. Size of particles in supernatants of **2a** and HPβCD-**2a** complex prepared by KM and PM. $C_{\mathbf{2a}} = 1$ mg/mL, $C_{\mathbf{HP\beta CD}} = 12$ mg/mL, pH 7.4.

Furthermore, the formation of the HPβCD-**2a** complex dramatically increased the intensity of the absorption maximum at ca. 265 nm, corresponding to **2a** in the UV spectra. The $S_{\mathbf{2a}}$ value (0.18 ± 0.02 mg/mL for free **2a**) increased up to 0.57 ± 0.05 mg/mL and 0.67 ± 0.04 mg/mL for **2a** in complexes prepared via PM and KM, respectively. As KM provided the highest $S_{\mathbf{2a}}$ value, we used this method for our further experiments.

3.4. Phase Solubility Studies

The phase solubility technique developed by Higuchi and Connons [24–26] was used to study the HPβCD-**2a** complex in order to elucidate how the concentration of HPβCD affected the guest compound solubility and to determine the host-guest molar ratio, as well as the value of K_c, the binding constant.

According to the measured phase-solubility profile, at pH 7.4, $S_{\mathbf{2a}}$ linearly rises at low HPβCD concentrations until saturation (A_N-type profile) (Figure 6, red curve). The decreased solubilization effect of CDs at higher concentrations can be attributed to the limited aqueous solubility of **2a**, the changes in viscosity and/or surface tension, or to self-association of CD molecules [24,42]. The highest $S_{\mathbf{2a}}$ value was determined at the HPβCD:**2a** molar ratio of 3:1, which might be explained by the saturation of all **2a** binding sites (all 3 aromatic fragments interact with CDs). We achieved an almost 4-fold increase of **2a** solubility (~0.2 mg/mL compared to 0.67 mg/mL).

The formation of ternary complexes might provide the enhancement of inclusion affinity [43]. We used ethanol as a third component that might also increase the $S_{\mathbf{2a}}$ value by the decrease in the medium polarity (Figure 6, blue curve). Indeed, ethanol (10 vol%) increased the solubility of **2a**, though the effect is not significant. The K_c values were determined by analyzing the linear ranges of the isotherms for 1:1 stoichiometry of complexation [44,45]: $K_c = 235 \pm 8$ M^{-1} (pH 7.4) and $K_c = 277 \pm 11$ M^{-1} (pH 7.4 + 10 vol%

EtOH). The determined K_c correspond to a range of values (ca. $50 \div 104\ \mathrm{M}^{-1}$) reported for the complexes with β-CDs with biologically active molecules [46–49].

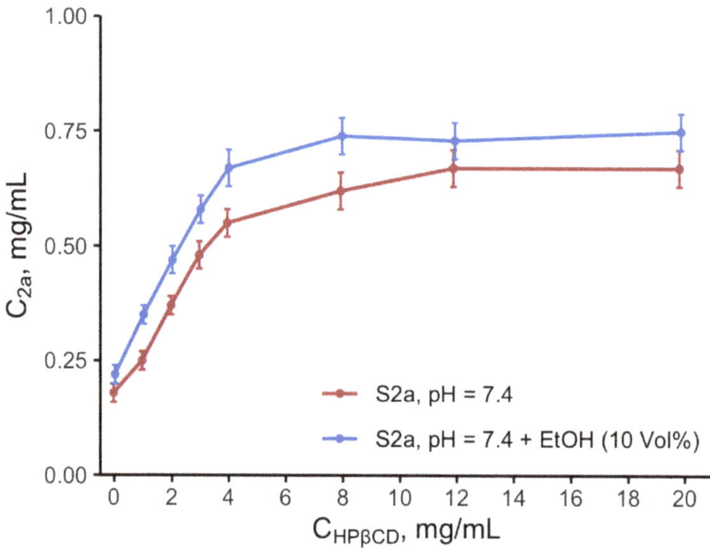

Figure 6. Phase-solubility profiles for HPβCD-**2a** complex in sodium phosphate buffer (pH 7.4) (red curve) and in sodium phosphate buffer (pH 7.4) with EtOH (10 vol%) (blue curve), C_{2a} =1 mg/mL, shake-flask method.

3.5. Influence of Substituents at β-CDs on SCO Solubility

The nature of substituents in the CDs might also influence the solubility of the guest molecule. For example, a similar effect was revealed for β-CD complexes with fluoroquinolones, wherein the substituents in the β-CDs additionally interacted with guest molecules, increasing the efficiency of complexation [47].

To reveal the effect of the substituents in β-CDs on their complexation with **2a**, two additional common β-CDs were examined: methyl-β-CD (MβCD) and sulfobutyl ether β-CD (SBEβCD) [17,26]. In terms of overall substituent polarity, the examined β-CDs can be rated as follows: SBEβCD > HPβCD > MβCD. We found that varying β-CDs had no noticeable effect on the type of phase-solubility profiles or ranges of saturation. Nevertheless, differences in complexation efficiency at low β-CDs molar excess were detected: $K_c = 235 \pm 8\ \mathrm{M}^{-1}$ (HPβCD-**2a**), $K_c = 294 \pm 11\ \mathrm{M}^{-1}$ (MβCD-**2a**), $K_c = 245 \pm 9\ \mathrm{M}^{-1}$ (SBEβCD-**2a**).

As MβCD provided the highest solubility for **2a**, we also investigated the MβCD-**2b** complex. As the intrinsic S_{2b} value was found to be almost five times higher than that of S_{2a} (Table 1), we could expect a higher K_c value for MβCD-**2b** vs. MβCD-**2a**. Indeed, the K_c value of the MβCD-**2b** complex was $574 \pm 12\ \mathrm{M}^{-1}$, ca. 2 times higher than that for MβCD-**2a**. Notably, for MβCD-**2b**, saturation was achieved at an MβCD:**2b** molar ratio of ca. 2:1, whereas for MβCD-**2a**, the ratio was ca. 3:1. As CDs mostly affect poorly soluble guest molecules, corresponding to Class II Drugs, according to the Biopharmaceutics Classification System [50], the limited effect of MβCD on the solubility of **2b** might be attributed to the high initial S_{2b} value.

Complex formation might change not only the solubility of the samples, but also the dissolution rate. The effect of stirring time on the equilibrium solubility is reasonable to be investigated during first 6 h [23]. Figure 7 demonstrates that MβCD pronouncedly increases the **2b** dissolution rate after 2 h of incubation. At 6 h, $S_{\mathrm{MβCD\text{-}2b}}$ is higher than S_{2b} on 15%.

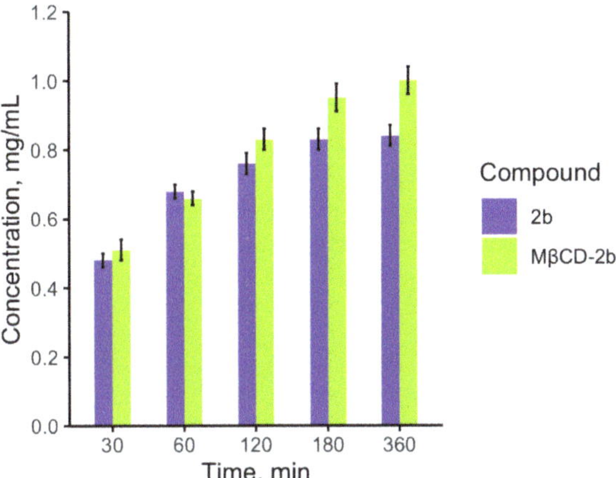

Figure 7. The dissolution rate of **2b** and MβCD-**2b**, sodium phosphate buffer (pH 7.4), shake-flask method.

3.6. Characterization of Inclusion Complexes

3.6.1. PXRD Analysis

To determine the degree of crystallinity for SCOs **2a,b** and their complexes with β-CDs, we used powder X-ray diffraction (PXRD) [51,52]. Narrow intense peaks in the PXRD patterns of **2a** and **2b** point to the predominance of crystalline forms (Figure 8a,d). The PXRD patterns for MβCD mainly represent an amorphous state, agreeing with reported data [53]. The formation of the β-CD-SCO complex affects the PXRD pattern: a halo appears, corresponding to a decrease in the degree of crystallinity (Figure 8b,c,e). This agrees well with the data reported for other β-CD complexes [47].

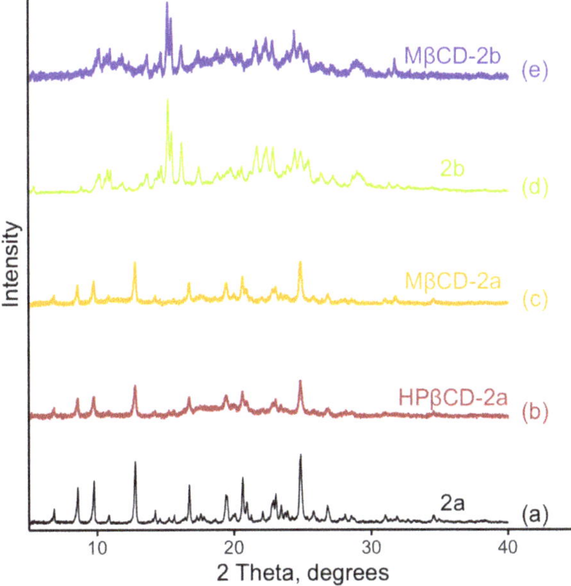

Figure 8. PXRD patterns for (**a**) **2a**; (**b**) HPβCD-**2a**; (**c**) MβCD-**2a**; (**d**) **2b**; (**e**) MβCD-**2b**. No signals were observed at 40−80°.

The degree of crystallinity is a crucial factor in drug development. For instance, the amorphous intraconazole formulation exhibited significantly higher systemic bioavailability via pulmonary administration than the nanocrystalline drug form [54]. Therefore, the decrease in crystallinity for the β-CD-SCO complexes might improve the biological activity of SCO.

3.6.2. FTIR Microscopy

The structures of the β-CD-SCO complexes were also studied via FTIR microscopy. This allowed us to detect changes in the microenvironments of the functional groups in molecules upon complexation. Moreover, macrostructure FTIR microscopy provides a pathway to determining the distribution of the guest molecules and the ratio of components in the complexes [55].

The main analytically significant absorption bands in the FTIR spectrum of HPβCD are located at 1220–950 cm^{-1} [56]. The most intense bands at 1032, 1083, and 1172 cm^{-1} correspond to the valence vibrations of C–O–C, C–H, and C–O–H groups, respectively.

In our FTIR spectrum of **2a** (Figure 9c, Table 2), the broad peaks at 2935 and 2840 cm^{-1} correspond to C-H$_{Alk}$ [57–59], while the intense peaks at 1697 and 1613 cm^{-1} correspond to amide I and II, respectively. The peaks in the 1430–1650 cm^{-1} range correspond to the C=C bonds in the aromatic rings.

All of these bands were observed in the FTIR spectra of the HPβCD-**2a** complex, as well (Figure 9c, Table 2). The intensity ratio for the peaks corresponding to HPβCD:**2a** was preserved for all the examined regions in the sample (Figure 9b, green circles), leading us to the conclusion that **2a** was uniformly distributed throughout the sample. The overall decrease in the intensity for the **2a** peaks might indicate complexation, as a similar effect was observed in the FTIR spectra of other β-CD-guest complexes [18].

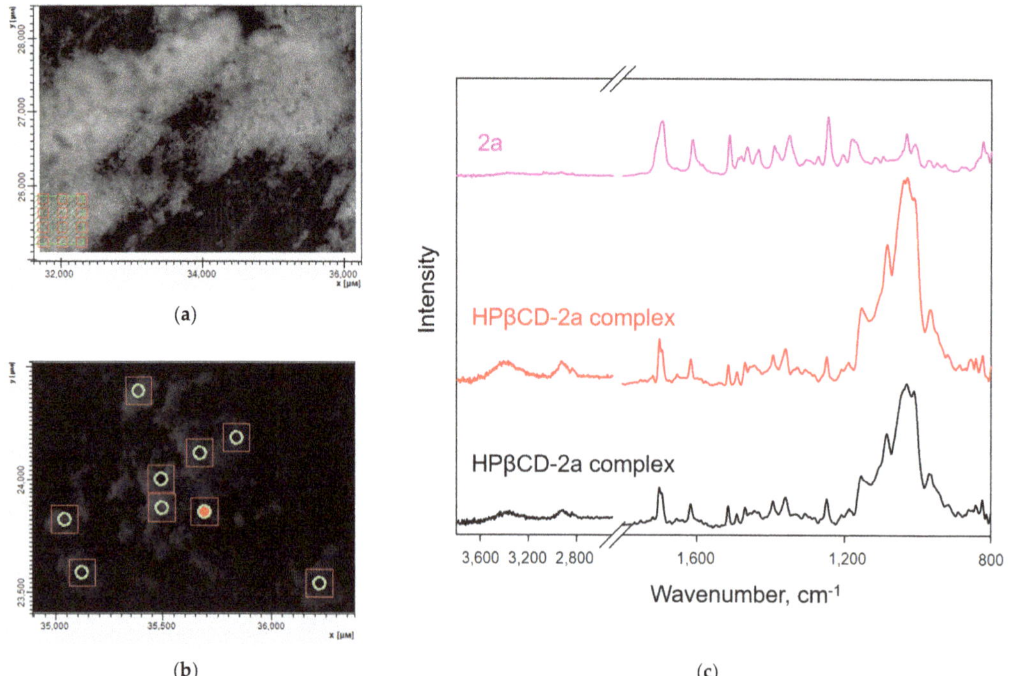

Figure 9. Microscopy photo of (**a**) **2a** and (**b**) HPβCD-**2a** complex. (**c**) FTIR spectra of **2a** (pink curve) and HPβCD-**2a** [red and black curves correspond to red and black areas circled in light-green in the photo (**b**)].

Table 2. Peaks in FTIR spectra of **2a** and HPβCD-**2a**, cm^{-1}.

	2a	HPβCD-2a
C-H$_{Alk}$	2935 ± 0.5	2935 ± 0.5
	2840 ± 0.5	2840 ± 0.5
Amide I (C=O)	1697 ± 0.5	1701 ± 0.5
Amide II (N-C=O)	1613 ± 0.5	1617 ± 0.5
C$_{Ar}$-H	1481 ± 0.5	-
C-O-C$_{Ar}$	1246 ± 0.5	1248 ± 0.5
C$_{Ar}$-Cl	1031 ± 0.5	1030 ± 0.5

In order to clarify the structure of HPβCD-**2a**, we took a closer look at the shifts in the positions of the initial **2a** bands (Table 2). The high-frequency shifts of the peaks at 1697, 1613, and 1650–1430 cm^{-1} uncovered that the N-C=O group and the aromatic rings were involved in complexation. As for the peaks corresponding to C-Cl (1031 cm^{-1}) and C-O-C$_{Ar}$ (1246 cm^{-1}) in **2a**, the former did not change its position, whereas the latter underwent a high-frequency shift that could point to the PMB group being involved in complexation. We could not determine whether the CH$_2$ groups participated in complexation because the C-HAlk vibrations region of 3050–2700 cm^{-1} is less informative due to the broadening and the decrease in the intensity of the bands. Thus, the FTIR results pointed to the formation of an HPβCD-**2a** inclusion complex, wherein the PMB group of **2a** was captured by the hydrophobic cavity of HPβCD, with the cyclopropane and *o*-chlorophenyl fragments sticking out.

3.6.3. Two-Dimensional NMR Spectroscopy: ^{1}H-^{1}H ROESY Experiments

An ^{1}H-^{1}H ROESY NMR spectrum was detected for the HPβCD-**2b** complex to support the complexation hypothesis. The cross-peaks between the signals assigned to the H atoms of the PMB group in **2b** and the H-3 and H-5 atoms of HPβCD (Figure 10a, circled in red) indicated the capture of the PMB moiety by the hydrophobic cavity of HPβCD (Figure 10b). These results agree with those of the FTIR experiments quite nicely.

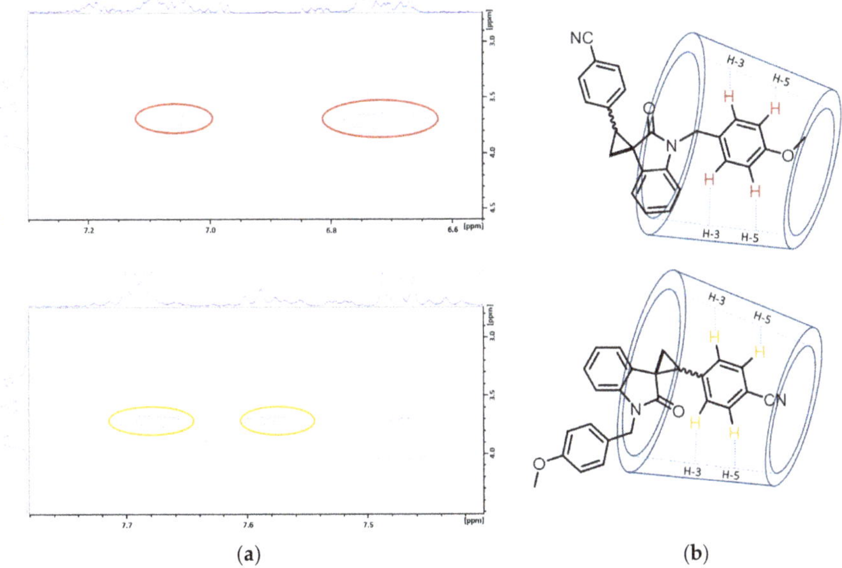

(**a**)   (**b**)

Figure 10. (**a**) Fragment of ^{1}H-^{1}H ROESY NMR spectrum of the HPβCD-**2b** complex; (**b**) possible inclusion modes of HPβCD-**2b**.

Meanwhile, the less intensive cross-peaks between the signals of the H atoms in the *p*-cyanophenyl ring and the H-3 and H-5 atoms of HPβCD were also detected (Figure 10a, circled in yellow). This pointed to the alternative possibility of complexation via insertion of the *p*-cyanophenyl group into the HPβCD cavity (Figure 10b).

3.6.4. Molecular Modeling

As of this writing, no experimental structures have been reported for β-CD-SCO complexes. We carried out molecular modeling studies of the MβCD-**2a,b** complexes to determine the main β-CD-**2a,b** interactions and predict the stability of the corresponding complexes.

First, all **2b** stereoisomers were docked into the MβCD cavity. Three possible binding modes (Type I-III) were predicted for the MβCD-**2b** complex (Figure 11).

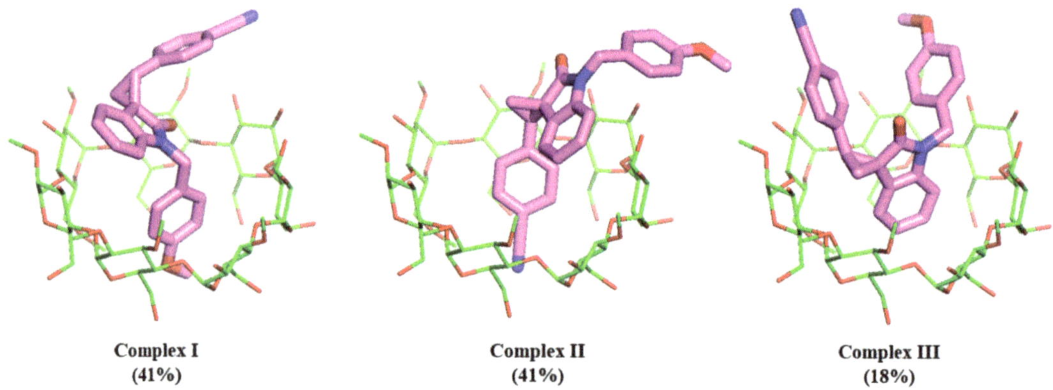

Figure 11. Three predicted MβCD-**2b** complex types.

The Type I and II conformations shared elongated geometries. On the one hand, this allowed them to enter the MβCD cavity with their PMB or *p*-cyanophenyl groups, respectively, resulting in hydrophobic interactions with the backbone atoms and the substituents in MβCD. On the other hand, the 3D configuration of the spiro-center in **2** oriented the substituent at the opposite side of the molecule to align it parallel to the MβCD backbone, forming numerous van der Waals contacts. Additionally, the CN and MeO groups were oriented towards the narrow rim of the MβCD torus and the water molecules. In turn, the water molecules were linked with the MeO groups in MβCD by fluctuating hydrogen bonds.

For the Type III conformation, **2b** adopted a U-shaped geometry, with the oxindole scaffold deeply buried in the MβCD cavity. Notably, the PMB and *p*-cyanophenyl moieties only formed a few hydrophobic contacts and hydrogen bonds with the water molecules of the wide MβCD rim.

MD simulations were performed to identify the favored binding mode, with the discovered Type I-III structures as initial ones.

The root-mean-square deviation (RMSD) and the distance between the center of mass for **2b** and MβCD were monitored to quantitatively assess the structural fluctuations of each binding mode from the resulting trajectories. The Type I complex exhibited the most stable conformation throughout the entire dynamic trajectory (Figure 12), which agrees with the NMR results, supporting primary complexation via the interaction of β-CD with the PMB group in **2b**.

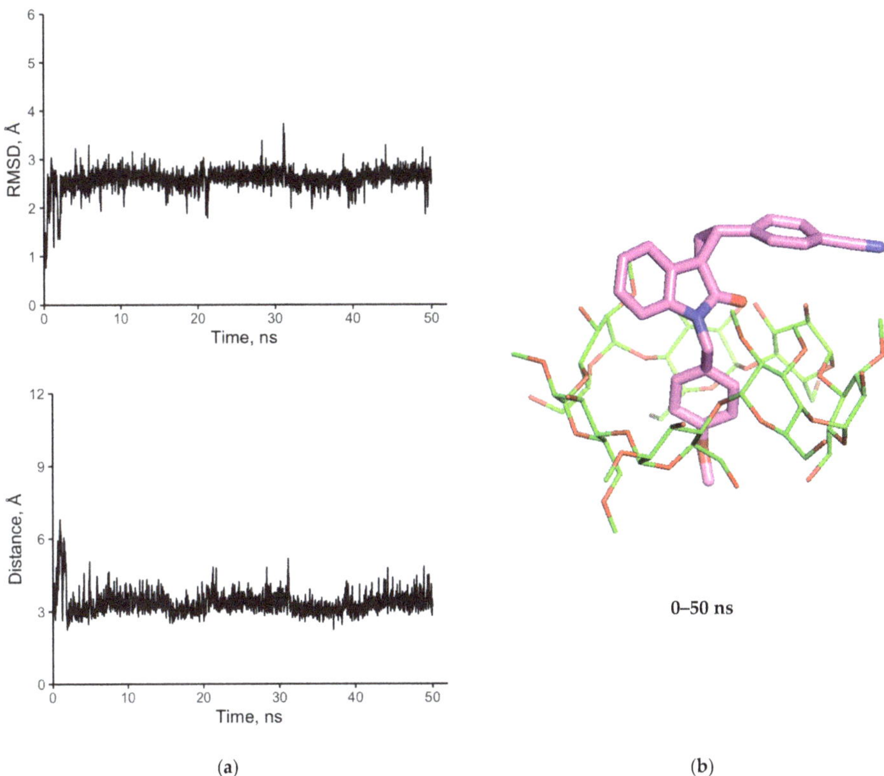

Figure 12. (**a**) Root-mean-square deviation (RMSD) and distance between the MβCD and **2b** centers of geometry (Type I complex). (**b**) Type I complex structure.

At the same time, the Type III conformation with the highest docking score was stable for the first 16 ns of the molecular dynamics trajectory. In our simulation, the complex dissociated between 16 and 20 ns (Figure 13a) to form a new stable Type II geometry, with the *p*-cyanophenyl group deep in the MβCD cavity (Figure 13b).

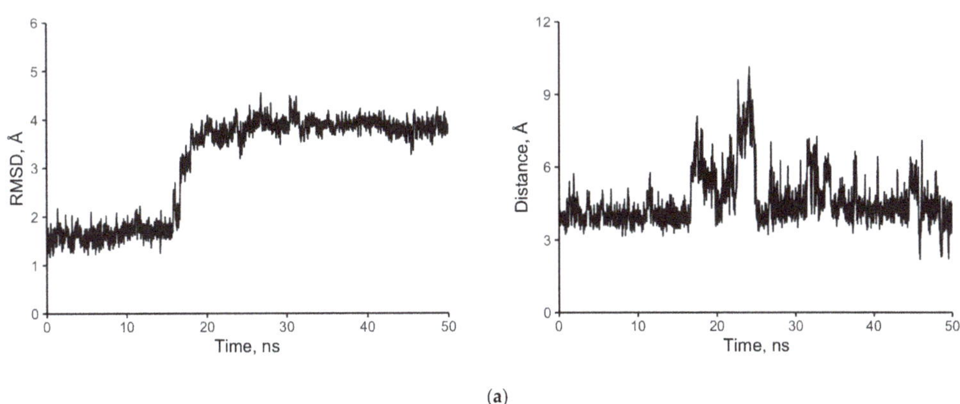

Figure 13. *Cont.*

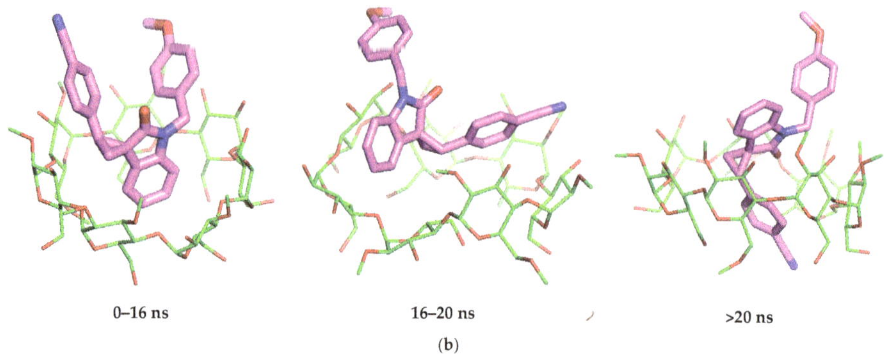

Figure 13. (**a**) Root-mean-square deviation (RMSD) and distance between the MβCD and **2b** centers of geometry (Type III complex). (**b**) Type III complex structure transformation into Type II geometry.

Molecular docking also revealed that the **2a** isomers bind MβCD similarly to the **2b** isomers, forming three types of complexes via the MβCD cavity, capturing one of the three available aromatic fragments. The elongated conformations of the **2a** isomers readily formed complexes, wherein the PMB group was deeply buried in the MβCD cavity (Figure 14a, complex I). This binding mode is in accordance with the FTIR spectroscopic results. The molecular dynamics trajectory for the Type I complex did not show any significant perturbations for the ligand conformation (Figure 14b), possibly pointing to the stability of this type.

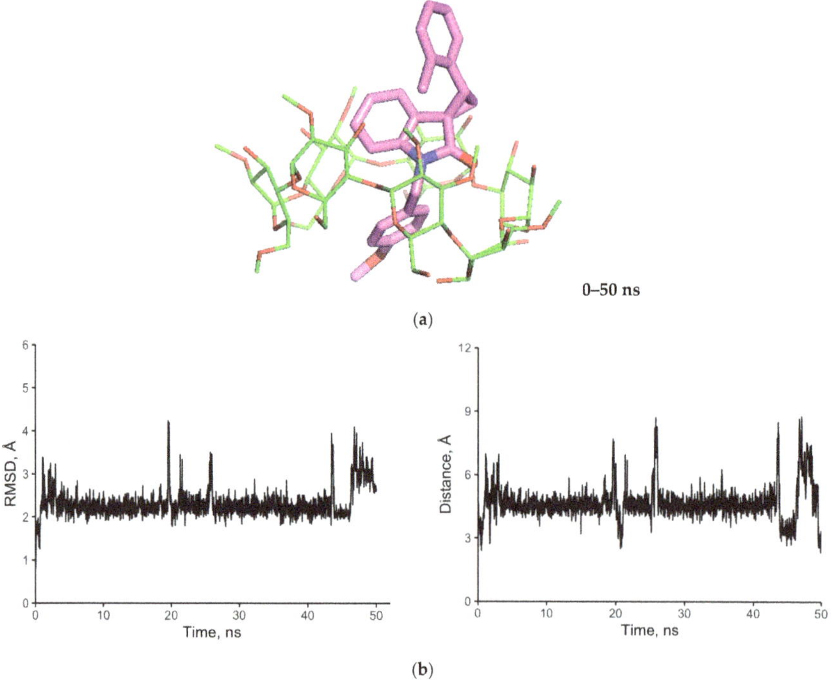

Figure 14. (**a**) Type I complex conformation; (**b**) MβCD and **2a** heavy atoms positions root-mean-square deviation (RMSD) and distance between the MβCD and **2a** centers of geometry (Type I complex).

3.7. Biological Activity of SCOs In Vitro

We tested the potential in vitro activity of **2a,b** SCOs against the gram-negative *E.coli* ATCC 25922 strain.

The minimum inhibition concentration (MIC) was determined via the agar well diffusion method (Figure 15), a fast and robust technique [27,51]. Both **2a** and **2b** inhibited bacteria growth (MIC_{2a}~1000 µg/mL; MIC_{2b}~3 µg/mL) (Table 3), with dose dependency characterizing their antibacterial effect. The significant difference between the MIC values might be associated with differences between the S_{2a} and S_{2b} values.

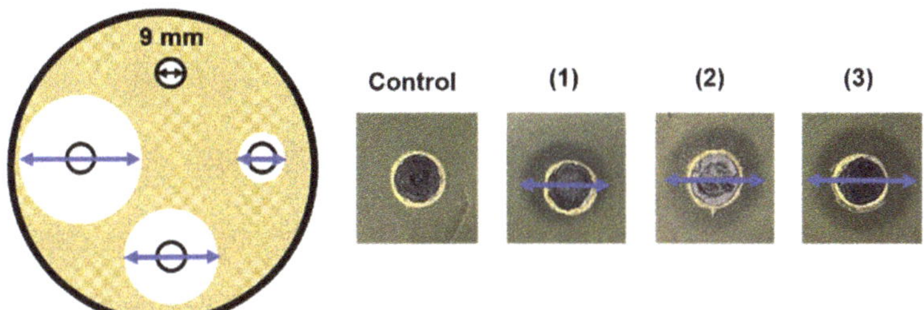

Figure 15. The scheme of the agar well diffusion method. The inhibition zones on Petri dishes appeared after treatment of (1) **2b** 5 µg/mL; (2) **2b** 7 µg/mL; (3) HPβCD-**2b** 10 µg/mL; pH 7.4 (0.01 M sodium phosphate buffer), 37 °C, 24 h of incubation. Blue arrows demonstrate the diameter of the inhibition zone.

Table 3. The MIC values of different samples, pH 7.4 (0.01 M PBS), 37 °C.

MIC, µg/mL	CD	2a	2b
Without CD		1000 ± 35	3.2 ± 0.3
HPβCD	–	150 ± 20	3.0 ± 0.4
MβCD	–	140 ± 23	3.4 ± 0.4

As expected, both HPβCD and MβCD proved to be non-toxic and biodegradable [11,28]. As CDs can decrease the MIC values [51,60], we studied the antibacterial activity of **2a** and **2b** complexes with βCDs. Both HPβCD and MβCD decreased the MIC_{2a} values sevenfold. Nevertheless, the MIC_{2b} values remained the same, despite complexation. Apparently, this is related to a significant increase in S_{2a} via complexation with βCDs, whereas complexation affects S_{2b} only slightly.

4. Conclusions

In conclusion, the strategy of increasing the water solubility of poorly soluble small molecules via complexation with CDs was successfully applied for a promising class of organic molecules, spiro[cyclopropane-1,3′-oxindoles], which are currently under active development in preclinical and clinical trials.

The complexation of spiro[cyclopropane-1,3′-oxindoles] with different β-CDs was first evaluated by phase solubility and optical microscopy studies. The PXRD analysis was also conducted, confirming the crystal size reduction. These results indicate a significant influence of β-CDs on the biopharmaceutical properties of synthesized SCO.

Then, the binding patterns of the observed SCO-βCD interaction were established by FTIR, 2D NMR, and molecular modeling experiments, proving the entrapment of SCO aromatic rings into the hydrophobic cavity of CD. The revealed data are in good agreement in all the cases, providing the most probable mechanism of SCO-βCD complexation.

Furthermore, it has been evidenced that SCO-βCDs were capable of inhibiting bacterial growth. In addition, complexation allowed a significant MIC decrease in the case of SCO with low intrinsic solubility and subsequently revealed an antibacterial effect. These facts elucidate that SCOs are perspective antibacterial agents, and their complexation with CDs is a promising strategy to enhance the water solubility, biological activity, and biopharmaceutical properties of spirooxindole derivatives.

Supplementary Materials: The following supplementary materials can be downloaded at: https://www.mdpi.com/article/10.3390/pharmaceutics15010228/s1, Figure S1: Influence of HPβCD on 2a solubility; Figure S2: RMSD and Distance between the centers of geometry for MβCD-2 (all complexes are shown); Table S1: Molecular formula strings, IUPAC names and docking scores.

Author Contributions: Conceptualization: A.A.K. and A.A.S.; experimental work: A.A.K., A.A.S. and A.S.M.; data analysis and interpretation: A.A.K., A.A.S. and A.S.M.; Writing—Original draft preparation: A.A.K. and A.A.S.; Writing—Review and editing: A.A.K., A.A.S., A.S.M., I.M.L.-D., E.V.K. and E.M.B.; supervision: E.M.B., I.M.L.-D. and E.V.K. All authors have read and agreed to the published version of the manuscript.

Funding: This research received no external funding.

Institutional Review Board Statement: Not applicable.

Informed Consent Statement: Not applicable.

Data Availability Statement: All data generated or analyzed during this study are included in this published article and its Supplementary Information.

Conflicts of Interest: The authors declare no conflict of interest.

References

1. Molvi, K.I.; Haque, N.; Awen, B.Z.S.; Zameeruddin, M. ChemInform abstract: Synthesis of spiro compounds as medicinal agents; New opportunities for drug design and discovery. Part I: A review. *World J. Pharm. Pharm. Sci.* **2014**, *3*, 536–563. [CrossRef]
2. Zhou, L.-M.; Qu, R.-Y.; Yang, G.-F. An overview of spirooxindole as a promising scaffold for Novel drug discovery. *Expert. Opin. Drug Discov.* **2020**, *15*, 603–625. [CrossRef] [PubMed]
3. Talele, T.T. The "Cyclopropyl Fragment" is a versatile player that frequently appears in preclinical/clinical drug molecules. *J. Med. Chem.* **2016**, *59*, 8712–8756. [CrossRef] [PubMed]
4. ClinicalTrials.gov. Available online: https://clinicaltrials.gov/ct2/results?term=CFI-400945&age_v=&gndr=&type=&rslt=&phase=1&phase=2&phase=3&Search=Apply (accessed on 6 November 2022).
5. ClinicalTrials.gov. Available online: https://clinicaltrials.gov/ct2/results?term=RV-521&age_v=&gndr=&type=&rslt=&phase=1&phase=2&phase=3&Search=Apply (accessed on 6 November 2022).
6. Jiang, T.; Kuhen, K.L.; Wolff, K.; Yin, H.; Bieza, K.; Caldwell, J.; Bursulaya, B.; Tuntland, T.; Zhang, K.; Karanewsky, D.; et al. Design, synthesis, and biological evaluations of novel oxindoles as HIV-1 non-nucleoside reverse transcriptase inhibitors. Part 2. *Bioorg. Med. Chem. Lett.* **2006**, *16*, 2109–2112. [CrossRef]
7. Hardee, D.; Brewer, J.; Hasvol, L.; Liu, D.; MCDaniel, K.; Schrimpf, M.; Shepard, G. Bromodomain Inhibitors. WO2018188047 A1, 18 October 2018.
8. Fensome, A.; Mccomas, C.C.; Melensky, E.G.; Marella, M.A.; Wrobel, J.E.; Grubb, G.S. Progesterone Receptor Modulators Comprising Pyrrole-Oxindole Derivates and Uses Thereof. WO2006023109 A1, 2 March 2006.
9. Beghyn, T.; Deprez, B.; Belouzard, S.; Brodin, P. A Compound As a Thyroid Hormone Beta Receptor Agonist and Use Thereof. WO2021/43185 A1, 11 March 2021.
10. Chen, L.; Feng, L.; He, Y.; Huang, M.; Yun, H. Spiro Indole-Cyclopropane Indolinones Useful as Ampk Modulators. WO2011070039 A1, 16 June 2011.
11. Becker, D.P.; Flynn, D.L.; Villamil, C.I. Indolones Useful as Serotonergic Agents. US5399562A, 21 March 1995.
12. Wurster, J.A. 3-Spyrocyclopropyl2-Oksindole Kinase Inhibitors. WO2007008664 A1, 18 January 2007.
13. Elder, D.; Holm, R. Aqueous solubility: Simple predictive methods (in silico, in vitro and bio-relevant approaches). *Int. J. Pharm.* **2013**, *453*, 3–11. [CrossRef]
14. Davis, M.E.; Brewster, M.E. Cyclodextrin-based pharmaceutics: Past, present and future. *Nat. Rev. Drug Discov.* **2004**, *3*, 1023–1035. [CrossRef]
15. Duchêne, D.; Bochot, A. Thirty years with cyclodextrins. *Int. J. Pharm.* **2016**, *514*, 58–72. [CrossRef]
16. Uekama, K.; Hirayama, F.; Irie, T. Cyclodextrin drug carrier systems. *Chem. Rev.* **1998**, *98*, 2045–2076. [CrossRef]
17. Gong, L.; Li, T.; Chen, F.; Duan, X.; Yuan, Y.; Zhang, D.; Jiang, Y. An inclusion complex of eugenol into β-Cyclodextrin: Preparation, and physicochemical and antifungal characterization. *Food Chem.* **2016**, *196*, 324–330. [CrossRef]
18. Skuredina, A.A.; Kopnova, T.Y.; Le-Deygen, I.M.; Kudryashova, E.V. Physical and chemical properties of the guest–host inclusion complexes of cyprofloxacin with β-cyclodextrin derivatives. *Mosc. Univ. Chem. Bull.* **2020**, *75*, 218–224. [CrossRef]

19. Řezanka, M. Synthesis of substituted cyclodextrins. *Environ. Chem. Lett.* **2019**, *17*, 49–63. [CrossRef]
20. Corey, E.J.; Chaykovsky, M. Dimethyloxosulfonium methylide (($CH_3)_2SOCH_2$) and dimethylsulfonium methylide ((CH3)2SCH2). Formation and application to organic synthesis. *J. Am. Chem. Soc.* **1965**, *87*, 1353–1364. [CrossRef]
21. Fraser, W.; Suckling, C.J.; Wood, H.C.S. Latent Inhibitors. Part 7. Inhibition of dihydro-orotate dehydrogenase by spirocyclo-propanobarbiturates. *J. Chem. Soc. Perkin 1* **1990**, 3137. [CrossRef]
22. Zaytsev, S.V.; Ivanov, K.L.; Skvortsov, D.A.; Bezzubov, S.I.; Melnikov, M.Y.; Budynina, E.M. Nucleophilic ring opening of donor–acceptor cyclopropanes with the cyanate ion: Access to spiro[pyrrolidone-3,3′-oxindoles]. *J. Org. Chem.* **2018**, *83*, 8695–8709. [CrossRef] [PubMed]
23. Baka, E.; Comer, J.E.A.; Takács-Novák, K. Study of equilibrium solubility measurement by saturation shake-flask method using hydrochlorothiazide as model compound. *J. Pharm. Biomed. Anal.* **2008**, *46*, 335–341. [CrossRef] [PubMed]
24. Brewster, M.E.; Loftsson, T. Cyclodextrins as Pharmaceutical Solubilizers. *Adv. Drug Deliv. Rev.* **2007**, *59*, 645–666. [CrossRef]
25. Wang, L.; Yan, J.; Li, Y.; Xu, K.; Li, S.; Tang, P.; Li, H. The influence of hydroxypropyl-β-cyclodextrin on the solubility, dissolution, cytotoxicity, and binding of riluzole with human serum albumin. *J. Pharm. Biomed. Anal.* **2016**, *117*, 453–463. [CrossRef] [PubMed]
26. Kicuntod, J.; Sangpheak, K.; Mueller, M.; Wolschann, P.; Viernstein, H.; Yanaka, S.; Kato, K.; Chavasiri, W.; Pongsawasdi, P.; Kungwan, N.; et al. Theoretical and experimental studies on inclusion complexes of pinostrobin and β-cyclodextrins. *Sci. Pharm.* **2018**, *86*, 5. [CrossRef]
27. Balouiri, M.; Sadiki, M.; Ibnsouda, S.K. Methods for in vitro evaluating antimicrobial activity: A Review. *J. Pharm. Anal.* **2016**, *6*, 71–79. [CrossRef]
28. Roos, K.; Wu, C.; Damm, W.; Reboul, M.; Stevenson, J.M.; Lu, C.; Dahlgren, M.K.; Mondal, S.; Chen, W.; Wang, L.; et al. OPLS3e: Extending force field coverage for drug-like small molecules. *J. Chem. Theory Comput.* **2019**, *15*, 1863–1874. [CrossRef]
29. Gurrath, M.; Müller, G.; Höltje, H.-D. Pseudoreceptor modelling in drug design: Applications of yak and PRGEN. *Perspect. Drug Discov. Des.* **1998**, *12*, 135–157. [CrossRef]
30. Friesner, R.A.; Banks, J.L.; Murphy, R.B.; Halgren, T.A.; Klicic, J.J.; Mainz, D.T.; Repasky, M.P.; Knoll, E.H.; Shelley, M.; Perry, J.K.; et al. Glide: A new approach for rapid, accurate docking and scoring. 1. Method and assessment of docking accuracy. *J. Med. Chem.* **2004**, *47*, 1739–1749. [CrossRef] [PubMed]
31. Wang, J.; Wolf, R.M.; Caldwell, J.W.; Kollman, P.A.; Case, D.A. Junmei Wang, Romain M. Wolf, James W. Caldwell, Peter A. Kollman, and David A. Case, "Development and Testing of a General Amber Force Field" Journal of Computational Chemistry(2004) 25(9) 1157–1174. *J. Comput. Chem.* **2005**, *26*, 114. [CrossRef]
32. Vassetti, D.; Pagliai, M.; Procacci, P. Assessment of GAFF2 and OPLS-AA general force fields in combination with the water models TIP3P, SPCE, and OPC3 for the solvation free energy of druglike organic molecules. *J. Chem. Theory Comput.* **2019**, *15*, 1983–1995. [CrossRef]
33. Jakalian, A.; Bush, B.L.; Jack, D.B.; Bayly, C.I. Fast, efficient generation of high-quality atomic charges. AM1-BCC Model: I. Method. *J. Comput. Chem.* **2000**, *21*, 132–146. [CrossRef]
34. Sousa da Silva, A.W.; Vranken, W.F. ACPYPE–Antechamber python parser interface. *BMC Res. Notes* **2012**, *5*, 367. [CrossRef]
35. Jorgensen, W.L.; Chandrasekhar, J.; Madura, J.D.; Impey, R.W.; Klein, M.L. Comparison of simple potential functions for simulating liquid water. *J. Chem. Phys.* **1983**, *79*, 926–935. [CrossRef]
36. Berendsen, H.J.C.; van der Spoel, D.; van Drunen, R. GROMACS: A message-passing parallel molecular dynamics implementation. *Comput. Phys. Commun.* **1995**, *91*, 43–56. [CrossRef]
37. Sampson, P.B.; Liu, Y.; Li, S.-W.; Forrest, B.T.; Pauls, H.W.; Edwards, L.G.; Feher, M.; Patel, N.K.B.; Laufer, R. Guohua Pan Kinase Inhibitors and Method of Treating Cancer with Same. WO2011123946 A8, 13 October 2011.
38. Wang, L.; Li, Z.; Lu, L.; Zhang, W. Synthesis of spiro[furan-3,3′-indolin]-2′-ones by PET-catalyzed [3+2] reactions of spiro[indoline-3,2′-oxiran]-2-ones with electron-Rich olefins. *Tetrahedron* **2012**, *68*, 1483–1491. [CrossRef]
39. Shinada, N.K.; de Brevern, A.G.; Schmidtke, P. Halogens in protein–ligand binding mechanism: A structural perspective. *J. Med. Chem.* **2019**, *62*, 9341–9356. [CrossRef]
40. Wang, Y.; Du, Y.; Huang, N. A survey of the role of nitrile groups in protein–ligand interactions. *Future Med. Chem.* **2018**, *10*, 2713–2728. [CrossRef]
41. Sukhoverkov, K.V.; Le-Deygen, I.M.; Egorov, A.M.; Kudryashova, E.V. Physicochemical properties of the inclusion complex of moxifloxacin with hydroxypropyl-β-cyclodextrin synthesized by RESS. *Russ. J. Phys. Chem. B* **2018**, *12*, 1193–1204. [CrossRef]
42. Jansook, P.; Ogawa, N.; Loftsson, T. Cyclodextrins: Structure, physicochemical properties and pharmaceutical applications. *Int. J. Pharm.* **2018**, *535*, 272–284. [CrossRef]
43. Méndez, S.G.; Otero Espinar, F.J.; Alvarez, A.L.; Longhi, M.R.; Quevedo, M.A.; Zoppi, A. Ternary complexation of benzoic acid with β-cyclodextrin and aminoacids. Experimental and theoretical studies. *J. Incl. Phenom. Macrocycl. Chem.* **2016**, *85*, 33–48. [CrossRef]
44. McIntosh, M.P.; Schwarting, N.; Rajewski, R.A. In vitro and in vivo evaluation of a sulfobutyl ether B-cyclodextrin Enabled etomidate formulation. *J. Pharm. Sci.* **2004**, *93*, 2585–2594. [CrossRef]
45. del Valle, E.M.M. Cyclodextrins and their uses: A review. *Process Biochem.* **2004**, *39*, 1033–1046. [CrossRef]
46. Crupi, V.; Ficarra, R.; Guardo, M.; Majolino, D.; Stancanelli, R.; Venuti, V. UV–vis and FTIR–ATR spectroscopic techniques to study the inclusion complexes of genistein with β-cyclodextrins. *J. Pharm. Biomed. Anal.* **2007**, *44*, 110–117. [CrossRef]

47. Le-Deygen, I.M.; Skuredina, A.A.; Uporov, I.V.; Kudryashova, E.V. Thermodynamics and molecular insight in guest–host complexes of fluoroquinolones with β-cyclodextrin derivatives, as revealed by ATR-FTIR spectroscopy and molecular modeling experiments. *Anal. Bioanal. Chem.* **2017**, *409*, 6451–6462. [CrossRef] [PubMed]

48. Barman, S.; Barman, B.K.; Roy, M.N. Preparation, characterization and binding behaviors of host-guest inclusion complexes of metoclopramide hydrochloride with α- and β-cyclodextrin molecules. *J. Mol. Struct.* **2018**, *1155*, 503–512. [CrossRef]

49. Upadhyay, S.K.; Kumar, G. NMR and molecular modelling studies on the interaction of fluconazole with β-cyclodextrin. *Chem. Cent. J.* **2009**, *3*, 9. [CrossRef]

50. Loftsson, T.; Moya-Ortega, M.D.; Alvarez-Lorenzo, C.; Concheiro, A. Pharmacokinetics of cyclodextrins and drugs after oral and parenteral administration of drug/cyclodextrin complexes. *J. Pharm. Pharmacol.* **2016**, *68*, 544–555. [CrossRef]

51. Skuredina, A.A.; Tychinina, A.S.; Le-Deygen, I.M.; Golyshev, S.A.; Kopnova, T.Y.; Le, N.T.; Belogurova, N.G.; Kudryashova, E.V. Cyclodextrins and their polymers affect the lipid membrane permeability and increase levofloxacin's antibacterial activity in vitro. *Polymers* **2022**, *14*, 4476. [CrossRef]

52. Sala, A.; Hoossen, Z.; Bacchi, A.; Caira, M.R. Two crystal forms of a hydrated 2:1 β-cyclodextrin fluconazole complex: Single crystal X-ray structures, dehydration profiles, and conditions for their individual isolation. *Molecules* **2021**, *26*, 4427. [CrossRef]

53. Kohut, A.; Demchuk, Z.; Kingsley, K.; Voronov, S.; Voronov, A. Dual role of methyl-β-cyclodextrin in the emulsion polymerization of highly hydrophobic plant oil-based monomers with various unsaturations. *Eur. Polym. J.* **2018**, *108*, 322–328. [CrossRef]

54. Yang, W.; Johnston, K.P.; Williams, R.O. Comparison of bioavailability of amorphous versus crystalline itraconazole nanoparticles via pulmonary administration in rats. *Eur. J. Pharm. Biopharm.* **2010**, *75*, 33–41. [CrossRef] [PubMed]

55. Skuredina, A.A.; Tychinina, A.S.; Le-Deygen, I.M.; Golyshev, S.A.; Belogurova, N.G.; Kudryashova, E.V. The formation of quasi-regular polymeric network of cross-linked sulfobutyl ether derivative of β-cyclodextrin synthesized with moxifloxacin as a template. *React. Funct. Polym.* **2021**, *159*, 104811. [CrossRef]

56. Skuredina, A.A.; Danilov, M.R.; Le-Deygen, I.M.; Kudryashova, E.V. Adsorption Properties of mesoporous silica gel with β-cyclodextrin as a pore-forming agent relative to moxifloxacin. *Mosc. Univ. Chem. Bull.* **2018**, *73*, 192–198. [CrossRef]

57. Palomba, M.; Rossi, L.; Sancineto, L.; Tramontano, E.; Corona, A.; Bagnoli, L.; Santi, C.; Pannecouque, C.; Tabarrini, O.; Marini, F. A new vinyl selenone-based domino approach to spirocyclopropyl oxindoles endowed with anti-HIV rt activity. *Org. Biomol. Chem.* **2016**, *14*, 2015–2024. [CrossRef]

58. Kavyani, S.; Baharfar, R. Design and characterization of Fe_3O_4/GO/Au-Ag nanocomposite as an efficient catalyst for the green synthesis of spirooxindole-dihydropyridines. *Appl. Organomet. Chem.* **2020**, *34*, e5560. [CrossRef]

59. Allahresani, A.; Taheri, B.; Nasseri, M.A. A green synthesis of spirooxindole derivatives catalyzed by SiO_2@g-C_3N_4 nanocomposite. *Res. Chem. Intermed.* **2018**, *44*, 1173–1188. [CrossRef]

60. Liang, H.; Yuan, Q.; Vriesekoop, F.; Lv, F. Effects of cyclodextrins on the antimicrobial activity of plant-derived essential oil compounds. *Food Chem.* **2012**, *135*, 1020–1027. [CrossRef] [PubMed]

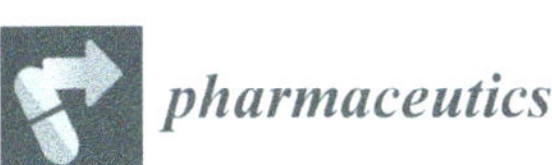

pharmaceutics

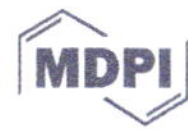

Article

In Situ Co-Amorphization of Olanzapine in the Matrix and on the Coat of Pellets

Nuno F. da Costa [1,†], Raquel F. Azevedo [1,†], João A. Lopes [1], Ana I. Fernandes [2,*] and João F. Pinto [1]

1   iMed.ULisboa—Research Institute for Medicines, Faculdade de Farmácia, Universidade de Lisboa, Av. Prof. Gama Pinto, 1649-003 Lisboa, Portugal
2   CiiEM—Interdisciplinary Research Center Egas Moniz, Instituto Universitário Egas Moniz, Monte de Caparica, 2829-511 Caparica, Portugal
*   Correspondence: aifernandes@egasmoniz.edu.pt; Tel.: +351-212946823
†   These authors contributed equally to this work.

Abstract: In situ amorphization is a promising approach, considered in the present work, to enhance the solubility and dissolution rate of olanzapine, while minimizing the exposure of the amorphous material to the stress conditions applied during conventional processing. The production of pellets by extrusion/spheronization and the coating of inert beads were investigated as novel methods to promote the co-amorphization of olanzapine, a poorly water-soluble drug, and saccharin. Samples were characterized using differential scanning calorimetry, X-ray powder diffraction, Fourier-transform infrared spectroscopy and scanning electron microscopy, and dissolution and stability testing. The co-amorphous produced were compared with crystalline olanzapine, or physical mixture of olanzapine and saccharin. Results suggested that the addition of water to mixtures containing olanzapine and saccharin during the production of pellets, and the coating of inert beads, induced the in situ co-amorphization of these substances. The coating of inert beads enhanced the solubility and dissolution rate of olanzapine, especially when compared to pellets coated with the crystalline drug, but also with pellets containing the co-amorphous entity in the matrix of beads. Nine months stability tests (23 °C/60% RH) confirmed the preservation of the solid-state properties of the co-amorphous form on/in pellets. Overall, results highlighted the feasibility and benefits of in situ co-amorphization, either when the drug was entrapped in the pellets matrix, or preferentially applied directly on the surface of pellets.

Keywords: (co-)amorphous; dissolution testing; in situ (co-)amorphization; olanzapine; pellets; solubility; stability

Citation: da Costa, N.F.; Azevedo, R.F.; Lopes, J.A.; Fernandes, A.I.; Pinto, J.F. In Situ Co-Amorphization of Olanzapine in the Matrix and on the Coat of Pellets. *Pharmaceutics* **2022**, *14*, 2587. https://doi.org/10.3390/pharmaceutics14122587

Academic Editor: Hisham Al-Obaidi

Received: 18 October 2022
Accepted: 22 November 2022
Published: 24 November 2022

Publisher's Note: MDPI stays neutral with regard to jurisdictional claims in published maps and institutional affiliations.

1. Introduction

Poor water solubility of drugs, including that of many novel drug candidates, remains a major impairment on drugs' bioavailability compromising therapeutic effectiveness [1,2]. To enhance the aqueous solubility of crystalline solids, multiple strategies are available. Among these, the formation of co-crystals has been described as a valuable strategy to enhance the water solubility and bioavailability of poorly water-soluble drugs [3,4]. However, additional strategies are warranted to further enhance the solubility of drugs and reduce the solubility concerns during the pharmaceutical development process. Disruption of the crystalline lattice, stabilization of the amorphous content, using polymers [5], or low molecular mass compounds—to produce the co-amorphous systems (CAMs) [6–8]—are amongst these strategies, which have been implemented with various degrees of success. Unfortunately, the high fraction of polymer commonly required to stabilize amorphous drugs (up to 90% w/w) [9] may result in the production of massive dosage forms, thus negatively impacting patient compliance [10]. In this regard, CAMs may be particularly useful for the pharmaceutical industry since higher drug loads can be used in formulations (up to 60–80% w/w) without compromising the stability of amorphous drugs [11], or the size amenable to patient administration. The formation of CAMs can be ascertained by diffractometry and calorimetry characterization methods. Diffractograms of CAMs present a characteristic halo pattern and the absence of crystalline diffraction peaks, unlike the typical diffractograms of crystalline materials (e.g., co-crystals). Additionally, thermograms of CAMs present a single glass transition temperature (T_g), indicating miscibility of the compounds, and the absence of melting events, a feature indicative of the crystallinity of samples [12]. Olanzapine (OLZ, pK_a = 4.69 and 7.37 [13], Figure 1A), the model drug used in this study, is an atypical antipsychotic substance commonly administered in the treatment of schizophrenia, depression, or bipolar disorder [14]. As shown previously [15], OLZ benefits from co-amorphization with saccharin (SAC, pK_a = 1.6 [16], Figure 1B), both in terms of solubility (5896 vs. 41 mg/L for OLZ-CAM and pure crystalline OLZ, respectively) and dissolution rate of the drug (88.7 vs. 25.2% of drug release for OLZ-CAM and pure crystalline OLZ, respectively). Both olanzapine [17] and saccharine [18] are reportedly stable under the conditions used for co-amorphization [15]. The formation of a stable CAM between OLZ and SAC was explained by salification, rather than hydrogen or π-π bonds, which was supported by the huge difference between the pK_a of OLZ and SAC (ΔpK_a = 6.06) [15]. The positive impact of the establishment of intermolecular interactions, particularly salt formation, on the physical stability of CAMs is well described in the literature [10,19–22]. Accordingly, the higher solubility and dissolution rate of OLZ in the CAM may foresee an improved bioavailability of the drug in the amorphous form, as compared to its crystalline counterpart [15].

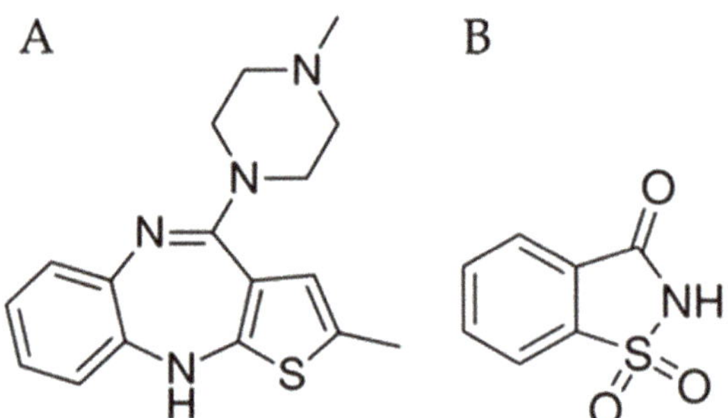

Figure 1. Chemical structure of olanzapine (**A**) and saccharin (**B**).

At the industrial scale, traditional techniques used to produce amorphous and CAMs drugs include spray-drying, freeze-drying and hot-melt extrusion [1,23–25]. Amorphous or CAMs prepared using these techniques are often blended with pharmaceutical excipients to enhance processability during manufacture (e.g., glidants), drug release (e.g., disintegrants), acceptability/compliance (e.g., sweeteners, colorants) and handling (e.g., fillers) by the patient. Additional pharmaceutical unit operations, such as dry or wet granulation, and pelletization, are often considered to improve the flowability of materials, if required [26–28]. However, the stress conditions (e.g., pressure, temperature, or moisture sorption) imposed to the system during these operations may result in instability and recrystallization of the amorphous content, negatively impacting drugs' bioavailability [29–32] and introducing product variability. Previous studies, performed by Joshi et al. [30], also reported the instability associated with the use of amorphous forms of celecoxib during compaction, resulting in the devitrification of the drug regardless of the compression pressure (between 27.4–137.5 MPa) applied to produce the compacts. These findings also hold when amorphous celecoxib was stabilized by polyvinyl pyrrolidone and meglumine, although the degree of recrystallization during compaction was substantially reduced to a value below 15% of crystallinity content [30]. Similar results were obtained by Thakral et al. [32] who prepared tablets containing amorphous indomethacin. At high compression pressures, the recrystallization of the model drug was evident immediately after the preparation of tablets [32].

Therefore, the development of strategies to induce the conversion of the crystalline into the (co-)amorphous form of drugs, and maintenance of such state, is of paramount importance. The conversion may be achieved directly during the manufacture of the dosage form, the so-called in situ amorphization, which may be advantageous to minimize the long-term stability concerns [29,33–35]. In addition to stabilization, in situ amorphization techniques offer the possibility to discard the production of amorphous solid dispersions prior to the manufacture of oral dosage forms, thus resulting in manufacturing savings and reduced logistic restrictions. Examples of investigations on in situ co-amorphization include carvedilol [36], furosemide, and indomethacin [33] by immersion of tablets coated with a gastro-resistant and water permeable polymer in acidic medium (0.1 M HCl). The use of radiation (e.g., microwave [37] or laser [38]) has been considered to avoid the pre-formation of the co-amorphous species prior to its downstreaming into dosage forms. Previous studies published by our research group [28,29] have reported the in situ co-amorphization of OLZ and SAC during tableting. In this respect, the extent of co-amorphization was proportional to the compression pressure and the dwell time applied to produce the compacts.

The present work aimed at the in situ co-amorphization of OLZ and SAC, present either in the matrix, or on the surface of pellets, to simultaneously enhance the OLZ solubility and dissolution rate, with the advantage of circumventing the preparation of the CAMs prior to the dosage form manufacturing process. The work also aimed at identifying the boundaries within which the in situ co-amorphization occurs.

2. Materials and Methods

2.1. Materials

OLZ (polymorphic form I, Rampex Labs Pvt. Ltd., Telangana, India), SAC (Sigma-Aldrich, Steinheim, Germany), and dichloromethane (Biochem Chemopharma, Cosne sur Loire, France) were used to prepare the OLZ-CAM. Microcrystalline cellulose (Avicel PH-101, FMC Corp., Cork, Ireland), polyvinyl pyrrolidone (K25, BASF, Ludwigshafen, Germany) and dibasic calcium phosphate anhydrous (DI-CAFOS® A60, Budenheim, Budenheim, Germany), were used in the production of the pellets. Demineralized water (Destillo 2 apparatus, Herco, Freiberg am Neckar, Germany) and dichloromethane (Biochem Chemopharma, Cosne sur Loire, France) were used as granulation liquids. Hard gelatin capsules (size 0, Lonza, Basel, Switzerland) were manually filled with the pellets produced. In the preparation of the pH 8.0 phosphate buffer for the dissolution studies, sodium hydroxide (Eka Chemicals Inc., Marietta, GA, USA), and potassium phosphate monobasic (Carlo Erba Reagents, Val de Reuil, France) were used.

2.2. Methods

2.2.1. Preparation of Powdered Co-Amorphous Olanzapine: Saccharin

OLZ-CAM was prepared by rapidly evaporating dichloromethane from a solution containing OLZ and SAC, in a 1:1 molar ratio (40 °C, 650 mbar, R-100, Buchi Rotavapor, Flawil, Switzerland). To ensure the total removal of the solvent, the product was left under vacuum for 24 h, after solvent evaporation [15]. Considering a maximum daily dose of 20 mg of OLZ, the dose of saccharin delivered to patients would be 12 mg, which is well below the acceptable human daily intake of 2.5 mg per kg of body weight [39].

2.2.2. Characterization of Powdered Co-Amorphous Olanzapine: Saccharin

To ensure particle size homogeneity before further characterization, as described below, OLZ-CAM was gently milled in a mortar (to ensure maintenance of the solid state; monitored by diffractometry, calorimetry and infrared spectroscopy), and sieved through a 180 μm mesh. Preliminary studies have shown that when the same gentle process of milling imposed to the co-amorphous was applied to the respective crystalline blends of raw materials, co-amorphization of the latter was not observed.

X-ray Powder Diffraction (XRPD): XRPD measurements were conducted in a PANalytical X-ray diffractometer (X'Pert PRO, PANalytical, Almelo, The Netherlands), using a CuKα source of radiation (λ = 1.54 Å, at 40 kV and 30 mA). Analysis (approximately 500 mg of sample) were performed in the range 7–35 °2θ, at a step size of 0.017 °2θ and counting time of 50 s. Spectragryph software (Spectragryph, version 1.2.13, 2019, Oberstdorf, Germany) was used in data analysis and treatment.

Modulated Differential Scanning Calorimetry (DSC): A calorimeter (Q200, TA Instruments, New Castle, DE, USA) was used in the thermal analysis. Samples (5–10 mg) were analyzed in hermetic aluminum pans (THEPRO GbR, Heinsberg, Germany) in the −20 to 250 °C temperature range (heating rate of 5 °C/min, amplitude of 0.796 °C and 60 s period). The proprietor software (Universal Analysis 2000, version 4.7A, 2009, TA Instruments, New Castle, DE, USA) was used to analyze the thermograms. The midpoint of the change in the heat capacity baseline was taken as the T_g of the amorphous materials.

Fourier-transform Infrared (FTIR) Spectroscopy: a spectrometer (Alpha II, Bruker, Billerica, MA, USA) fitted with a diamond ATR accessory (Platinum ATR, Bruker, Billerica, MA, USA) was used. Samples (n = 3, approximately 50 mg) were scanned (wavenumber interval 4000–700 cm^1, at a 4 cm^{-1} resolution), 24 times. Spectragryph software (Spectragryph, version 1.2.13, 2019, Oberstdorf, Germany) was used to analyze the data.

2.2.3. Production of Pellets via Extrusion-Spheronization

Crystalline OLZ, crystalline OLZ:SAC, and OLZ-CAM were blended (10 min), with the excipients (Table 1) in a planetary mixer (Chef, Kenwood, New Lane, UK); demineralized water or dichloromethane (30% w/w on a dry basis) were used as granulation liquids. OLZ was included, at a constant fraction of 5% w/w, in both formulations I and II. After wetting of powders, materials were blended for an additional 10 min and stored in air-tight polyethylene bags for 24 h. A universal testing machine (LR50K Plus, Lloyd Instruments, Largo, FL, USA) fitted with a 50 kN load cell was used for extrusion (die length to diameter ratio of 4.0; test speed 200 mm/min). The load applied to masses was recorded as a function of the displacement of the cell using the proprietary software (Nexygen Plus, version 3.0, 2013, Largo, FL, USA). Spheronization was then conducted (1000 rpm for 20 min) on the extrudates in a radial plate spheronizer (230, Caleva, Dorset, UK). Pellets were oven-dried (40 °C) to constant mass (UM 100, Memmert, Schwabach, Germany). Pellets (200 mg, equivalent to 10 mg of OLZ) were weighted and used to fill size 0 hard gelatin capsules. Placebo pellets, without OLZ and SAC, were also produced for comparison purposes (formulation P, Table 1).

Table 1. Composition of formulations (% w/w) used in the study.

		Formulation	
Material	**P**	**I**	**II ***
OLZ	-	5	5
SAC	-	-	3
Dibasic calcium phosphate anhydrous	75	71	69
Microcrystalline cellulose	20	19	18
Polyvinylpyrrolidone	5	5	5

* the proportion of 5 OLZ: 3 SAC represents a 1:1 molar ratio.

2.2.4. Coating of Pellets

A fluidized bed coater (Strea 1, Aeromatic AG, Muttenz, Switzerland) equipped with a single spray nozzle was used to coat pellets using a dichloromethane or demineralized water solution/suspension of OLZ and SAC, in a 1:1 molar ratio. The drying temperature was set at 40 °C and the capacity of the fan was set at 11 units. An atomization pressure of 0.5 bar and a spay rate of 3 g/min were applied. After drying, pellets were oven dried (UM 100, Memmert, Schwabach, Germany) at 40 °C for 24 h.

2.2.5. Characterization of Pellets

To gain an insight into the solid-state and solution-state properties, pellets were characterized immediately after preparation. In addition to the methods described below, XRPD, DSC, and FTIR were also used to investigate the solid-state arrangement of OLZ in samples obtained after processing and performed, as described previously (Section 2.2.2).

Drug content: physical mixtures or pellets (n = 10, 100 mg of mixtures or pellets, equivalent to 5 mg of OLZ) were placed in phosphate buffer pH 8.0 (1000 mL). After 24 h (no solid residues were visually observed), samples were diluted and drug content was estimated by using ultraviolet photometry (λ = 254 nm, U-1900, Hitachi, Tokyo, Japan).

Water content: samples (approximately 500 mg) were crushed and heated at 80 °C until constant weight. The weight variation, before and after heating, was recorded and used to determine the water content, according to Equation (1), where W_B and W_A represent the weight of powder before and after the drying cycle.

$$\text{Water Content } (\%) = \frac{W_B - W_A}{W_B} \times 100 \tag{1}$$

Crushing Strength: to measure the crushing strength of pellets, a texture analyzer equipped with a cylinder probe (TA.XT Plus, Stable Micro Systems, Surrey, UK) was used at a testing speed of 100 mm/min (n = 10 pellets).

Dissolution Tests: dissolution studies (paddle method, 100 rpm), were conducted in a dissolution apparatus (AT7, Sotax, Aesch, Switzerland). Approximately 200 or 2000 mg of powdered mixtures or pellets—equivalent to 10 mg (sink conditions), or 100 mg of OLZ (non-sink conditions), respectively—were placed in 1000 mL phosphate buffer pH 8.0 (to ensure that the drug is predominantly unionized), pre-heated to 37 $\pm$ 0.5 °C. At pre-defined times (0, 5, 10, 15, 30, 60, 120, 180, 240, 360, 480, 720, 960, 1200, and 1440 min), a sample of 4 mL of dissolution media was withdrawn, passed through a 0.22 μm MCE filter (Merck, Boston, MA, USA), and OLZ quantified using ultraviolet spectrophotometry, as before, to determine the fraction of OLZ released over time. Fresh dissolution medium was added to the dissolution vessel after each sample collection to maintain the dissolution volume constant throughout the test.

Scanning Electron Microscopy (SEM): the morphology of pellets was evaluated using an electron microscope (JEOL-JSM-S200LV, JOEL, Peabody, MA, USA), equipped with a secondary electron detector, at a magnification of 35×. Prior to analysis, pellets were gold coated in a sputtering chamber (JEOL JFC-1200, JOEL, Peabody, MA, USA).

Gas Chromatography (GC): the content of residual solvent (dichloromethane) was determined by injecting approximately 10 μL of sample into a gas chromatographer (Clarus® 690 GC Perkin Elmer, Waltham, MA, USA) fitted with a highly sensitive ionization detector (FID).

Olanzapine solubility: approximately 300 mg of pellets (equivalent to 15 mg of OLZ) were added to eppendorfs containing 1 mL of the phosphate-buffered solution pH 8.0 pre-set at 37 °C and left to rest for 24 h (n = 3). Eppendorfs were centrifuged at 17,320× *g* for 60 min (Z 233M, Hermle, Wehingen, Germany) and filtered through a 0.22 μm MCE filter (Darmstadt, Germany). Afterwards, the filtered solution was diluted to a UV measurable concentration (λ = 254 nm, U-1900, Hitachi, Tokyo, Japan), taken as the solubility of OLZ-CAM.

2.2.6. Principal Component Analysis

Principal component analysis was applied to the analysis of the FTIR spectra, pre-processed using the multiplicative scatter correction method (Matlab software, R2015a, 2015, MathWorks, Sherborn, MA, USA).

2.2.7. Statistical Analysis

Data analysis was conducted using the one-way ANOVA and when statistical significance was found the post hoc Tukey's test was performed for comparison purposes (SPSS

Statistics, version 27.0.1.0, 2020, IBM, New York, NY, USA). Statistical significance was considered at $p < 0.05$.

2.2.8. Stability Studies

Powdered mixtures and pellets were stored in open glass vials for 9 months under room conditions (23 ± 2 °C/60 ± 5%RH) in a climatic chamber (Vötsch, VC2023, Balingen, Germany) and analyzed by XRPD to evaluate if recrystallization of OLZ-CAM had occurred.

3. Results

3.1. Differential Scanning Calorimetry and X-ray Powder Diffraction

DSC is a thermoanalytical characterization technique applied to analyze the thermal transitions of materials (e.g., glass transitions and melting) as a function of the temperature, and hence to provide evidence of the amorphization and co-amorphization of materials [40]. The co-amorphization of a drug substance and co-amorphous stabilizers can be detected by the observation of a single T_g and the absence of melting events in thermograms [10]. Thermograms of pure crystalline OLZ (Figure 2A, orange) presented a single endothermic event at 192.4 °C, confirming the use of the polymorphic form I of the drug [41]. Similarly, thermograms of SAC presented a single endothermic peak at 224.8 °C (Figure 2A, yellow), in good agreement with the literature [42,43]. In contrast, the evaporation of dichloromethane from a solution containing OLZ and SAC, in a 1:1 molar ratio, resulted in a powdered sample presenting a single T_g, at approximately 100.8 °C, and the absence of melting events (Figure 2A, blue), suggesting the co-amorphization of both compounds.

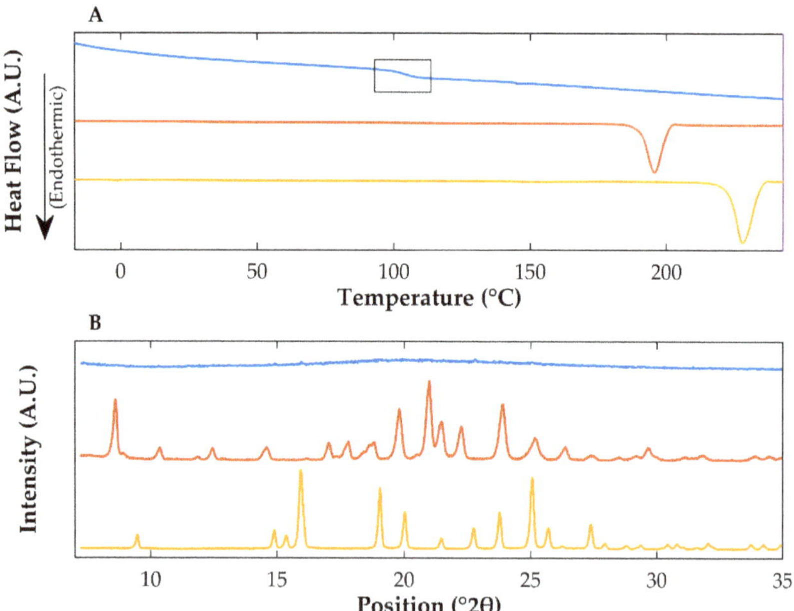

Figure 2. Differential scanning calorimetry thermograms (**A**) and X-ray powder diffractograms (**B**) of powdered crystalline saccharin (yellow), crystalline olanzapine (orange), and co-amorphous olanzapine:saccharin (blue). The glass transition of co-amorphous olanzapine:saccharin is highlighted in (**A**).

XRPD studies were run to support the aforementioned results. Diffractograms of pure crystalline OLZ presented characteristic diffraction peaks at 8.62, 19.81, 21.00, 21.08,

22.27, and 23.89 °2θ (Figure 2B, orange), comparable to diffractograms available in the literature [41] for the polymorphic form I of OLZ. Diffractograms of pure SAC presented diffraction peaks at 16.01, 19.09, 22.75, 23.86, and 25.07 °2θ (Figure 2B, yellow), also aligned with those published in the literature [7,44]. In contrast, after solvent evaporation, diffractograms of OLZ and SAC samples, presented the typical halo pattern of amorphous materials and the absence of diffraction peaks (Figure 2B, blue), which are characteristic of crystalline solids. Therefore, the combination of XRPD and DSC confirmed the co-amorphization of OLZ and SAC by evaporation of dichloromethane.

3.2. Fourier-Transform Infrared Spectroscopy

During the preparation of CAMs, intermolecular interactions may be established between drug(s) and co-amorphous stabilizer(s), enhancing stability of CAMs, as compared to pure amorphous drugs [45]. In this respect, FTIR spectroscopy was conducted on samples to investigate the intermolecular interactions established between OLZ and SAC. Pure crystalline OLZ presented characteristic peaks at 3218 cm^{-1} (N-H stretching), 2931 and 2791 cm^{-1} (C-H stretching), 1583 cm^{-1} (N-H stretching), 1289 cm^{-1} (C-N stretching), 965 cm^{-1} (C-S stretching) and 745 cm^{-1} (C-H out of the plan deformation) (Figure 3). Pure crystalline SAC presented peaks at 3093 cm^{-1} (N-H stretch), 1717 cm^{-1} (C=O stretch) and 1333 cm^{-1} (S=O stretching vibration). Due to the dilution of both substances, equivalent peaks were observed in the physical mixture (containing both crystalline OLZ and SAC, in a 1:1 molar ratio) spectrum but with lower intensity (Figure 3). The major difference in the spectrum of the CAM, compared to the spectrum of the respective crystalline physical mixture, was the inexistence of the C=O peak of SAC at 1717 cm^{-1}, suggesting the formation of a salt (OLZ saccharinate) between the compounds, which is supported by the difference in pK$_a$ between OLZ and SAC (ΛpK$_a$ > 5 units) [1,10], and reported before as the mechanism of formation of these CAMs [15]. Salification is expected to promote a more stable entity than hydrogen bonds. Salt formation between OLZ and SAC is likely to prevent the recrystallization of the amorphous content, since for the recrystallization to occur, the interactions established between the compounds need to be disrupted to enable the formation and growth of crystalline nuclei [45].

3.3. Manufacture of Pellets Containing Olanzapine

The downstream processing of formulations containing amorphous and CAMs constitutes the last hurdle to overcome during the industrial development of novel drug products containing poorly water-soluble drugs. As discussed before, during the production of conventional oral dosage forms (e.g., tablets or pellets), stress conditions imposed on materials are likely to promote the recrystallization of the amorphous content and thus the reduction of solubility and dissolution rate. Therefore, close monitoring of the stability of CAMs during the manufacture of oral drug products is mandatory. To circumvent such problem, the in situ co-amorphization of drugs during the manufacture of pellets, or directly on the surface of inert beads during coating, is regarded as extremely advantageous. With such approach, the stress conditions to which the CAMs are exposed to are minimized, as is the risk of recrystallization. In this respect, the manufacture of pellets containing OLZ:SAC in the matrix and on the surface of inert beads was investigated in this study. For comparison purposes, pellets containing OLZ, either in the matrix or on the surface of pellets, were produced and characterized.

3.3.1. Preparation of Pellets Containing Olanzapine in the Matrix

Physical mixtures were wet using dichloromethane or water, and stored for 24 h prior to extrusion. Extrusion of masses wetted with dichloromethane failed to produce extrudates possibly due to the evaporation of the solvent during storage and the high force required to extrude the masses (>50 kN). In contrast, the use of water enabled the production of extrudates which were subsequently used to produce pellets. Ranking of the force of extrusion of the formulations (P > I > II), could be related to the content in calcium phosphate.

In fact, the placebo formulation P was mainly composed of anhydrous dibasic calcium phosphate (75% w/w), which is recognized by its brittle behavior during compaction. The reduction of the fraction of calcium phosphate in formulations containing OLZ, alone (71%, formulation I) or with SAC (69% w/w, formulation II), may have increased the plasticity of formulations, thus lowering the force required to extrude masses [46]. These results are in line with those of Pinto et al. [47], who have demonstrated that the use of higher ratios of microcrystalline cellulose:lactose in formulations containing indomethacin, decreased the force needed to extrude the wet masses through the die, due to the increased plasticity of formulations. Extrudates were subsequently radial plate-spheronized to produce pellets. Content uniformity analysis indicated that regardless of the formulation considered, all samples presented an average content of OLZ within the range 99.91–100.81% ($p > 0.05$, Table 2). Worth mentioning is that no individual samples contained a content of OLZ outside the limits established by the Ph. Eur. (<85 and >115%) [48], confirming the uniformity of the drug in the pellets. Additionally, the water content was below 2% (w/w) in all samples.

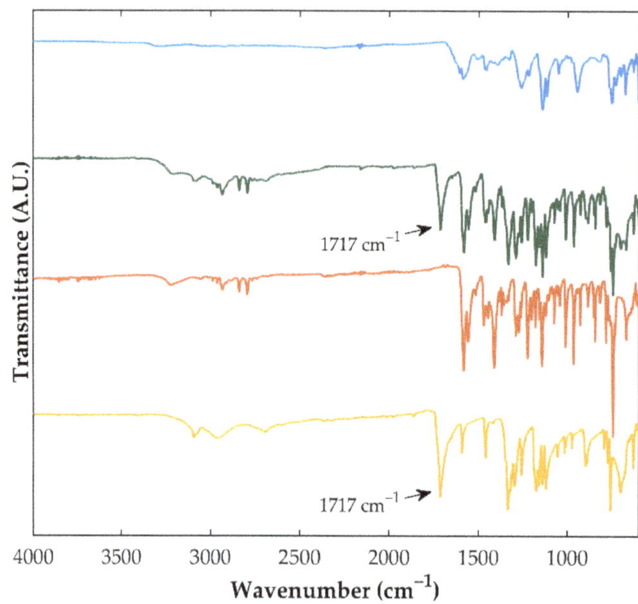

Figure 3. Fourier-transform infrared spectra of pure crystalline saccharin (yellow), pure crystalline olanzapine (orange), the physical mixture containing crystalline olanzapine and saccharin (green), and the co-amorphous system produced using both compounds (blue).

Table 2. Properties of pellets containing OLZ, or OLZ and SAC, in the matrix or on the surface.

	Matrix			Surface	
	OLZ	**OLZ:SAC**	**CAM**	**OLZ**	**OLZ:SAC**
OLZ content (% w/w)	100.19 ± 4.71	100.02 ± 6.79	99.91 ± 2.22	100.48 ± 8.20	100.81 ± 7.92
Crushing Strength (N)	23.97 ± 2.84 **	33.61 ± 2.44 ##	36.38 ± 2.02 ##	23.76 ± 3.18 **	24.67 ± 2.47 **
$t_{50\%}$ (min) [1]	70.71 ± 3.35 **	31.36 ± 4.28 ##	39.25 ± 3.90 ##,*	35.37 ± 3.30 ##	6.72 ± 1.78 ##,**
$t_{75\%}$ (min) [1]	252.86 ± 22.99 **	88.77 ± 8.95 ##	102.17 ± 10.04 ##	58.89 ± 4.29 ##,*	13.96 ± 1.15 ##,**

[1] t_{50} and t_{75} represent the time required to achieve a drug release of 50 and 75%, respectively (under sink conditions, 10 mg/L of OLZ); ## $p < 0.01$ vs. pellets containing OLZ in the matrix (crystalline OLZ, as starting material); * $p < 0.05$ and ** $p < 0.01$ vs. pellets containing OLZ and SAC in the matrix (crystalline OLZ and SAC, as starting material).

Samples were characterized using DSC and XRPD to investigate the solid-state of OLZ in extrudates and pellets. Unfortunately, DSC thermograms have not shown any thermal events in the temperature interval considered possibly due to the low fraction of OLZ in formulations (5% *w/w*). On the other hand, the diffractograms of the physical mixture containing crystalline OLZ or crystalline OLZ and SAC presented diffraction peaks at 8.7, 19.2, and 21.1 °2θ, which were absent in the diffractograms of the physical mixture of the placebo formulation (Figure 4). Comparison of these diffractograms with those of pure crystalline OLZ and SAC allowed association of the diffraction peaks at 8.7 and 21.1 °2θ with OLZ, whilst the peak at 19.2 °2θ was associated with the presence of crystalline SAC (Figure 4). As a result, these peaks were used as indicators of OLZ and SAC.

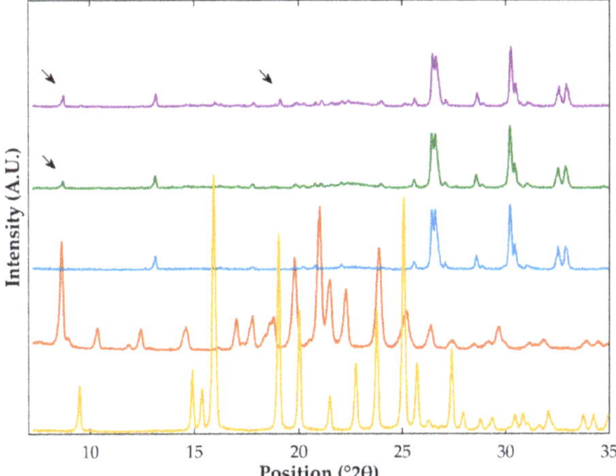

Figure 4. Diffractograms of crystalline saccharin (yellow), crystalline olanzapine (orange), and the physical mixtures obtained from the placebo formulation P (blue) and blends containing crystalline olanzapine (green, formulation I) or olanzapine and saccharin (purple, formulation II). Arrows highlight the peaks present in diffractograms, which could be related to either crystalline olanzapine or saccharin.

Extrusion and spheronization of formulation I (containing the crystalline form I of OLZ as starting material) produced samples whose diffractograms exhibited the most relevant diffraction peaks associated with OLZ (in the same position compared to the diffractograms of pure crystalline OLZ and the physical mixture prepared). Therefore, it may be assumed that no-solid state modifications of the drug have occurred during the production of extrudates and pellets (Supplementary Material—Figure S1). The same conclusions hold also true for the powder blend containing the OLZ-CAM (formulation II). Therefore, the high stability of OLZ-CAM when exposed to the different stress conditions considered in this study (e.g., solvent or drying temperature) is highlighted. In contrast, extrudates and pellets produced using formulation II (containing crystalline OLZ and SAC as starting materials) failed to show the presence of diffraction peaks related to either OLZ or SAC. These results suggest the co-amorphization of both compounds during processing (Figure 5). Water-induced co-amorphization of OLZ was previously reported by the authors [49].

To confirm the XRPD results, FTIR spectroscopy was conducted. FTIR spectra of extrudates and pellets prepared using formulation I failed to show noticeable variations, as compared to the spectrum of the physical mixture. Similar observations were made for samples containing the OLZ-CAM as starting material. Hence, FTIR spectroscopy supported the XRPD results, regarding the maintenance of the solid-state of OLZ during processing.

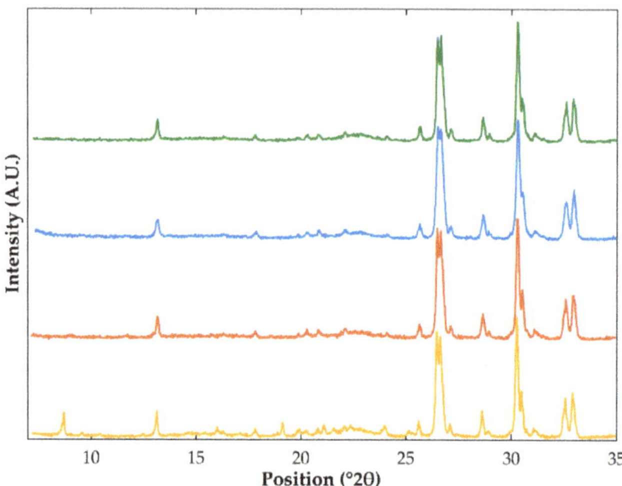

Figure 5. Diffractograms of samples prepared using crystalline olanzapine and saccharin (as starting material) obtained from the physical mixtures (yellow), extrudates (orange), and pellets (blue). The diffractogram of the physical mixture prepared using the co-amorphous olanzapine was plotted (green) for comparison purposes.

When samples prepared using crystalline OLZ and SAC as starting materials (formulation II) were considered, FTIR spectroscopy has shown considerable differences in the spectra of extrudates or pellets, as compared to those of the respective physical mixture. As pointed out above, the most notorious variations in the spectra of crystalline vs. OLZ-CAM were detected in the wavenumber interval 1750–1450 cm^{-1}, which are likely due to the formation of a salt between both compounds (Figure 3).

Principal component analysis was conducted to gain a better insight on these differences. The principal component analysis was conducted using the wavenumber interval 1750–1450 cm^{-1}, where the most relevant differences were detected. The scores plot clearly shows the clustering of samples prepared using the placebo-based formulation (Figure 6, green). Similar clustering of samples was observed for samples prepared using crystalline OLZ (Formulation I, Figure 6, blue) or OLZ-CAM (Formulation II, Figure 6, yellow), as starting material. The incorporation of SAC in formulations, as a physical mixture, resulted only in minor variations in scores, in the wavenumber interval considered, as illustrated by the clustering of these samples together with those of formulations containing the crystalline form of the drug (in the absence of SAC). Inversely, the processing of this blend resulted in spectra with high similarity with formulation II containing the OLZ-CAM as starting material. In conclusion, by combining the results obtained using FTIR spectroscopy and XRPD, it may be assumed that co-amorphization of both OLZ and SAC has occurred during the production of extrudates and pellets.

Crushing strength measurements were conducted to determine the compressive load at which the structure of pellets is broken. Results have shown that the incorporation of OLZ alone in formulations (formulation I) slightly decreased the resistance of pellets (27.73 ± 1.65 vs. 23.97 ± 2.84 N for pellets produced using formulations P and I, respectively). Inversely, the addition of SAC to OLZ-containing formulations resulted in a substantial enhancement of the crushing strength of pellets ($p < 0.01$, by comparison with pellets containing OLZ in the matrix) (Table 2). These results are in line with previous publications which reported that tablets containing CAMs presented higher crushing strength values, as compared to those prepared using the respective crystalline counterparts [27,28,50]. This may be explained by the higher cohesiveness of OLZ in the CAM form [27,28,50] which may have increased the number and/or intensity of bonds established in the matrix of pellets.

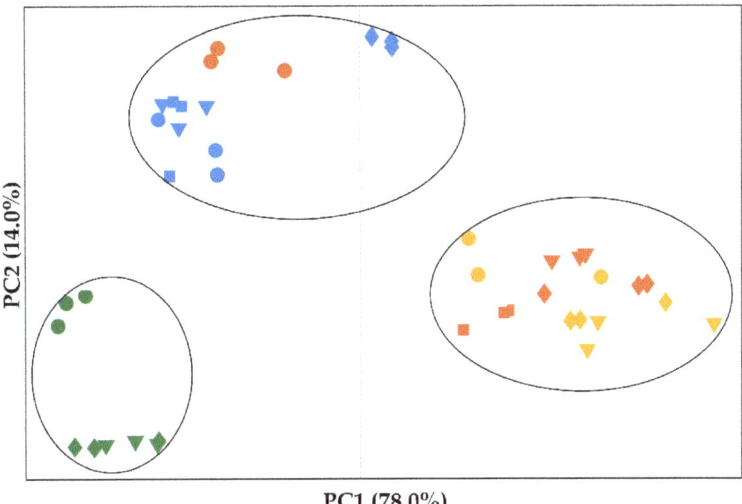

Figure 6. Scores plot from the principal component analysis conducted on the FTIR spectra of samples prepared using the placebo-based formulation (Formulation P, green), formulation I (blue) or formulation II, using the crystalline (orange) or the co-amorphous (yellow) form of olanzapine and saccharin, as starting material. Markers reflect the nature of samples: physical mixtures (circles), extrudates (diamonds), uncoated pellets (triangles), or pellets coated with olanzapine or olanzapine and saccharin (squares).

Concomitantly, dissolution studies were conducted, under sink and non-sink conditions (to reflect the poor solubility of crystalline OLZ, by contrast to amorphous OLZ), to evaluate the rate and extent of OLZ release. Dissolution profiles of samples, under sink conditions (10 mg/L of OLZ, equivalent to 200 mg of pellets), indicated that all samples released the entire quantity of the drug into the dissolution media after 24 h of test, as expected. Particularly, pellets containing OLZ in the matrix (formulation I) resulted in dissolution profiles presenting a slow release of the drug from the structure of pellets (Figure 7, yellow). The dissolution rate of OLZ from samples was considerably enhanced by introducing SAC in formulations, as reflected by the reduction of the time required to release 75% of the drug (89 vs. 253 min for pellets containing crystalline OLZ:SAC and crystalline OLZ, respectively; $p < 0.01$; Table 2). Interestingly, pellets of formulation II containing OLZ-CAM in the matrix exhibited a slightly slower release of the drug when compared to pellets prepared using the crystalline OLZ:SAC as starting material (t_{50} of 39 and 31 min for pellets containing OLZ-CAM and crystalline OLZ:SAC; $p < 0.05$; Table 2). The slower release of the drug in the CAM from pelletized samples may be related to the higher crushing strength of pellets containing OLZ-CAM (Table 2); the penetration of water into the matrix of the beads may have been hampered by the more compact structure, thus slowing down the release of the drug. Nevertheless, pellets containing OLZ-CAM in the matrix have shown to significantly enhance the drug dissolution rate by comparison with pellets without the co-amorphous stabilizer (SAC, Table 2, $p < 0.01$). Inversely, dissolution tests conducted under non-sink conditions (100 mg/L of OLZ, equivalent to 2 g of pellets) on formulation I-based samples have shown the stabilization of the release of the drug at approximately 40%, in line with the solubility of the crystalline drug in the dissolution media (41 mg/L, at 37 °C) which guaranteed the maintenance of the non-sink conditions throughout the test. Both the co-amorphization of OLZ and SAC, by solvent evaporation (prior to the manufacture of pellets) or in situ (during the production of pellets), increased the equilibrium concentration of the drug. Therefore, based on the higher dissolution rate and equilibrium concentration of OLZ-CAM in pellets, one may expect enhanced oral bioavailability of the drug and maximization of the therapeutic effectiveness of the treatment. Noteworthy is that the dissolution profiles of studies performed at pH > 8.0 did not show significant differences. At lower pH, the solubility of the drug, even in the absence of SAC, was significantly increased and so was release rate and dissolution, thus not guaranteeing the required non-sink conditions.

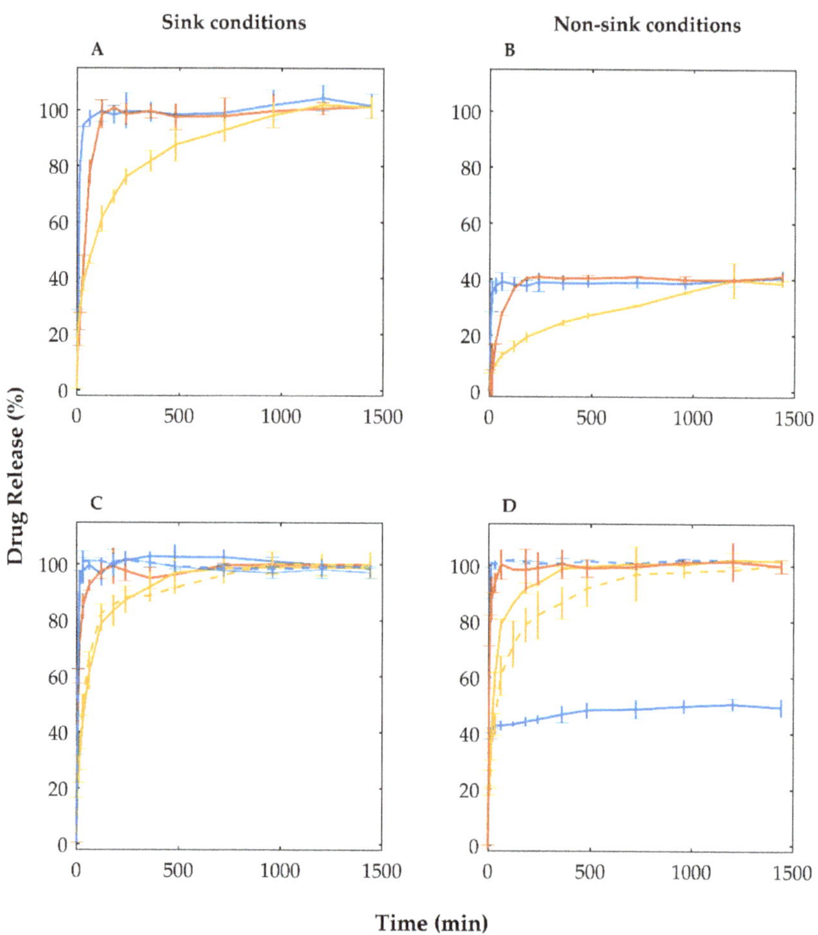

Figure 7. Dissolution profiles under sink (10 mg/L of OLZ, **A,C**) and non-sink conditions (100 mg/L of OLZ, **B,D**), of formulations I (**A,B**) and II (using the crystalline—solid line—or the co-amorphous form—dashed line—of olanzapine and saccharin, as starting materials) (**C,D**). Colors reflect the state of samples: physical mixtures (blue), uncoated pellets (yellow), and coated pellets (orange).

3.3.2. Preparation and Characterization of Pellets Containing Olanzapine on the Surface

After the manufacture of placebo-based pellets, beads were film-coated using solutions of dichloromethane and OLZ or OLZ:SAC, or water suspensions of OLZ or OLZ:SAC. Unfortunately, spraying of water suspensions, clogged the atomization nozzle and the pellets produced presented an OLZ content of approximately 54% (equivalent to 2.7% *w/w* of OLZ in pellets), well below the drug content of OLZ aimed. On the contrary, the use of solutions of OLZ, or OLZ and SAC, in dichloromethane, resulted in the manufacture of pellets presenting the desired content of the drug ($100.48 \pm 8.20\%$ or $100.81 \pm 7.92\%$, respectively). SEM microphotographs (Figure 8) indicated that the coating of placebo-based pellets, using a solution of OLZ or OLZ:SAC, resulted in pellets presenting a rough surface (Figure 8B,C) with an outer layer of approximately 20 µm thick (readers are recommended to the Supplementary Material to observe the cross section of pellets; Figure S2). In contrast, pellets containing the model drug in the matrix presented a clean and smooth surface (Figure 8D–F). Since dichloromethane may result in safety concerns for patients, gas chromatography analysis was conducted on coated pellets to determine the concentration of the solvent. Results have shown that for all samples dichloromethane was present in pellets at a concentration lower than 200 ppm, thus well below the maximum concentration of residual solvents imposed by the ICH Q3C (<600 ppm) [51]. Furthermore, considering the maximum daily intake of OLZ (20 mg), the quantity of solvent administered to the patients lies well below the permissible daily exposure established by the guideline (<6 mg/day) [51].

As before, the solid-state arrangement of OLZ in samples was investigated using XRPD and FTIR spectroscopy. Diffractograms of samples obtained from pellets coated using the dichloromethane OLZ solution, presented the diffraction peaks of OLZ at 8.7 and 21.1 °2θ (Supplementary Material—Figure S1), in line with the polymorphic form I of the drug (as discussed in Section 3.3.1). Likewise, the FTIR spectra of samples obtained from pellets containing OLZ on the surface did not show any noticeable modifications, when compared to those of the physical mixture and pellets containing OLZ in the matrix. Therefore, one may conclude that OLZ recrystallized during the coating of inert beads.

On the other hand, the incorporation of SAC into the spraying solution resulted in the production of coated pellets, whose diffractograms failed to present the diffraction peaks of both OLZ and SAC. Worth highlighting here, that no additional peaks were observed in diffractograms and those present therein were related to the excipients used to produce the pellets. Furthermore, the FTIR spectra of pellets coated with OLZ and SAC did not present the peak characteristic of the C=O group of SAC (at approximately 1717 cm^{-1}), suggesting the interaction of OLZ and SAC in the solid-state. Consequently, co-amorphization of OLZ and SAC is suggested by the results of both techniques.

Multivariate analysis (Figure 6) allowed identification of clustering of samples obtained from pellets coated with OLZ and SAC with those prepared using the OLZ-CAM, previously prepared by solvent evaporation, as starting material. The high similarity of the spectra of both samples was thus ascertained. Consequently, FTIR spectroscopy reinforces the co-amorphization of OLZ and SAC during the coating of inert beads. In fact, the low boiling temperature of dichloromethane (40 °C, [52]) and the atomization of solutions into small droplets may have resulted in a rapid evaporation of the solvent and hence a short time available for the arrangement of molecules.

Measurements of the crushing strength of pellets have shown that the coating of beads using solutions containing OLZ or OLZ:SAC had no significant impact on the internal resistance of the pellets as compared to the values obtained for placebo-based pellets and pellets containing OLZ in the matrix ($p > 0.05$, Table 2). These results are expected since the pellets coated by either OLZ or OLZ:SAC presented the same common matrix (placebo-based pellets). In contrast, the internal resistance of the pellets coated with OLZ or OLZ:SAC was significantly reduced by comparison with the pellets containing OLZ:SAC in the matrix (Table 2).

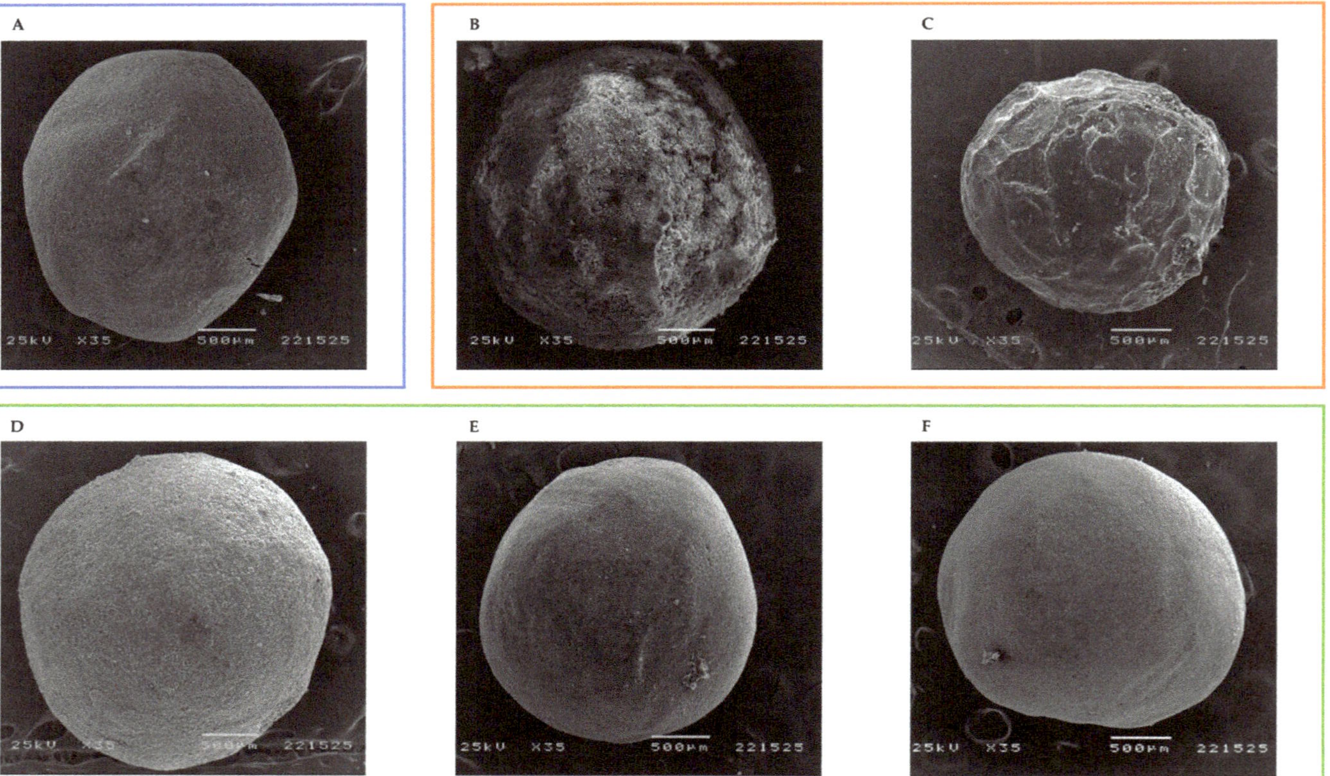

Figure 8. Scanning electron microphotographs of placebo-based pellets (**A**), pellets containing olanzapine (**B**) or olanzapine and saccharin (**C**) on the surface and pellets containing olanzapine in the matrix of the bead—formulation I (**D**) and formulation II, using olanzapine and saccharin in the crystalline (**E**) or the co-amorphous (**F**) form, as starting materials.

Deposition of OLZ or OLZ:SAC on the surface of pellets considerably enhanced the dissolution rate of the drug as compared to samples containing OLZ in the matrix ($p < 0.01$). Dissolution of pellets containing OLZ on the surface has shown that at 1 h of test more than 75% of the drug was already dissolved in the dissolution media (Table 2). This represents a 4-fold enhancement in the drug dissolution rate compared to samples containing OLZ in the matrix. Dissolution tests, under non-sink conditions (100 mg/L of OLZ, equivalent to 2 g of pellets), showed the stabilization of the drug release at approximately 40%, equivalent to 40 mg/L, aligned with the solubility of the polymorphic form I of the drug, as discussed before.

Pellets containing OLZ and SAC on the surface of beads released the drug faster—approximately 75% of the drug in 14 min, which stands for a 6- and 7-fold enhancement compared to pellets containing OLZ:SAC or the CAM, as starting materials, in the matrix of pellets, respectively. The higher dissolution rate of OLZ from the surface of pellets was also observed in dissolution tests conducted under non-sink conditions (Figure 7D). Under non-sink conditions, it was also shown that the pellets coated with OLZ:SAC in dichloromethane, released the total amount of OLZ inserted in the dissolution vessel (100 mg of OLZ/L). In fact, the solubility of OLZ-CAM in pellets has shown to be considerably enhanced to values (5897.5 $\pm$ 194.9 mg/L for pellets containing OLZ:SAC on the surface, and 5903.3 $\pm$ 279.1 and 5847.9 $\pm$ 281.7 mg/L for pellets containing OLZ:SAC and OLZ:CAM in the matrix, respectively) way above that of the crystalline counterpart. It is worth highlighting that no statistical differences were found for the solubility of OLZ from pellets containing OLZ:SAC on the surface, or pellets containing OLZ:SAC and OLZ:CAM in the matrix ($p > 0.05$). The results obtained stand for about a 145-fold enhancement in the solubility of OLZ and are aligned with previous works [15].

These results highlighted the value of coating as a novel preparation technique to generate CAMs of poorly water soluble drugs directly during the production of dosage forms. Compared to conventional manufacture methods using CAMs, this technique precludes the prior preparation of the CAMs, thus reducing the number of unit operations required in the manufacturing process and the associated costs; stability concerns, such as the recrystallization of the amorphous content due to the exposure to stress conditions (e.g., temperature or humidity), are also minimized. In addition, coating of inert beads has proven to considerably enhance the solubility and dissolution rate of the drug from pellets, as compared to conventional pellets in which drugs are present in the matrix, thus anticipating a higher oral bioavailability.

3.4. Evaluation of the Stability of Co-Amorphous Olanzapine in Pellets

Stability studies were run for 9 months at 23 °C/60% of relative humidity (shelf storage conditions) to evaluate the extent of recrystallization of OLZ-CAM in pellets. At the end of the stability test, diffractograms of samples (Figure 9) did not show any noticeable variations, when compared to diffractograms of recently manufactured samples, suggesting the maintenance of OLZ in the co-amorphous form during the storage time considered. The formation of OLZ saccharinate by salification may have prevented the reorganization of molecules, explaining the high stability of the OLZ-CAM. These results are aligned with previous studies, which reported that the CAM containing OLZ and SAC was stable for more than 3 years, at 23 °C/65% RH [28]. The storage of samples for longer periods of time is recommended to compare the rate of recrystallization of OLZ-CAM from samples containing the drug in the matrix or on the surface of pellets.

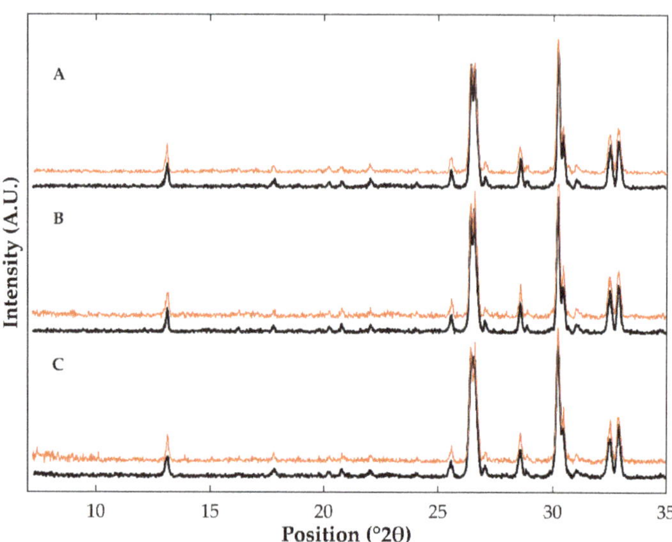

Figure 9. Diffractograms of samples obtained from pellets containing olanzapine and saccharin on the surface (**A**) or in the matrix of the beads, using the crystalline (**B**) or the co-amorphous form (**C**), as starting materials. Colors reflect the storage time: 0 (black) or 9 months (orange).

4. Conclusions

The production of pellets containing OLZ in the highly soluble co-amorphous form, either in the matrix, or on the surface of pellets, was achieved. The stability of OLZ-CAMs throughout the manufacture of pellets was confirmed, since no signs of drug recrystallization were detected. Water-induced in situ co-amorphization of crystalline OLZ and SAC, during the production of pellets, resulted in solubility increase and a faster release of the drug from the matrix ($t_{75\%}$ < 89 min vs. $t_{75\%}$ > 252 min, for pellets containing crystalline OLZ in the matrix). Conversely, coating of inert beads, using an organic solution of OLZ and SAC (1:1 molar ratio), was established as a novel method to prepare CAMs in situ, both enhancing the solubility and the dissolution rate ($t_{75\%}$ < 14 min) of the drug. Compared to the conventional methods of pellet production from CAMs, the co-amorphization of OLZ achieved directly on the surface of beads, not only minimizes the recrystallization risk but also is likely to reduce the production costs and time, since no previous production of CAMs is needed. The added-value of the coating-induced co-amorphization, as a novel preparation technique to generate CAMs, was confirmed in this work. In the future, the same approach should be extended to other poorly water-soluble drugs, combinations of drugs and co-amorphous stabilizers (e.g., amino acids) and considered in tailoring drug release, once long-term stability has been proved for such new entities.

Supplementary Materials: The following supporting information can be downloaded at: https://www.mdpi.com/article/10.3390/pharmaceutics14122587/s1, Figure S1: Diffractograms of samples obtained from placebo formulations (**A**), and formulations containing olanzapine (**B**) or olanzapine:saccharin in the crystalline (**C**) or the co-amorphous (**D**) form, as starting materials; Figure S2: Scanning electron microphotographs of the cross sectional area of pellets containing olanzapine (formulation I, **A**) or olanzapine and saccharin (formulation II, **B**) on the surface of the bead.

Author Contributions: Conceptualization, N.F.d.C. and J.F.P.; methodology, N.F.d.C. and R.F.A.; formal analysis, N.F.d.C., R.F.A. and J.F.P.; investigation, N.F.d.C. and R.F.A.; data curation, N.F.d.C. and R.F.A.; writing—original draft preparation, N.F.d.C. and R.F.A.; writing—review and editing, A.I.F., J.A.L. and J.F.P.; supervision, A.I.F. and J.F.P.; project administration, A.I.F. and J.F.P.; funding acquisition, A.I.F. and J.F.P. All authors have read and agreed to the published version of the manuscript.

Funding: This research was funded by Fundação para a Ciência e a Tecnologia, Lisbon, Portugal (PTDC/CTM-BIO/3946/2014 and SFRH/BD/137080/2018).

Data Availability Statement: All data generated or analyzed during this study is included in this published article [and its Supplementary Information Files].

Acknowledgments: Luisa Mateus is acknowledged for conducting the gas chromatography analysis and Telmo Nunes for performing the SEM analysis. Rampex Labs Pvt. Ltd. (Telangana, India) and Budenheim (Budenheim, Germany) are acknowledged for the generous gifts of OLZ and dibasic calcium phosphate anhydrous (DI-CAFOS® A60), respectively.

Conflicts of Interest: Authors declared no competing interest.

References

1. Liu, J.; Grohganz, H.; Löbmann, K.; Rades, T.; Hempel, N.-J.J. Co-Amorphous Drug Formulations in Numbers: Recent Advances in Co-Amorphous Drug Formulations with Focus on Co-Formability, Molar Ratio, Preparation Methods, Physical Stability, In Vitro and In Vivo Performance, and New Formulation Strategies. *Pharmaceutics* **2021**, *13*, 389. [CrossRef] [PubMed]
2. Chen, X.; Li, D.; Zhang, H.; Duan, Y.; Huang, Y. Co-amorphous systems of sinomenine with nonsteroidal anti-inflammatory drugs: A strategy for solubility improvement, sustained release, and drug combination therapy against rheumatoid arthritis. *Int. J. Pharm.* **2021**, *606*, 120894. [CrossRef] [PubMed]
3. Karimi-Jafari, M.; Padrela, L.; Walker, G.M.; Croker, D.M. Creating cocrystals: A review of pharmaceutical cocrystal preparation routes and applications. *Cryst. Growth Des.* **2018**, *18*, 6370–6387. [CrossRef]
4. Batisai, E. Solubility Enhancement of Antidiabetic Drugs Using a Co-Crystallization Approach. *ChemistryOpen* **2021**, *10*, 1260–1268. [CrossRef] [PubMed]
5. Wilson, V.R.; Lou, X.; Osterling, D.J.; Stolarik, D.A.F.; Jenkins, G.J.; Nichols, B.L.B.; Dong, Y.; Edgar, K.J.; Zhang, G.G.Z.; Taylor, L.S. Amorphous solid dispersions of enzalutamide and novel polysaccharide derivatives: Investigation of relationships between polymer structure and performance. *Sci. Rep.* **2020**, *10*, 18535. [CrossRef]
6. Löbmann, K.; Grohganz, H.; Laitinen, R.; Strachan, C.; Rades, T. Amino acids as co-amorphous stabilizers for poorly water soluble drugs—Part 1: Preparation, stability and dissolution enhancement. *Eur. J. Pharm. Biopharm.* **2013**, *85*, 873–881. [CrossRef]
7. Gao, Y.; Liao, J.; Qi, X.; Zhang, J. Coamorphous repaglinide—Saccharin with enhanced dissolution. *Int. J. Pharm.* **2013**, *450*, 290–295. [CrossRef]
8. Zhang, M.; Xiong, X.; Suo, Z.; Hou, Q.; Gan, N.; Tang, P.; Ding, X.; Li, H. Co-amorphous palbociclib-organic acid systems with increased dissolution rate, enhanced physical stability and equivalent biosafety. *RSC Adv.* **2019**, *9*, 3946–3955. [CrossRef]
9. Lino, P.; Henriques, J. Amorphous Solid Dispersions-Increasing Solubility from API to Tablets. Available online: https://drug-dev.com/amorphous-solid-dispersions-increasing-solubility-from-api-to-tablets/ (accessed on 6 July 2022).
10. Karagianni, A.; Kachrimanis, K.; Nikolakakis, I. Co-Amorphous Solid Dispersions for Solubility and Absorption Improvement of Drugs: Composition, Preparation, Characterization and Formulations for Oral Delivery. *Pharmaceutics* **2018**, *10*, 98. [CrossRef]
11. Han, J.; Wei, Y.; Lu, Y.; Wang, R.; Zhang, J.; Gao, Y.; Qian, S. Co-amorphous systems for the delivery of poorly water-soluble drugs: Recent advances and an update. *Expert Opin. Drug Deliv.* **2020**, *17*, 1411–1435. [CrossRef]
12. Chavan, R.B.; Thipparaboina, R.; Kumar, D.; Shastri, N.R. Co amorphous systems: A product development perspective. *Int. J. Pharm.* **2016**, *515*, 403–415. [CrossRef] [PubMed]
13. Fini, A.; Cavallari, C.; Ceschel, G.; Rabasco, A.M. Bimodal Release of Olanzapine from Lipid Microspheres. *J. Pharm. Sci.* **2010**, *99*, 4251–4260. [CrossRef] [PubMed]
14. Balbão, M.S.; Hallak, J.E.C.; Nunes, E.A.; de Mello, M.H.; Triffoni-Melo, A.T.; Ferreira, F.I.S.; Chaves, C.; Durão, A.M.S.; Ramos, A.P.P.; Crippa, J.A.S.; et al. Olanzapine, weight change and metabolic effects: A naturalistic 12-month follow up. *Ther. Adv. Psychopharmacol.* **2014**, *4*, 30–36. [CrossRef] [PubMed]
15. da Costa, N.F.; Santos, I.A.; Fernandes, A.I.; Pinto, J.F. Sulfonic acid derivatives in the production of stable co-amorphous systems for solubility enhancement. *J. Pharm. Sci.* **2022**, *111*, 3327–3339. [CrossRef] [PubMed]
16. Aparnathi, K.D. Chemistry and Use of Artificial Intense Sweeteners. *Int. J. Curr. Microbiol. Appl. Sci.* **2017**, *6*, 1283–1296. [CrossRef]
17. Shah, C.R.; Suhagia, B.N.; Shah, N.J.; Patel, D.R.; Patel, N.M. Stability-indicating simultaneous HPTLC method for olanzapine and fluoxetine in combined tablet dosage form. *Indian J. Pharm. Sci.* **2008**, *70*, 251–255. [CrossRef]
18. Mahmood, A.A.R.; Al-Juboori, S.B. A Review: Saccharin Discovery, Synthesis, and Applications. *Ibn AL- Haitham J. Pure Appl. Sci.* **2020**, *33*, 43–61. [CrossRef]
19. Jensen, K.T.; Blaabjerg, L.I.; Lenz, E.; Bohr, A.; Grohganz, H.; Kleinebudde, P.; Rades, T.; Löbmann, K. Preparation and characterization of spray-dried co-amorphous drug-amino acid salts. *J. Pharm. Pharmacol.* **2016**, *68*, 615–624. [CrossRef]
20. Wu, W.; Löbmann, K.; Rades, T.; Grohganz, H. On the role of salt formation and structural similarity of co-formers in co-amorphous drug delivery systems. *Int. J. Pharm.* **2018**, *535*, 86–94. [CrossRef] [PubMed]
21. Narala, S.; Nyavanandi, D.; Srinivasan, P.; Mandati, P.; Bandari, S.; Repka, M.A. Pharmaceutical Co-crystals, Salts, and Co-amorphous Systems: A novel opportunity of hot-melt extrusion. *J. Drug Deliv. Sci. Technol.* **2021**, *61*, 102209. [CrossRef]

22. Allu, S.; Suresh, K.; Bolla, G.; Mannava, M.K.C.; Nangia, A. Role of hydrogen bonding in cocrystals and coamorphous solids: Indapamide as a case study. *CrystEngComm* **2019**, *21*, 2043. [CrossRef]

23. Lenz, E.; Löbmann, K.; Rades, T.; Knop, K.; Kleinebudde, P. Hot Melt Extrusion and Spray Drying of Co-amorphous Indomethacin-Arginine With Polymers. *J. Pharm. Sci.* **2017**, *106*, 302–312. [CrossRef] [PubMed]

24. Wlodarski, K.; Sawicki, W.; Paluch, K.J.; Tajber, L.; Grembecka, M.; Hawelek, L.; Wojnarowska, Z.; Grzybowska, K.; Talik, E.; Paluch, M. The influence of amorphization methods on the apparent solubility and dissolution rate of tadalafil. *Eur. J. Pharm. Sci.* **2014**, *62*, 132–140. [CrossRef] [PubMed]

25. Paudel, A.; Meeus, J.; Mooter, G. Van den Structural Characterization of Amorphous Solid Dispersions. In *Amorphous Solid Dispersions*; Shah, N., Sandhu, H., Choi, D.S., Chokshi, H., Malick, A.W., Eds.; Springer: New York, NY, USA, 2014; pp. 421–485. ISBN 9781493915989.

26. Ploeger, K.J.M.; Adack, P.; Sundararajan, P.; Valente, P.C.; Henriques, J.G.; Rosenberg, K.J. Spray drying and amorphous dispersions. In *Chemical Engineering in the Pharmaceutical Industry*; Ende, D.J.A., Ende, M.T.A., Eds.; John Wiley & Sons, Inc.: Hoboken, NJ, USA, 2019; pp. 267–292. ISBN 9781119600800.

27. da Costa, N.F.; Pinto, J.F.; Fernandes, A.I. Cohesiveness of Powdered Co-Amorphous Olanzapine and Impact on Tablet Production. *Med. Sci. Forum* **2021**, *5*, 2. [CrossRef]

28. da Costa, N.F.; Daniels, R.; Fernandes, A.I.; Pinto, J.F. Downstream Processing of Amorphous and Co-Amorphous Olanzapine Powder Blends. *Pharmaceutics* **2022**, *14*, 1535. [CrossRef]

29. da Costa, N.F.; Fernandes, A.I.; Pinto, J.F. Measurement of the amorphous fraction of olanzapine incorporated in a co-amorphous formulation. *Int. J. Pharm.* **2020**, *588*, 119716. [CrossRef] [PubMed]

30. Joshi, A.B.; Patel, S.; Kaushal, A.M.; Bansal, A.K. Compaction studies of alternate solid forms of celecoxib. *Adv. Powder Technol.* **2010**, *21*, 452–460. [CrossRef]

31. Démuth, B.; Farkas, A.; Balogh, A.; Bartosiewicz, K.; Kállai-Szabó, B.; Bertels, J.; Vigh, T.; Mensch, J.; Verreck, G.; Van Assche, I.; et al. Lubricant-Induced Crystallization of Itraconazole From Tablets Made of Electrospun Amorphous Solid Dispersion. *J. Pharm. Sci.* **2016**, *105*, 2982–2988. [CrossRef]

32. Thakral, N.K.; Mohapatra, S.; Stephenson, G.A.; Suryanarayanan, R. Compression-induced crystallization of amorphous indomethacin in tablets: Characterization of spatial heterogeneity by two-dimensional X-ray diffractometry. *Mol. Pharm.* **2015**, *12*, 253–263. [CrossRef]

33. Petry, I.; Löbmann, K.; Grohganz, H.; Rades, T.; Leopold, C.S. In situ co-amorphisation of arginine with indomethacin or furosemide during immersion in an acidic medium—A proof of concept study. *Eur. J. Pharm. Biopharm.* **2018**, *133*, 151–160. [CrossRef]

34. Huang, C.; Klinzing, G.; Procopio, A.; Yang, F.; Ren, J.; Burlage, R.; Zhu, L.; Su, Y. Understanding Compression-Induced Amorphization of Crystalline Posaconazole. *Mol. Pharm.* **2019**, *16*, 825–833. [CrossRef] [PubMed]

35. Doreth, M.; Hussein, M.A.; Priemel, P.A.; Grohganz, H.; Holm, R.; de Diego, H.L.; Rades, T.; Löbmann, K. Amorphization within the tablet: Using microwave irradiation to form a glass solution in situ. *Int. J. Pharm.* **2017**, *519*, 343–351. [CrossRef] [PubMed]

36. Petry, I.; Löbmann, K.; Grohganz, H.; Rades, T.; Leopold, C.S. In situ co-amorphisation in coated tablets—The combination of carvedilol with aspartic acid during immersion in an acidic medium. *Int. J. Pharm.* **2019**, *558*, 357–366. [CrossRef] [PubMed]

37. Kim, D.H.; Kim, Y.W.; Tin, Y.Y.; Soe, M.T.P.; Ko, B.H.; Park, S.J.; Lee, J.W. Recent technologies for amorphization of poorly water-soluble drugs. *Pharmaceutics* **2021**, *13*, 1318. [CrossRef] [PubMed]

38. Qiang, W.; Löbmann, K.; McCoy, C.P.; Andrews, G.P.; Zhao, M. Microwave-induced in situ amorphization: A new strategy for tackling the stability issue of amorphous solid dispersions. *Pharmaceutics* **2020**, *12*, 655. [CrossRef]

39. Rowe, R.C.; Sheskey, P.J.; Quinn, M.E.; Hoppu, P. Saccharin. In *Handbook of Pharmaceutical Excipients*; Rowe, R.C., Sheskey, P.J., Quinn, M.E., Eds.; Pharmaceutical Press: London, UK; the American Pharmacists Association: Chicago, IL, USA, 2009; pp. 605–607. ISBN 9780853697923.

40. Mainardes, R.M.; Gremião, M.P.D.; Evangelista, R.C. Thermoanalytical study of praziquantel-loaded PLGA nanoparticles. *Rev. Bras. Ciencias Farm. J. Pharm. Sci.* **2006**, *42*, 523–530. [CrossRef]

41. Polla, G.I.; Vega, D.R.; Lanza, H.; Tombari, D.G.; Baggio, R.; Ayala, A.P.; Filho, J.M.; Fernández, D.; Leyva, G.; Dartayet, G. Thermal behaviour and stability in Olanzapine. *Int. J. Pharm.* **2005**, *301*, 33–40. [CrossRef] [PubMed]

42. Basavoju, S.; Boström, D.; Velaga, S.P. Indomethacin-saccharin cocrystal: Design, synthesis and preliminary pharmaceutical characterization. *Pharm. Res.* **2008**, *25*, 530–541. [CrossRef]

43. Ferreira, P.O.; de Moura, A.; de Almeida, A.C.; dos Santos, É.C.; Kogawa, A.C.; Caires, F.J. Mechanochemical synthesis, thermoanalytical study and characterization of new multicomponent solid forms of norfloxacin with saccharin. *J. Therm. Anal. Calorim.* **2022**, *147*, 1985–1997. [CrossRef]

44. Gao, Y.; Zu, H.; Zhang, J. Enhanced dissolution and stability of adefovir dipivoxil by cocrystal formation. *J. Pharm. Pharmacol.* **2011**, *63*, 483–490. [CrossRef]

45. Dengale, S.J.; Grohganz, H.; Rades, T.; Löbmann, K. Recent advances in co-amorphous drug formulations. *Adv. Drug Deliv. Rev.* **2016**, *100*, 116–125. [CrossRef] [PubMed]

46. Erkoboni, D.F. Extrusion/Spheronization. In *Pharmaceutical Extrusion Technology*; Ghebre-Sellassie, I., Martin, C., Eds.; Marcel Dekker Incorporated: New York, NY, USA, 2003; pp. 249–290. ISBN 9780824755201.

47. Pinto, J.F.; Buckton, G.; Newton, J.M. The influence of four selected processing and formulation factors on the production of spheres by extrusion and spheronisation. *Int. J. Pharm.* **1992**, *83*, 187–196. [CrossRef]
48. European Directorate for the Quality of Medicines & HealthCare. *European Pharmacopoeia*, 10th ed.; Council of Europe: Strasbourg, France, 2021.
49. da Costa, N.F.; Daniels, R.; Fernandes, A.I.; Pinto, J.F. Amorphous and Co-Amorphous Olanzapine Stability in Formulations Intended for Wet Granulation and Pelletization. *Int. J. Mol. Sci.* **2022**, *23*, 10234. [CrossRef] [PubMed]
50. Lenz, E.; Jensen, K.T.; Blaabjerg, L.I.; Knop, K.; Grohganz, H.; Löbmann, K.; Rades, T.; Kleinebudde, P. Solid-state properties and dissolution behaviour of tablets containing co-amorphous indomethacin-arginine. *Eur. J. Pharm. Biopharm.* **2015**, *96*, 44–52. [CrossRef] [PubMed]
51. International Conference on Harmonisation (ICH) Committee for Medicinal Products for Human Use, ICH Harmonized Guideline Q3C (R8) on Impurities: Guideline for Residual Solvents. *ICH Expert Work. Gr.* **2021**, *31*. Available online: https://database.ich.org/sites/default/files/ICH_Q3C-R8_Guideline_Step4_2021_0422.pdf (accessed on 17 October 2022).
52. Yang, N. Dichloromethane. In *Encyclopedia of Toxicology*; Wexler, P., Ed.; Elsevier Inc.: London, UK, 2014; pp. 99–101. ISBN 9780123864543.

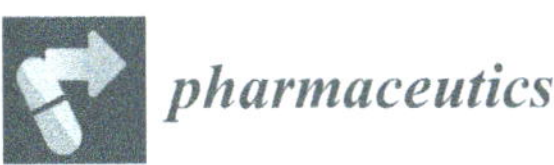

Article

Crystal Engineering of Ionic Cocrystals Sustained by Azolium···Azole Heterosynthons

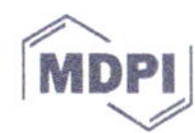

Maryam Rahmani, Vijith Kumar, Julia Bruno-Colmenarez and Michael J. Zaworotko *

Department of Chemical Sciences and Bernal Institute, University of Limerick, V94 T9PX Limerick, Ireland
* Correspondence: xtal@ul.ie

Abstract: Crystal engineering of multi-component molecular crystals, cocrystals, is a subject of growing interest, thanks in part to the potential utility of pharmaceutical cocrystals as drug substances with improved properties. Whereas molecular cocrystals (MCCs) are quite well studied from a design perspective, ionic cocrystals (ICCs) remain relatively underexplored despite there being several recently FDA-approved drug products based upon ICCs. Successful cocrystal design strategies typically depend on strong and directional noncovalent interactions between coformers, as exemplified by hydrogen bonds. Understanding of the hierarchy of such interactions is key to successful outcomes in cocrystal design. We herein address the crystal engineering of ICCs comprising azole functional groups, particularly imidazoles and triazoles, which are commonly encountered in biologically active molecules. Specifically, azoles were studied for their propensity to serve as coformers with strong organic (trifluoroacetic acid and p-toluenesulfonic acid) and inorganic (hydrochloric acid, hydrobromic acid and nitric acid) acids to gain insight into the hierarchy of $NH^+ \cdots N$ (azolium-azole) supramolecular heterosynthons. Accordingly, we combined data mining of the Cambridge Structural Database (CSD) with the structural characterization of 16 new ICCs (11 imidazoles, 4 triazoles, one imidazole-triazole). Analysis of the new ICCs and 66 relevant hits archived in the CSD revealed that supramolecular synthons between identical azole rings (A^+B^-A) are much more commonly encountered, 71, than supramolecular synthons between different azole rings (A^+B^-C), 11. The average $NH^+ \cdots N$ distance found in the new ICCs reported herein is 2.697(3) Å and binding energy calculations suggested that hydrogen bond strengths range from 31–46 kJ mol^{-1}. The azolium-triazole ICC (A^+B^-C) was obtained via mechanochemistry and differed from the other ICCs studied as there was no $NH^+ \cdots N$ hydrogen bonding. That the CNC angles in imidazoles and 1,2,4-triazoles are sensitive to protonation, the cationic forms having larger (approximately 4.4 degrees) values than comparable neutral rings, was used as a parameter to distinguish between protonated and neutral azole rings. Our results indicate that ICCs based upon azolium-azole supramolecular heterosynthons are viable targets, which has implications for the development of new azole drug substances with improved properties.

Keywords: crystal engineering; ionic cocrystals; charge-assisted hydrogen bond; azolium···azole; supramolecular heterosynthon

Citation: Rahmani, M.; Kumar, V.; Bruno-Colmenarez, J.; Zaworotko, M.J. Crystal Engineering of Ionic Cocrystals Sustained by Azolium···Azole Heterosynthons. *Pharmaceutics* **2022**, *14*, 2321. https://doi.org/10.3390/pharmaceutics14112321

Academic Editor: Hisham Al-Obaidi

Received: 13 September 2022
Accepted: 18 October 2022
Published: 28 October 2022

Publisher's Note: MDPI stays neutral with regard to jurisdictional claims in published maps and institutional affiliations.

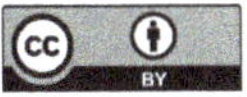

1. Introduction

Crystal engineering [1] is the field of chemistry that studies the design, properties, and applications of crystalline solids [2,3] and offers promise for the design of new materials with improved properties for a number of applications including porous materials gas separation and storage [4–6], polar crystals for non-linear optics [7,8], and the use of pharmaceutical cocrystals as improved drug substances [9–12]. With respect to pharmaceutical science, crystal engineering can also offer insight into other classes of crystalline drug substances including their propensity to form polymorphs and multi-component molecular crystals such as solvates, hydrates, and cocrystals [13,14]. Cocrystals, defined as "solids that are crystalline single phase materials composed of two or more different molecular and/or ionic compounds generally in a stoichiometric ratio which are neither solvates nor simple salts" [13], are of relevance to pharmaceutical science because they can modify the physicochemical properties of a drug molecule without changing its chemical structure. Cocrystals can thereby offer improved, sometimes greatly improved solubility [15,16], stability [17], dissolution rate [18], and bioavailability [19,20]. It is therefore unsurprising that the increased interest in the study of pharmaceutical cocrystals that started in the early 2000s [21–24] has resulted introduction of new drug products based upon pharmaceutical cocrystals [11,25].

Cocrystals can be classified as molecular cocrystals (MCCs) or ionic cocrystals (ICCs). MCCs are crystalline solids comprised of at least two neutral molecular compounds (coformers) sustained by noncovalent bonds, e.g., hydrogen [3] or halogen bonds [26], in a stoichiometric ratio. ICCs are comprised of at least one salt and a coformer [27] and typically sustained by charge-assisted supramolecular synthons or, if metals are present, coordination bonds (therefore ICCs and coordination networks may not be mutually exclusive) [17,28]. Indeed, the first cocrystal was an ICC of NaCl and urea reported 1783 by De I'Ise, who noted a change in morphology of NaCl crystals obtained from slow evaporation urea-containing solutions (e.g., urine) [29]. Subsequently, ICCs of NaCl and sugars were reported in the literature [30–33]. In the 1960s, the crystal structure of sodium chloride and urea was reported by Palm and MacGillivray, after Kleber detailed the morphology and optics of this compound [34]. In 2004, Childs et al. presented an early example of a pharmaceutical ICC that used carboxylic acid coformers to regulate the dissolution rate of fluoxetine hydrochloride (Prozac®) [23]. To describe the sodium bromide-barbituric acid cocrystal, Braga coined the term "ionic cocrystal" in 2010 [27]. This nomenclature however is not universal, with terms such as "complex salts", "metal salt complexes", "acid salts", "salt-cocrystals", "adducts", and "hybrid salt-cocrystals" also being used for ionic cocrystals [35–39]. Most recently, systematic studies of ICCs have been conducted by our group through the study of phenol-phenolate ICCs sustained by PhOH···PhO⁻ supramolecular heterosynthons [40] and phosphoric acid-dihydrogen phosphate ICCs [41].

ICCs are almost always sustained by charge-assisted hydrogen bonding, which can be advantageous as they are typically shorter and stronger than hydrogen bonds formed between two neutral groups [42]. That they are necessarily comprised of three or more components means that ICCs also offer greater compositional diversity than MCCs, e.g., A^+B^-C, where A^+ = cation, B^- = anion and C = neutral coformer. This contrasts with MCCs, most of which are 2-component AB cocrystals. There is also the possibility of ICCs in which a free base serves as a coformer with a salt of that free base or the free acid serves as a coformer with a salt of that acid, i.e., A^+B^-A or A^+B^-B, respectively. Such ICCs are attractive in pharmaceutical science since there would be a relatively high mass % of the drug compound, reducing the drug dosage. An FDA-approved cocrystal that comprises an A^+B^-B drug substance is Depakote®. In addition, there are pharmaceutical ICCs involving two different drug molecules that serve as coformers. Entresto® (a hydrated A^+B^-B'-co-crystal comprised of the sodium salts of sacubitril and valsartan) [43] and Seglentis® (an A^+B^-C co-crystal where C = celecoxib, an anti-inflammatory, A^+ = protonated tramadol, an analgesic, and B = chloride) [25,44]. Nevertheless, from a crystal engineering perspective, ICCs remain understudied as shown by an investigation into multicomponent crystal structures archived in the CSD by the Grothe group, which revealed that the number of such ICCs (2.1%) was much lower than MCCs (10.6%) [35]. As such, it is plausible to assert that ICCs are a long-known but understudied class of multicomponent crystals.

The design of cocrystals involves understanding of the hierarchy of supramolecular synthons as the strongest hydrogen bond donors-acceptors would be expected to dominate. This is one of Etter's rules [45,46]. In this regard, charge-assisted hydrogen bonds can drive the formation of supramolecular heterosynthons, including between chemical species that cocrystallize as conjugate acid-bases [47]. Whereas dicarboxylate salts, [COO-HOOC]⁻, are quite well studied [39], [N-H···N]⁺ hydrogen bonds are underexplored from a crystal engineering perspective, with pyridines being the most studied thus far [48,49]. The relative paucity of systematic crystal engineering studies is despite azole compounds being appealing targets due to their presence in biologically active compounds [50]. Our survey of the DrugBank database (v 5.1.7) [51] revealed that 12.8% (349/2721) of approved small molecule drug substances contain at least one azole moiety. There are three main types of azoles, N-, N/O-, and N/S-containing azoles, with N-azoles accounting for 246 drug substances (almost 70% of azole-based drug molecules). Imidazole and triazole derivatives offer a broad range of biological activity, including anti-fungal, anti-inflammatory, anti-platelet, anti-microbial, anti-mycobacterial, anti-tumoral, and antiviral properties [52–56], and form hydrogen bonds with drugs and proteins [57,58]. However, due to their poor aqueous solubility (many are BCS class II [59]), the bioavailability of this family of medicines can be a challenge. In this context, developing new salt forms of basic drug compounds has traditionally been the approach taken [60,61], although increasingly MCCs are being studied to improve key physicochemical properties such as solubility, bioavailability and stability [62–66]. ICCs comprising azolium compounds are of interest not just because their proven biological activity [67,68], they are also relevant to molecular sensors [69–71], catalysis [72,73], and energetic materials [74,75]. Indeed, to date most azolium⋯azole ICCs were studied in the context of energetic materials through ionic liquids and salts comprised of nitrogen-rich molecules [76,77]. Herein, we report a systematic crystal engineering study that evaluates the potential of azole compounds to reliably form ICCs.

2. Materials and Methods

All reagents and solvents were obtained commercially and utilized without additional purification.

2.1. Powder X-ray Diffraction (PXRD)

PXRD patterns were obtained using a PANalytical Empyrean™ diffractometer equipped with a PIXcel3D detector with the following experimental parameters: Cu Kα radiation (λ = 1.54056 Å); 40 kV and 40 mA; scan speed 8°/min; step size 0.05°, 2θ = 5–40°.

2.2. Single-Crystal X-ray Diffraction

SCXRD data for compounds 1–6, 10–12, 14 and 15 were collected using a Bruker Quest D8 Mo Sealed Tube equipped with CMOS camera and Oxford cryosystem with MoKα radiation (wavelength of λ = 0.7103 Å). SCXRD data for compounds 7, 8, 13, 16 and 17 were collected on a Bruker Quest D8 Cu Microfocus with CuKα radiation (wavelength of λ = 1.5418 Å). X-ray measurements were made using APEX 4 software, frames were integrated with Bruker SAINT [78] software and absorption corrections were performed using multi-scan methods. Crystal structures were solved by direct methods using OLEX2 [79] and anisotropic displacement parameters for non-hydrogen atoms were applied. Some hydrogen atoms were placed at calculated positions and treated using a riding model whereas other H-atoms were located in the Fourier difference maps and placed geometrically.

2.3. ICC Design (Coformer Selection)

Several criteria were applied for selecting coformers (Scheme 1): (i) imidazole and 1,2,4-triazole moieties should have sp^2 N acceptor atoms that are sterically accessible; (ii) only one azole group should be present to preclude intramolecular hydrogen bonding interactions after protonation; (iii) coformers should be free of competing protonation sites; (iv) organic and inorganic acid coformers (Scheme 1) must be acidic enough to prevent molecular cocrystal formation (ΔpK_a > 3.7) and contain just one acidic hydrogen. The ΔpK_a rule [80] was taken into account as the azole-based molecules and acids studied herein have ΔpK_a values from 6.17 to 21.06 ($\Delta pK_a \geq 3.7$), consistent with proton transfer with the selected acids (Table S1).

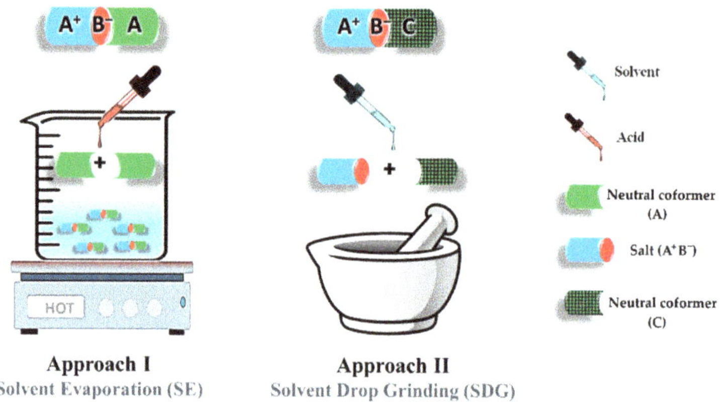

Scheme 1. Cocrystal formers studied herein and their corresponding abbreviations, along with the pK$_a$ values.

2.4. Synthesis of Ionic Cocrystals

To synthesize azolium-azole ICCs, two approaches were followed (Scheme 2). Details are presented in the Supplementary Materials (Section S1).

Scheme 2. Approaches I (crystallization) and II (mechanochemistry) were used to prepare ICCs.

2.4.1. Approach I (Solvent Evaporation)

Approach I relied on slow evaporation of solutions of each azole derivative (A or C) in a 2:1 stoichiometric molar ratio with an acid. In this study, several solvent systems were used for ICC screening (water, methanol, ethanol, and acetonitrile, or a combination of these solvents). Suitable single crystals for single crystal X-ray diffraction were isolated and bulk samples were tested using X-ray powder diffraction (see Table 1 and Table S1 for crystallographic details).

2.4.2. Approach II (Solvent-Drop Grinding)

ICCs were prepared using A⁺B⁻ salts with a 1:1 ratio of azole (A) and acid (B) (Table S2) that were subjected to solvent-drop grinding (SDG) by adding 1 molar ratio of azole as a coformer (A) to generate type A⁺B⁻ A cocrystals (comprising AH⁺···A supramolecular heterosynthons) or a different neutral coformer (C) to generate A⁺B⁻ C ICCs (comprising AH⁺···C supramolecular heterosynthons). PXRD was used to characterise the microcrystalline products (see Section S2, Figures S1–S15, of Supplementary Materials for comparison of calculated and experimental PXRD patterns, which are consistent with each other).

Table 1. Crystallographic data and structure refinement parameters for ICCs 1–17.

ICC ID	DMIHBA	BEPTEX	MPIHBA·2H$_2$O	MPINIA	MPINIA·2H$_2$O	MPITSA
formula	C$_{10}$H$_{17}$BrN$_4$	C$_{10}$H$_{17}$ClN$_4$	C$_{20}$H$_{24}$BrN$_4$O$_4$	C$_{20}$H$_{21.10}$N$_5$O$_{5.04}$	C$_{21}$H$_{25}$N$_4$O$_7$	C$_{27}$H$_{28}$N$_4$O$_5$S
crystal system	orthorhombic	orthorhombic	monoclinic	monoclinic	monoclinic	monoclinic
space group	$Pca2_1$	$Pca2_1$	$P2_1/c$	$C2/c$	$P2_1/n$	$P2_1/n$
a (Å)	13.7773(5)	13.6634(7)	8.292(1)	19.3498(8)	9.6840(3)	13.9274(18)
b (Å)	9.9093(4)	10.0618(5)	12.0213(16)	8.1285(3)	9.1315(2)	9.6125(8)
c (Å)	9.2692(4)	8.8159(4)	21.786(3)	12.4460(5)	23.9779(7)	19.599(3)
α (deg)	90	90	90	90	90	90
β (deg)	90	90	91.467(4)	91.468(1)	94.445(1)	103.497(3)
γ (deg)	90	90	90	90	90	90
vol (Å^3)	1265.46(9)	1214.81(10)	2170.94(5)	1956.92(13)	2113.97(10)	2551.39(8)
Z	4	4	4	4	4	4
T (K)	150(2)	150(2)	150(2)	150(2)	150(2)	173(2)
R$_1$	0.0201	0.0532	0.0445	0.0392	0.0487	0.0681
wR$_2$	0.0516	0.1050	0.1106	0.0960	0.1464	0.1330
GOF	1.059	1.235	1.009	1.023	1.023	1.062
CCDC#	2190303	BEPTEX	2190306	2190307	2190308	2190310

ICC ID	MPITFA	IMBHBA	NPIHBA	NPIHCA	NPINIA	NPITFA
formula	C$_{21}$H$_{21}$F$_3$N$_4$O$_5$S	C$_{40}$H$_{34}$Br$_2$N$_8$O$_4$	C$_{18}$H$_{15}$BrN$_6$O$_4$	C$_{18}$H$_{15}$ClN$_6$O$_4$	C$_{18}$H$_{14}$N$_7$O$_7$	C$_{19}$H$_{15}$F$_3$N$_6$O$_7$S
crystal system	monoclinic	monoclinic	triclinic	orthorhombic	monoclinic	triclinic
space group	$P2_1/c$	$C2/c$	$P\bar{1}$	$Pbca$	$C2$	$P\bar{1}$
a (Å)	13.8953(4)	32.9927(6)	8.0379(5)	7.0102(3)	32.372(2)	8.3095(3)
b (Å)	10.2973(3)	8.1315(2)	8.1504(5)	14.9429(8)	7.8860(5)	9.9778(3)
c (Å)	15.4543(4)	21.2172(5)	15.4708(9)	35.3795(17)	3.7236(2)	13.1516(4)
α (deg)	90	90	87.586(2)	90	90	93.2280(10)
β (deg)	98.310(2)	110.838(2)	88.707(2)	90	95.797(2)	100.0570(10)
γ (deg)	90	90	65.284(2)	90	90	94.8960(10)
vol (Å^3)	2188.05(11)	5319.83(7)	919.85(10)	3706.12(3)	945.71(10)	1066.91(6)
Z	4	8	2	8	4	2
T (K)	150(2)	150(2)	150(2)	186(2)	293(2)	100(2)
R$_1$	0.0564	0.0431	0.0258	0.0828	0.0476	0.0360
wR$_2$	0.1485	0.1125	0.0603	0.1252	0.1132	0.1021
GOF	1.051	1.046	1.090	1.022	1.168	1.034
CCDC#	2190309	2190304	2190315	2190316	2190317	2190318

ICC ID	MPTHBA	MPTHCA	MPTHCA·2H$_2$O	MPTTFA	MPIBMPT
formula	C$_{18}$H$_{19}$BrN$_6$O$_2$	C$_{18}$H$_{19}$ClN$_6$O$_2$	C$_{18}$H$_{24}$ClN$_6$O$_4$	C$_{19}$H$_{19}$F$_3$N$_6$O$_5$S	C$_{38}$H$_{38}$Cl$_2$N$_{10}$O$_4$
crystal system	triclinic	triclinic	triclinic	monoclinic	monoclinic
space group	$P\bar{1}$	$P\bar{1}$	$P\bar{1}$	$C2/c$	Cc
a (Å)	7.9413(13)	7.7313(4)	8.3338(2)	15.521(3)	7.0520(8)
b (Å)	8.6863(13)	8.5007(3)	11.5631(3)	21.124(3)	19.680(2)
c (Å)	14.233(2)	14.3868(7)	11.6282(3)	15.615(3)	13.6463(16)
α (deg)	83.211(5)	82.761(2)	73.6850(10)	90	90
β (deg)	83.831(6)	83.458(2)	69.9830(10)	117.825(7)	104.322(3)
γ (deg)	81.315(5)	81.233(2)	82.9500(10)	90	90
vol (Å^3)	959.72(3)	922.69(7)	1010.02(4)	4527.81(4)	1835.13(4)
Z	2	2	2	8	2
T (K)	150(2)	150(2)	150(2)	303(2)	150(2)
R$_1$	0.0411	0.0663	0.0505	0.0981	0.0664
wR$_2$	0.0936	0.1010	0.1352	0.3173	0.1577
GOF	0.995	0.959	1.076	1.206	1.033
CCDC#	2190311	2190312	2190313	2190314	2190305

2.5. Computational Methods

The intermolecular interaction energies of charge-assisted azolium-azole hydrogen bonds were calculated using monomer wavefunctions at the B3LYP/6-31G(d,p) level in the CrystalExplorer 17.5 [81] program package followed by geometry optimization carried out using the CASTEP module with GGA-type PBE functional contained in Materials Studio 8.0. The total interaction energy was divided into electronic (E_{ele}), polarization (E_{pol}), dispersion (E_{dis}), and repulsion (E_{rel}) components.

2.6. Cambridge Structural Database (CSD) Analysis

A CSD survey was conducted using ConQuest (v.5.43, November 2021) and the results were processed with Mercury (v.2021.3.0). Restrictions are detailed in Section 3 of the SI. ICC entries were manually filtered from the resultant hitlist (Scheme S1). The findings of the CSD search for azolium-azole heterosynthons are presented in Charts 1 and 2. The following parameters were evaluated: (i) azole ring arrangements in azolium-azole ICCs; (ii) charge assisted $NH^+\cdots N$ heterosynthons between identical ($AH^+\cdots A$) or different ($AH^+\cdots C$) azoles; (iii) average distances and angles for $NH^+\cdots N$ hydrogen bonds; (iv) average CNC angles within neutral and protonated imidazole or 1,2,4-triazole rings.

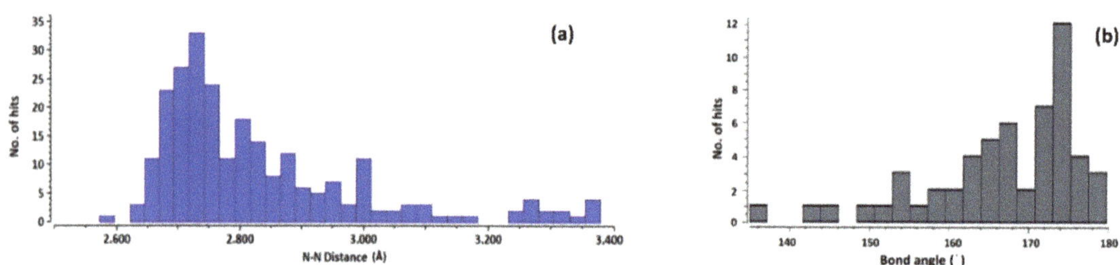

Chart 1. Histograms of hydrogen bond parameters in azolium-azole ICCs retrieved from the CSD revealed (**a**) an average bond length of 2.743(74) Å and (**b**) an average bond angle of 166.8(84).

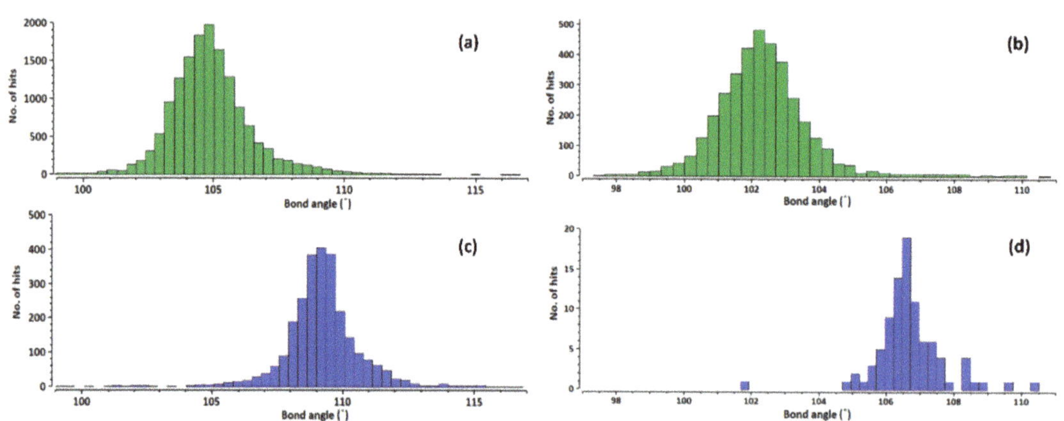

Chart 2. Histogram of CNC angles (θ_1/θ_2) in neutral (green) imidazoles (**a**) and 1,2,4-triazoles (**b**) and in protonated (blue) imidazoles (**c**) and 1,2,4-triazoles (**d**).

3. Results and Discussion

3.1. CSD Analysis of Azolium-Azole Supramolecular Heterosynthons

The CSD survey revealed 211 crystal structures of azole moieties that involve azolium$\cdots$azole supramolecular heterosynthons, 132 (63%) salts, 66 ICCs (31%) and 13 zwitterions (6%) (Scheme S1). 9-ethylguanine hemi-hydrochloric acid, the earliest azolium-azole ICC entry in the CSD, was reported in 1975 and exhibited the shortest $NH\cdots N$ hydrogen bond (2.637 Å) observed at the time [82]. When two or more azole groups are present in the same crystal structure, two types of $NH^+\cdots N$ supramolecular heterosynthons are possible, those involving the same azole, AH$^+$···A (56) or those involving different azoles, AH$^+$···C (10). Our analysis of the 40 imidazole-containing hits in the 66 archived ICCs (Scheme S1 and Table S3) revealed significantly more AH$^+$···A (38) than AH$^+$···C (2) supramolecular heterosynthons. Moreover, more AH$^+$···A (10) than AH$^+$···C (2) supramolecular heterosynthons were in the 12 hits involving 1,2,4-triazole rings. Despite there being hits for other azolium···azole interactions, as indicated in Scheme S1, their small quantity (e.g., 9 hits for pyrazolium-pyrazole and 1 hit for 1,2,3-triazolium-1,2,3-triazole) precludes statistical evaluation.

That 79% of previously reported azolium···azole ICCs are sustained by NH···N supramolecular heterosynthons involving imidazoles or 1,2,4-triazoles suggests that charge-assisted NH$^+$···N interactions could be generally suitable for ICC formation via the motif in Scheme 3; this is the primary focus of this contribution.

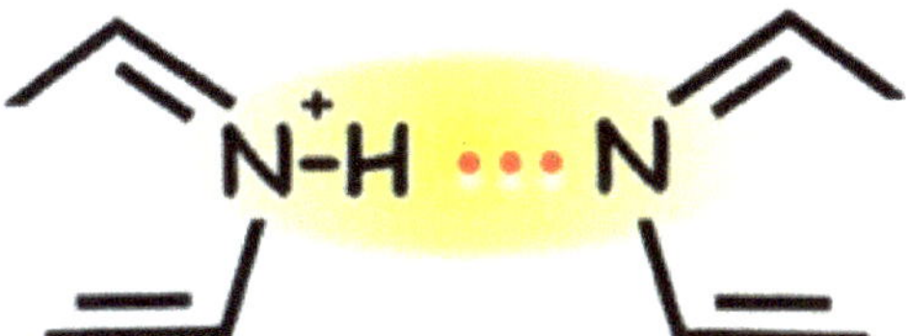

Scheme 3. The NH$^+$···N supramolecular heterosynthon.

3.2. Structural Parameters That Distinguish between Azole and Azolium Rings

The location of hydrogen atom positions can be disputed due to the low electron density of hydrogen atoms which means that determination of their coordinates by X-ray diffraction experiments is challenging. Fortunately, the hydrogen atom position in an NH$^+$···N supramolecular heterosynthon may be verified using the azole ring structural parameters, as shown by Rogers's and co-workers in their studies on imidazolium salts [83]. Further, our prior work on pyridines examined the use of the CNC angle in aromatic rings to distinguish between protonated and free base pyridines [84].

To address this issue, we identified key parameters in crystal structures of neutral and protonated imidazoles or 1,2,4-triazoles (Scheme 4) to distinguish between azole and azolium moieties.

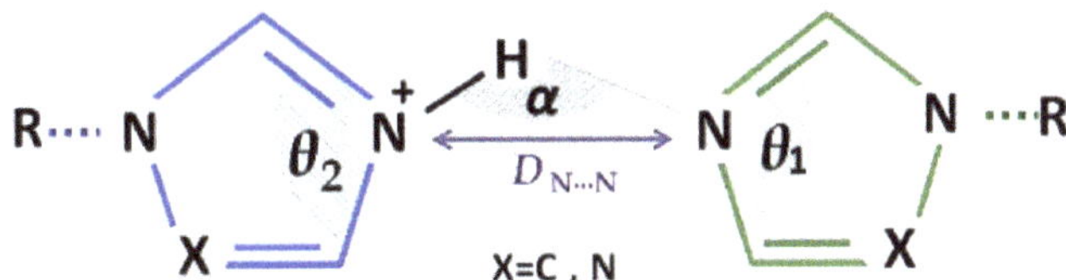

Scheme 4. Key parameters to evaluate azolium-azole heterosynthons in imidazoles and 1,2,4-triazoles.

Histograms of hydrogen bond parameters in azolium-azole ICCs and CNC angles in neutral and cationic (θ_1 and θ_2) imidazoles and 1,2,4-triazoles are given in Charts 1 and 2, respectively. For 11360 neutral imidazoles (θ_1), the average CNC angle was determined to be 104.9(10)°. In comparison, 1868 cationic imidazoles revealed a CNC angle (θ_2) averaging 109.2(8)°. The corresponding values were 102.3(9)° and 106.7(6)° for 1,2,4-triazole (2414 hits) and 1,2,4-triazolium (72 hits) rings, respectively. This difference in average θ_1 and θ_2 values (approximately 4 degrees) in imidazoles and 1,2,4-triazoles clearly illustrates that they are sensitive to protonation, and their cationic forms have higher values (around 4.4 degrees) than comparable neutral rings, allowing us to distinguish between protonated and neutral rings.

3.3. Crystal Structure Descriptions

SE and SDG approaches were applied to prepare seventeen ICCs (ICC 2 is previously reported in the CSD as BEPTEX [84]), 16 of which are A^+B^-A ICCs sustained by $NH^+\cdots N$ supramolecular heterosynthons. SDG (ICCs 1, 3–9, 11, 12, 14–16) and SE (ICCs 2, 4–16) approaches yielded similarly high success rates with respect to isolation of A^+B^-A ICCs (Table S1). Several cocrystals that did not form by SE were obtained by SDG in the same solvent, or vice versa. Table 1 lists the crystallographic parameters of all 17 ICCs obtained in this study and Figure 1 presents their ORTEP diagrams.

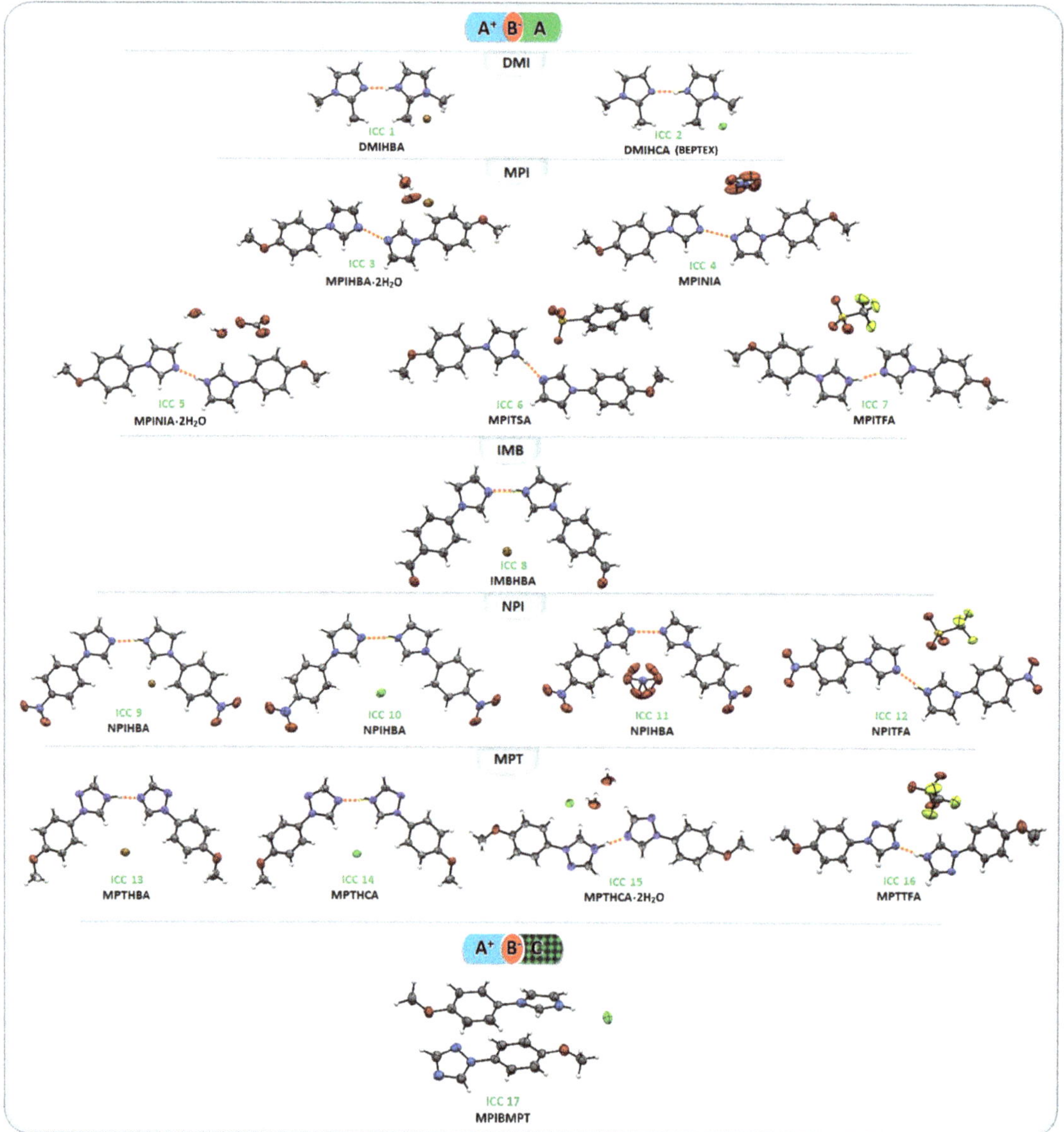

Figure 1. ORTEP diagrams of A^+B^-A ICCs 1–16 and A^+B^-C ICC 17 (50% probability).

3.3.1. ICCs Containing 1,2-Dimethylimidazole, DMI (1 and 2)

SCXRD revealed that the two ICCs obtained with DMI (**DMIHBA** and **BEPTEX**) are isostructural and that both crystallize in the orthorhombic space group $Pca2_1$ (Figure S16). As noted in Table 1, the crystal structure of **BEPTEX** was previously reported [84], however in order to do a detailed analysis on $NH^+\cdots N$ hydrogen bonds, we include it in this report. **DMIHBA** and **BEPTEX** contain one free DMI molecule, one protonated DMI^+ cation and one bromide or chloride anion, respectively. Charge-assisted $NH^+\cdots N$ supramolecular heterosynthons ($D_{N\cdots N}$, 2.712(3) in **DMIHBA**, and 2.699(4) Å in **BEPTEX**) are present in both ICCs. The CNC angles of the imidazolium and imidazole rings (Table 2) are 108.54(24)° and 106.02(23)° for **DMIHBA** and 108.83(37)° and 106.17(36)° for **BEPTEX**, enabling identification of which ring is protonated.

Table 2. Geometries of $NH^+\cdots N$ hydrogen bonding synthons for 1–16.

No	Code	d(N-H)/Å	d(H···N)/Å	d(N···N)/Å	$\alpha/°$	$\theta_1/°$	$\theta_2/°$
1	**DMIHBA**	0.936(33)	1.787(34)	2.712(3)	169.4(30)	106.02(23)	108.54(24)
2	**BEPTEX**	0.880(3)	1.829(3)	2.699(4)	169.4(2)	106.17(36)	108.83(37)
3	**MPIHBA·2H₂O**	0.791(66)	1.872(66)	2.662(4)	178.2(68)	107.50(24)	107.50(24)
				2.644(3)		105.88(27)	105.88(27)
4	**MPINIA**	0.907(38)	1.745(38)	2.652(1)	178.7(36)	107.29(12)	107.68(12)
5	**MPINIA·2H₂O**	1.030(19)	1.648(19)	2.678(1)	177.3(18)	105.79(10)	108.67(11)
6	**MPITSA**	0.924(39)	1.877(39)	2.791(4)	169.4(36)	104.90(31)	109.00(26)
7	**MPITFA**	0.997(45)	1.762(45)	2.748(3)	169.6(38)	105.44(22)	108.70(23)
8	**IMBHBA**	0.880(3)	1.823(3)	2.678(4)	163.2(2)	107.29(30)	108.25(30)
				2.658(4)		107.05(31)	107.04(31)
9	**NPIHBA**	0.880(1)	1.839(1)	2.686(2)	161.0(1)	106.08(17)	109.23(17)
10	**NPIHCA**	1.059(26)	1.634(24)	2.691(2)	175.3(25)	106.47(17)	108.70(16)
11	**NPINIA**	0.887(48)	1.798(48)	2.678(3)	171.1(47)	107.83(23)	107.83(23)
12	**NPITFA**	0.922(22)	1.911(21)	2.808(1)	163.6(18)	105.30(12)	109.11(12)
13	**MPTHBA**	1.038(43)	1.665(45)	2.690(3)	168.3(37)	103.41(24)	105.41(24)
14	**MPTHCA**	0.880(1)	1.814(1)	2.663(2)	161.2(1)	103.44(16)	106.36(16)
15	**MPTHCA·2H₂O**	1.046(39)	1.677(39)	2.723(3)	178.7(29)	103.42(20)	106.04(20)
16	**MPTTFA**	0.860(4)	1.844(4)	2.694(6)	169.1(3)	101.71(54)	105.70(52)

3.3.2. ICCs Containing 1-(4-Methoxyphenyl)-1H-Imidazole, MPI, 3–7

Cocrystallization of MPI was successful in all acids except for HCl, affording five new ICCs. HCl produced a physical mixture of MPI and related salt (Table S2). SCXRD revealed that the MPI cocrystals each formed monoclinic crystals. **MPIHBA·2H₂O** and **MPITFA** crystallized in $P2_1/c$, **MPINIA·2H₂O** and **MPITSA** crystallized in $P2_1/n$, while **MPINIA** crystallized in space group $C2/c$. Their $NH^+\cdots N$ supramolecular synthons and crystal packing are illustrated in Scheme 3. The proton positions in **MPIHBA·2H₂O** and **MPINIA** were found to be disordered between two imidazole rings, making it difficult to differentiate imidazole from imidazolium. While in other ICCs the θ_1 and θ_2 angles in MPI molecules support the proposed ionic nature of one of the MPI molecules, for **MPIHBA·2H₂O** and **MPINIA** this was not the case.

In **MPIHBA·2H₂O**, the $D_{N\cdots N}$ distances, 2.644(3) and 2.662(4) Å, are at the short end of the range of distances for this type of interaction. In **MPIHBA·2H₂O**, an isolated site hydrate ICC, water molecules interact with bromide anions through $R_4^2(8)$ and $R_6^4(12)$ graph set motifs (Figure S17). Two ICCs of MPI with nitric acid were isolated. **MPINIA** is an anhydrate with a disordered hydrogen atom in $NH^+\cdots N$ hydrogen bond, whereas **MPINIA·2H₂O** is an isolated site hydrate. The $D_{N\cdots N}$ in **MPIHCA** is 2.652(1) Å, which is shorter than the 2.678(1) Å length in **MPINIA·2H₂O**. In the crystal structure of **MPINIA·2H₂O**, the values of θ_1 and θ_2 in imidazole rings are 105.79(10)° and 108.67(11)°, respectively, allowing identification of the protonated ring, whereas in **MPINIA** there is no statistical difference between the two rings (Table 2). Water molecules in **MPINIA·2H₂O** form chains with nitrate anions ($C_3^3(8)$ motifs) along the crystallographic b-axis (Figure S18).

MPITSA and **MPITFA** are comprised of one MPI free base, one protonated MPI$^+$ and one anion (p-TSO$^-$/OTf$^-$), which are both sustained by NH$^+\cdots$N hydrogen bonds with distances of 2.791(4) and 2.748(3) Å, respectively. In **MPITSA**, the values of θ_1 and θ_2 in the imidazole rings are 104.90(31)° and 109.00(26)°, respectively, and 105.44(22)° and 108.70(23)° in **MPITFA**. The orientation of the imidazole ring in relation to the benzene moiety in **MPIHBA·2H$_2$O, MPINIA, MPINIA·2H$_2$O, MPITSA**, and **MPITFA** was determined to be 27.23(38)°, 44.38(24)°, 17.05(18)°, 17.58(43)°, and 24.50(21)°, respectively, suggesting that the MPI molecule in **MPINIA·2H$_2$O** has the most planar structure in the MPI-based ICCs, while **MPINIA** has the least (Figure 2). In addition, the orientation of the imidazole ring to the methoxy group in **MPIHBA·2H$_2$O** and **MPITFA** differs from that of others.

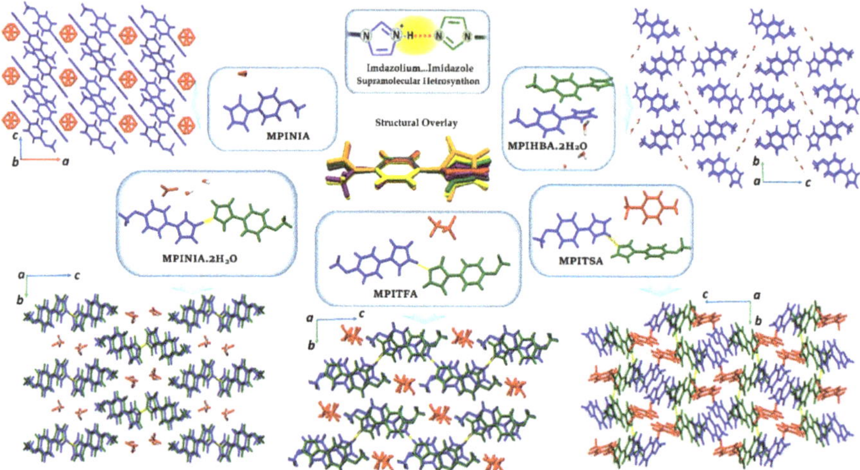

Figure 2. Crystal packing of MPI-based ICCs. Cations are colored blue, neutral coformers green and anions red. Structural overlay of free MPI is presented in the middle of the figure: Free MPI: green, MPIHBA·2H$_2$O: red, MPINIA: orange, MPINIA·2H$_2$O: purple, MPITSA: grey, MPITFA: yellow.

3.3.3. ICC Containing 4-(1H-Imidazol-1-yl) Benzaldehyde, IMB, 8

Attempts to prepare IMB ICCs resulted in the formation of only one ICC (**IMBHBA**), with most attempts resulting in a physical mixture of starting materials or new solid forms with poor-quality crystals. SCXRD revealed that **IMBHBA** crystallizes in a monoclinic space group $C2/c$ (Table 1), and the asymmetric unit comprises one IMB cation, one free IMB molecule and well as one-half of the anion (Br$^-$) and one IMB cation with a disordered hydrogen atom (Figure 3). In IMBHBA, $D_N\cdots N$ distances are 2.678(4) and 2.658(4) Å, and the values of θ_1 and θ_2 are 107.29(30)° and 108.25(30)° in one pair of IMBs, and 107.05(31)° in paired IMBs sustained by disordered NH$^+\cdots$N hydrogen bond.

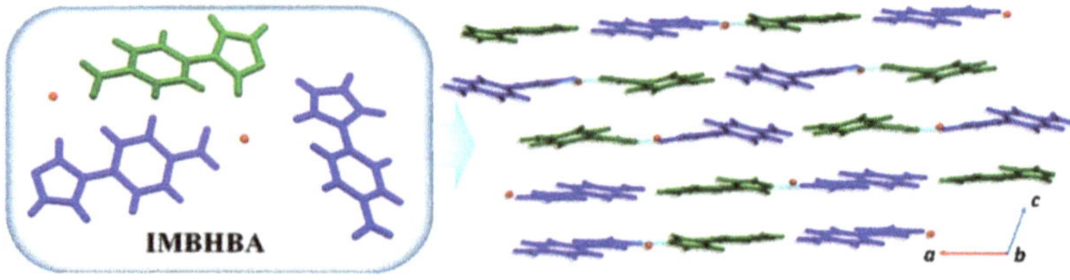

Figure 3. The asymmetric unit and crystal packing of IMBHBA (along b axis).

3.3.4. ICCs Containing 1-(4-Nitrophenyl)-1H-Imidazole, NPI, 9–12

NPIHBA crystallized in the triclinic space group $P\bar{1}$, the asymmetric unit comprising an NPI cation, a free NPI and one bromide anion. $D_N \cdots _N$ in **NPIHBA** is 2.686(2) Å and the CNC angles of the imidazolium and imidazole rings are 106.08(17)° and 109.23(17)°, respectively. SCXRD revealed that the **NPIHCA** asymmetric unit is comprised of one NPI cation, one free NPI molecule and one Cl^- anion. The value of $D_N \cdots _N$ in **NPIHCA** is 2.691(2) Å, while the values of θ_1 and θ_2 are 106.46(1)° and 108.71(1)°, respectively. **NPINIA** crystallized in the monoclinic space group $C2$ and its asymmetric unit is similar to **MPINIA**, comprising one INP molecule with disordered hydrogen atoms and half a disordered nitrate anion (Figure 4). The $D_N \cdots _N$ in **NPINIA** is 2.678(3) Å, shorter than the other ICCs that contain NPI molecules. As the hydrogen atom between the two imidazole rings is disordered, the imidazole angles θ_1 and θ_2 in this ICC are identical (107.83(23)°). When TFA was used as the acid, one free INP molecule, one INP cation and one triflate anion form the **NPITFA** asymmetric unit (Figure 4). In this structure, $D_N \cdots _N$ is 2.808(1) Å (the longest $D_N \cdots _N$ in this family of ICCs), and the 4 degree difference between θ_1 and θ_2 (105.30(12)° and 109.11(12)°, respectively) supports the ionic nature of one of the NPI molecules.

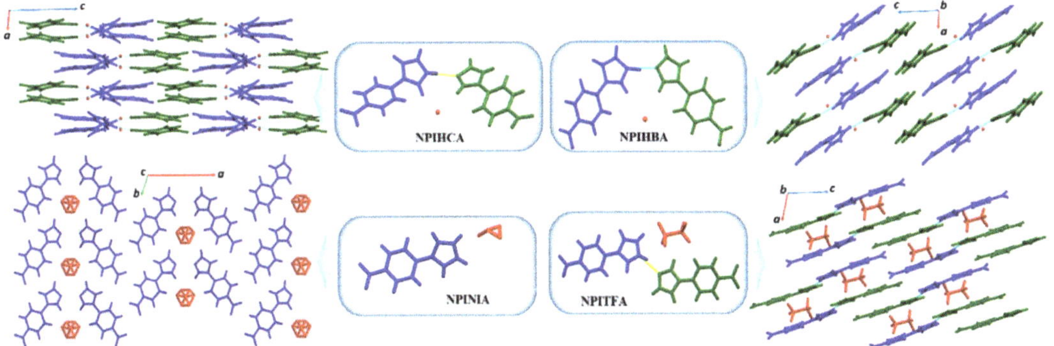

Figure 4. Chemical composition and crystal packing for ICCs involving NPI.

3.3.5. ICCs Containing 1-(4-Methoxyphenyl)-1H-1,2,4-Triazole, MPT, 13–16

Four ICCs were formed by MPT, a 1,2,4-triazole. **MPTHBA** and **MPTHCA** crystallized in the triclinic space group $P\bar{1}$, their asymmetric units comprising one MPT$^+$ cation, one MPT molecule and one bromide or chloride, respectively. In **MPTHBA** and **MPTHCA**, which are isostructural, NH$^+$$\cdots$N hydrogen bonds connect triazole and triazolium moieties at distances of 2.690(3) and 2.663(2) Å, respectively. **MPTHCA·2H$_2$O** is an isolated site hydrate form of **MPTHCA** harvested from a 5:1 EtOH/H$_2$O solution that crystallized in the triclinic space group $P\bar{1}$, with an asymmetric unit consisting of one MPT cation, one MPT molecule, one chloride anion, and two water molecules. Water molecules interact with chloride anions through $R_4^2(8)$ and $R_6^4(12)$ graph set-motifs (Figure S19). The $D_N \cdots _N$ in **MPTHCA** and **MPTHCA·2H$_2$O** are 2.663(2) and 2.723(3) Å. Moreover, the values of θ_1 and θ_2 are similar (103.44(16)° and 106.36(16)° in **MPTHCA**, 103.42(20)° and 106.04(20)° in **MPTHCA·2H$_2$O**). **MPTTFA** crystallized in the monoclinic space group $C2/c$ with one MPT$^+$, one MPT and one triflate anion in the asymmetric unit (Figure 5). The $D_N \cdots _N$ in this structure is 2.694(6) Å, and the values of θ_1 and θ_2 in triazole rings, 101.71(54)° and 105.70(52)°, allow identification of the protonated triazole.

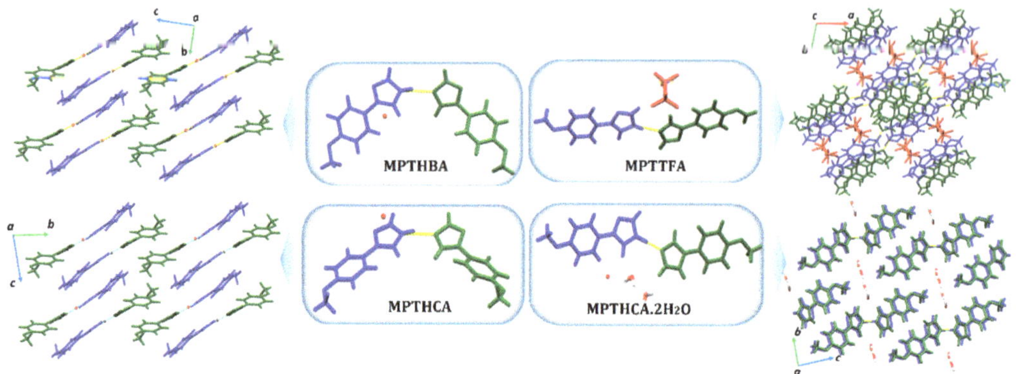

Figure 5. Local structure and crystal packing of ICCs containing MPT.

3.3.6. A⁺B⁻C Type ICCs

We also attempted to prepare azolium-azole ICCs comprised of different azoles (AH⁺···C). Such an approach could be useful to form ICCs containing azole-based APIs or pharmaceutical ICCs with azole coformers to improve physicochemical properties. Approaches I and II (Scheme 2) resulted in a very low success rate, compatible with the conclusions of our CSD survey. Solvent evaporation with a 1:1:1 ratio of coformer 1, coformer 2 and acid generally resulted in a physical mixture of azole and the salt of the more basic azole. In terms of using a salt as a coformer, just one attempt by SDG was successful in forming azolium-azole ICC between two different azole compounds (**MPIBMPT**). **MPIBMPT** crystallized in the monoclinic space group *Cc* with one MPI⁺ cation, one chloride anion and one MPT molecule in the asymmetric unit. The absence of a charge-assisted NH···N⁺ supramolecular heterosynthon in **MPIBMPT** distinguishes it from the other ICCs reported herein (Figure 6). Rather, the MPI⁺ cation was found to have formed a hydrogen bond with the chloride anion (N2⁺···Cl1⁻ = 3.036(5) Å). MPI⁺ cations and MPT molecules were observed to form infinite chains of alternating cations and molecules, thereby enabling head-to-tail π···π stacking of azole and phenyl rings (Figure 6). The CNC angle in the imidazole ring is 108.52(54)°, which is within the range of protonated imidazoles, and the CNC angle in the triazole ring is 101.94(52)°, confirming that the triazole ring in this structure is neutral.

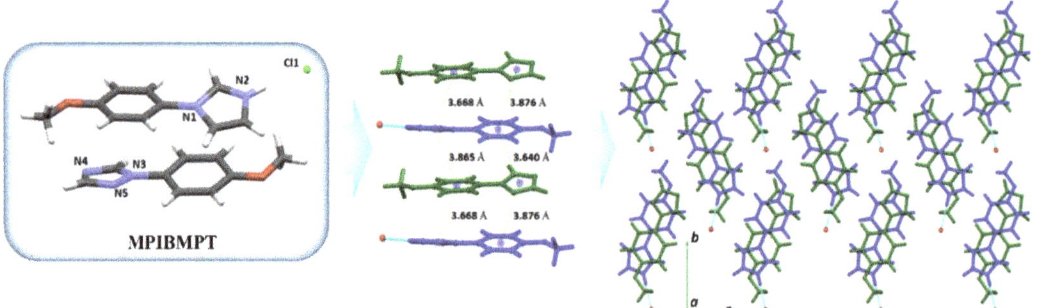

Figure 6. Illustration of the asymmetric unit and crystal packing in MPIBMPT.

3.4. Overall Analysis of Crystal Structures

Several ICCs reported herein were found to exhibit disordered hydrogen atoms between azoles, so-called 'confused protons', a term coined in previous research on azole compounds [83,85]. In such structures, distinguishing between protonated and neutral azole rings is problematic but this does not affect the overall reliability of the approach of exploiting the $NH^+\cdots N$ supramolecular heterosynthon for ICC formation. Figure 7 and Figure S20 compare hydrogen bond parameters in neutral $NH\cdots N$ hydrogen bonds with those of charge-assisted interactions ($NH^+\cdots N$) from the CSD and the ICCs reported in this study. The interactions observed in this study, with distances ranging from 2.644(3) to 2.808(1) Å and angles approaching 180° are consistently amongst the strongest based upon these structural parameters.

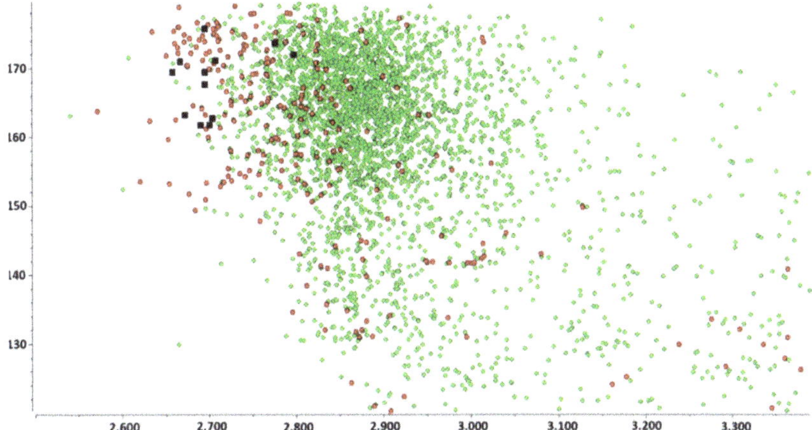

Figure 7. Bond distance vs. bond angle in 2129 neutral $NH\cdots N$ (green dots) and 211 charge-assisted $NH^+\cdots N$ (red spots) hydrogen bonds in azoles. Black squares represent the $NH^+\cdots N$ supramolecular heterosynthons reported herein.

3.5. Hydrogen-Bond Strengths

The calculated energies of azolium azole hydrogen bonds at the B3LYP/6–31g (d,p) level of theory are shown in Table 3 for 13 ICCs (in which the hydrogen atoms' positions in $NH^+\cdots N$ supramolecular heterosynthons were not disordered). The contributions to total energies from electrostatic, polarization, dispersion, and repulsion interactions for $NH^+\cdots N$ hydrogen bonds were also estimated. In terms of the azole rings involved in hydrogen bonds, the refined crystal structures of the ICCs described herein can consider two forms of hydrogen bonding, $NH^+\cdots N$ supramolecular heterosynthons in imidazolium-imidazole ICCs and triazolium-triazole ICCs.

Table 3. Interaction energies (E_{tot}) in kJ mol^{-1} calculated using B3LYP/6–31g (d,p).

Code	E_{ele}	E_{pol}	E_{dis}	E_{rep}	E_{tot}
DMIHBA	−74.9	−13.8	−13.9	71.6	−31.0
BEPTEX	−77.9	−14.5	−13.9	74.2	−32.1
MPINIA·2H$_2$O	−88.8	−15.9	−9.2	74.8	−39.1
MPITST	−66.3	−12.5	−8.6	47.9	−39.5
MPITFA	−74.5	−13.7	−8.8	58.3	−41.4
IMBHBA	−85.1	−16.4	−10.4	67.1	−44.8
NPIHBA	−83.8	−16.4	−9.8	65.0	−45.0
NPIHCA	−88.1	−17.4	−9.5	69.4	−45.6
NPITFA	−64.6	−13.5	−8.5	42.1	−44.5
MPTHBA	−84.3	−14.9	−9.4	67.0	−41.6
MPTHCA	−85.4	−15.0	−9.6	70.6	−39.4
MPTHCA·2H$_2$O	−79.6	−14.3	−8.4	62.2	−40.1
MPTTFA	−85.5	−15.6	−8.7	68.3	−41.5

These results indicate binding energies 31.0 to 45.6 kJ mol^{-1}, with **NPIHCA** showing the highest energy at 45.6 kJ mol^{-1}. Electrostatic energy (F_{ele}) has a stronger effect on E_{tot} than dispersion and polarization energies. Furthermore, the energies of imidazolium-imidazole and triazolium-triazole hydrogen bonding are comparable, as switching from imidazole in MPITFA (-41.4 kJ mol^{-1}) to triazole in MPTTFA (-41.5 kJ mol^{-1}) showed negligible impact. Conversely, substituting a methoxy group (**MPITFA**) for a nitro group in **NPITFA** (-44.6 kJ mol^{-1}) had a more substantial impact. The azolium-azole dimer strength in ICCs containing the same coformers suggest that the impact of anions on binding energy is low (around 1–2 kJ mol^{-1}), even when replacing inorganic anions with larger organic anions. The greater binding energies calculated for IMB/NPI-containing ICCs suggest that electronegative substituents may result in stronger NH$\cdots$N hydrogen bonds. With hydrated ICCs in mind, we were curious to examine the energy of these interactions in the two ICCs that afforded both hydrate and anhydrate forms. The analysis in **MPINIA** failed due to disorder. By calculating the energy of NH$^{+}\cdots$N interactions in **MPTHCA** and **MPTHCA·2H$_2$O**, despite the energies of the anhydrate form (-39.4 kJ mol^{-1}) and hydrate ICC (-40.1 kJ mol^{-1}) being almost comparable, formation of the hydrate ICC can lead to stronger interactions. However, it seems that estimations of lattice stabilization energy of ICCs may require deeper analysis.

4. Conclusions

Azole-containing compounds with varying biological activity have comprised 12.8% of approved small-molecule medicines, despite often having poor physicochemical and/or pharmacokinetic properties. Our CSD study reveals that multicomponent crystals based on the azolium-azole supramolecular heterosynthon are understudied. The synthesis and single crystal structures of 16 new ICCs based on imidazole and 1,2,4-triazole are presented herein to highlight the strong potential of azole groups to exhibit NH$^{+}\cdots$N supramolecular heterosynthons that can be exploited to generate ICCs. Whereas we attempted to isolate two kinds of ICCs, A^{+}B^{-}A and A^{+}B^{-}C, formation of ICCs based upon AH$^{+}\cdots$A supramolecular heterosynthons was more generally successful, consistent with CSD statistics of ICCs. Our CSD analysis showed that in imidazoles and 1,2,4-triazoles, the CNC angles are sensitive to protonation, and their cationic forms display larger values than those of the equivalent neutral rings, which is confirmed by the findings of this study. Three of the seventeen ICCs investigated herein formed isolated site hydrate ICCs, with two of them exhibiting both hydrate and anhydrate forms, both of which were sustained by charge-assisted NH$^{+}\cdots$N supramolecular heterosynthons. Analysis of calculated binding energies revealed that protonated azolium moieties offer a thermodynamically favourable NH$^{+}\cdots$N binding energy of 31.0 to 46 kJ mol^{-1}. In this study mechanochemistry has proven to be a reliable and efficient method for synthesizing new ICCs using salts as a coformer. Application of this technique and others paves the way for the systematic construction of the robust and underexplored NH$^{+}\cdots$N supramolecular networks for the formation of ionic cocrystals of azole-based APIs to improve their physicochemical properties.

Overall, our results indicate that many parameters can be varied, including solvent, method, acids to enable isolation of azolium . . . azole ICCs. Furthermore, charge-assisted NH$\cdots$N hydrogen bonding in A^{+}B^{-}A ICCs when the cation and neutral azole moiety are the same are not only statistically more likely, were calculated to offer more favourable energetic interactions. While the findings of this study are limited to ICCs of model coformers studied, they suggest that crystal engineering of azolium . . . azole ICCs for various purposes, including pharmaceutical products, is a viable crystal engineering strategy.

Supplementary Materials: The following supporting information can be downloaded at: https://www.mdpi.com/article/10.3390/pharmaceutics14112321/s1. Section S1: Synthesis of ionic cocrystals reported herein; Section S2: Comparison of experimental and calculated PXRD patterns; Section S3: Cambridge Structural Database (CSD) analysis; Section S4: Crystal structure analysis; Section S5: Hydrogen bond analysis.

Author Contributions: Conceptualization, M.J.Z. and M.R.; methodology, M.R.; software, M.R. and J.B.-C.; formal analysis, M.R.; investigation, M.R.; data curation, M.R.; writing—original draft preparation, M.R. and V.K.; writing—review and editing, M.J.Z. and V.K.; supervision, M.J.Z.; project administration, M.R.; funding acquisition, M.J.Z. All authors have read and agreed to the published version of the manuscript.

Funding: This research was funded by Science Foundation Ireland (SFI) through Synthesis and Solid State Pharmaceutical Centre (SSPC), 12/RC/2275_P2 and 16/IA/4624.

Institutional Review Board Statement: Not applicable.

Informed Consent Statement: Not applicable.

Data Availability Statement: The data presented in this study are available on request from the corresponding authors.

Acknowledgments: The authors would like to thank Yassin H. Andaloussi and Sanaz Khorasani for review and editing the manuscript and helpful discussion on crystal structure collection and solution. The authors gratefully acknowledge SFI and SSPC for financial supports.

Conflicts of Interest: The authors declare no conflict of interest.

References

1. Desiraju, G.R. Supramolecular synthons in crystal engineering—A new organic synthesis. *Angew. Chem. Int. Ed. Engl.* **1995**, *34*, 2311–2327. [CrossRef]
2. Moulton, B.; Zaworotko, M.J. From Molecules to Crystal Engineering: Supramolecular Isomerism and Polymorphism in Network Solids. *Chem. Rev.* **2001**, *101*, 1629–1658. [CrossRef] [PubMed]
3. Bhattacharya, S.; Peraka, K.S.; Zaworotko, M.J. The role of hydrogen bonding in co-crystals. In *Co-Crystals: Preparation, Characterization and Applications*; The Royal Society of Chemistry: Croydon, UK, 2018; pp. 33–79.
4. Zhang, J.-P.; Zhang, Y.-B.; Lin, J.-B.; Chen, X.-M. Metal Azolate Frameworks: From Crystal Engineering to Functional Materials. *Chem. Rev.* **2012**, *112*, 1001–1033. [CrossRef] [PubMed]
5. Mukherjee, S.; Zaworotko, M.J. Crystal Engineering of Hybrid Coordination Networks: From Form to Function. *Trends Chem.* **2020**, *2*, 506–518. [CrossRef]
6. Gao, M.-Y.; Song, B.-Q.; Sensharma, D.; Zaworotko, M.J. Crystal engineering of porous coordination networks for C3 hydrocarbon separation. *SmartMat* **2021**, *2*, 38–55. [CrossRef]
7. Evans, O.R.; Lin, W. Crystal Engineering of Nonlinear Optical Materials Based on Interpenetrated Diamondoid Coordination Networks. *Chem. Mater.* **2001**, *13*, 2705–2712. [CrossRef]
8. Wong, M.S.; Bosshard, C.; Günter, P. Crystal engineering of molecular NLO materials. *Adv. Mater.* **1997**, *9*, 837–842. [CrossRef]
9. Bolla, G.; Nangia, A. Pharmaceutical cocrystals: Walking the talk. *Chem. Commun.* **2016**, *52*, 8342–8360. [CrossRef]
10. Duggirala, N.K.; Perry, M.L.; Almarsson, Ö.; Zaworotko, M.J. Pharmaceutical cocrystals: Along the path to improved medicines. *Chem. Commun.* **2016**, *52*, 640–655. [CrossRef]
11. Kavanagh, O.N.; Croker, D.M.; Walker, G.M.; Zaworotko, M.J. Pharmaceutical cocrystals: From serendipity to design to application. *Drug Discov. Today* **2019**, *24*, 796–804. [CrossRef]
12. Bolla, G.; Sarma, B.; Nangia, A.K. Crystal Engineering of Pharmaceutical Cocrystals in the Discovery and Development of Improved Drugs. *Chem. Rev.* **2022**, *122*, 11514–11603. [CrossRef]
13. Aitipamula, S.; Banerjee, R.; Bansal, A.K.; Biradha, K.; Cheney, M.L.; Choudhury, A.R.; Desiraju, G.R.; Dikundwar, A.G.; Dubey, R.; Duggirala, N.; et al. Polymorphs, Salts, and Cocrystals: What's in a Name? *Cryst. Growth Des.* **2012**, *12*, 2147–2152. [CrossRef]
14. Berry, D.J.; Steed, J.W. Pharmaceutical cocrystals, salts and multicomponent systems; intermolecular interactions and property based design. *Adv. Drug Deliv. Rev.* **2017**, *117*, 3–24. [CrossRef] [PubMed]
15. Smith, A.J.; Kavuru, P.; Wojtas, L.; Zaworotko, M.J.; Shytle, R.D. Cocrystals of Quercetin with Improved Solubility and Oral Bioavailability. *Mol. Pharm.* **2011**, *8*, 1867–1876. [CrossRef] [PubMed]
16. Kumari, N.; Bhattacharya, B.; Roy, P.; Michalchuk, A.A.L.; Emmerling, F.; Ghosh, A. Enhancing the Pharmaceutical Properties of Pirfenidone by Mechanochemical Cocrystallization. *Cryst. Growth Des.* **2019**, *19*, 6482–6492. [CrossRef]
17. Duggirala, N.K.; Smith, A.J.; Wojtas, Ł.; Shytle, R.D.; Zaworotko, M.J. Physical Stability Enhancement and Pharmacokinetics of a Lithium Ionic Cocrystal with Glucose. *Cryst. Growth Des.* **2014**, *14*, 6135–6142. [CrossRef]
18. Shiraki, K.; Takata, N.; Takano, R.; Hayashi, Y.; Terada, K. Dissolution Improvement and the Mechanism of the Improvement from Cocrystallization of Poorly Water-soluble Compounds. *Pharm. Res.* **2008**, *25*, 2581–2592. [CrossRef]
19. Shan, N.; Perry, M.L.; Weyna, D.R.; Zaworotko, M.J. Impact of pharmaceutical cocrystals: The effects on drug pharmacokinetics. *Expert Opin. Drug Metab. Toxicol.* **2014**, *10*, 1255–1271. [CrossRef]
20. Nangia, A.K.; Desiraju, G.R. Heterosynthons, Solid Form Design and Enhanced Drug Bioavailability. *Angew. Chem.* **2022**, *134*, e202207484. [CrossRef]

21. Remenar, J.F.; Morissette, S.L.; Peterson, M.L.; Moulton, B.; MacPhee, J.M.; Guzmán, H.R.; Almarsson, Ö. Crystal engineering of novel cocrystals of a triazole drug with 1, 4-dicarboxylic acids. *J. Am. Chem. Soc.* **2003**, *125*, 8456–8457. [CrossRef]
22. Walsh, R.D.B.; Bradner, M.W.; Fleischman, S.; Morales, L.A.; Moulton, B.; Rodríguez-Hornedo, N.; Zaworotko, M.J. Crystal engineering of the composition of pharmaceutical phases. *Chem. Commun.* **2003**, *2*, 186–187. [CrossRef] [PubMed]
23. Childs, S.L.; Chyall, L.J.; Dunlap, J.T.; Smolenskaya, V.N.; Stahly, B.C.; Stahly, G.P. Crystal Engineering Approach To Forming Cocrystals of Amine Hydrochlorides with Organic Acids. Molecular Complexes of Fluoxetine Hydrochloride with Benzoic, Succinic, and Fumaric Acids. *J. Am. Chem. Soc.* **2004**, *126*, 13335–13342. [CrossRef] [PubMed]
24. Fleischman, S.G.; Kuduva, S.S.; McMahon, J.A.; Moulton, B.; Bailey Walsh, R.D.; Rodríguez-Hornedo, N.; Zaworotko, M.J. Crystal Engineering of the Composition of Pharmaceutical Phases: Multiple-Component Crystalline Solids Involving Carbamazepine. *Cryst. Growth Des.* **2003**, *3*, 909–919. [CrossRef]
25. Salaman, C.R.P.; Tesson, N. Co-Crystals of Tramadol and Coxibs. U.S. Patent 8598152B2, 21 April 2015.
26. Christopherson, J.C.; Topić, F.; Barrett, C.J.; Friščić, T. Halogen-Bonded Cocrystals as Optical Materials: Next-Generation Control over Light–Matter Interactions. *Cryst. Growth Des.* **2018**, *18*, 1245–1259. [CrossRef]
27. Braga, D.; Grepioni, F.; Maini, L.; Prosperi, S.; Gobetto, R.; Chierotti, M.R. From unexpected reactions to a new family of ionic co-crystals: The case of barbituric acid with alkali bromides and caesium iodide. *Chem. Commun.* **2010**, *46*, 7715–7717. [CrossRef]
28. Sanii, R.; Andaloussi, Y.H.; Patyk-Kaźmierczak, E.; Zaworotko, M.J. Polymorphism in Ionic Cocrystals Comprising Lithium Salts and l-Proline. *Cryst. Growth Des.* **2022**, *22*, 3786–3794. [CrossRef]
29. de l'Isle, J.R. *Cristallographie, ou Description des Forms Propres À Tous les Corps du Regne Minéral*, 2nd ed.; Édition de L'imprimerie de Monsieur Paris: Paris, France, 1783; Volume 2, pp. 29–50.
30. Kobell, F. Krystallographische Beobachtungen. *J. Für. Prakt. Chem.* **1843**, *28*, 489–491. [CrossRef]
31. Gill, C.H. XVI.—On some saline compounds of cane-sugar. *J. Chem. Soc.* **1871**, *24*, 269–275. [CrossRef]
32. Wood, R.A.; James, V.J.; Mills, J.A. 2,5-O-Methylene-D-Mannitol Sodium-Chloride, $C_7H_{14}O_6$·Nacl. *Cryst. Struct. Commun.* **1976**, *5*, 207–210.
33. Ferguson, G.; Kaitner, B.; Connett, B.E.; Rendle, D.F. Structure of the [alpha]-d-glucose-sodium chloride-water complex (2/1/1). *Acta Crystallogr. Sect. B* **1991**, *47*, 479–484. [CrossRef]
34. Palm, J.H.; MacGillavry, C.H. Habit modification in the system rocksalt-urea-water. *Acta Crystallogr.* **1963**, *16*, 963–968. [CrossRef]
35. Grothe, E.; Meekes, H.; Vlieg, E.; ter Horst, J.H.; de Gelder, R. Solvates, Salts, and Cocrystals: A Proposal for a Feasible Classification System. *Cryst. Growth Des.* **2016**, *16*, 3237–3243. [CrossRef]
36. Grifasi, F.; Chierotti, M.R.; Gaglioti, K.; Gobetto, R.; Maini, L.; Braga, D.; Dichiarante, E.; Curzi, M. Using Salt Cocrystals to Improve the Solubility of Niclosamide. *Cryst. Growth Des.* **2015**, *15*, 1939–1948. [CrossRef]
37. Childs, S.L.; Stahly, G.P.; Park, A. The Salt–Cocrystal Continuum: The Influence of Crystal Structure on Ionization State. *Mol. Pharm.* **2007**, *4*, 323–338. [CrossRef] [PubMed]
38. Barbas, R.; Font-Bardia, M.; Paradkar, A.; Hunter, C.A.; Prohens, R. Combined Virtual/Experimental Multicomponent Solid Forms Screening of Sildenafil: New Salts, Cocrystals, and Hybrid Salt–Cocrystals. *Cryst. Growth Des.* **2018**, *18*, 7618–7627. [CrossRef]
39. Clare Speakman, J. Acid salts of carboxylic acids, crystals with some "very short" hydrogen bonds. In *Structure and Bonding*; Springer: Berlin/Heidelberg, Germany, 1972; pp. 141–199.
40. Jin, S.; Sanii, R.; Song, B.-Q.; Zaworotko, M.J. Crystal Engineering of Ionic Cocrystals Sustained by the Phenol–Phenolate Supramolecular Heterosynthon. *Cryst. Growth Des.* **2022**, *22*, 4582–4591. [CrossRef]
41. Haskins, M.M.; Lusi, M.; Zaworotko, M.J. Supramolecular Synthon Promiscuity in Phosphoric Acid–Dihydrogen Phosphate Ionic Cocrystals. *Cryst. Growth Des.* **2022**, *22*, 3333–3342. [CrossRef]
42. Steiner, T. The Hydrogen Bond in the Solid State. *Angew. Chem. Int. Ed.* **2002**, *41*, 48–76. [CrossRef]
43. Desai, A.S.; McMurray, J.J.V.; Packer, M.; Swedberg, K.; Rouleau, J.L.; Chen, F.; Gong, J.; Rizkala, A.R.; Brahimi, A.; Claggett, B.; et al. Effect of the angiotensin-receptor-neprilysin inhibitor LCZ696 compared with enalapril on mode of death in heart failure patients. *Eur. Heart J.* **2015**, *36*, 1990–1997. [CrossRef]
44. Cebrecos, J.; Carlson, J.D.; Encina, G.; Lahjou, M.; Sans, A.; Sust, M.; Vaqué, A.; Morte, A.; Gascón, N.; Plata-Salamán, C. Celecoxib-tramadol co-crystal: A Randomized 4-Way Crossover Comparative Bioavailability Study. *Clin. Ther.* **2021**, *43*, 1051–1065. [CrossRef]
45. Etter, M.C.; MacDonald, J.C.; Bernstein, J. Graph-set analysis of hydrogen-bond patterns in organic crystals. *Acta Crystallogr. Sect. B* **1990**, *46*, 256–262. [CrossRef] [PubMed]
46. Etter, M.C. Encoding and decoding hydrogen-bond patterns of organic compounds. *Acc. Chem. Res.* **1990**, *23*, 120–126. [CrossRef]
47. Khan, M.; Enkelmann, V.; Brunklaus, G. Heterosynthon mediated tailored synthesis of pharmaceutical complexes: A solid-state NMR approach. *CrystEngComm* **2011**, *13*, 3213–3223. [CrossRef]
48. Li, C.; Campillo-Alvarado, G.; Swenson, D.C.; MacGillivray, L.R. Photoreactive salt cocrystal: N+–H···N hydrogen bond and cation–π interactions support a cascade-like photodimerization of a 4-stilbazole. *CrystEngComm* **2021**, *23*, 1071–1074. [CrossRef]
49. Fabry, J. A long symmetric N . . . H . . . N hydrogen bond in bis(4-aminopyridinium)(1+) azide(1-): Redetermination from the original data. *Acta Crystallogr. Sect. E* **2017**, *73*, 1344–1347. [CrossRef] [PubMed]
50. Sharma, M.; Prasher, P. An epigrammatic status of the 'azole'-based antimalarial drugs. *RSC Med. Chem.* **2020**, *11*, 184–211. [CrossRef]

51. Wishart, D.S.; Feunang, Y.D.; Guo, A.C.; Lo, E.J.; Marcu, A.; Grant, J.R.; Sajed, T.; Johnson, D.; Li, C.; Sayeeda, Z.; et al. DrugBank 5.0: A major update to the DrugBank database for 2018. *Nucleic Acids Res.* **2017**, *46*, D1074–D1082. [CrossRef] [PubMed]

52. Klose, W.; Boettcher, I. Antiinflammatory imidazole derivatives. U.S. Patent US4585771A, 29 April 1986.

53. Sheehan, D.J.; Hitchcock, C.A.; Sibley, C.M. Current and emerging azole antifungal agents. *Clin. Microbiol. Rev.* **1999**, *12*, 40–79. [CrossRef]

54. Maertens, J.A. History of the development of azole derivatives. *Clin. Microbiol. Infect.* **2004**, *10*, 1–10. [CrossRef]

55. Maddila, S.; B Jonnalagadda, S. New class of triazole derivatives and their antimicrobial activity. *Lett. Drug Des. Discov.* **2012**, *9*, 687–693. [CrossRef]

56. El-Sebaey, S. Recent Advances in 1, 2, 4-Triazole Scaffolds as Antiviral Agents. *ChemistrySelect* **2020**, *5*, 11654–11680. [CrossRef]

57. Banfi, E.; Scialino, G.; Zampieri, D.; Mamolo, M.G.; Vio, L.; Ferrone, M.; Fermeglia, M.; Paneni, M.S.; Pricl, S. Antifungal and antimycobacterial activity of new imidazole and triazole derivatives. A combined experimental and computational approach. *J. Antimicrob. Chemother.* **2006**, *58*, 76–84. [CrossRef] [PubMed]

58. Mojaddami, A.; Sakhteman, A.; Fereidoonnezhad, M.; Faghih, Z.; Najdian, A.; Khabnadideh, S.; Sadeghpour, H.; Rezaei, Z. Binding mode of triazole derivatives as aromatase inhibitors based on docking, protein ligand interaction fingerprinting, and molecular dynamics simulation studies. *Res. Pharm. Sci.* **2017**, *12*, 21–30. [CrossRef] [PubMed]

59. Amidon, G.L.; Lennernäs, H.; Shah, V.P.; Crison, J.R. A Theoretical Basis for a Biopharmaceutic Drug Classification: The Correlation of in Vitro Drug Product Dissolution and in Vivo Bioavailability. *Pharm. Res.* **1995**, *12*, 413–420. [CrossRef]

60. Gould, P.L. Salt selection for basic drugs. *Int. J. Pharm.* **1986**, *33*, 201–217. [CrossRef]

61. Bharate, S.S. Recent developments in pharmaceutical salts: FDA approvals from 2015 to 2019. *Drug Discov. Today* **2021**, *26*, 384–398. [CrossRef] [PubMed]

62. Vasilev, N.A.; Surov, A.O.; Voronin, A.P.; Drozd, K.V.; Perlovich, G.L. Novel cocrystals of itraconazole: Insights from phase diagrams, formation thermodynamics and solubility. *Int. J. Pharm.* **2021**, *599*, 120441. [CrossRef]

63. Martin, F.; Pop, M.; Kacso, I.; Grosu, I.G.; Miclăuş, M.; Vodnar, D.; Lung, I.; Filip, G.A.; Olteanu, E.D.; Moldovan, R.; et al. Ketoconazole-p-aminobenzoic Acid Cocrystal: Revival of an Old Drug by Crystal Engineering. *Mol. Pharm.* **2020**, *17*, 919–932. [CrossRef]

64. Chen, J.-M.; Wang, Z.-Z.; Wu, C.-B.; Li, S.; Lu, T.-B. Crystal engineering approach to improve the solubility of mebendazole. *CrystEngComm* **2012**, *14*, 6221–6229. [CrossRef]

65. Bolla, G.; Nangia, A. Novel pharmaceutical salts of albendazole. *CrystEngComm* **2018**, *20*, 6394–6405. [CrossRef]

66. Sanphui, P.; Mishra, M.K.; Ramamurty, U.; Desiraju, G.R. Tuning Mechanical Properties of Pharmaceutical Crystals with Multicomponent Crystals: Voriconazole as a Case Study. *Mol. Pharm.* **2015**, *12*, 889–897. [CrossRef]

67. Vlahakis, J.Z.; Lazar, C.; Crandall, I.E.; Szarek, W.A. Anti-Plasmodium activity of imidazolium and triazolium salts. *Bioorg. Med. Chem.* **2010**, *18*, 6184–6196. [CrossRef] [PubMed]

68. Schrekker, H.S.; Donato, R.K.; Fuentefria, A.M.; Bergamo, V.; Oliveira, L.F.; Machado, M.M. Imidazolium salts as antifungal agents: Activity against emerging yeast pathogens, without human leukocyte toxicity. *MedChemComm* **2013**, *4*, 1457–1460. [CrossRef]

69. Yoon, J.; Kim, S.K.; Singh, N.J.; Kim, K.S. Imidazolium receptors for the recognition of anions. *Chem. Soc. Rev.* **2006**, *35*, 355–360. [CrossRef] [PubMed]

70. Xu, Z.; Kim, S.K.; Yoon, J. Revisit to imidazolium receptors for the recognition of anions: Highlighted research during 2006–2009. *Chem. Soc. Rev.* **2010**, *39*, 1457–1466. [CrossRef]

71. Byrne, S.; Mullen, K.M. Sensing anions on surfaces: Tethering triazolium based anion receptors to polymer resins. *RSC Adv.* **2016**, *6*, 33880–33887. [CrossRef]

72. Vaishya, V.; Patider, S.; Pilania, M. Imidazolium/triazolium based NHC–Palladium complexes and their application in catalysis. *Mater. Today Proc.* **2021**, *43*, 3181–3187. [CrossRef]

73. Comès, A.; Poncelet, R.; Pescarmona, P.P.; Aprile, C. Imidazolium-based titanosilicate nanospheres as active catalysts in carbon dioxide conversion: Towards a cascade reaction from alkenes to cyclic carbonates. *J. CO$_2$ Util.* **2021**, *48*, 101529. [CrossRef]

74. Gutowski, K.E.; Rogers, R.D.; Dixon, D.A. Accurate Thermochemical Properties for Energetic Materials Applications. II. Heats of Formation of Imidazolium-,1,2,4-Triazolium-, and Tetrazolium-Based Energetic Salts from Isodesmic and Lattice Energy Calculations. *J. Phys. Chem. B* **2007**, *111*, 4788–4800. [CrossRef]

75. Singh, R.; Singh, H.J.; Sengupta, S.K. Computational studies on 1,2,4-Triazolium-based salts as energetic materials. *J. Chem. Sci.* **2015**, *127*, 1099–1107. [CrossRef]

76. Ren, J.; Zhang, W.; Zhang, T.; Li, Z.; Zeng, Q.; Zhang, T. A simple and efficient strategy for constructing nitrogen-rich isomeric salts and cocrystal through pKa calculation. *J. Mol. Struct.* **2021**, *1223*, 128955. [CrossRef]

77. Fu, X.; Liu, X.; Sun, P.; Zhang, S.; Yang, Q.; Wei, Q.; Xie, G.; Chen, S.; Fan, X. A new family of insensitive energetic copolymers composed of nitro and nitrogen-rich energy components: Structure, physicochemical property and density functional theory. *J. Anal. Appl. Pyrolysis* **2015**, *114*, 79–90. [CrossRef]

78. Bruker, A. *SAINT Software Reference Manual*; Scientific Research Publishing: Madison, WI, USA, 1998; p. 5465.

79. Dolomanov, O.V.; Bourhis, L.J.; Gildea, R.J.; Howard, J.A.; Puschmann, H. OLEX2: A complete structure solution, refinement and analysis program. *J. Appl. Crystallogr.* **2009**, *42*, 339–341. [CrossRef]

80. Cruz-Cabeza, A.J. Acid–base crystalline complexes and the p K a rule. *CrystEngComm* **2012**, *14*, 6362–6365. [CrossRef]

81. Turner, M.; McKinnon, J.; Wolff, S.; Grimwood, D.; Spackman, P.; Jayatilaka, D.; Spackman, M. *CrystalExplorer17*; The University of Western Australia: Perth, Australia, 2017.
82. Mandel, G.S.; Marsh, R.E. 9-Ethylguanine hemihydrochloride: A short asymmetric N-H . . . N hydrogen bond. *Acta Crystallogr. Sect. B* **1975**, *31*, 2862–2867. [CrossRef]
83. Kelley, S.P.; Narita, A.; Holbrey, J.D.; Green, K.D.; Reichert, W.M.; Rogers, R.D. Understanding the Effects of Ionicity in Salts, Solvates, Co-Crystals, Ionic Co-Crystals, and Ionic Liquids, Rather than Nomenclature, Is Critical to Understanding Their Behavior. *Cryst. Growth Des.* **2013**, *13*, 965–975. [CrossRef]
84. Bis, J.A.; Zaworotko, M.J. The 2-Aminopyridinium-carboxylate Supramolecular Heterosynthon: A Robust Motif for Generation of Multiple-Component Crystals. *Cryst. Growth Des.* **2005**, *5*, 1169–1179. [CrossRef]
85. Easton, M.E.; Li, K.; Titi, H.M.; Kelley, S.P.; Rogers, R.D. Controlling the Interface between Salts, Solvates, Co-crystals, and Ionic Liquids with Non-stoichiometric Protic Azolium Azolates. *Cryst. Growth Des.* **2020**, *20*, 2608–2616. [CrossRef]

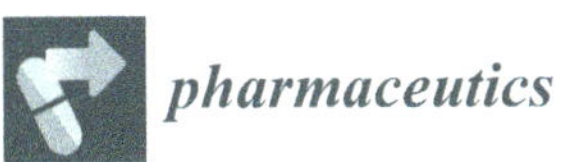

pharmaceutics

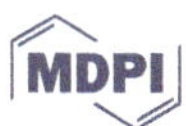

Article

Insight into the Formation of Cocrystal and Salt of Tenoxicam from the Isomer and Conformation

Yifei Xie [1,†], Penghui Yuan [2,†], Tianyu Heng [2], Lida Du [3], Qi An [2], Baoxi Zhang [2], Li Zhang [2,4,*], Dezhi Yang [2,*], Guanhua Du [1] and Yang Lu [2,*]

1   Beijing City Key Laboratory of Drug Target and Screening Research, National Center for Pharmaceutical Screening, Institute of Materia Medica, Chinese Academy of Medical Sciences and Peking Union Medical College, Beijing 100050, China
2   Beijing City Key Laboratory of Polymorphic Drugs, Center of Pharmaceutical Polymorphs, Institute of Materia Medica, Chinese Academy of Medical Sciences and Peking Union Medical College, Beijing 100050, China
3   Shandong Soteria Pharmaceutical Co., Ltd., Laiwu 271100, China
4   Laboratory of Xinjiang Uygur Medical Research, Xinjiang Institute of Materia Medica, Urumqi 830004, China
*   Correspondence: zhangl@imm.ac.cn (L.Z.); ydz@imm.ac.cn (D.Y.); luy@imm.ac.cn (Y.L.)
†   These authors contributed equally to this work.

Abstract: Tenoxicam (TNX) is a new non-steroidal anti-inflammatory drug that shows a superior anti-inflammatory effect and has the advantages of a long half-life period, a fast onset of action, a small dose, complete metabolism, and good tolerance. Some compounds often have tautomerism, and different tautomers exist in different crystalline forms. TNX is such a compound and has three tautomers. TNX always exists as the zwitterionic form in cocrystals. When the salt is formed, TNX exists in the enol form, which exhibits two conformations depending on whether a proton is gained or lost. Currently, the crystal structure of the keto form is not in the Cambridge Structural Database (CSD). Based on the analysis of existing crystal structures, we derived a simple rule for what form of TNX exists according to the pKa value of the cocrystal coformer (CCF) and carried out validation tests using three CCFs with different pKa values, including *p*-aminosalicylic acid (PAS), 3,5-dinitrobenzoic acid (DNB), and 2,6-dihydroxybenzoic acid (DHB). The molecular surface electrostatic potential (MEPS) was combined with the pKa rule to predict the interaction sites. Finally, two new cocrystals (TNX-PAS and TNX-DNB) and one salt (TNX-DHB) of TNX were obtained as expected. The differences between the cocrystals and salt were distinguished by X-ray diffraction, vibration spectra, thermal analysis, and dissolution measurements. To further understand the intermolecular interactions in these cocrystals and salt, the lattice energy and energy decomposition analysis (EDA) were used to explain them from the perspective of energy. The results suggest that the melting point of the CCF determines that of the cocrystal or salt, the solubility of the CCF itself plays an important role, and the improvement of the solubility after salt formation is not necessarily better than that of API or its cocrystals.

Keywords: tenoxicam; cocrystal; salt; conformation; pKa; theoretical calculation

Citation: Xie, Y.; Yuan, P.; Heng, T.; Du, L.; An, Q.; Zhang, B.; Zhang, L.; Yang, D.; Du, G.; Lu, Y. Insight into the Formation of Cocrystal and Salt of Tenoxicam from the Isomer and Conformation. *Pharmaceutics* **2022**, *14*, 1968. https://doi.org/10.3390/pharmaceutics14091968

Academic Editors: Hisham Al-Obaidi and Andrea Erxleben

Received: 16 July 2022
Accepted: 15 September 2022
Published: 19 September 2022

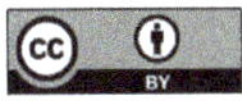

1. Introduction

Tenoxicam (TNX) is a non-steroidal anti-inflammatory drug developed by Roche in 1976 and first listed in Switzerland in March 1987 under the trade name Tihotil. It exerts pharmacological effects by inhibiting cyclooxygenase, reducing the synthesis of local prostaglandins, and inhibiting the chemotaxis of leukocytes and the release of lysosomal enzymes [1]. Its anti-inflammatory effect is superior to that of aspirin, mefenamic acid, and naproxen, and its efficacy is equal to that of piroxicam [2]. Its clinical dosage forms are tablets and suppositories [3], which have the advantages of a long half-life period (70~90 h), a fast onset of action, a small dose (20 mg/d), complete metabolism, hydrophilicity, and good tolerance. It is clinically used to treat arthritis, acute gout, frozen shoulder, etc. [4–7]. TNX is a Biopharmaceutics Classification System (BCS) class II drug that possesses a low solubility and high permeability [8]. Therefore, improving its solubility is an important way to improve bioavailability. The available methods include the formation of different polymorphs, salts/cocrystals, and other solid forms [9–14]. At present, there are five polymorphs and seven solvates of TNX that have been reported [15,16]. Conformation is an important factor leading to the polymorphism of TNX. There are three conformations of TNX: the enol form, keto form, and zwitterionic form, but TNX is mainly in the enol or zwitterionic form in known crystal structures (see Figure 1). The solubilities of different crystal forms are different according to Reference [17], and the orders are form II > form IV > form III > form I, and dioxane solvate > n, n-dimethylformamide solvate > acetonitrile solvate. Forms I and IV conform well with the keto form, while III conforms with the enol form in infrared spectra (IR), according to Reference [18]. However, a single-crystal X-ray diffraction analysis showed that form III and solvates of TNX exist in the zwitterionic form.

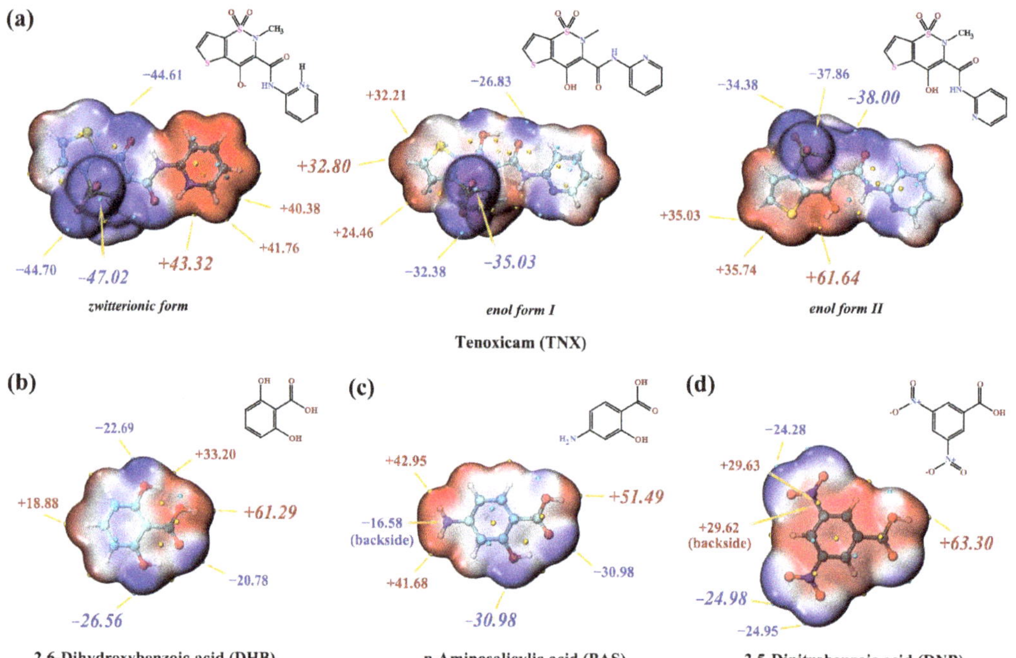

Figure 1. Molecular structures and MEPS of API (**a**) and CCFs (**b–d**).

Pharmaceutical cocrystals and salts are both a kind of multicomponent drug system. Some physicochemical properties of API, such as solubility and thermal stability, can be significantly improved by forming cocrystals or salts with the proper coformer. Moreover, cocrystals and salts likely possess the advantage of multiple or synergistic pharmacological effects when the coformer has pharmacological activities. There are currently 11 cocrystals and salts reported in the CSD of the Cambridge Crystallographic Data Center (CCDC) database [19,20]. The main coformer types of salts or cocrystals are phenolic and benzoic acid compounds. All TNX exists in the zwitterionic form in cocrystals and in the enol form in salts, whereas there are two conformations, namely, enol form I and enol form II, in this work (see Figure 1). This is an interesting phenomenon, and Arkhipov et al. [21] analyzed why TNX was more likely to appear in the zwitterionic form rather than the keto or enol form in different crystal and cocrystal structures based on the role of the S bond. In this work, we obtained a similar result and further analyzed the reason from the perspective of the pKa of the coformer compound and the interaction energy. We derived a rough rule; that is, if the coformer compound is an acidic compound and its pKa value is less than 2, or the coformer compound is an alkaline compound and its pKa value is greater than 9, the salt will be formed in enol form I or enol form II, while with pKa values outside of this range, the cocrystal will usually be formed in the zwitterionic form. This simple rule helps explain why several phenolic compounds (pKa > 9) listed in Table 1 form cocrystals but not salt with TNX [22,23]. Detailed information on the crystals/salts of TNX is listed in Table 2.

Table 1. The melting point, pKa, and ΔpKa of different CCFs and TNX cocrystals.

CCF	Melting Point	Cocrystal Melting Point	pKa [i] Value	ΔpKa Value	Conformation of TNX
Glycolic acid (GLA)	77.1	137.2	3.74	0.76	Unknown
4-Hydroxybenzoic acid (HBA)	215.4	205.2	4.57	0.07	Unknown
α-Ketoglutaric acid (KLA)	114.5	139.3	2.38	2.12	Unknown
Succinic acid (SNA)	187.6	194	4.24	0.26	Unknown
Maleic acid (MLA)	144.1	164.2	2.39	2.11	Unknown
Malonic acid (MNA)	134.9	154	2.92	2.11	Unknown
Oxalic acid (OLA)	191.7	203.6	1.38	1.58	Unknown
Saccharin (SCR)	228.1	237.1	1.60	3.12	Unknown
Benzoic acid (BZA)	122	185	4.20	1.49	A
Salicylic acid (SCA)	159	200	3.01	0.30	A
Pyrocatechol (PRC)	105	174	9.50	5.00	A
Resorcinol (RSC)	110	190	9.45	4.95	A
Pyrogallol (PRG)	131	180	9.28	4.78	A
Piperazine (PPZ)	106	190	9.55	5.05	B
Hydrochloric acid (HCA)	—	198	−8	12.50	B
Methanesulfonic acid (MSA)	—	209	1.75	2.75	B
p-Aminosalicylic acid (PAS)	143.4	200.5	3.58	0.92	A
3,5-Dinitrobenzoic acid (DNB)	205.9	209.3	2.77	1.73	A
2,6-Dihydroxybenzoic acid (DHB)	169.3	206.4	1.30	3.20	B

[i]: The melting points and pKa values in the table were obtained from SciFinder. "A" represents the zwitterionic form, and "B" represents enol form I or enol form II. —: The coformer compound is liquid.

Table 2. Crystal Cell Parameters and Structure Refinement of the Cocrystals or Salt of TNX.

	TNX-PAS	TNX-DNB	TNX-DHB
Formula	$C_{13}H_{11}N_3O_4S_2 \cdot C_7H_7NO_3$	$C_{13}H_{11}N_3O_4S_2 \cdot C_7H_4N_2O_6$	$C_{13}H_{11}N_3O_4S_2 \cdot C_7H_6O_4$
Description	flake	flake	flake
Crystal system	monoclinic	triclinic	monoclinic
Space group	$P\,2_1$	$P\,\bar{1}$	$C\,2/c$
	9.220 (1)	9.578 (1)	21.516 (1)
	20.215 (1)	10.721 (1)	7.731 (1)
Unit cell parameters	11.617 (1)	11.617 (1)	26.440 (1)
(Å, °)	90	93.248 (3)	90
	97.98 (1)	107.587 (3)	104.070 (10)
	90	99.406 (2)	90
Volume (Å^3)	2144.65 (2)	1114.75 (6)	4266.37 (11)
Z	4	2	2
Density (g/cm^3)	1.519	1.637	1.530
Theta range for data collection	3.84~72.14	4.01~71.55	3.42~72.16
Independent reflections	7115	4187	4166
Reflections with I > 2σ(I)	6192	3814	3694
R (I > 2σI)	R = 0.052	R = 0.0404	R = 0.0571
	wR$_2$ = 0.147	wR$_2$ = 0.1146	wR$_2$ = 0.1599
Goodness-of-fit on F^2	1.066	1.086	1.025
Completeness	99.3	97.6	99.7
Deposition number	2174287	2174286	2174285

Based on the above analysis, we selected *p*-aminosalicylic acid (PAS), 3,5-dinitrobenzoic acid (DNB), and 2,6-dihydroxybenzoic acid (DHB) as coformer compounds to prepare new cocrystals or salt to verify the rule. PAS possesses anti-inflammatory and antibacterial activity [24]. DNB also exhibits antibacterial activity [25]. They have great potential to improve or extend the pharmacological activity of TNX by forming a cocrystal or salt with the parent drug. DHB, as a phenolic compound, has poor biological performance [26], but it still possesses important meaning to verify the rule we derived. Moreover, all three coformers are commonly used coformers in pharmaceutical cocrystal and salt research due to their relatively high stability and solubility. The structural formulas of coformer compounds are shown in Figure 1. Two cocrystals and one salt were obtained by grinding under slurry conditions and using solvent evaporation methods as expected. The cocrystals and salt were characterized by single-crystal X-ray diffraction (SXRD), powder X-ray diffraction (PXRD), differential scanning calorimetry (DSC), infrared spectroscopy (IR), and Raman spectroscopy. In addition, theoretical calculations based on density functional theory (DFT) were used to predict the interaction sites using the molecular electrostatic potential surface (MEPS) and analyze the hydrogen bonding motifs and intermolecular interactions of cocrystals and salts, thus providing valuable insights for further cocrystal/salt research on TNX.

2. Materials and Methods

2.1. Materials

TNX (purity > 98%) was purchased from Xi'an Kechuang Pharmaceutical Co., Ltd. (Xi'an, China). PAS (purity > 98%), DNB (purity > 98%), and DHB (purity > 98%) were purchased from Hubei Wande Chemical Co., Ltd. (Wuhan, China). All analytical-grade solvents were purchased from Beijing Chemical Works (Beijing, China).

2.2. Methods

2.2.1. Preparation

TNX-PAS and TNX-DNB Cocrystals and TNX-DHB salt were prepared for characterization and evaluation by grinding under slurry conditions [27–30] as follows: TNX (169 mg, 0.5 mol) and PAS (77 mg, 0.5 mol), DNB (106 mg, 0.5 mmol), and DHB (77 mg, 0.5 mmol) in a stoichiometric ratio of 1:1 were each weighed into a clean mortar and ground thoroughly with 1 mL of methanol for about 10 min, and then yellow powder samples were obtained.

2.2.2. Crystallization

Crystals of the above cocrystals and salt for SXRD analysis were prepared by the slow solvent evaporation (SSE) method at room temperature as follows: TNX (169 mg, 0.5 mmol) mixed with PAS (77 mg, 0.5 mmol), DNB (106 mg, 0.5 mmol), or DHB (77 mg, 0.5 mmol) was dissolved in 30 mL of methanol and stirred for two hours. Then, the solutions were filtered and left to stand at room temperature for about two weeks, and flaked yellow crystals were obtained.

2.3. Powder X-ray Diffraction (PXRD) Analysis

PXRD experiments were performed on a Rigaku SmartLab 9 KW diffractometer with Cu Kα radiation ($\lambda = 1.54178$ Å) (Rigaku, Tokyo, Japan). The powder samples were scanned continuously with a coverage of 3–40° at a constant rate of 8°/min. Simulated PXRD patterns were calculated using Mercury software (v 4.1.0, Cambridge Crystallographic Data Center, Cambridge, UK) at a starting angle of 3°, a final angle of 40°, a step size of 0.02°, and a full width at half maximum of 0.15°.

2.4. Single-Crystal X-ray Diffraction (SXRD) Analysis

SXRD experiments were performed on a Rigaku MicroMax-002+ CCD diffractometer with Cu Kα radiation ($\lambda = 1.54178$ Å) (Rigaku, Americas, The Woodlands, TX, USA). Intensity data were collected at 293 K. Absorption correction and integration of the collected data were performed using the CrystalClear software package. Crystal structures were solved and refined through full-matrix least-square methods, which were performed using Olex2 and SHELXL crystallography software [31–33]. All non-hydrogen atoms were refined anisotropically. Hydrogen atoms linked to carbon atoms were fixed in geometrically constrained positions, whereas hydrogen atoms associated with nitrogen and oxygen atoms were located through the difference Fourier method [34,35].

2.5. Differential Scanning Calorimetry (DSC) Analysis

DSC thermograms were recorded with DSC 1 (Mettler Toledo, Greifensee, Switzerland) and STARe Evaluation software 16.0. Approximately 3–5 mg was weighed into an aluminum crucible and heated at a constant rate of 10 °C/min over a temperature range of 30−300 °C under atmospheric conditions.

2.6. Infrared Spectroscopy (IR) Analysis

IR experiments were performed on a Spectrμm 400 Fourier transform infrared spectrometer (PerkinElmer, Waltham, MA, USA). Experimental conditions included an attenuated total reflection accessory, a spectral scanning range of 4000–650 cm^{-1}, a resolution of 4.000 cm^{-1}, and a scan number of 16.

2.7. Raman Analysis

All FT-Raman spectra in this paper were recorded at room temperature in the range of 4000–100 cm^{-1} with a 3 s integration time using a Horiba HR Evolution FT-Raman spectrometer equipped with a 532 nm Nd and YAG laser beam for spectral acquisition.

2.8. Theoretical Computation

The B3LYP-D3/6-311G + (d, p) level was employed for all hydrogen atom geometry optimizations, while all heavy atoms were observed at the original X-ray coordinates, and the same level was used for frequency and single-energy calculations using the Gaussian 16 package [36] based on density functional theory (DFT). The lattice energy calculations were carried out on the cocrystals and salt using CRYSTAL17 software [37] at the B3LYP/6-31G (d, p) level based on single-crystal structures. The EDA of the intermolecular interactions of the cocrystals and salt was carried out based on the generalized Kohn–Sham EDA (GKS-EDA) method by using the XEDA program [38–40]. The Multiwfn 3.8 package was used for all wave function analyses [41].

2.9. Dissolution Measurements

Dissolution measurements were investigated by the basket method by using an RC12AD dissolution instrument (Tianjin Tianda Tianfa Technology Co., Ltd., Tianjin, China). According to a previous study [42], it is necessary that all of the particle sizes of TNX, cocrystals, and salt are at the same level when the same operation is performed on these samples. To do so, the powder samples of TNX, two cocrystals, and one salt were milled and sieved through 100-mesh sieves to minimize the size influence on the results. The temperature and rotation speed were set to 37 °C and 160 r·min^{-1}. The dissolution mediums were water (pH 7.0), phosphate buffer (pH 6.8), acetate buffer (pH 4.5), and hydrochloric buffer (pH 1.2). Accurately weighed samples (containing 60 mg of TNX) were each added to 900 mL of dissolution mediums. The sampling points were at 5, 10, 15, 20, 30, 45, 60, 90, 120, 180, 240, 360, 480, 600, and 720 min. The concentrations of TNX were quantified on an Agilent 1200 Series HPLC system (Agilent Technologies, Santa Clara, USA) with a Sil-Green C_{18} HPLC column (4.6 mm × 250 mm, 5μm) and a UV detector at a wavelength of 257 nm. The mobile phase was methanol–0.04% formic acid aqueous solution (61:39). The flow rate and column temperature were set to 1 mL·min^{-1} and 25 °C.

3. Results and Discussion

3.1. Prediction of Interaction Sites

Based on the structural analysis of TNX cocrystals in CSD, TNX exists in the zwitterionic form in cocrystals. During salt formation, TNX can act as either an acid (proton donor) or a base (proton acceptor). As a base, the conformation of TNX is usually in the form of enol form I, and as an acid, it is usually in the form of enol form II. According to the results of previous studies [43–45], the MEPS of a compound with different conformations also shows differences, which will lead to different intermolecular interaction sites. Therefore, we calculated the MEPS of CCFs and different conformations of TNX and carried out a prediction analysis of the interaction sites combined with the pKa rule.

The pKa of TNX is 4.50, and the pKa values of CCFs, including DHB, PAS, and DNB, are listed in Table 1. According to the derived pKa rule, the pKa of PAS and DNB is 3.58 and 2.77, which indicates cocrystal formation because their pKa values are more than 2. The pKa of DHB is 1.30, which indicates salt formation because its pKa is less than 2, and TNX acts as a base.

The MEPS of the zwitterionic form of TNX showed that the electron-rich region was on the left side, and the electron-deficient region was on the right side. Due to electrostatic attraction, two TNX molecules tend to form a dimer side by side in opposite directions. Thus, due to the existence of a local minimum point (-44.61 kcal/mol) near the hydroxyl oxygen where proton transfer occurred, it can interact with the global maximum point existing in the MEPS of PAS ($+51.49$ kcal/mol) or DNB ($+63.30$ kcal/mol) molecules to form hydrogen bonds. Only one proton acceptor site exists at the MEPS of enol form I of TNX, i.e., the nitrogen of the pyridine ring. Although there are three proton donors in DHB, the hydroxyl proton in the carboxyl group is more active ($+61.29$ kcal/mol) and will be preferentially transferred. At the MEPS of enol form II of TNX, the hydroxyl proton on the thiazine ring is more active ($+61.64$ kcal/mol) and will be preferentially transferred. Due to proton transfer, the distribution of molecular electron density changes, and the MEPS also changes, so the possible action sites of the salt cannot be predicted according to the MEPS in Figure 1.

3.2. Single-Crystal X-ray Diffraction (SXRD) Analysis

The structural details of two cocrystals and one salt were revealed by X-ray crystallography. All crystallographic data were deposited in CSD with deposition numbers 2174285–2174287. The main crystallographic data of the three novel crystals are summarized in Table 2.

Based on SXRD analysis, the hydrogen bonding network in all crystals was systematically investigated. The hydrogen bonding parameters are listed in Table 3. The TNX-DNB cocrystal was crystallized in the triclinic space group $P\bar{1}$, and the asymmetric unit contained one TNX molecule and one DNB molecule. In this cocrystal, the TNX molecule also existed in zwitterionic form, having two intramolecular N-H ... O hydrogen bonds (N_2-H_2 ... O_1; N_3-H_3 ... O_4). Two TNX molecules were linked by intermolecular N-H ... O hydrogen bonds (N_3-H_3 ... O_4) to form a centrosymmetric dimer with the $R_2^2(4)$ graph set notation. Two 3,5-dinitrobenzoic acid molecules were connected on each side through O-H ... O hydrogen bonds (O_{2D}-H_{2D} ... O_1) to form a centrosymmetric tetramer. The tetramers were linked together through weak C-H ... O interactions to form an approximately planar structure. The planes were linked by weak C-H ... O interactions and S-S interactions to form a three-dimensional layered structure (Figure 2a). The TNX-PAS cocrystal was crystallized in the monoclinic space group $P2_1$, and the asymmetric unit contained two TNX and two PAS molecules. The TNX molecule existed in the zwitterionic form in this cocrystal. There were two intramolecular N-H ... O hydrogen bonds (N_2-H_2 ... O_1 and N_3-H_3 ... O_4) in the motif $S_1^1(6)$ in the TNX molecule. Two TNX molecules were connected by intermolecular N-H ... O hydrogen bonds ($N_3$$-$$H_3$ ... O_8; $N_6$$-$$H_6$ ... O_4) to form a centrosymmetric dimer with the $R_2^2(4)$ graph set notation. Similar to the TNX-DNB cocrystal, in the TNX-PAS cocrystal, two TNX dimers linked two PAS molecules, respectively, through O-H ... O (O_{1A}-H_{1A} ... O_1; O_{4A}-H_{4A} ... O_5) hydrogen bonds to form a tetramer. The tetramer extends infinitely on each side to form a planar structure through N-H ... O (N_{1A}-H_{1AB} ... O_3; N_{2A}-H_{2AA} ... O_7) hydrogen bonds. Each plane was connected by O-H ... O (O_{3A}-H_{3AA} ... O_6; O_{6A}-H_{6A} ... O_2) hydrogen bonds to form a three-dimensional layered structure (Figure 2b). The TNX-DHB salt was crystallized in the monoclinic space group *C*2/c, and the asymmetric unit contained one TNX molecule and one DNB molecule. Unlike the cocrystals, the TNX molecule existed as enol form I with intramolecular O-H ... O hydrogen bonds (O_1-H_1 ... O_4). Two TNX molecules were linked by intermolecular O-H ... O hydrogen bonds (O_1-H_1 ... O_4) to form a centrosymmetric dimer with the $R_2^2(4)$ graph set notation. Two DHB molecules were connected on each side through N-H ... O hydrogen bonds (N_2-H_2 ... O_5; N_3-H_{3A} ... O_6) to form a centrosymmetric tetramer. The tetramer formed a curved surface structure, and every two tetramers were interlaced face to face through weak C-H ... O interactions. This structure extended indefinitely to form a three-dimensional network (Figure 2c). The result of SXRD analysis shows that the arrangements of cocrystals with the same TNX conformation were similar, but the arrangement of the salt was quite different from that of the cocrystals due to the change in the TNX conformation.

Table 3. Parameters (Å, °) of Main Hydrogen Bonds for Cocrystals and Salt of TNX.

Cocrystal/Salt	D–H ... A	D ... A (Å)	∠DHA (°)
TNX-PAS	N_2-H_2 ... O_1	2.607	140.28
	N_3-H_3 ... O_4	2.651	131.79
	N_3-H_3 ... O_8 [a]	2.894	139.58
	N_{1A}-H_{1AB} ... O_3	3.017	152.46
	O_{1A}-H_{1A} ... O_1 [b]	2.572	160.00
	O_{3A}-H_{3AA} ... O_{2A}	2.624	137.63
TNX-DNB	N_2-H_2 ... O_1	2.637	138.40
	N_3-H_3 ... O_4 (intra-)	2.585	133.03
	N_3-H_3 ... O_4 [c] (inter-)	2.991	135.57
	O_{2D}-H_{2D} ... O_1	2.572	166.51
	N_2-H_2 ... O_5	3.018	168.02
	N_3-H_{3A} ... O_6	2.593	157.48
TNX-DHB	O_1-H_1 ... O_4 (intra-)	2.559	142.82
	O_1-H_1 ... O_4 [d] (inter-)	2.886	122.41
	O_7-H_7 ... O_6	2.529	146.91
	O_8-H_8 ... O_5	2.568	147.81

Symmetry Codes: [a] x + 1, y, z; [b] x + 1, y, z − 1; [c] −x + 2, −y + 1, −z + 1; [d] −x + 1, y, −z + 1/2.

3.3. Powder X-ray Diffraction (PXRD) Analysis

The experimental PXRD patterns of the cocrystals and salt are shown in Figure 3, which differ from those of API and CCFs, indicating the formation of new phases. The simulated PXRD patterns colored in gray corresponding to the crystal structures were calculated using Mercury software. The experimental PXRD patterns of the cocrystals and salt agree well with the simulated ones. Their consistency indicates that the phase purities of the solid forms were good, and they can be used in other characterizations.

3.4. Infrared Spectroscopy (IR) Analysis

Vibrational spectroscopy is a reliable technique for characterizing hydrogen bonding and crystal packing in solids [46,47]. Changes in hydrogen bonding will lead to vibrational frequency shifts. The carbonyl stretching frequency of PAS (1611 cm^{-1}), DNB (1698 cm^{-1}), and DHB (1666 cm^{-1}) was shifted to 1631 cm^{-1} in TNX-PAS, 1725 cm^{-1} in TNX-DNB, and 1646 cm^{-1} in TNX-DHB, revealing the influence of intermolecular O-H ... O and N-H ... O hydrogen bond formation, as shown in Figure 4 and Table 3.

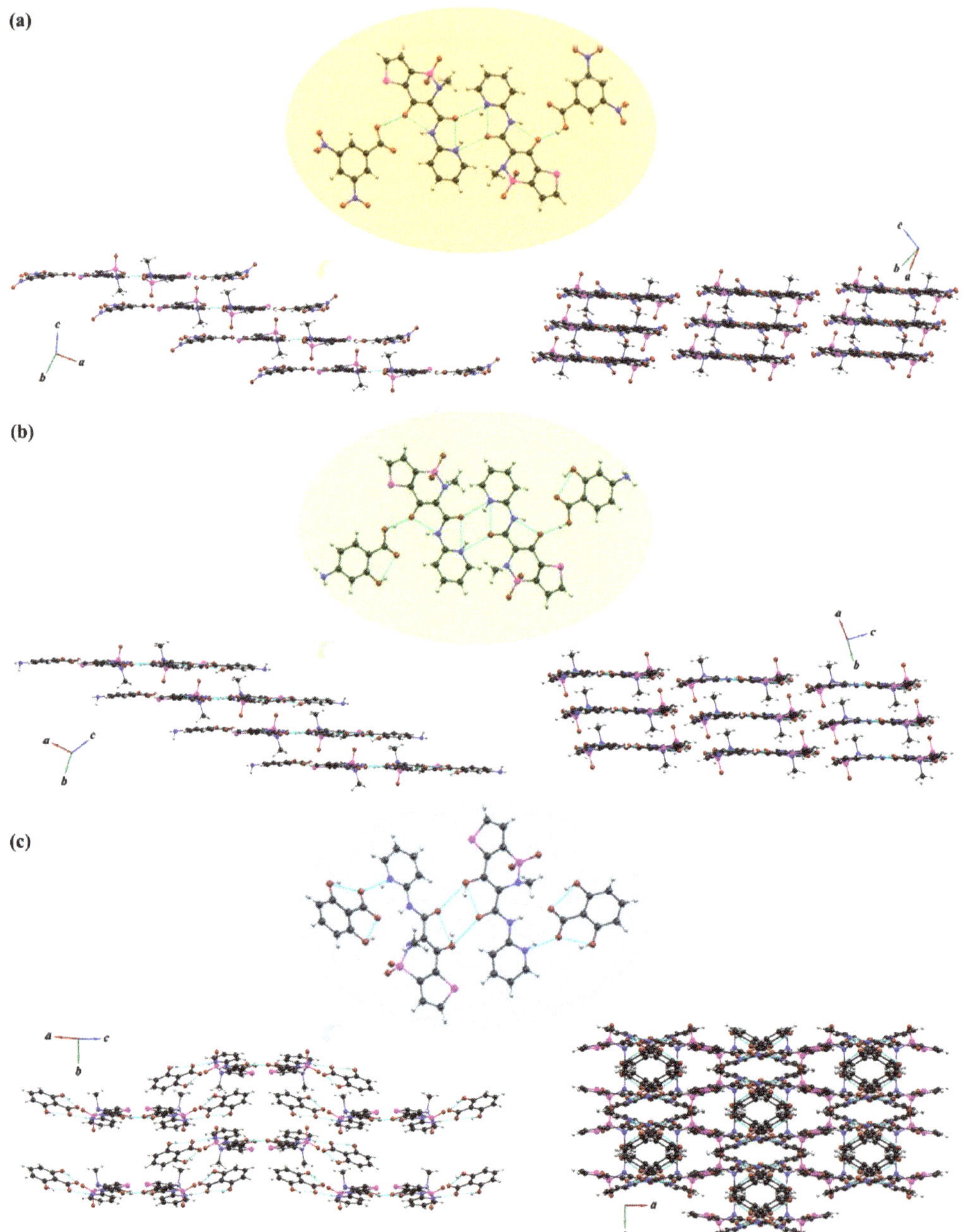

Figure 2. Hydrogen bond motifs and molecular stacking mode of (**a**) TNX-DNB, (**b**) TNX-PAS, and (**c**) TNX-DHB.

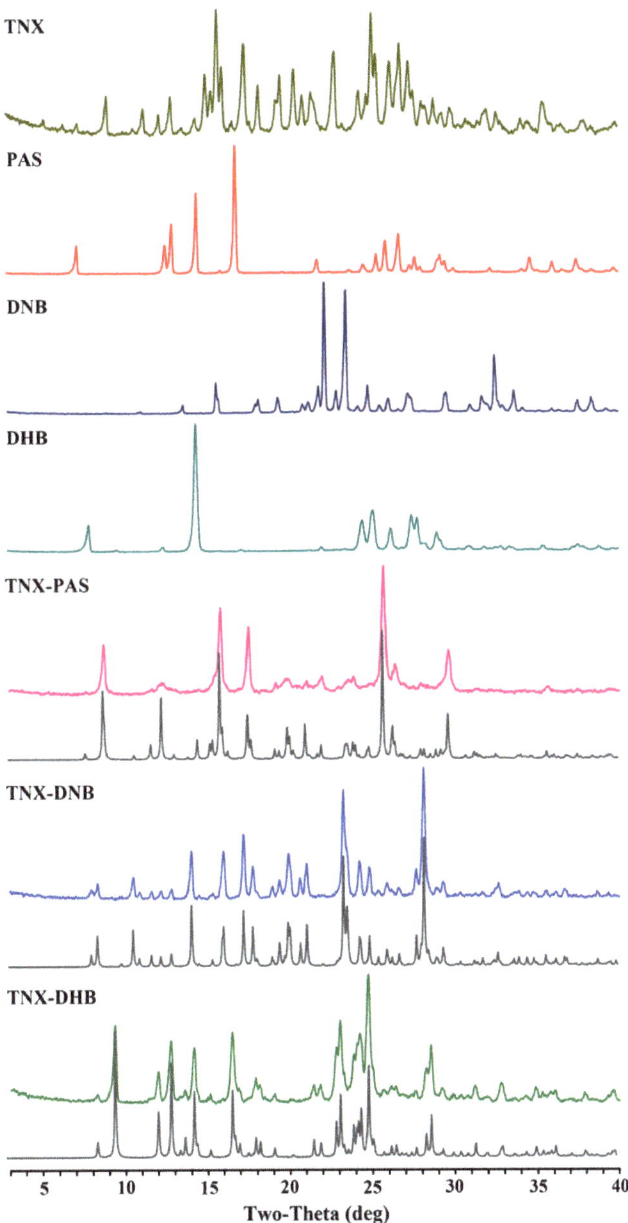

Figure 3. PXRD patterns of TNX, CCFs, and the corresponding cocrystals/salt.

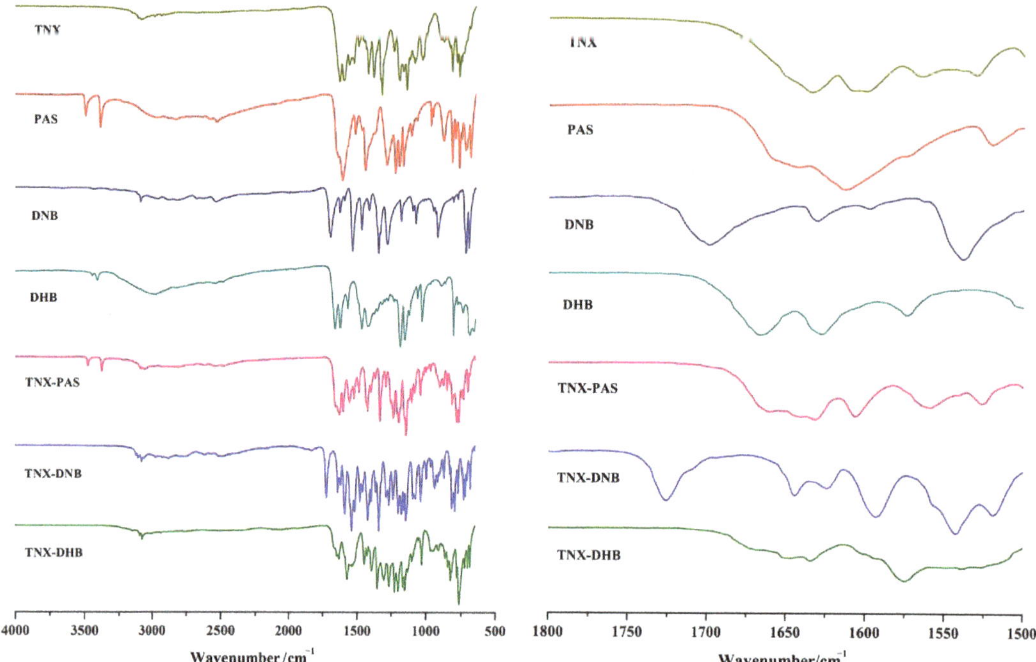

Figure 4. IR spectra of TNX, CCFs, and the corresponding cocrystals/salt (**left**); the region for OH stretch in IR spectra of TNX, CCFs, and the corresponding cocrystals/salt (**right**).

3.5. Raman Analysis

Raman spectroscopy is generated by changes in the polarization rate of molecules and is advantageous for identifying non-polar groups in molecules. This method can provide valid evidence to determine the form of tenoxicam and provide assistance in distinguishing between cocrystals and salts. Figure 5 shows the different Raman spectra between TNX, CCFs, and the corresponding cocrystals/salts. NH_2-Ar exists in the PAS molecule, and there is a characteristic peak of $\nu_{N\text{-}H}$ at 3412 cm^{-1}, but no such peak appears in the spectrum of TNX-PAS, indicating that NH_2 participates in eutectic formation. DNB and DHB are both derivatives of benzoic acid. There is a $\nu_{C\text{-}H}$ vibration of the benzene ring between 2800–3100 cm^{-1} on the ring. The characteristic peaks at 3114 cm^{-1} and 3101 cm^{-1} in the Raman spectra of TNX-DNB and TNX-DHB disappear, indicating that there is π-π accumulation in the participating structure of the benzene ring. There is a strong peak of 1561 cm^{-1} in TNX-DHB because the carbonyl group on the six-membered ring of TNX is converted into the enol structure, showing strong $\nu_{C\,=\,C}$. In addition, tenoxicam has three different states. The torsion of the C-H bond used in this paper is an important indicator to distinguish between the cocrystal and salt of TNX. In the Raman spectra of TNX-PAS and TNX-DNB cocrystals, TNX is composed of dimers in the zwitterionic form. In the Raman spectra of the TNX-DHB salt, there are two sharp characteristic peaks at 1262 cm^{-1} and 1299 cm^{-1}, indicating that due to the interaction between DHB and TNX, the C-H structure in the TNX structure is twisted, and the hydrogen on the carboxyl of DHB is transferred to the N of the pyridine ring of TNX. An ionic bond between N-H and C-O was formed, and a hydrogen bond between N-H and C-O was formed. However, there was no such characteristic peak in TNX-PAS and TNX-DNB. Therefore, Raman spectroscopy can effectively distinguish between the TNX eutectic and salt. TNX exists in three different forms, and the reversal of the C-H bond used in this study is an important marker to distinguish the cocrystal from the salt. The two sharp peaks appear at 1262 cm $^{-1}$ and 1299 cm $^{-1}$ in the Raman spectra of TNX-DHB, which shows that the C-H structure of TNX was reversed due to the interaction between DHB and TNX. The hydrogen on the carboxyl group of DHB was transferred to the N of the pyridine ring belonging to TNX, which formed ionic bonds between N-H and C-O and hydrogen bonds between N-H and C=O. However, no such peaks existed in TNX-PAS and TNX-DNB. Therefore, Raman spectroscopy is an effective method to distinguish between the cocrystal and salt of TNX.

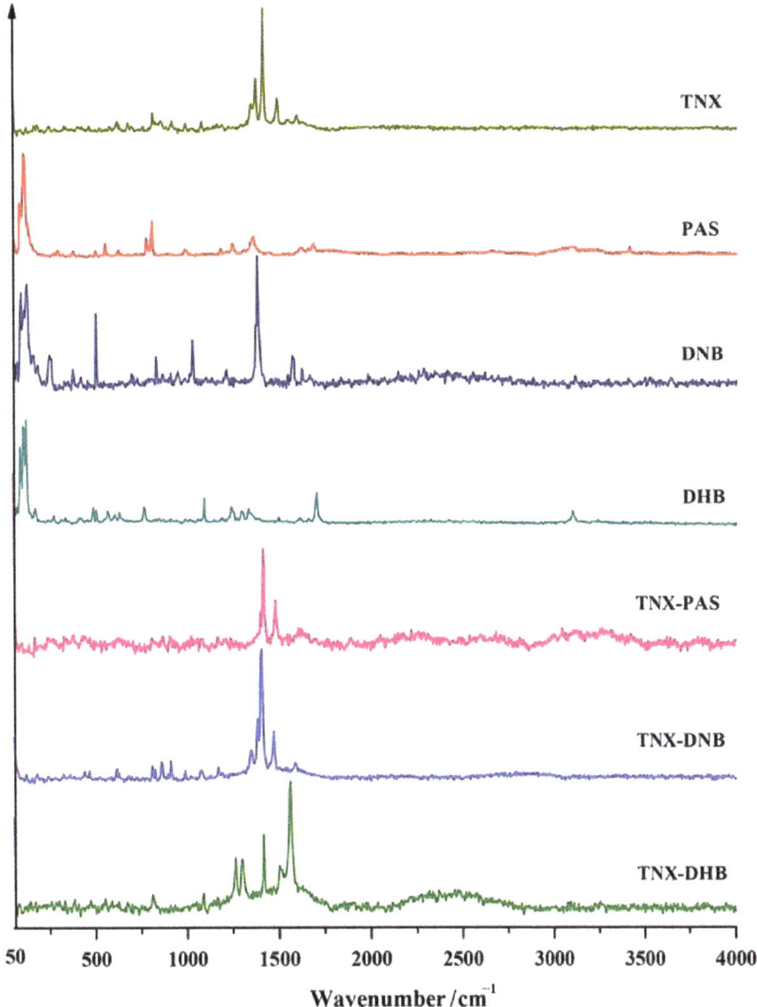

Figure 5. Raman spectra of TNX, CCFs, and the corresponding cocrystals/salt.

3.6. Differential Scanning Calorimetry (DSC) Analysis

DSC analysis was performed to determine the melting points of the cocrystals/salts and to study their thermal behavior, as shown in Figure 6. TNX-PAS, TNX-DNB, and TNX-DHB showed sharp endothermic peaks at 200.48 °C, 209.26 °C, and 206.38 °C, respectively, which are different from those of API and CCFs, indicating the formation of new phases. The order of peak values from high to low is TNX-DNB > TNX-DHB > TNX-PAS, which is consistent with the order of the melting points of CCF and the crystal density of the cocrystals and salts. It is speculated that lower crystal density results in looser crystal packing and weaker interactions, thus leading to lower melting points [48]. We plotted the melting points of the cocrystals or salts and CCFs listed in Table 1 (Figure 7), and the results show that although the trends of the melting points of cocrystals and salts are not consistent with those of CCFs from low to high, the CCF of the cocrystal with the lowest melting point also had the lowest melting point, and the CCF of the cocrystal with the highest melting point also had the highest melting point. It can be seen that the thermal stability of CCFs has a great influence on the thermal stability of the cocrystal and salt of TNX. In addition, TNX-PAS, TNX-DNB, and TNX-DHB decomposed immediately after melting, similar to the melting behavior of TNX (Figure S1). Although the melting points of the cocrystals and salt were lower than that of TNX, they still showed features of melting decomposition. This indicates that TNX might have decomposed at lower temperatures, but the formation of different crystals delayed the process to varying degrees.

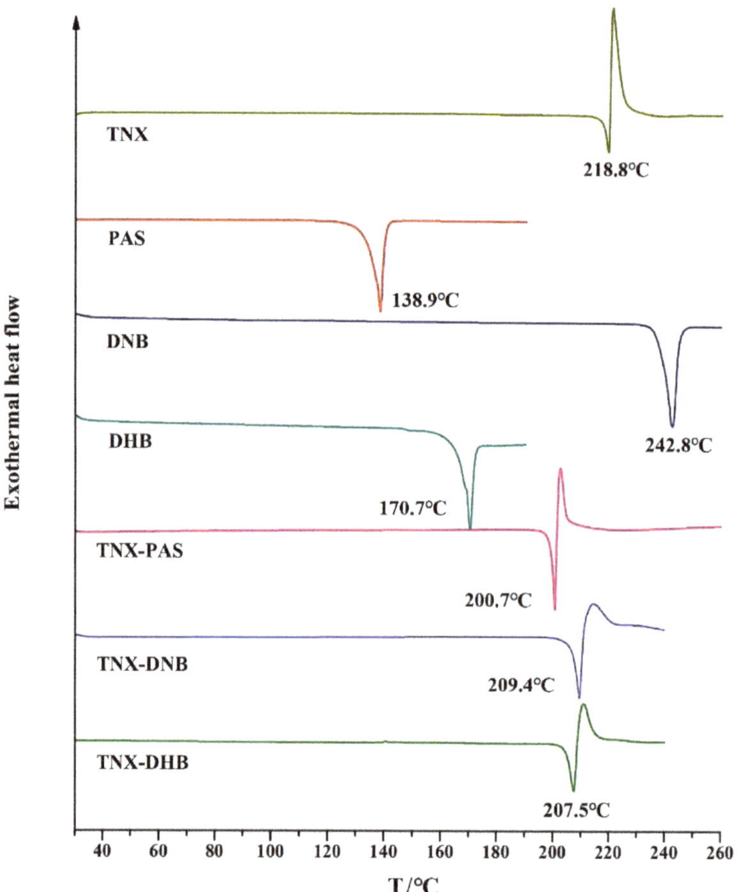

Figure 6. DSC profiles of TNX, CCFs, and the corresponding cocrystals/salt.

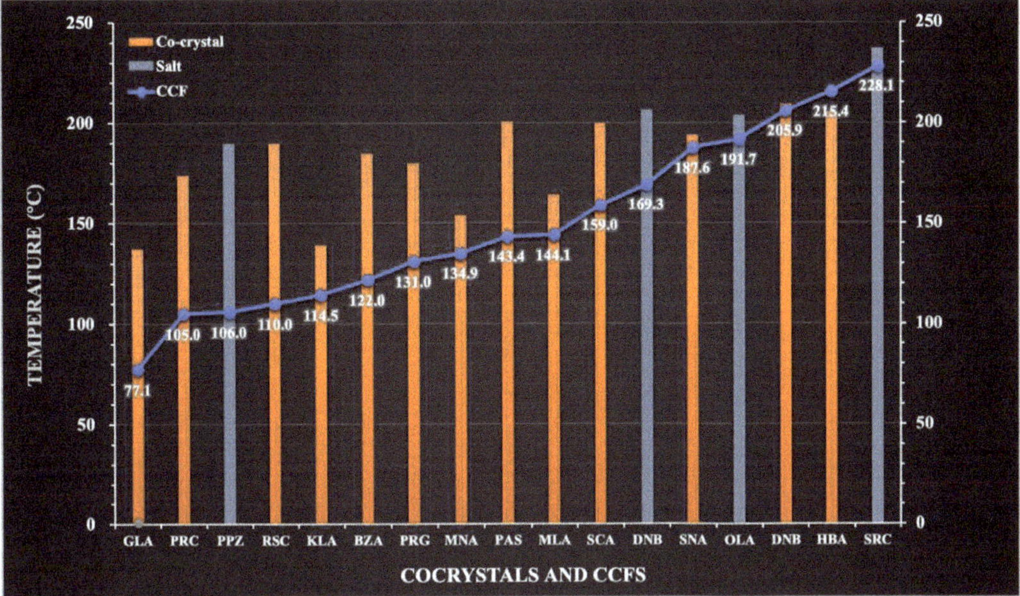

Figure 7. Melting point trend diagram of cocrystal/salt and CCF.

3.7. Lattice Energy Analysis

Lattice energy can be used to compare the thermodynamic stability of crystal structures to a certain extent. The higher the value is, the more stable the structure is. In this work, the lattice energies of TNX-PAS, TNX-DNB, and TNX-DHB are −43.25, −48.72, and −125.82, respectively. The enthalpy-of-fusion values of TNX-PAS, TNX-DNB, and TNX-DHB determined by DSC are −498.11 mJ, −965.18 mJ, and −144.31 mJ, respectively. For the two cocrystals, because they all belong to molecular crystals, TNX-DNB is more stable than TNX-PAS due to its higher lattice energy, which is consistent with the DSC analysis results. For the TNX-DHB salt belonging to ionic crystals, its lattice energy is usually larger than that of the molecular crystal, so it is not suitable for direct comparison with the molecular crystal. The enthalpy-of-fusion values of three TNX solid forms also proved this point.

3.8. Energy Decomposition Analysis (EDA)

Energy decomposition is an important component of the analytical method of quantum chemistry, and this process can decompose the total interaction energy between molecules into energy terms of physical significance to investigate the nature of the interaction [49–51]. Generalized Kohn–Sham EDA (GKS-EDA) decomposes the total interaction energy of the complex (ΔE^{total}) into five parts, i.e., the electrostatic energy (ΔE^{ele}), the exchange energy (ΔE^{ex}), the repulsion energy (ΔE^{rep}), the polarization energy (ΔE^{pol}), and the electron correlation energy (ΔE^{disp}). In this study, GSK-EDA was used to analyze the total interactions of the tetramers (constitutional repeating unit) in the cocrystals and salt (shown in Figure 2) to comprehensively understand the multi-body interaction.

Because the compositions of TNX-PAS, TNX-DNB, and TNX-DHB were different, it was not possible to judge the strength of the intermolecular interactions of different complexes by directly comparing the total interaction energy. However, by using EDA, differences in the components of interactions among these complexes can be revealed. The results of EDA showed that attractive intermolecular interactions of the fragments in the cocrystals and salt were dominated by ΔE^{ele} and ΔE^{ex}. For the two cocrystals, the electrostatic interactions were the manifestation of intermolecular hydrogen bonds, and they were attractive energy. For the salt, the electrostatic interactions were the electrostatic attraction between opposite ions and the electrostatic repulsion between like ions. ΔE^{EA} is the energy contribution of orbital relaxation from monomers to the supermolecule, and it can be seen that the exchange energy of the salt is higher than that of the cocrystal because of proton transfer in the salt. Similarly, the proportion of polarization energy in the salt as the attractive energy was larger than that in the cocrystals. The dispersion energy was the minimum, but its effect cannot be ignored. The three-dimensional structures of the crystals are based on the interactions of these kinds of energies. The results of the GSK-EDA of the cocrystals and salt of TNX are plotted as a three-dimensional line chart in Figure 8, and data are listed in Tables S1–S3 in the Supplementary Materials.

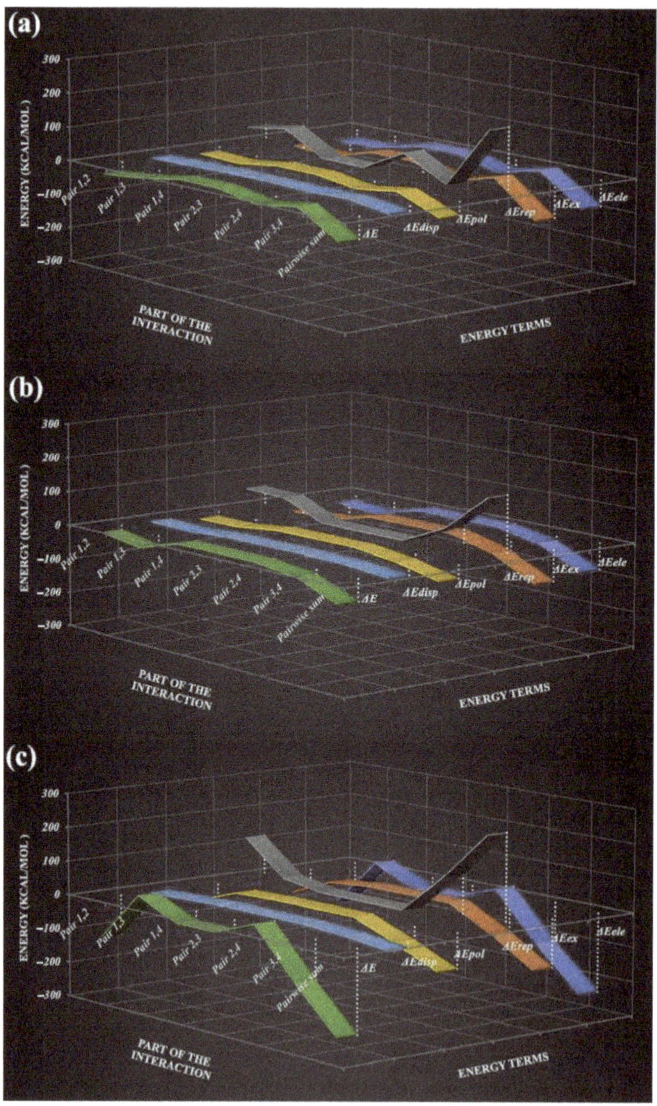

Figure 8. GSK-EDA of the cocrystals and salt of TNX, (**a**) TNX-DNB, (**b**) TNX-PAS, and (**c**) TNX-DHB.

3.9. Dissolution Measurement Analysis

Figure 9 shows the results of dissolution measurements of TNX, TNX-PAS, TNX-DNB, and TNX-DHB in four buffers. TNX-PAS had similar solubility features to TNX, and its solubility was slightly higher than that of TNX at pH 1.2 and 6.8, but there were no solubility differences, relatively. The solubility of TNX-DNB was lower than those of TNX, TNXPAS, and TNX-DHB at pH 1.2 and 6.8 and slightly higher than that of TNX-DHB at pH 7.0. TNX-DHB also had similar solubility characteristics to TNX, which was slightly lower. In general, the solubility of the three samples was not improved compared to API, which may be related to the solubility of CCFs.

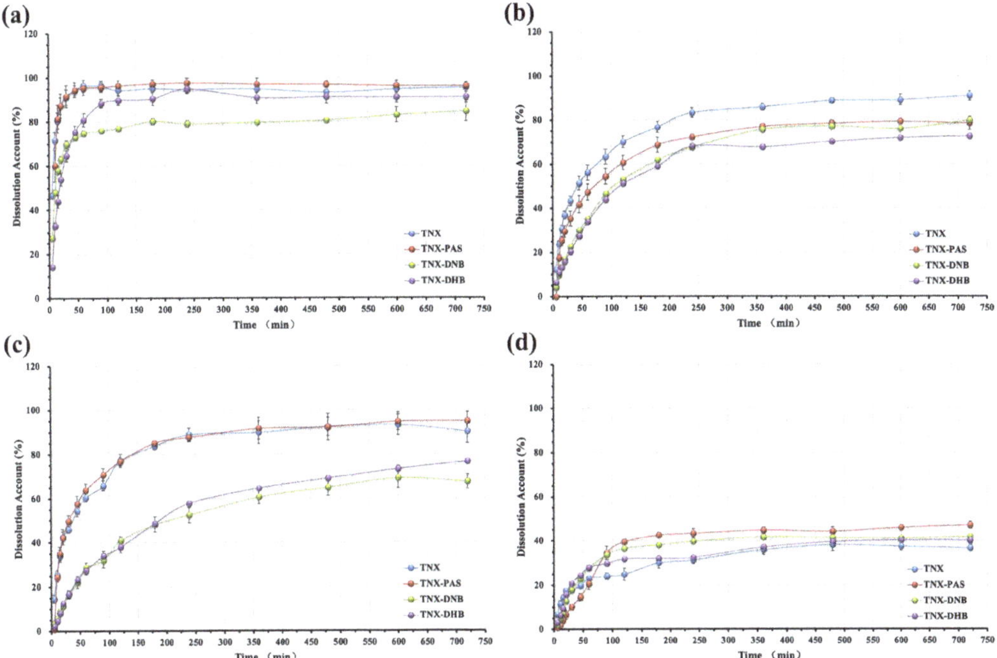

Figure 9. Powder dissolution profiles of the cocrystals and salt of TNX in four solvent systems. (**a**) Hydrochloric buffer (pH 1.2); (**b**) acetate buffer (pH 4.5); (**c**) phosphate buffer (pH 6.8); and (**d**) water (pH 7.0).

4. Conclusions

In this work, different solid forms that existed in the cocrystals and salt of TNX were carefully investigated, and a simple rule was derived as follows: when the CCF is an acidic compound and the pKa value is less than 2, or the CCF is a basic compound and its pKa value is greater than 9, the salt will be formed, and TNX will exist in enol form I or II, respectively; when the pKa value of the CCF is out the range mentioned above, the cocrystal will be formed, and TNX will exist in the zwitterionic form. According to this rule, two cocrystals and one salt of TNX were synthesized for the first time. In the thermal analysis, we found that the melting point of CCF determined that of the cocrystal or salt, and the thermal stability of TNX was determined. In addition, theoretical calculations, such as lattice energy and energy decomposition, were performed to analyze the intermolecular interactions in the cocrystals and salt, which made the strength of intermolecular forces clearer and the difference between the salt and cocrystal more intuitive. Finally, although neither the cocrystals nor the salt can improve the solubility of TNX, the results suggest that the solubility of the CCF itself plays an important role, and the improvement of solubility after salt formation is not necessarily better than that of API or its cocrystals.

Supplementary Materials: The following supporting information can be downloaded at: https://www.mdpi.com/article/10.3390/pharmaceutics14091968/s1. Table S1: GSK-EDA of the TNX-PAS cocrystal; Table S2: GSK-EDA of the TNX-DNB cocrystal; Table S3: GSK-EDA of the TNX-DHB salt; Figure S1: DSC and TG profiles of TNX, CCFs, and the corresponding cocrystals/salt.

Author Contributions: Conceptualization, L.Z., D.Y. and Y.L.; methodology, Y.X. and P.Y.; investigation, Y.X. and P.Y.; formal analysis, Y.X., P.Y. and T.H.; software, L.D. and Q.A.; validation, L.D. and Q.A.; data curation, B.Z.; writing—original draft preparation, Y.X. and P.Y.; writing—review and editing, L.Z. and D.Y.; supervision, L.Z., D.Y., G.D. and Y.L.; project administration, L.Z., D.Y. and Y.L.; funding acquisition, L.Z., D.Y. and Y.L. All authors have read and agreed to the published version of the manuscript.

Funding: This work was funded by the Key R&D Program of Shan Dong Province (No. 2019JZZY020909), the Fundamental Research Funds for the Central Universities (2021-RW350-001), the Chinese Pharmacopoeia Commission Drug Standard Promoting Fund (Grant No. 2022Y14), and CAMS Innovation Fund for Medical Sciences (Grant No. 2022-I2M-JB-011).

Institutional Review Board Statement: Not applicable.

Informed Consent Statement: Not applicable.

Data Availability Statement: CCDC 2174285, 2174286, and 2174287 contain the supplementary crystallographic data for this paper. These data can be obtained free of charge via www.ccdc.cam.ac.uk/data_request/cif (accessed on 1 September 2022) or by emailing data_request@ccdc.cam.ac.uk or by contacting The Cambridge Crystallographic Data Centre, 12 Union Road, Cambridge, CB2 1EZ, UK; Fax: +441223-336033.

Acknowledgments: The authors are thankful to the Key R&D Program of Shan Dong Province, the Fundamental Research Funds for the Central Universities, and the Chinese Pharmacopoeia Commission Drug Standard Promoting Fund for financial support.

Conflicts of Interest: The authors declare no conflict of interest. The company had no role in the design of the study; in the collection, analyses, or interpretation of data; in the writing of the manuscript, and in the decision to publish the results.

References

1. Eren, O.T.; Armağan, R.; Talmaç, M.A. Nonsteroidal Anti-inflammatory Drugs (NSAIDs) and Corticosteroids. In *Musculoskeletal Research and Basic Science*; Korkusuz, F., Ed.; Springer: Cham, Switzerland, 2016; pp. 683–693, ISBN 978-3-319-20777-3.
2. Gonzalez, J.P.; Todd, P.A. Tenoxicam. *Drugs* **1987**, *34*, 289–310. [CrossRef]
3. Chopade, S.S.; Gaikwad, E.; Jadhav, A.; Patil, N.; Payghan, S. Formulation and Evaluation of Fast Disintegrating Tenoxicam Tablets and The Comparison with Marketed Product. *Asian J. Res. Pharm. Sci.* **2020**, *10*, 257–263. [CrossRef]
4. Qiu, L.; Xue, S.; Liu, Z.; Liu, Y. Study on pharmacokinetics and bioavailability of tenoxicam in human. *Her. Med.* **2007**, *26*, 1282–1283. [CrossRef]
5. Ashri, L.Y.; Amal El Sayeh, F.; Ibrahim, M.A.; Alshora, D.H.; Naguib, M.J. Optimization and evaluation of chitosan buccal films containing tenoxicam for treating chronic periodontitis: In vitro and in vivo studies. *J. Drug Deliv. Sci. Technol.* **2020**, *57*, 101720. [CrossRef]
6. Elakkad, Y.E.; Younis, M.K.; Allam, R.M.; Mohsen, A.F.; Khalil, I.A. Tenoxicam loaded hyalcubosomes for osteoarthritis. *Int. J. Pharm.* **2021**, *601*, 120483. [CrossRef] [PubMed]
7. Gaydukova, I.Z.; Aparkina, A.V.; Khondkaryan, E.V.; Rebrov, A.P. Effectiveness of the tenoxicam in patients with ankylosing spondylitis. *Zhurnal Nevrol. I Psikhiatrii Im. SS Korsakova* **2018**, *118*, 35–39. [CrossRef]
8. Lipinski, C. Poor aqueous solubility-an industry wide problem in drug discovery. *Am. Pharm. Rev.* **2002**, *5*, 82–85.
9. Patel, J.R.; Carlton, R.A.; Needham, T.E.; Chichester, C.O.; Vogt, F.G. Preparation, structural analysis, and properties of tenoxicam cocrystals. *Int. J. Pharm.* **2012**, *436*, 685–706. [CrossRef]
10. Patel, J.R.; Carlton, R.A.; Yuniatine, F.; Needham, T.E.; Wu, L.; Vogt, F.G. Preparation and structural characterization of amorphous spray-dried dispersions of tenoxicam with enhanced dissolution. *J. Pharm. Sci.* **2012**, *101*, 641–663. [CrossRef]
11. Albadri, A.A.; Jihad, M.I.; Radhi, Z.A. Preparation, Characterization, and In-Vitro Evaluation of Tenoxicam-Paracetamol Cocrystal. *Int. J. Drug Deliv. Technol.* **2021**, *10*, 542–546. [CrossRef]
12. Salahuddin, N.; Gaber, M.; Elneanaey, S.; Snowdon, M.R.; Abdelwahab, M.A. Co-delivery of norfloxacin and tenoxicam in Ag-TiO2/poly (lactic acid) nanohybrid. *Int. J. Biol. Macromol.* **2021**, *180*, 771–781. [CrossRef] [PubMed]
13. Bawazeer, S.; El-Telbany, D.F.A.; Al-Sawahli, M.M.; Zayed, G.; Keed, A.A.A.; Abdelaziz, A.E.; Abdel-Naby, D.H. Effect of nanostructured lipid carriers on transdermal delivery of tenoxicam in irradiated rats. *Drug Deliv.* **2020**, *27*, 1218–1230. [CrossRef] [PubMed]

14. Khattab, A.; Abouhussein, D.M.N. Development of injectable tenoxicam in situ forming microparticles based on sesame oil and poly-DL-lactide: Characterization, efficacy and acute toxicity. *J. Drug Deliv. Sci. Technol.* **2019**, *51*, 682–694. [CrossRef]
15. Caira, M.R.; Nassimbeni, L.R.; Timme, M. Zwitterionic Nature of Tenoxicam: Crystal Structures and Thermal Analyses of a Polymorph of Tenoxicam and a 1: L Tenoxicam: Acetonitrile Solvate. *J. Pharm. Sci.* **1995**, *84*, 884–888. [CrossRef]
16. Cantera, R.G.; Leza, M.G.; Bachiller, C.M. Solid phases of tenoxicam. *J. Pharm. Sci.* **2002**, *91*, 2240–2251. [CrossRef]
17. Nabulsi, L.; Owais, L.; Arafat, T.A.; AIkaysi, H.; Sheikh Salem, M.; Badwan, A.A. Tenoxicam polymorphic modifications. In Proceedings of the Sixth International Conference on Pharmaceutical Technology, Paris, France, 2–4 June 1992; pp. 203–212.
18. Jiao, L.T.; Yang, D.Z.; Zhang, L.; Yang, S.Y.; Du, G.H.; Lu, Y. Salt solvates of quinolones and oxicams: Theoretical computation, structural characterization and dissolution studies. *J. Mol. Struct.* **2021**, *1223*, 128865. [CrossRef]
19. Bolla, G.; Sanphui, P.; Nangia, A. Solubility Advantage of Tenoxicam Phenolic Cocrystals Compared to Salts. *Cryst. Growth Des.* **2013**, *13*, 1988–2003. [CrossRef]
20. Arkhipov, S.G.; Sherin, P.S.; Kiryutin, A.S.; Lazarenko, V.A.; Tantardini, C. The role of S-bond in tenoxicam keto-enolic tautomerization. *CrystEngComm.* **2019**, *21*, 5392–5401. [CrossRef]
21. Childs, S.L.; Stahly, G.P.; Park, A. The salt-cocrystal continuum: The influence of crystal structure on ionization state. *Mol. Pharm.* **2007**, *4*, 323–338. [CrossRef]
22. Allu, S.; Bolla, G.; Tothadi, S.; Nangia, A.K. Novel pharmaceutical cocrystals and salts of bumetanide. *Cryst. Growth Des.* **2020**, *20*, 793–803. [CrossRef]
23. Wang, W.; Zhang, W.; Jiang, Y.; Wang, X.; Zhang, X.; Liu, H.; Zhang, T. Preparation of ursolic acid-phospholipid complex by solvent-assisted grinding method to improve dissolution and oral bioavailability. *Pharm. Dev. Technol.* **2020**, *25*, 68–75. [CrossRef] [PubMed]
24. Grossjohann, C.; Serrano, D.R.; Paluch, K.J.; O'Connell, P.; Vella-Zarb, L.; Manesiotis, P.; McCabe, T.; Tajber, L.; Corrigan, O.I.; Healy, A.M. Polymorphism in sulfadimidine/4-aminosalicylic acid cocrystals: Solid-state characterization and physicochemical properties. *J. Pharm. Sci.* **2015**, *104*, 1385–1398. [CrossRef] [PubMed]
25. Dhivya, C.; Vandarkuzhali, S.A.A.; Radha, N. Antimicrobial activities of nanostructured polyanilines doped with aromatic nitro compounds. *Arab. J. Chem.* **2019**, *12*, 3785–3798. [CrossRef]
26. Santoso, S.P.; Ismadji, S.; Angkawijaya, A.E.; Soetaredjo, F.E.; Go, A.W.; Ju, Y.H. Complexes of 2, 6-dihydroxybenzoic acid with divalent metal ions: Synthesis, crystal structure, spectral studies, and biological activity enhancement. *J. Mol. Liq.* **2016**, *221*, 617–623. [CrossRef]
27. Friščić, T.; Childs, S.L.; Rizvi, S.A.A.; Jones, W. The role of solvent in mechanochemical and sonochemical cocrystal formation: A solubility-based approach for predicting cocrystallisation outcome. *CrystEngComm.* **2009**, *11*, 418–426. [CrossRef]
28. Friščić, T. New opportunities for materials synthesis using mechanochemistry. *J. Mater. Chem.* **2010**, *20*, 7599–7605. [CrossRef]
29. Solares-Briones, M.; Coyote-Dotor, G.; Páez-Franco, J.C.; Zermeño-Ortega, M.R.; de la O. Contreras, C.M.; Canseco-González, D.; Avila-Sorrosa, A.; Morales-Morales, D.; Germán-Acacio, J.M. Mechanochemistry: A green approach in the preparation of pharmaceutical cocrystals. *Pharmaceutics* **2021**, *13*, 790. [CrossRef]
30. Haskins, M.M.; Zaworotko, M.J. Screening and Preparation of Cocrystals: A Comparative Study of Mechanochemistry vs Slurry Methods. *Cryst. Growth Des.* **2021**, *21*, 4141–4150. [CrossRef]
31. Dolomanov, O.V.; Bourhis, L.J.; Gildea, R.J.; Howard, J.A.; Puschmann, H. OLEX2: A complete structure solution, refinement and analysis program. *J. Appl. Crystallogr.* **2009**, *42*, 339–341. [CrossRef]
32. Sheldrick, G.M. A short history of SHELX. *Acta Crystallogr. A* **2008**, *64*, 112–122. [CrossRef]
33. Sheldrick, G.M. Crystal structure refinement with SHELXL. *Acta Crystallogr. C* **2015**, *71*, 3–8. [CrossRef] [PubMed]
34. Yang, D.; Wang, R.; Jin, G.; Zhang, B.; Zhang, L.; Lu, Y.; Du, G. Structural and computational insights into cocrystal interactions: A case on cocrystals of antipyrine and aminophenazone. *Cryst. Growth Des.* **2019**, *19*, 347–361. [CrossRef]
35. Yuan, Y.; Li, D.; Wang, C.; Chen, S.; Kong, M.; Deng, Z.; Zhang, H. Structural features of sulfamethizole and its cocrystals: Beauty within. *Cryst. Growth Des.* **2019**, *19*, 7185–7192. [CrossRef]
36. Frisch, M.; Trucks, G.; Schlegel, H.; Scuseria, G.; Robb, M.; Cheeseman, J.; Scalmani, G.; Barone, V.; Petersson, G.; Nakatsuji, H. *Gaussian 16, Revision A.03*; Gaussian Inc.: Wallingford, CT, USA, 2016.
37. Palatinus, L.; Brázda, P.; Boullay, P.; Perez, O.; Klementová, M.; Petit, S.; Eignerm, V.; Zaarour, M.; Mintova, S. Hydrogen positions in single nanocrystals revealed by electron diffraction. *Science* **2017**, *355*, 166–169. [CrossRef]
38. Schmidt, M.W.; Baldridge, K.K.; Boatz, J.A.; Elbert, S.T.; Gordon, M.S.; Jensen, J.H.; Koseki, S.; Matsunaga, N.; Nguyen, K.A.; Su, S.J.; et al. General atomic and molecular electronic structure system. *J. Comput. Chem.* **1993**, *14*, 1347–1363. [CrossRef]
39. Su, P.; Jiang, Z.; Chen, Z.; Wu, W. Energy Decomposition Scheme Based on the Generalized Kohn-Sham Scheme. *J. Phys. Chem. A* **2014**, *118*, 2531–2542. [CrossRef]
40. Su, P.; Tang, Z.; Wu, W. Generalized Kohn-Sham energy decomposition analysis and its applications. *Wiley Interdiscip. Rev. Comput. Mol. Sci.* **2020**, *10*, e1460. [CrossRef]
41. Lu, T.; Chen, F. Multiwfn: A multifunctional wavefunction analyzer. *J. Comput. Chem.* **2012**, *33*, 580–592. [CrossRef] [PubMed]
42. Ren, S.; Jiao, L.; Yang, S.; Zhang, L.; Song, J.; Yu, H.; Wang, J.R.; Lv, T.T.; Sun, L.; Lv, Y.; et al. A novel co-crystal of bexarotene and ligustrazine improves pharmacokinetics and tissue distribution of bexarotene in SD rats. *Pharmaceutics* **2020**, *12*, 906. [CrossRef]
43. Yang, D.; Cao, J.; Heng, T.; Xing, C.; Du, G. Theoretical calculation and structural analysis of the cocrystals of three flavonols with praziquantel. *Cryst. Growth Des.* **2021**, *21*, 2292–2300. [CrossRef]

44. Yang, D.; Wang, H.; Liu, Q.; Yuan, P.; Chen, T.; Zhang, L.; Yang, S.; Zhou, Z.; Lu, Y.; Du, G. Structural landscape on a series of rhein: Berberine cocrystal salt solvates: The formation, dissolution elucidation from experimental and theoretical investigations. *Chin. Chem. Lett.* **2022**, *10*, 43. [CrossRef]
45. Wang, H.; Yang, D.; Zhang, W.; Song, J.; Gong, N.; Yu, M.; Yang, S.; Zhang, B.; Liu, Q.; Du, G. An innovative rhein-matrine cocrystal: Synthesis, characterization, formation mechanism and pharmacokinetic study. *Chin. Chem. Lett.* **2022**. [CrossRef]
46. Silverstein, R.M. *Spectrometric Identification of Organic Compounds*, 6th ed.; Webster, F.X., Ed.; John-Wiley: New York, NY, USA, 2002; pp. 71–143.
47. Romero, S.; Escalera, B.; Bustamante, P. Solubility behavior of polymorphs I and II of mefenamic acid in solvent mixtures. *Int. J. Pharm.* **1999**, *178*, 193–202. [CrossRef]
48. Babu, N.J.; Reddy, L.S.; Nangia, A. Amide−n-oxide heterosynthon and amide dimer homosynthon in cocrystals of carboxamide drugs and pyridine n-oxides. *Mol. Pharm.* **2007**, *4*, 417–434. [CrossRef] [PubMed]
49. Hopffgarten, M.V.; Frenking, G. Energy decomposition analysis. *Wiley Interdiscip. Rev. Comput. Mol. Sci.* **2012**, *2*, 43–62. [CrossRef]
50. Gao, W.; Feng, H.; Xuan, X.; Chen, L. The assessment and application of an approach to noncovalent interactions: The energy decomposition analysis (EDA) in combination with DFT of revised dispersion correction (DFT-D3) with Slater-type orbital (STO) basis set. *J. Mol. Model.* **2012**, *18*, 4577–4589. [CrossRef] [PubMed]
51. Zhao, L.; von Hopffgarten, M.; Andrada, D.M.; Frenking, G. Energy decomposition analysis. *Wiley Interdiscip. Rev. Comput. Mol. Sci.* **2018**, *8*, e1345. [CrossRef]

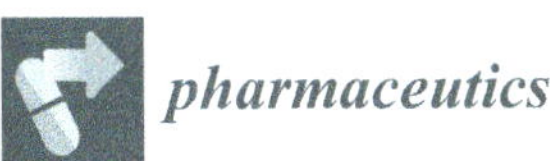

pharmaceutics

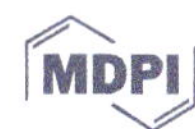

Article

Varied Bulk Powder Properties of Micro-Sized API within Size Specifications as a Result of Particle Engineering Methods

Zijian Wang [1], Marina Solomos [2], Stephanus Axnanda [3], Chienhung Chen [3], Margaret Figus [3], Luke Schenck [2,*] and Changquan Calvin Sun [1,*]

[1] Pharmaceutical Materials Science and Engineering Laboratory, Department of Pharmaceutics, College of Pharmacy, University of Minnesota, Minneapolis, MN 55455, USA
[2] Process Research & Development Merck & Co., Inc., Rahway, NJ 07065, USA
[3] Analytical Research & Development Merck & Co., Inc., Rahway, NJ 07065, USA
* Correspondence: luke.schenck@merck.com (L.S.); sunx0053@umn.edu (C.C.S.)

Abstract: Micronized particles are commonly used to improve the content uniformity (CU), dissolution performance, and bioavailability of active pharmaceutical ingredients (API). Different particle engineering routes have been developed to prepare micron-sized API in a specific size range to deliver desirable biopharmaceutical performance. However, such API particles still risk varying bulk powder properties critical to successful manufacturing of quality drug products due to different particle shapes, size distribution, and surface energetics, arising from the anisotropy of API crystals. In this work, we systematically investigated key bulk properties of 10 different batches of Odanacatib prepared through either jet milling or fast precipitation, all of which meet the particle size specification established to ensure equivalent biopharmaceutical performance. However, they exhibited significantly different powder properties, solid-state properties, dissolution, and tablet CU. Among the 10 batches, a directly precipitated sample exhibited overall best performance, considering tabletability, dissolution, and CU. This work highlights the measurable impact of processing route on API properties and the importance of selecting a suitable processing route for preparing fine particles with optimal properties and performance.

Keywords: particle size; particle engineering; bulk properties; surface anisotropy; contact angle

Citation: Wang, Z.; Solomos, M.; Axnanda, S.; Chen, C.; Figus, M.; Schenck, L.; Sun, C.C. Varied Bulk Powder Properties of Micro-Sized API within Size Specifications as a Result of Particle Engineering Methods. *Pharmaceutics* **2022**, *14*, 1901. https://doi.org/10.3390/pharmaceutics14091901

Academic Editor: Hisham Al-Obaidi

Received: 27 July 2022
Accepted: 1 September 2022
Published: 8 September 2022

Publisher's Note: MDPI stays neutral with regard to jurisdictional claims in published maps and institutional affiliations.

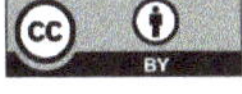

1. Introduction

Particle size plays a crucial role in the performance of pharmaceutical products. For example, the dissolution behavior of an active pharmaceutical ingredient (API) depends on particle size, where larger specific surface area of smaller API particles yields faster dissolution according to the theory of the Noyes-Whitney equation [1]. Smaller API particles in the sub-micron range may also exhibit higher solubility [2]. Therefore, micron-sized or nano-sized API particles have been commonly employed to improve bioavailability of poorly soluble APIs [3]. Tabletability is also affected by particle size, where a larger surface area available for bonding between particles in a tablet contributes to higher tabletability [4]. Conversely, larger particle size favors flowability [5]. Blend and tablet content uniformity (CU) may be improved from a purely statistical standpoint by micronizing API [6,7], but CU is also affected by segregation or agglomeration of API particles during manufacturing [8]. For poorly soluble APIs, e.g., biopharmaceutical classification system (BCS) class II and IV APIs, it is imperative to enhance their dissolution and bioavailability [9]. To this end, several particle engineering techniques have been used to prepare micron-sized APIs in the pharmaceutical industry [10]. Among them, milling is representative of the "top-down" methods, where large particles are reduced into micron-sized particles through breakage by mechanical impact, and precipitation is representative of the "bottom-up" methods, where API molecules in solution assemble into micron-sized particles.

Milling can be performed either dry or in a liquid medium. Compared to dry milling, wet milling (e.g., media milling or high pressure homogenization) usually produces smaller and smoother particles with a lower tendency to agglomerate, though filtering and isolating wet-milled particles can be difficult [10,11]. Among available dry milling processes, air-jet milling is preferred in pharmaceutical industry over ball milling [12], pin milling [13], and hammer milling [14], due to its high efficiency and the absence of moving parts. During jet milling, fast air flow moves particles and causes collision, attrition, shear, and compression to reduce particle size [15]. The high energy input of this method may result in a disordered crystal lattice, potentially leading to the formation of amorphous content, or polymorphic transition [10,16–18]. There is also the risk of product contamination by fine metal particles shed during milling.

In the classic "bottom-up" precipitation method, a high concentration API solution in a solvent is mixed with a miscible anti-solvent, resulting in high supersaturation and fast precipitation of fine particles. Particle size of precipitated API can be controlled by changing crystallization parameters and solvent systems [19]. However, rapidly formed small crystals also tend to aggregate, resulting in a broad particle size distribution (PSD). In addition to size, crystal morphology may be affected by experimental conditions and solvent system, resulting in different surface area, dissolution, flowability, and tabletability of an API even when a similar PSD is maintained [20–23]. Moreover, different faces of molecular crystals may have different surface properties due to the presence of different functional groups. Such surface anisotropy may lead to different wettability and dissolution behavior of the same API solid form prepared through different routes [18,20,24–26].

This work sought to systematically investigate how different particle engineering routes, while reaching equivalent biopharmaceutical performance of an API, may impact key bulk powder properties. Such knowledge informs the selection of a route to meet the target particle size specifications while optimizing powder properties. Odanacatib, an inhibitor of cathepsin K [27], was selected as a model API. The particle size specifications <6 μm (M_v) was established through semi-mechanistic pharmacokinetic/pharmacodynamic (PK/PD) models and *in vivo* data to demonstrate bioequivalence criteria based on AUC and C_{max}. Jet milling and liquid anti-solvent precipitation approaches were selected to prepare 10 batches of fine API with particle size in the target range. In addition, jet milling with processing aids to reduce milling induced disorder was assessed for possible impact on dissolution.

2. Materials and Methods

2.1. Materials

Various lots of Odanacatib were obtained from Merck & Co., Inc. (Rahway, NJ, USA). Ethanol (200 proof) was purchased from Decon Labs, Inc. (King of Prussia, PA, USA). DMF and acetone were used to prepare precipitated samples and were purchased from Fisher Scientific (Fair Lawn, NJ, USA). Pharmaceutical excipients used in this work, i.e., Avicel PH102 (MCC; FMC Biopolymers; Newark, DE, USA), spray-dried lactose monohydrate (LM; Foremost; Baraboo, WI, USA), Kollidon VA64 (Crospovidone; BASF; Ludwigshafen, Germany), sodium stearyl fumarate (SSF; JRS Pharma; Patterson, NY, USA) magnesium stearate (MgSt; Covidien, Dublin, Ireland) were used as received.

2.2. Methods

2.2.1. Preparation of Samples

A bulk sample of Odanacatib, referred to as Sample A, was re-crystallized from an acetone and water mixed solvent system. Odanacatib was suspended in 8 volumes of a 1:2 acetone–water mixed solvent. The slurry was agitated with mixing to just suspend solids and heated to 45 °C over 60 min to partially dissolve it and held at 45 °C for 15 min before cooling to 20 °C over 10 h. This heating–cooling cycle was repeated a second time. Solids were filtered, washed with water, and dried.

Sample A was separately jet milled at 300 kg scale to create Samples A1 and A2. Samples A3, A(S) and A(M) were all milled starting from Sample A using a spiral mill (Jet

Pulverizer 2″ Micron Master). Sample A3 was generated by milling 100 g of Sample A with an injection pressure of 100–120 psi, and a grinding pressure of 50 psi. Sample A(S) was first prepared by blending 99 g of Sample A with 1 g of sodium stearyl fumarate (SSF) on a LabRam acoustic mixer at 60 Hz for 10 min, generating a 1 wt% coated SSF sample. The blend was then milled using conditions scaled down from milling Samples A1 and A2, with an injection pressure of 100–120 psi, and a grinding pressure of 50 psi. Similarly, Sample A(M) was prepared by first blending 99 g of Sample A with 1 g of magnesium stearate (MgSt) on a LabRam acoustic mixer at 60 Hz for 10 min, generating a 1 wt% coated MgSt sample. The blend was then milled with an injection pressure of 100–120 psi, and a grinding pressure of 50 psi. Processing aids, MgSt (hydrophobic) and SSF (hydrophilic), were used to alleviate possible disorders introduced by milling. To remove amorphous content, A2 was annealed at 40 °C and 75% relative humidity for 3 weeks (Sample A2 (3 wks)) and 5 weeks (Sample A2 (5 wks)).

Sample P1 and Sample P2 were prepared from high shear direct precipitation. A rotor/stator wet mill was used to achieve a high shear environment for precipitation. The following parameters were used: (1) Quadro HV0 with 6 mm/3 mm emulsion tooling operating at 70 m/s; (2) Solvent to antisolvent volume ratios for precipitation were consistently 1:10, with addition of solvent to the mill head at an approximate flow rate 10% of the flow rate of the antisolvent. Sample P1 was prepared by dissolving Sample A in 2.5 volumes of DMF and precipitating in 25 volumes deionized (DI) water pre-cooled to 0.2 °C and seeded with 1 wt% of A1. Precipitation was completed over 90 s using a tip speed of 70 m/s. The slurry was aged for 72 h at room temperature before filtration, followed by washing with antisolvent, and drying using a nitrogen sweep applied across a filter funnel until ICH residual solvent specifications were met. Sample P2 was prepared by dissolving Sample A in 3.85 volumes of a 9:1 acetone-water mixed solvent system and precipitating in 38.5 volumes of DI water pre-cooled to 0.2 °C and seeded with 1 wt% of A1. Precipitation was completed over 90 s using a tip speed of 70 m/s. The slurry was aged for 4 h at 50 °C before being filtered, washed with antisolvent, and dried.

To investigate effects of starting API morphology on properties of milled Odanacatib, Sample B was obtained from recrystallization in acetone and methyl tert-butyl ether (MTBE). Odanacatib was suspended in 20 volumes of 3:2 acetone–MTBE mixed solvent system and heated to 50 °C to dissolve all solids. The batch was held at 50 °C for 10 min, then cooled to 37 °C over 15 min, and 2 wt% Sample A1 was added as seeds. The seeded batch was aged for 60 min at 37 °C, then 16 volumes of MTBE was dosed over 5 h. The batch was cooled to 20 °C over 10 h and subsequently filtered and dried to generate Sample B. Sample B1 was generated by milling 100 g of Sample B with an injection pressure of 100–120 psi, and a grinding pressure of 50 psi. These samples are summarized in Scheme 1 for easy comparison.

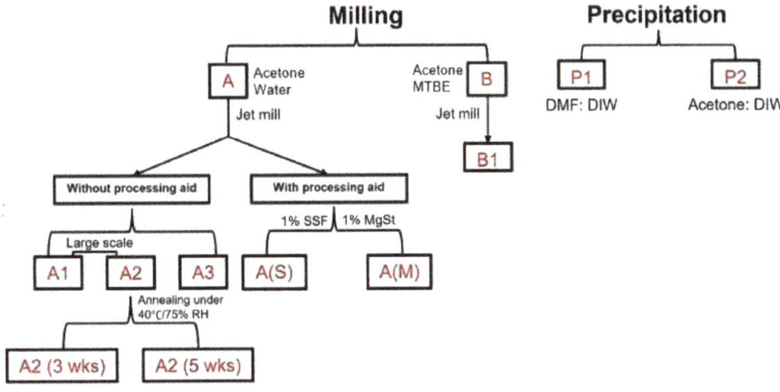

Scheme 1. Genealogy of different lots of API in this work.

2.2.2. Particle Size Distribution

Particle size distribution (PSD) measurements were made using a laser diffraction particle size analyzer (Microtrac S3500, York, PA, USA) having a detector system located at a distance from the point where the particles interact with the light. The laser light (λ = 780 nm) allows for measurement of particles by detecting the light scattered over an angular range of 0.02° to approximately 45° angle. The instrument was set for measuring irregular solid API particles, using a refractive index of 1.51. The circulating media was Isopar-G with refractive index of 1.42. Volume distribution of particles was used in reported particle size data. For each measurement, the sample was sonicated at 30 W for 120 s to disperse particle aggregates.

2.2.3. X-ray Diffractometry

Powder X-ray diffractometry (XRD) and tablet XRD were collected on a powder X-ray diffractometer (PANalytical X'pert pro, Westborough, MA, USA), using Cu Kα radiation (1.54056 Å). Samples were scanned with a step size of 0.02° and 1 s/step dwell time from 5° to 35° 2θ. The tube voltage and amperage were 45 kV and 40 mA, respectively. Tablets for XRD were prepared at a compaction pressure of 400 MPa for 1 min on a material testing machine (model 1485; Zwick/Roell, Ulm, Germany).

2.2.4. Scanning Electron Microscopy (SEM)

Samples were sputter-coated with gold using a sputter coater (Electron Microscopy Service Q150R, Hatfield, PA, USA) and images were taken using a scanning electron microscope (Hitachi SU-3400, Dallas, TX, USA). Each image was obtained using the secondary electron detector with 2 keV accelerating voltage under high vacuum.

2.2.5. Surface Area Analysis

Specific surface area of each API lot was obtained from analyzing low-temperature nitrogen adsorption-desorption isotherms (at 77 K) collected using a TriStar II analyzer (Micromeritics Instrument Corp., Norcross, GA, USA). Each material was loaded into a sample tube and degassed under nitrogen at 35 °C for 1 h before analysis. After cooling to room temperature, the tube was weighed and placed into the adsorption port of the instrument. A static adsorption mode was used including full equilibration after each adsorbate load. The adsorption isotherms were measured over a relative pressure, p/p_o, range of 0.001–0.995. Desorption isotherms were measured over a relative pressure range of 0.995–0.015. Surface area was calculated via the Brunauer–Emmett–Teller (BET) method using the relative pressure range from 0.1 to 0.30 [28].

2.2.6. Tabletability

Tabletability is the capacity of a powder to be transformed into a tablet of specified strength under the effect of compaction pressure [29]. An API powder with poor tabletability cannot be made into sufficiently strong tablets by compaction. Thus, an appropriate formulation must be developed to enable successful manufacturing of tablets. A compaction simulator (Styl'One, Medelpharm, Beynost, France) was used to prepare tablets for the powder tabletability study. Forces on the upper and lower punches were captured with force sensors (strain gauges), while punch displacements were monitored using incremental sensors. Round (8 mm diameter) flat-faced punches were used for all compaction experiments. For each powder, a series of compacts were obtained in the compaction pressure range of 20 to 350 MPa. All compaction experiments were performed at a speed corresponding to a 103 ms dwell time. MgSt spray (Styl'One Mist) was used to lubricate the die wall and punch tips.

All tablets were relaxed for at least 24 h before measuring their diameters and thicknesses using a digital caliper. Diametrical breaking force was determined using a texture analyzer (TA-XT2i, Texture Technologies Corp., Scarsdale, NY, USA) at a speed of 0.001 mm/s with a 5 g trigger force. Tablet tensile strength was calculated from the maximum breaking force and tablet dimensions using Equation (1).

$$\sigma = \frac{2F}{\pi DT} \tag{1}$$

where F is breaking force, D is diameter, and T is thickness.

2.2.7. Shear Cell Testing

A ring shear cell tester (RST-XS, Dietmar Schulze, Wolfenbüttel, Germany), with a 10 mL cell, was used to perform powder flow testing ($n = 3$) at pre-shear normal stress of 3 kPa by following a standard 230 method [30,31]. To perform a shear test, a shear cell was overfilled with a powder of interest and excess powder was gently scraped off using a spatula to obtain a surface flush with the upper edge of the shear cell. Care was taken to avoid compression or shaking of the powder bed.

2.2.8. Intrinsic Dissolution Rate

Intrinsic dissolution rate (IDR) was measured using a rotating disc method [32]. Each powder was compressed at a pressure of 400 MPa for 1 min by a material testing machine (model 1485; Zwick/Roell, Ulm, Germany) with a custom-made stainless-steel die, against a flat stainless steel disc for 2 min to prepare a pellet (6.39 mm in diameter). A range of compaction pressures were assessed, but this pressure was necessary to avoid shedding of micronized particles from the faces of the compacts, which would convolute the dissolution performance. The obtained pellet had a visually smooth surface that was coplanar with the surface of the die. While rotating at 300 rpm, the die was immersed in 300 mL of pure ethanol in a water-jacketed beaker. An UV-vis fiber optic probe (Ocean Optics, Dunedin, FL, USA) was used to continuously monitor the UV absorbance of the solution at 267 nm, which was converted to a concentration–time profile based on a previously constructed concentration–absorbance standard curve. The initial linear part of the dissolution curve was used for calculating the dissolution rate.

2.2.9. Contact Angle

Compacts of each sample were prepared by a Styl'One compaction simulator at 300 MPa to attain an essentially pore-free surface for measuring contact angle by the sessile drop method using a goniometer (DM-CE1; Kyowa Interface Science Co. Ltd., Niiza, Japan). A drop of 2 μL of DI water was placed on the surface using a syringe dispenser. The equilibrium contact angle, θ, between the sample surface and the tangent line at the edge of the drop was determined from the captured images using the software (FAMAS, Kyowa Interface Science, Niiza, Japan). Three measurements made on different tablets of each API sample were used to calculate the mean and standard deviation.

2.2.10. Content Uniformity (CU)

Samples A, A1, B1, P1 and P2 were selected to study the CU of a generic formulation consisting of 1% API, 27% MCC, 66% lactose monohydrate, 5% crospovidon, and 1% MgSt. To maximize uniformity, blends (50 g batch size) were prepared by layering ingredients in a bottle in the following order: LM, API, crospovidon, MCC. The powder was then mixed on a shaker mixer (Turbula T2F, Glen Mills Inc., Clifton, NJ, USA) for 10 min at 49 rpm. Then, MgSt was added to the blend and further mixed for 2 min. A total of 100 tablets (300 mg tablet weight) of each formulation were prepared at a compaction pressure of 200 MPa on Styl'One, and 10 out of the 100 tablets were randomly selected to determine API amount for assessing CU measurement by following USP <905> [33].

Each tablet was weighed and ground into a powder. Subsequently, the powder was transferred into 100 mL of pure ethanol to dissolve API and passed through a syringe filter with a 0.45 μm membrane. Then, 2 mL of the filtered solution was diluted to 10 mL with ethanol. The concentration of the resulting solution was determined from absorbance at 267 nm (UV-vis fiber optic probe) using a previously constructed calibration curve.

2.2.11. Statistical Analysis

To assess statistical significance of difference, the one-way analysis of variance (ANOVA) and Tukey's multiple comparisons test were performed for all API samples, at a $p < 0.05$ level [34].

3. Results and Discussion

3.1. Solid-State Characterization

3.1.1. Particle Size Distribution and Specific Surface Area

The two starting API lots for jet milling, Samples A and B, were much larger in particle size than all milled samples (Table 1), suggesting the effectiveness of particle size reduction by jet milling. The PSDs of the three milled API lots from A are similar (Table 1). Crystals in Sample B1 are clearly smaller than those of A1, A2, and A3 lots. The use of processing aids led to smaller particles in both A(S) and A(M) than those processed without using a processing aid. It is possible that lubricated API particles agglomerated to a lesser extent and could travel with the nitrogen jet at a higher speed, leading to a more effective size reduction due to a higher energy of impact. The Sample P2 contained particles larger than those in Sample P1, indicating a clear impact of desaturation kinetics on the precipitation process. Importantly, the particle sizes of all engineered API samples (Table 1) meet the size specifications, i.e., $M_v < 6$ μm, which was deemed sufficient for equivalent clinical biopharmaceutical performance of Odanacatib. Thus, despite their different mechanisms, both jet milling and fast precipitation could generate fine particles meeting the size specifications. This opens an opportunity for investigating potentially different powder properties of such biopharmaceutically equivalent API lots, and their impact on tablet CU.

Table 1. Particle size distributions, specific surface area (SSA), and descriptions of Odanacatib samples.

Sample	Particle Size Distribution (μm)				Span	SSA (m^2/g)
	d_{10}	d_{50}	d_{90}	M_v		
A	**10.2**	**21.8**	**49.2**	**26.6**	**2.4**	**0.9 ± 0.03**
A1	1.4	3.4	6.8	3.9	1.6	4.3 ± 0.06
A2	1.0	3.2	8.6	4.6	2.4	6.8 ± 0.02
A2 (t = 3 wks)	1.2	3.5	8.5	4.5	2.1	N/R
A2 (t = 5 wks)	1.2	3.4	8.0	4.2	2.0	N/R
A3	2.2	4.9	7.8	5.0	1.1	7.5 ± 0.02
A(S)	0.8	1.9	3.9	2.2	1.6	7.9 ± 0.02
A(M)	1.1	2.6	4.8	2.8	1.4	6.6 ± 0.02
B	**4.1**	**15.8**	**102.5**	**40.9**	**10.7**	**2.8 ± 0.11**
B1	0.7	1.6	2.9	1.7	1.4	8.1 ± 0.03
P1	0.8	2.7	8.2	3.9	2.7	6.3 ± 0.03
P2	2.6	4.9	9.9	5.7	1.5	2.6 ± 0.03

As expected, all milled API samples had larger specific surface area (SSA) than their respective parent API (Table 1). Sample A1 had smaller SSA than A2 and A3, which is consistent with the overall smaller M_v of A1 (Table 1). Sample A(S) had significantly larger SSA than A(M). This was attributed to the overall smaller particles in A(S). The precipitated Sample P2 had SSA about 50% of that of P1, which is consistent with the overall larger particles in Sample P2 (Table 1). Among the milled samples, A1 had a broader PSD as suggested by its larger span. Similarly, among the two precipitated samples, P1 exhibited a broader PSD than P2 (Table 1).

3.1.2. Crystal Morphology

SEM images of all samples were obtained to compare their crystal morphologies. Crystals in the unmilled Sample A were rod-like while crystals in Sample B were needle-like, with a much higher aspect ratio than Sample A (Figure 1). All engineered samples, however, had a comparable crystal morphology.

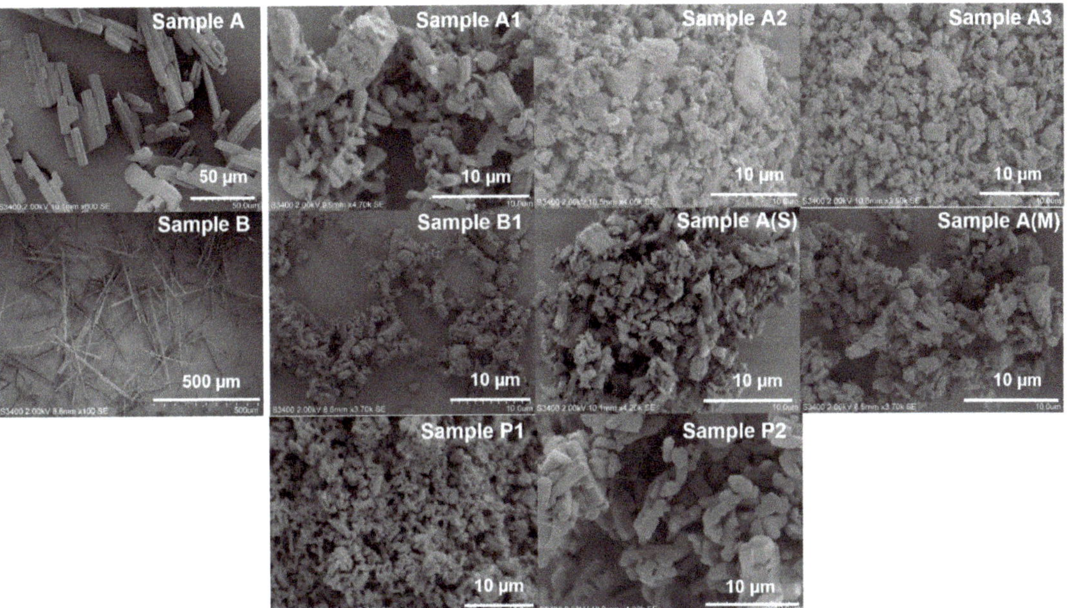

Figure 1. SEM images of crystal morphologies of all Odanacatib samples.

3.2. Crystallinity and Bulk Powder Properties

The PXRD patterns of all engineered samples were consistent with the calculated pattern from single crystal data. However, the parent API lots, A and B, exhibited visible differences in the range of 17 to 21 degrees (Figure 2a), which may be attributed to the preferred orientation effect due to their elongated crystal morphologies. This hypothesis gained support from the observation that milled lots of both materials exhibited similar XRD patterns that conform to the calculated XRD pattern (Figure 2a), suggesting that all milled and precipitated samples were the same solid form.

As all the XRD data were normalized to minimize the possible impact of different sample size and variations in X-ray experimental parameters, the degree of crystallinity of samples is better assessed by peak width than peak intensity [35,36]. The tablet XRD of all samples showed clearly broader peaks than corresponding powder XRD patterns (Figure 2b), suggesting inherent sensitivity of Odanacatib crystals to mechanical stresses. This is consistent with the observation that peaks are sharper in the two unmilled API lots, A and B, than peaks in milled samples (Figure 2a). Among milled samples, A2 exhibited broadest peaks with the poorest resolution of neighboring peaks (Figure 2a). All these observations establish the sensitivity of Odanacatib crystals to external mechanical stresses, which are encountered during both milling and compaction.

The tabletability plots of all samples are markedly different (Figure 2c). Sample A, with larger crystals, exhibited better tabletability than all of its corresponding milled samples, which could not form intact tablets due to severe lamination. We speculate that air entrapment could have caused the different tableting behaviors, since milled API materials are more cohesive and it is more difficult for air to escape the die during the course of compression. Consequently, the expansion of entrapped air during decompression led to lamination of tablets [37,38]. This hypothesis is supported by the observation that intact tablets of all samples could be obtained using a slow tableting speed when preparing specimens for IDR and contact angle measurements. The air entrapment mechanism is also consistent with the fact that it is more difficult for air to escape from the cotton-ball-like Sample B, which consisted of long entangled needles and laminated upon tablet ejection. The better tabletability of P2 powder compared to Sample A can be explained by the fact that, in the absence of lamination by entrapped air, the smaller size of P2 led to stronger tablets than A due to a larger bonding surface area of P2.

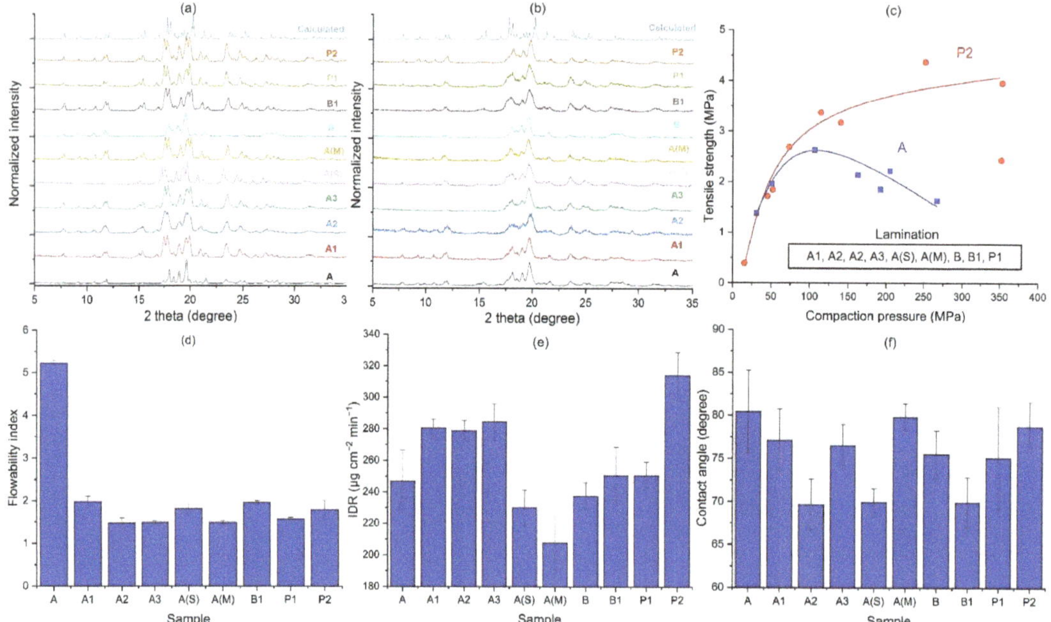

Figure 2. Solid-state properties and bulk powder properties of all Odanacatib samples. (**a**) Powder XRD; (**b**) tablet XRD; (**c**) tabletability; (**d**) flowability; (**e**) intrinsic dissolution rate; (**f**) contact angle.

All micro-sized API samples were very cohesive based on their flowability index (FFC) values (Figure 2d) [39], which is characteristic of fine particles. With a larger particle size, unmilled Sample A exhibited a better flowability than all corresponding milled samples (Figure 2d), which is expected [40]. The flowability of Sample B could not be measured by shear cell, because it consisted of large cotton-ball like agglomerates of crystals, and a flat sample surface could not be prepared.

The significantly different tabletability and flowability ($p < 0.0001$) of the investigated API powders could be attributed, in part, to the slightly different particle sizes (Table 1). However, the different surface energies arising from surface anisotropy is also expected to play an important role. To confirm the possible differences in surface energy, we studied their IDR as this property is independent of the particle size of the API. We also directly assessed differences in surface energy by contact angle measurement.

Because of the low aqueous solubility of Odanacatib, our attempts to measure IDR in aqueous media was unsuccessful due to poor precision. Hence, pure ethanol was used as a dissolution medium for IDR testing. However, ethanol could not be used for contact angle measurement due to difficulty with delivering a drop onto the sample surface. As a result, we used DI water to probe wettability. Significant differences among the IDR (Figure 2e, $p < 0.0001$) and the contact angle (Figure 2f, $p = 0.0009$) data of all engineered samples were observed, suggesting their different surface energetics. Thus, differential surface energy is a factor when explaining the different bulk properties of these API samples. To gain a better understanding of how the preparation routes affected the bulk properties of API powders, we have systematically examined effects of various process variables in a pair-wise fashion in the following section.

3.3. Comparison of Various Process Variables

3.3.1. Inherent Process Variability of Jet Milling (A1 vs. A2)

A1 and A2 were different batches prepared by jet milling Sample A at a commercial manufacturing scale under the same set of processing conditions. However, A2 has significantly lower crystallinity than A1, as suggested by broader peaks in the powder XRD pattern of A2 (Figure 3a). For example, adjacent peaks at ~15, 17.5 and 20 degrees could barely be distinguished in the PXRD pattern of A2 due to peak broadening, but these peaks were clearly resolved in the PXRD pattern of A1. The different crystallinities could have been caused by (1) a higher amorphous content generated in Sample A2 during jet milling, and (2) more of the amorphous content in Sample A1 crystallized during the storage. Since both samples had been stored at ambient conditions for several years, it is more likely that the first factor was responsible for the different crystallinity, i.e., external stresses applied onto crystals were somehow lower when preparing A1 by milling. This is supported by the observation that differences in crystallinity between A1 and A2 were diminished after compression at 400 MPa (Figure 3a), i.e., A2 tablet only showed a slightly lower crystallinity than that of A1. This can be explained by the compaction pressure being higher than the stresses during milling. Hence, the crystallinity of the tablets was more affected by compaction, which was the same for the two samples, rather than milling. This is consistent with the observation that their IDRs are not significantly different (Figure 3c), despite the higher amorphous content in A2 powder. The water contact angle of A1 tablet is also not significantly different from A2 (Figure 3d). A1 exhibited significantly better flowability than A2 (Figure 3b, $p = 0.0003$). However, differences in the tabletability of A1 and A2 could not be demonstrated, because neither powder could form intact tablets under high-speed compression. The differences in amorphous content between A1 and A2 highlight inherent variability in a full-scale jet milling process.

Thus, the seemingly same set of jet milling parameters did not guarantee the same properties of milled API, suggesting potential milling parameters not robustly controlled, or perhaps storage conditions of the two samples in time following milling were different.

3.3.2. Effects of Starting Material on Jet-Milled API (A3 vs. B1)

To assess the impact of starting materials on the milled API, two batches of morphologically different Odanacatib (A and B) were jet milled at laboratory scale under identical milling conditions to obtain A3 and B1. The control of milling parameters at the laboratory scale was expected to be robust. Hence, we assumed that the differences between A3 and B1 were mostly due to the differences in the starting materials. However, contributions from process variations cannot be excluded. Under given milling conditions, the fracture of crystals depends on the presence of energetically weak cleavage planes, size, and aspect ratio. Fracture along cleavage planes is energetically favored for crystals in A because of the relatively lower aspect ratio. However, breaking crystals along the long dimension for B crystals is statistically preferred. If such fracture surfaces are not the same as the cleavage plane, the distributions of exposed crystal surfaces in the two milled samples could be different even if their milled crystals have closely similar size and shape (Figure 1 and Table 1).

Although powder XRD patterns of A3 and B1 are comparable, the XRD peaks of the B1 tablet in the 17–20 degrees region were broader than those of A3 tablet (Figure 4a and Figure S1, Table S1), suggesting that the crystals in Sample B1 were more prone to stress-induced disorders during compaction. The flowability of A3 was significantly worse than B1 (Figure 4b, $p = 0.0002$). Since crystals in A3 were larger than those in B1 (Table 1), difference in flowability cannot be explained by differences in size. Hence, we attribute it to different surface energies of these milled samples. Compared to B1, A3 showed a higher IDR (Figure 4c) and a larger contact angle by water (Figure 4d), but the differences were not statistically significant. This suggests that differences in surface energies, which led to different flow properties between the two API lots, were largely reduced by compaction.

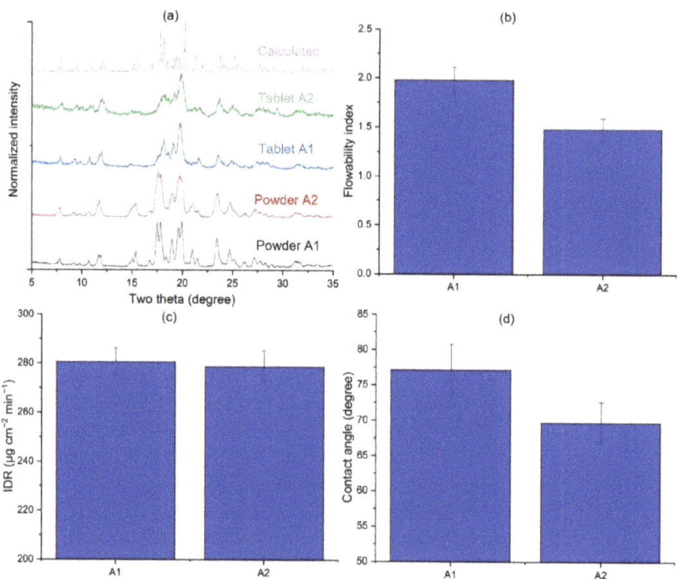

Figure 3. Solid-state characterization, bulk properties of Samples A1 and A2. (**a**) X-ray diffraction; (**b**) flowability (**c**) intrinsic dissolution rate; (**d**) contact angle.

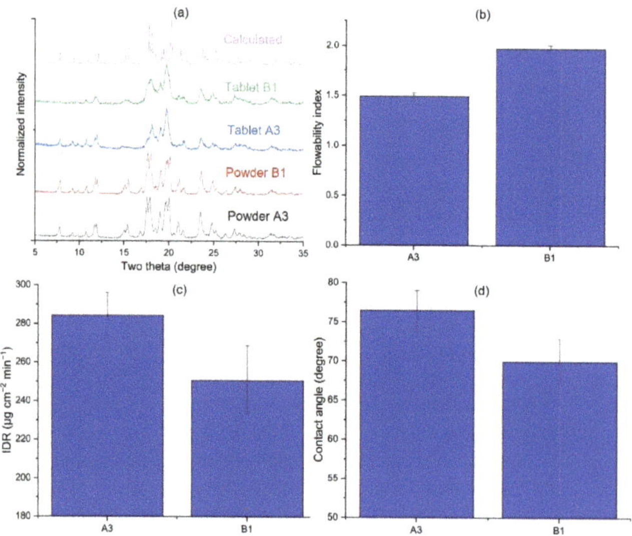

Figure 4. Solid-state characterization, bulk properties of Samples A3 and B1. (**a**) X-ray diffraction; (**b**) flowability; (**c**) intrinsic dissolution rate; (**d**) contact angle.

3.3.3. Effects of the Milling Scale (A1 vs. A3)

Successful scale-up is a challenge in the development of drug products [41,42]. Potential effects of the scale of jet milling were assessed in this study by comparing A1 to A3, which were generated from the same starting material at an industrial scale and a laboratory scale, respectively.

The crystallinity, IDR, and contact angle of A1 and A3 did not significantly differ (Figure 5a,c,d). However, A1 exhibited a statistically better flowability than A3 (Figure 5b, $p = 0.0002$), despite the smaller sizes of crystals in A1 (Table 1). This observation suggests that materials generated by jet milling at different scale can exhibit different powder properties, likely due to different external stresses during milling, leading to differences in exposed surfaces in the milled materials. Overall, the impact of scale effects are less than the effects caused by different starting materials discussed in the preceding section.

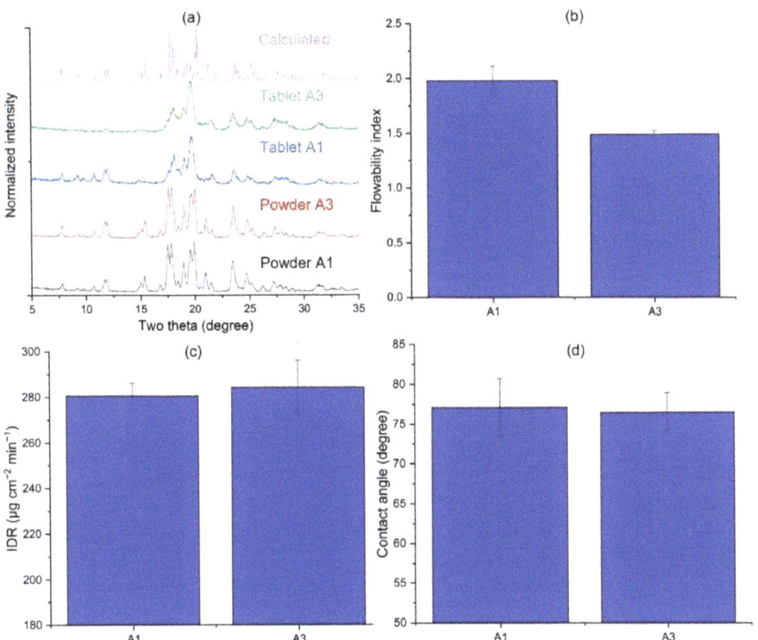

Figure 5. Solid-state characterization, bulk properties of Samples A1 and A3. (**a**) X-ray diffraction; (**b**) flowability (**c**) intrinsic dissolution rate; (**d**) contact angle.

3.3.4. Jet-Milled vs. Precipitated Samples (A3 vs. P2)

To assess the extent of the impact of particle engineering techniques on bulk properties of micro-sized particles, we compared jet-milled Sample A3 to precipitated P2. Jet milling produces fine particles from large ones by mechanical stresses (top-down). Fast precipitation produces fine particles from the solution through fast nucleation and growth (bottom-up). Given the significantly different preparation mechanisms, different crystal surfaces are generated, exhibiting different surface energetics and powder properties. We chose P2, instead of P1, for the pair-wise comparison, because its PSD is closer to that of A3 (identical d_{50} and overlapping PSD, Table 1).

Both powder and tablet XRD patterns of the two samples revealed no detectable differences (Figure 6a). However, P2 could form intact and strong tablets in the entire pressure range investigated but no intact tablet of A3 could be obtained (Figure 6b). The difference in tabletability was attributed to their different surface properties, since they exhibit comparable crystallinity and PSD (Table 1). In fact, crystals in P2 appear to have smoother surfaces than those in A3. Rougher particle surfaces generally lead to more difficult air escape from a powder bed during compaction. This explains why intact tablets could not be prepared from A3 under fast compression but could be prepared under a slower compression speed when preparing pellets for contact angle measurements. The rougher crystal surfaces in A3 also explain its significantly worse flowability than P2 (Figure 6c, $p = 0.0216$). The IDRs and contact angles of the two samples differed but the differences are not statistically significant (Figure 6d,e). Again, any differences in surface properties would have been minimized by the process of compaction, which amorphized both powders to about the same extent (Figure 6a).

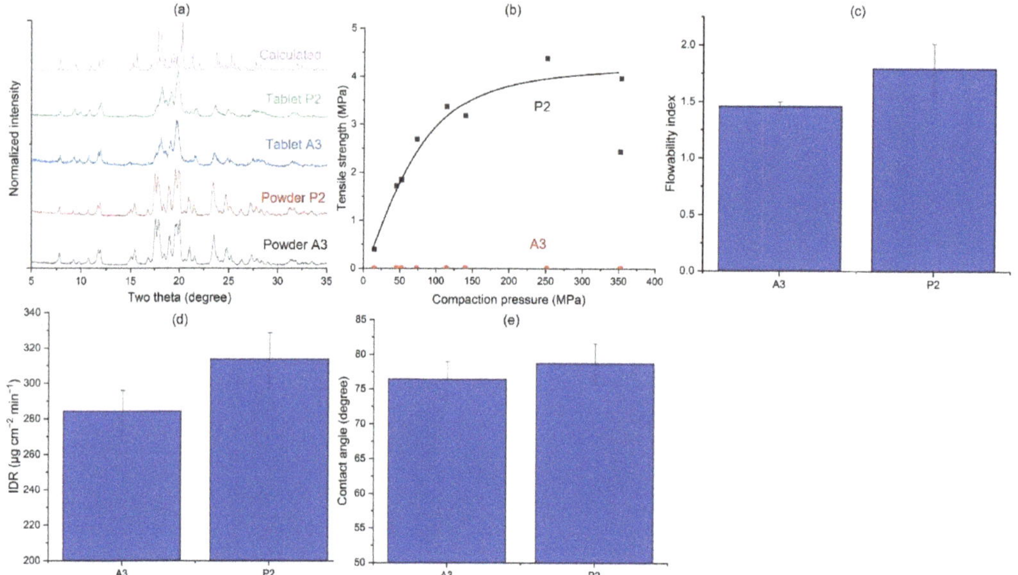

Figure 6. Solid-state characterization, bulk properties of Samples A3 and P2. (**a**) X-ray diffraction; (**b**) tabletability; (**c**) flowability; (**d**) intrinsic dissolution rate; (**e**) contact angle.

3.3.5. Effects of Solvent Systems in the Precipitation Route (P1 vs. P2)

The properties of an API powder from a fast precipitation process, such as crystallinity, particle size and particle morphologies, are known to be affected by process factors such as ratio of solvent to anti-solvent, mixing rate, desaturation kinetics, and type of solvent/anti-solvent pair [10]. The selection of the solvent systems is typically based on three factors, i.e., miscibility between the pair of solvents, viscosity ratio between the solvent pair (less than 3), and a solubility phase diagram that favors anti-solvent precipitation [43]. Thus, we have evaluated effects of solvent systems on material properties using DMF/water (P1) and acetone/water (P2) solvent pairs.

Powder XRD patterns revealed no major differences between the two samples (Figure 7a), suggesting negligible impact of solvent type on crystallinity of precipitated API. However, crystallinity of P1 tablet is lower than that of P2 tablet, as suggested by the broader diffraction peaks of P1 tablet (Figure S2, Table S2). P2 exhibited significantly better tabletability than P1 (Figure 7b), which can be attributed to the smaller sizes of crystals in P1 (Table 1, Figure 1). For the same material, smaller particles lead to more cohesive powders, exhibiting higher porosity. Thus, there was more air in the P1 powder that needed to escape during compaction. Additionally, air escape from a powder bed consisting of smaller particles is also less efficient [37]. Taken together, severe lamination of P1 tablets was observed when compressed at a high speed, where little time was available for air to escape the powder bed. Similar to the tableting behavior of A3, P1 powder could form intact tablets when compressed at a slower speed to form pellets for contact angle experiments.

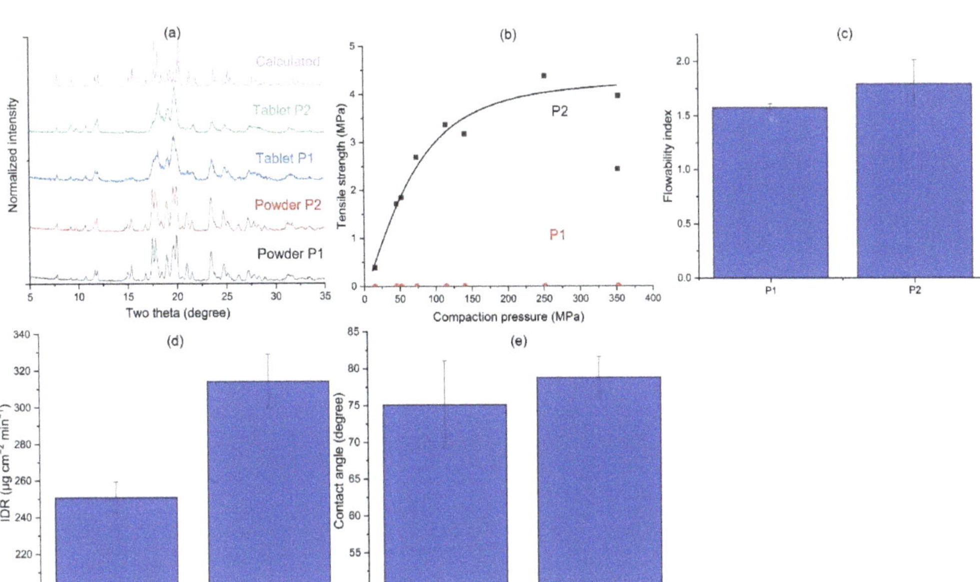

Figure 7. Solid-state characterization, bulk properties of Samples P1 and P2. (**a**) X-ray diffraction; (**b**) tabletability; (**c**) flowability; (**d**) intrinsic dissolution rate; (**e**) contact angle.

The smaller particle size of P1 was expected to cause poor flowability. However, no significant difference was observed (Figure 7c). This was likely because any differences are masked by the slightly large variability in the measured flowability of P2. P2 exhibited faster dissolution rate than P1 (Figure 7d, $p = 0.0002$), indicating more favorable surface characteristics for wetting by ethanol. This was because tablet XRD suggested lower crystallinity of the P2 tablet, which favors faster dissolution because of the higher free energy of a more disordered solid. However, both samples did not show a statistically significant difference of contact angle with water (Figure 7e). It is likely that any difference in contact angle was masked by the relatively high degree of variability in the measured contact angle value of P1.

3.3.6. Effects of Crystallinity

The previous pairwise comparison could not rule out potential effects of different particle sizes on powder properties. The less crystalline Sample A2 provides an opportunity to study the impact of crystallinity on powder properties without significant impact from different particle sizes. This was done by annealing A2 at 40 °C and 75% relative humidity for different lengths of time to obtain API with increasing degrees of crystallinities through inducing crystallization of amorphous domains [44,45]. Longer annealing time led to higher crystallinity (Figure 8a), as expected. Upon compression, a more crystalline powder also formed tablets with higher crystallinity (Figure 8a).

The results show that higher crystallinity corresponded to better flowability (Figure 8b), which is consistent with the earlier observation that more crystalline A1 exhibited significantly better flowability than A2 (Figure 3d). Although both IDR and contact angle are expected to differ among the three samples of different degrees of crystallinity, observed differences were not statistically significant (Figure 8c,d), which may be a result of compression induced amorphization.

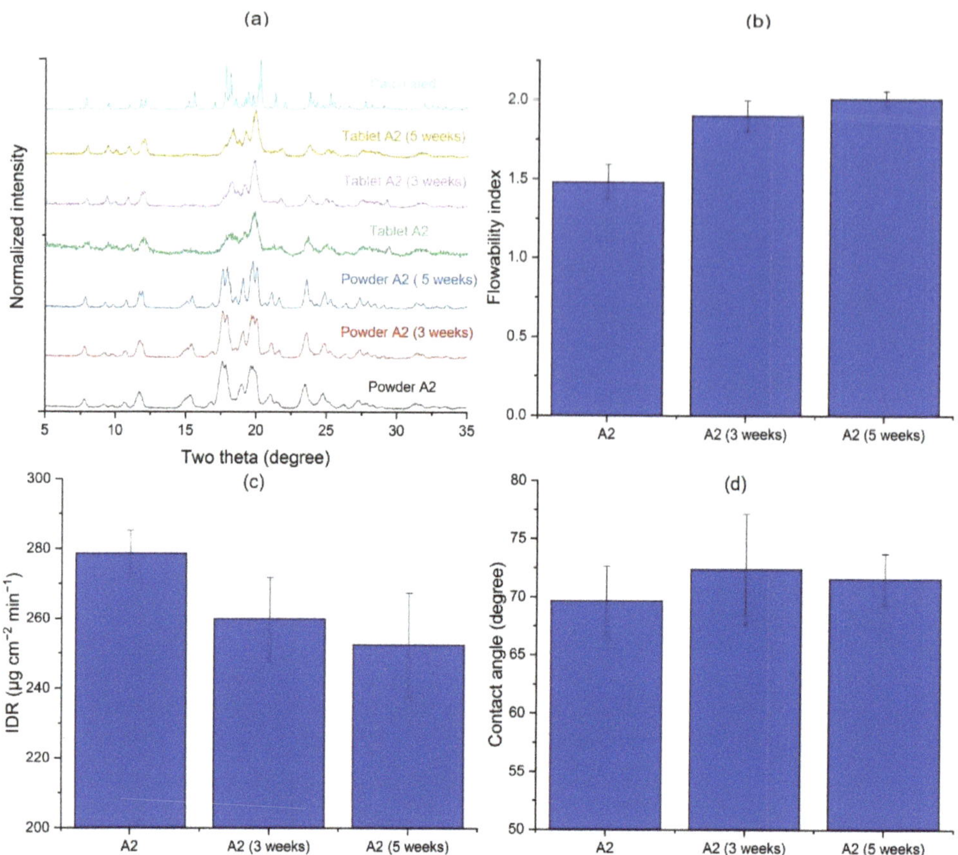

Figure 8. Solid-state characterization, bulk properties of Samples A2 with different annealing times. (**a**) X-ray diffraction; (**b**) flowability; (**c**) intrinsic dissolution rate; (**d**) contact angle.

3.3.7. Effects of Processing Aids during Jet Milling (A3 vs. A(S) vs. A(M))

Given the observed sensitivity of Odanacatib to external stresses, processing aids with known lubricating functionality were used to reduce the amorphous content in jet-milled API. A(S) was jet-milled Sample A with 1% SSF, a hydrophilic lubricant, and Sample A(M) was prepared by milling Sample A with 1% MgSt, a hydrophobic lubricant. A jet-milled lot without any processing aid, A3, was used as a reference sample to evaluate the impact of processing aid on bulk properties.

All three samples were highly crystalline based on their powder XRD patterns. Based on peaks within the range of 17 to 21 degrees, crystallinity of A(M) and A(S) were both higher than A3 (Figure S3, Table S3). Thus, the use of processing aids did alleviate milling-induced amorphization of Odanacatib. We note that diffraction peaks at 2Θ below 16 degrees were unexpectedly much less intense for A(S) than A(M) (Figure 9a). Although a clear explanation for this observation is elusive, preferred orientation is unlikely due to the small crystal sizes in both samples and the relatively low aspect ratios of crystals (Figure 1). However, tablets of all three powders exhibited significantly lower crystallinity, again confirming the stress sensitivity of Odanacatib crystals (Figure 9a).

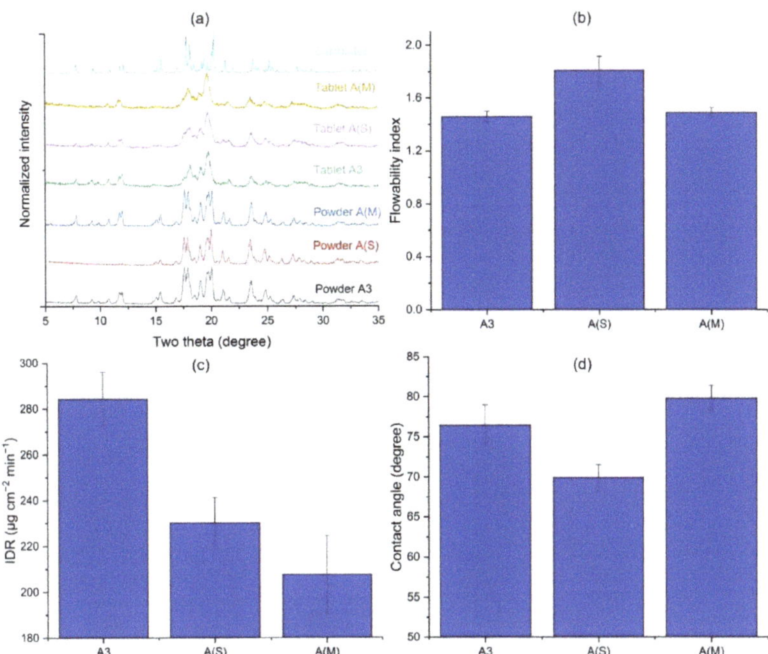

Figure 9. Solid-state characterization, bulk properties of Samples A3, A(S) and A(M). (**a**) X-ray diffraction; (**b**) flowability; (**c**) intrinsic dissolution rate; (**d**) contact angle.

A(S) showed significantly better flowability than the other two samples (Figure 9b), despite its smaller particle size (Table 1). Thus, the presence of SSF not only reduced amorphization but also improved powder flowability. However, the use of MgSt as a processing aid did not improve flowability as reported for other materials [46]. The use of a processing aid; however, significantly reduced the IDR (Figure 9c). The extent of reduction was more significant by the hydrophobic lubricant, MgSt, which is expected because wetting would be more difficult with MgSt present on the tablet surface. In addition, the coverage of API particle surfaces by lubricant particles would also have led to slower dissolution. Wettability by water followed a descending order of A(S) > A3 > A(M) (Figure 9d). This is expected as SSF is hydrophilic, but MgSt is hydrophobic.

The result indicated that, when a processing aid is needed to reduce the extent of amorphization of API by milling, a hydrophilic processing aid is preferred.

3.4. Impact on Content Uniformity in Tablets

So far, it is clear that Odanacatib batches using different particle engineering routes, while meeting size specifications for biopharmaceutical performance, exhibited different powder properties and processability. If the API loading is high, such differences are expected to impact corresponding properties of final blends. When the API loading is low, such differences may influence tablet CU. The latter effect was investigated using tablet formulations with 1% API loading. Since CU is typically sensitive to particle size but the PSDs of these API samples varied, two samples from each particle engineering technique covering a wide range of PSD were studied. Sample A with larger particle size was also selected as a control.

Among all five formulations prepared, the formulation of Sample A surprisingly exhibited the best CU (Figure 10a). At a constant 1% API loading, from a purely statistical perspective, smaller API particles should lead to better CU, provided API particles are uniformly distributed in the blend. This counterintuitive observation was attributed to the lowest agglomeration tendency of the A formulation during storage. Micro-sized API formed large agglomerates during storage to different extents (Figure 10b). In general, higher agglomeration tendency correlates with poorer flowability (Figure 2d).

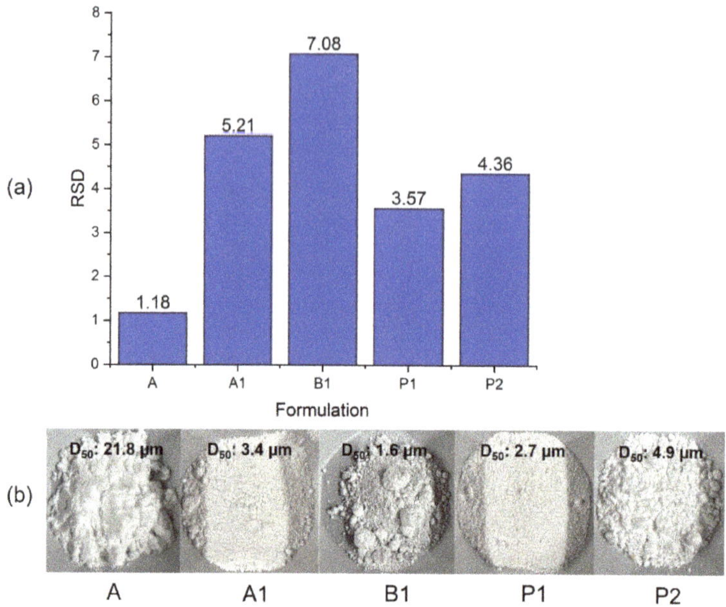

Figure 10. (**a**) Relative standard deviation of API loading of each formulation, which is an indicator of content uniformity ($n = 10$); (**b**) bulk powders of 5 API batches used in the content uniformity study.

Among the micro-sized API batches, CU of tablets containing API generated by milling (A1 and B1) was poorer than that of those by precipitation (P1 and P2) (Figure 10a). This was likely due to the fact that, compared to precipitation, the milling process led to API crystals with higher surface energy, and subsequently a higher agglomeration tendency. Compared to A1 and B1, P1 and P2 agglomerates were also weaker and could be broken without applying a large force. Thus, agglomerates observed in Sample P2 could have been broken during powder feeding and mixing immediately before compression.

Based on all results in this study, API lots prepared through different engineering routes exhibited significantly different powder properties, which impact performance when used in a tablet formulation. Among these Odanacatib batches, P2 has the overall best powder properties and performance for tablet manufacturing.

4. Conclusions

This study showed that, while different engineering routes can be used to produce Odanacatib lots that meet the target Mv, they do have a measurable impact on a range of pharmaceutical properties, including solid-state properties, powder properties, dissolution, and content uniformity. While many more subtle trends can be deduced from the data set, general avoidance of fines seems a key consideration. Samples with higher d_{10} (A3, P2) showed fastest IDR, reasonable compression performance and flow, while the samples with the lowest d_{10} showed poor flow and slowest IDR (not accounting for samples milled with lubricants). While the addition of processing aids may reduce disorder during milling, this had a detrimental impact on IDR, and did not appreciably improve flow. Hence, beyond API size specifications based on biopharmaceutical considerations, properties influencing robust manufacturability and drug product performance should also be considered when selecting a particle engineering route for drug substance manufacturing. For Odanacatib, the direct precipitated Sample P2 exhibited overall best performance (tabletability, dissolution, and content uniformity) relative to the other processed samples. The new insights attained from this work help the selection of an optimal processing route for preparing micronized Odanacatib. This systematic methodology for evaluating the performance of a diverse range of engineered particles can be applied to other active pharmaceutical ingredients to ensure a globally optimum process and product.

Supplementary Materials: The following supporting information can be downloaded at: https://www.mdpi.com/article/10.3390/pharmaceutics14091901/s1, Figure S1. XRD overlap of Samples A3 and B1. (Enlargement of Figure 4a). Figure S2. XRD overlap of Samples P1 and P2. (Enlargement of Figure 7a). Figure S3. XRD overlap of Samples A3, A(S) and A(M). (Enlargement of Figure 9a). Table S1. Full width at half maximum (FWHM) analysis of tablets XRD of Samples A3 and B1. Table S2. Full width at half maximum (FWHM) analysis of tablets XRD of Samples P1 and P2. Table S3. Full width at half maximum (FWHM) analysis of tablets XRD of Samples A3, A(S), and A(M).

Author Contributions: Conceptualization, L.S. and C.C.S.; Formal analysis, Z.W., C.C. and M.F.; Investigation, Z.W., M.S., S.A., C.C. and M.F.; Methodology, Z.W. and C.C.S.; Project administration, C.C.S., S.A. and L.S.; Resources, C.C.S., M.S., C.C. and M.F.; Writing—original draft, Z.W.; Writing—review & editing, M.S., S.A., L.S. and C.C.S. All authors have read and agreed to the published version of the manuscript.

Funding: This research was supported by a grant from Merck.

Institutional Review Board Statement: Not applicable.

Informed Consent Statement: Not applicable.

Data Availability Statement: The data presented in this study are available upon request.

Acknowledgments: The authors would like to thank Alex Coelho for assistance with spiral milling, James Corry for help compiling historical data, as well as Aaron Cote, Anisha Patel and Lorenzo Codan for careful review and comments.

Conflicts of Interest: The authors declare no conflict of interest. The company had no role in the design of the study; in the collection, analyses, or inter-pretation of data; in the writing of the manuscript; or in the decision to publish the results.

References

1. Williams, H.D.; Trevaskis, N.L.; Charman, S.A.; Shanker, R.M.; Charman, W.N.; Pouton, C.W.; Porter, C.J.H. Strategies to Address Low Drug Solubility in Discovery and Development. *Pharmacol. Rev.* **2013**, *65*, 315–499. [CrossRef] [PubMed]
2. Buckton, G.; Beezer, A.E. The Relationship between Particle Size and Solubility. *Int. J. Pharm.* **1992**, *82*, R7–R10. [CrossRef]
3. Noyes, A.A.; Whitney, W.R. The rate of solution of solid substances in their own solutions. *J. Am. Chem. Soc.* **1897**, *19*, 930–934. [CrossRef]
4. Sun, C.C. On the Mechanism of Reduced Tabletability of Granules Prepared by Roller Compaction. *Int. J. Pharm.* **2008**, *347*, 171–172. [CrossRef]
5. Fu, X.; Huck, D.; Makein, L.; Armstrong, B.; Willen, U.; Freeman, T. Effect of Particle Shape and Size on Flow Properties of Lactose Powders. *Particuology* **2012**, *10*, 203–208. [CrossRef]
6. Yalkowsky, S.H.; Bolton, S. Particle Size and Content Uniformity. *Pharm. Res. Off. J. Am. Assoc. Pharm. Sci.* **1990**, *7*, 962–966. [CrossRef]
7. Rohrs, B.R.; Amidon, G.E.; Meury, R.H.; Secreast, P.J.; King, H.M.; Skoug, C.J. Particle Size Limits to Meet USP Content Uniformity Criteria for Tablets and Capsules. *J. Pharm. Sci.* **2006**, *95*, 1049–1059. [CrossRef]
8. Jakubowska, E.; Ciepluch, N. Blend Segregation in Tablets Manufacturing and Its Effect on Drug Content Uniformity—A Review. *Pharmaceutics* **2021**, *13*, 1909. [CrossRef]
9. Wuelfing, W.P.; El Marrouni, A.; Lipert, M.P.; Daublain, P.; Kesisoglou, F.; Converso, A.; Templeton, A.C. Dose Number as a Tool to Guide Lead Optimization for Orally Bioavailable Compounds in Drug Discovery. *J. Med. Chem.* **2022**, *65*, 1685–1694. [CrossRef]
10. Kumar, R.; Thakur, A.K.; Chaudhari, P.; Banerjee, N. Particle Size Reduction Techniques of Pharmaceutical Compounds for the Enhancement of Their Dissolution Rate and Bioavailability. *J. Pharm. Innov.* **2021**, *17*, 333–352. [CrossRef]
11. Kumar, D.; Worku, Z.A.; Gao, Y.; Kamaraju, V.K.; Glennon, B.; Babu, R.P.; Healy, A.M. Comparison of Wet Milling and Dry Milling Routes for Ibuprofen Pharmaceutical Crystals and Their Impact on Pharmaceutical and Biopharmaceutical Properties. *Powder Technol.* **2018**, *330*, 228–238. [CrossRef]

12. Salah, N.; Habib, S.S.; Khan, Z.H.; Memic, A.; Azam, A.; Alarfaj, E.; Zahed, N.; Al-Hamedi, S. High-Energy Ball Milling Technique for ZnO Nanoparticles as Antibacterial Material. *Int. J. Nanomed.* **2011**, *6*, 863–869. [CrossRef]

13. Bonakdar, T.; Ghadiri, M. Analysis of Pin Milling of Pharmaceutical Materials. *Int. J. Pharm.* **2018**, *552*, 394–400. [CrossRef]

14. Yeung, C.C.; Hersey, J.A. Powder Homogenization Using a Hammer Mill. *J. Pharm. Sci.* **1979**, *68*, 721–724. [CrossRef]

15. Saleem, I.; Smyth, H. Micronization of a Soft Material: Air-Jet and Micro-Ball Milling. *AAPS PharmSciTech* **2010**, *11*, 1642–1649. [CrossRef]

16. Latreche, M.; Willart, J.-F.; Guerain, M.; Hédoux, A.; Danède, F. Using Milling to Explore Physical States: The Amorphous and Polymorphic Forms of Sulindac. *J. Pharm. Sci.* **2019**, *108*, 2635–2642. [CrossRef]

17. Elisei, E.; Willart, J.-F.; Danède, F.; Siepmann, J.; Siepmann, F.; Descamps, M. Crystalline Polymorphism Emerging From a Milling-Induced Amorphous Form: The Case of Chlorhexidine Dihydrochloride. *J. Pharm. Sci.* **2018**, *107*, 121–126. [CrossRef]

18. Chikhalia, V.; Forbes, R.T.; Storey, R.A.; Ticehurst, M. The Effect of Crystal Morphology and Mill Type on Milling Induced Crystal Disorder. *Eur. J. Pharm. Sci.* **2006**, *27*, 19–26. [CrossRef]

19. Thorat, A.A.; Dalvi, S.V. Liquid Antisolvent Precipitation and Stabilization of Nanoparticles of Poorly Water Soluble Drugs in Aqueous Suspensions: Recent Developments and Future Perspective. *Chem. Eng. J.* **2012**, *181–182*, 1–34. [CrossRef]

20. Modi, S.R.; Dantuluri, A.K.R.; Puri, V.; Pawar, Y.B.; Nandekar, P.; Sangamwar, A.T.; Perumalla, S.R.; Sun, C.C.; Bansal, A.K. Impact of Crystal Habit on Biopharmaceutical Performance of Celecoxib. *Cryst. Growth Des.* **2013**, *13*, 2824–2832. [CrossRef]

21. Modi, S.R.; Dantuluri, A.K.R.; Perumalla, S.R.; Sun, C.C.; Bansal, A.K. Effect of Crystal Habit on Intrinsic Dissolution Behavior of Celecoxib Due to Differential Wettability. *Cryst. Growth Des.* **2014**, *14*, 5283–5292. [CrossRef]

22. Chattoraj, S.; Sun, C.C. Crystal and Particle Engineering Strategies for Improving Powder Compression and Flow Properties to Enable Continuous Tablet Manufacturing by Direct Compression. *J. Pharm. Sci.* **2018**, *107*, 968–974. [CrossRef] [PubMed]

23. Chen, H.; Xu, H.; Wang, C.; Kang, H.; Haynes, C.L.; Mahanthappa, M.K.; Sun, C.C. Novel Quasi-Emulsion Solvent Diffusion-Based Spherical Cocrystallization Strategy for Simultaneously Improving the Manufacturability and Dissolution of Indomethacin. *Cryst. Growth Des.* **2020**, *20*, 6752–6762. [CrossRef]

24. Bartkowiak, T.; Berglund, J.; Brown, C.A. Multiscale Characterizations of Surface Anisotropies. *Materials* **2020**, *13*, 3028. [CrossRef]

25. Jain, T.; Sheokand, S.; Modi, S.R.; Ugale, B.; Yadav, R.N.; Kumar, N.; Nagaraja, C.M.; Bansal, A.K. Effect of Differential Surface Anisotropy on Performance of Two Plate Shaped Crystals of Aspirin Form I. *Eur. J. Pharm. Sci.* **2017**, *99*, 318–327. [CrossRef]

26. Dirba, I.; Li, J.; Sepehri-Amin, H.; Ohkubo, T.; Schrefl, T.; Hono, K. Anisotropic, Single-Crystalline SmFe12-Based Microparticles with High Roundness Fabricated by Jet-Milling. *J. Alloys Compd.* **2019**, *804*, 155–162. [CrossRef]

27. Gauthier, J.Y.; Chauret, N.; Cromlish, W.; Desmarais, S.; Duong, L.T.; Falgueyret, J.-P.; Kimmel, D.B.; Lamontagne, S.; Léger, S.; LeRiche, T.; et al. The Discovery of Odanacatib (MK-0822), a Selective Inhibitor of Cathepsin K. *Bioorg. Med. Chem. Lett.* **2008**, *18*, 923–928. [CrossRef]

28. Brunauer, S.; Emmett, P.H.; Teller, E. Adsorption of Gases in Multimolecular Layers. *J. Am. Chem. Soc.* **1938**, *60*, 309–319. [CrossRef]

29. Sun, C.; Grant, D.J.W. Influence of Crystal Structure on the Tableting Properties of Sulfamerazine Polymorphs. *Pharm. Res.* **2001**, *18*, 274–280. [CrossRef]

30. Standard Shear Test Method for Bulk Solids Using the Schulze Ring Shear Tester. Available online: https://www.astm.org/d6773-08.html (accessed on 4 June 2022).

31. Shi, L.; Feng, Y.; Sun, C.C. Origin of Profound Changes in Powder Properties during Wetting and Nucleation Stages of High-Shear Wet Granulation of Microcrystalline Cellulose. *Powder Technol.* **2011**, *208*, 663–668. [CrossRef]

32. Wang, C.; Perumalla, S.R.; Lu, R.; Fang, J.; Sun, C.C. Sweet Berberine. *Cryst. Growth Des.* **2016**, *16*, 933–939. [CrossRef]

33. United States Pharmacopeia Convention. *USP 37 NF 32, USP General Chapter <905> Uniformity of Dosage Units*.

34. Keselman, H.J.; Rogan, J.C. The Tukey Multiple Comparison Test: 1953–1976. *Psychol. Bull.* **1977**, *84*, 1050–1056. [CrossRef]

35. Watanabe, S.; Akahori, T. Determination of Crystallinity in Cellulose Fibers by X-Ray Diffraction. *J. Soc. Chem. Ind. Jpn.* **1969**, *72*, 1565–1572. [CrossRef]

36. Surana, R.; Suryanarayanan, R. Quantitation of Crystallinity in Substantially Amorphous Pharmaceuticals and Study of Crystallization Kinetics by X-Ray Powder Diffractometry. *Powder Diffr.* **2000**, *15*, 2–6. [CrossRef]

37. Vreeman, G.; Sun, C.C. Air Entrapment during Tablet Compression—Diagnosis, Impact on Tableting Performance, and Mitigation Strategies. *Int. J. Pharm.* **2022**, *615*, 121514. [CrossRef]

38. Mazel, V.; Busignies, V.; Diarra, H.; Tchoreloff, P. Lamination of Pharmaceutical Tablets Due to Air Entrapment: Direct Visualization and Influence of the Compact Thickness. *Int. J. Pharm.* **2015**, *478*, 702–704. [CrossRef]

39. Schulze, D. *Powders and Bulk Solids: Behavior, Characterization, Storage and Flow*; Springer International Publishing: Cham, Switzerland, 2021. [CrossRef]

40. Hou, H.; Sun, C.C. Quantifying Effects of Particulate Properties on Powder Flow Properties Using a Ring Shear Tester. *J. Pharm. Sci.* **2008**, *97*, 4030–4039. [CrossRef]

41. Bell, T.A. Challenges in the Scale-up of Particulate Processes—An Industrial Perspective. *Powder Technol.* **2005**, *150*, 60–71. [CrossRef]

42. Paliwal, R.; Babu, R.J.; Palakurthi, S. Nanomedicine Scale-up Technologies: Feasibilities and Challenges. *AAPS PharmSciTech* **2014**, *15*, 1527–1534. [CrossRef]

43. Ramakers, L.A.I.; McGinty, J.; Beckmann, W.; Levilain, G.; Lee, M.; Wheatcroft, H.; Houson, I.; Sefcik, J. Investigation of Metastable Zones and Induction Times in Glycine Crystallization across Three Different Antisolvents. *Cryst. Growth Des.* **2020**, *20*, 4935–4944. [CrossRef]
44. Marchese, P.; Celli, A.; Fiorini, M.; Gabaldi, M. Effects of Annealing on Crystallinity and Phase Behaviour of PET/PC Block Copolymers. *Eur. Polym. J.* **2003**, *39*, 1081–1089. [CrossRef]
45. Simmons, H.; Tiwary, P.; Colwell, J.E.; Kontopoulou, M. Improvements in the Crystallinity and Mechanical Properties of PLA by Nucleation and Annealing. *Polym. Degrad. Stab.* **2019**, *166*, 248–257. [CrossRef]
46. Horio, T.; Yasuda, M.; Matsusaka, S. Measurement of Flowability of Lubricated Powders by the Vibrating Tube Method. *Drug Dev. Ind. Pharm.* **2013**, *39*, 1063–1069. [CrossRef] [PubMed]

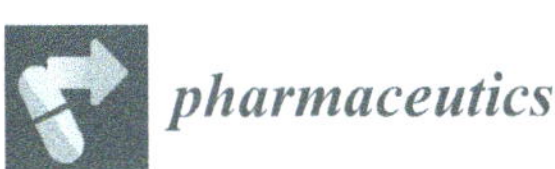

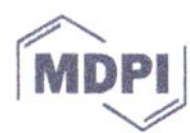

Article

Crystallization Thermodynamics of α-Lactose Monohydrate in Different Solvents

Youliang Guan [1], Zujin Yang [1,*], Kui Wu [2] and Hongbing Ji [3,*]

1 School of Chemical Engineering and Technology, Sun Yat-sen University, Zhuhai 519082, China
2 School of Chemistry and Chemical Engineering, Jinggangshan University, Ji'an 343009, China
3 School of Chemistry, Sun Yat-sen University, Guangzhou 510275, China
* Correspondence: yangzj3@mail.sysu.edu.cn (Z.Y.); jihb@mail.sysu.edu.cn (H.J.)

Citation: Guan, Y.; Yang, Z.;
Wu, K.; Ji, H. Crystallization
Thermodynamics of α-Lactose
Monohydrate in Different Solvents.
Pharmaceutics **2022**, *14*, 1774.
https://doi.org/10.3390/
pharmaceutics14091774

Academic Editor: Hisham
Al-Obaidi

Received: 29 July 2022
Accepted: 19 August 2022
Published: 25 August 2022

Abstract: It is common to find that some of the lactose in dairy powders and pharmaceutical tablets is present in the unstable amorphous state. Therefore, their crystallization thermodynamics in different solvents are particularly important. In this paper, the solubility of α-lactose monohydrate (α-LM) in 15 mono-solvents such as ethanol, isopropanol, methanol, 1-propanol, 1-butanol, 2-butanol, isobutanol, 1-pentanol, isoamylol, 1-hexanol, 1-heptanol, 1-octanol, propanoic acid, acetonitrile, and cyclohexanone was evaluated by using the gravimetric method in the temperature ranges from 274.05 K to 323.05 K at constant pressure (1 atm). In the given temperature range, the solubility of α-LM in these solvents increased with the rising of temperature, the highest solubility of α-LM was found in methanol (2.37×10^4), and the lowest was found in 1-hexanol (0.80×10^5). In addition, the increase of α-LM solubility in isopropanol was the largest. The sequence at 298.15 K was: methanol > 1-butanol > isopropanol > ethanol > 1-propanol > 1-heptanol > isobutanol > propionic acid > 1-pentanol > 1-octanol > acetonitrile > isoamylol > 2-butanol > cyclohexanone > 1-hexanol. Solvent effect analysis shows that the properties of α-LM are more important than those of solvents. The Apelblat equation, λh equation, Wilson model, and NRTL model were used to correlate the experimental values. The root-mean-square deviation ($RMSD$) and relative average deviation (RAD) of all models were less than 2.68×10^{-2} and 1.41×10^{-6}, respectively, implying that the fitted values of four thermodynamic models all agreed well with the experimental values. Moreover, the thermodynamic properties of the dissolution process (i.e., dissolution Gibbs free energy ($\Delta_{dis}G$), molar enthalpy ($\Delta_{dis}H$), and molar entropy ($\Delta_{dis}S$)) for α-LM in selected solvents were determined. The results indicate that $\Delta_{dis}H/(\text{J/mol})$ (from 0.2551 to 6.0575) and $\Delta_{dis}S/(\text{J/mol/K})$ (from 0.0010 to 0.0207) of α-LM in these solvents are all positive, and the values of $\Delta_{dis}H$ and $\Delta_{dis}S$. $\Delta_{dis}G/(\text{J/mol})$ (from -0.0184 to -0.6380) are all negative. The values were observed to decrease with rising temperatures, implying that α-LM dissolution is an endothermic, entropy-driven, and spontaneous process. The solid–liquid equilibrium data and dissolution thermodynamics of α-LM were obtained, which provide a basis for industrial production.

Keywords: α-lactose monohydrate; solubility models; solvent effect; dissolution thermodynamics

1. Introduction

Lactose (4-O-β-D-galactopyranosyl-D-glucopyranose), a by-product of the milk industry, is produced from the solution crystallization of whey [1,2]. Due to the different orientation of -OH groups in glucose unit, lactose molecule has two different isomers (i.e., α and β anomers) [3]. The α-lactose monohydrate ($C_{12}H_{22}O_{11}\cdot H_2O$, molar mass 360.31 g·mol^{-1}, CAS No. 5989-81-1, abbreviated as α-LM, the chemical structure shown in Figure 1), the most stable form of lactose, is widely used as sweetener, stabilizer, and excipient in food and pharmaceutical excipient because of its excellent texture, taste, and adhesion [4–6]. However, α-lactose products usually exist as a mixture of α and β-lactose in the aqueous solution with a ratio of 60:40 [7]. Altamimi et al. used a new H^1-NMR to analyze a group of 19 commercial lactose samples to establish a library, implying the isomer content of a large number of lactose products, because a change of more than 10% in the isomer content of the α-lactose monohydrate sample may affect the bioavailability of the final preparation [8]. Therefore, the purity of α-LM in the production process will significantly affect its functions, so it is necessary to purify the food and drug additive, and the solubility of the additive in various pure solvents can provide a theoretical basis for the food and drug crystallization process. Different methods such as anti-solvent crystallization [4,5], micro-fluidic spray drying [9], ultrasonic crystallization [10,11], and solvated crystallization [12] have been used to improve the yield and the desired shape, size, and polymorphic form of α-LM crystals. Industrial production of α-LM is an energy-intensive process. Optimized solvents can recover α-LM from the mixture of α- and β-lactose, which can save stringent energy and help regulate the nucleation, growth, and polymorphism of α-LM crystals. López-Pablos et al. proposed a method to prepare pure anhydrous β-lactose (β-L) by static reaction of α-LM in alkaline alcohol solution under the condition of controlling temperature [13]. Therefore, obtaining the solubility data of α-LM in different solvents helps choose the appropriate crystallization solvent and production process. Majd et al. measured the solubility of lactose in 70–90% alcohol-aqueous solution, which guided the recovery of lactose crystals [14]. Choscz et al. discussed the effects of different whey salts and mixed salts on the solubility of lactose in aqueous solution (20–50 °C), and proposed a semi-predictive modeling method based on EPC-SAFT model [15]. Machado et al. obtained the solubility of α-lactose in water–ethanol mixed solvents (25, 40 and 60 °C, with concentrations ranging from 0 to 100 wt.% water), and correlated and predicted it using the UNIQUAC model [16]. But there have been few relevant reports on the solubility distribution of α-LM in different pure solvents, solvent effect, and thermodynamic properties of the dissolution process in previous literature.

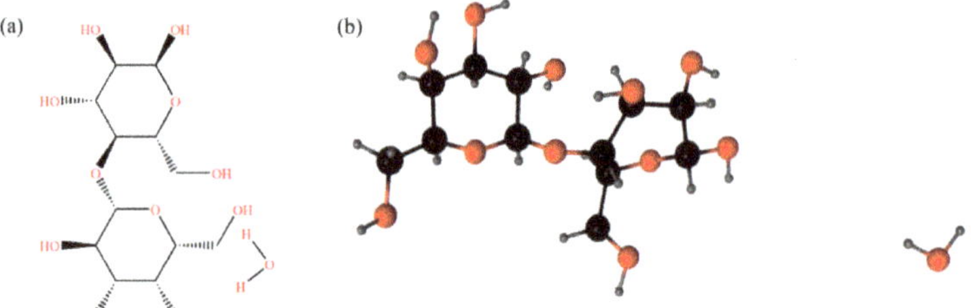

Figure 1. Structure of α-LM: (**a**) chemical molecular; (**b**) ball and stick model.

Alcohols, ketones, and hydrocarbons are commonly used organic solvents in industrial operations (including chemical reactions, preparation and separation). From various lengths of the carbon chain to different types of isomerism, multiple homologous alcohols exist and different alcohols show different hydrophilic and hydrophobic propensities. Most organic solvents are usually volatile, and therefore solution crystallization does not need too-high temperatures; solubility data in a temperature range 0–60 °C is enough for daily use. Thus, the purpose of this work was to accurately determine the solid–liquid equilibrium data of α-LM in 15 pure solvents, including methanol, ethanol, 1-propanol, isopropanol, 1-butanol, 2-butanol, isobutanol, 1-pentanol, isoamylol, 1-hexanol, 1-heptanol, 1-octanol, propanoic acid, acetonitrile, and cyclohexanone from $T = 274.05$ to $T = 323.05$ K at 1 atm. Four thermodynamic phase equilibrium models (Apelblat equation, λh equation, NRTL model, and Wilson model) were used to correlate the experimental data. The relationship between the solubility of α-LM and the selected solvent parameters was analyzed by the KAT-LSER model. The dissolution enthalpy, entropy, and Gibbs free energy of α-LM in these solvents would be determined.

2. Experimental Section

2.1. Materials

The α-LM with a purity of 0.990 in the mass fraction was purchased from Sigma-Aldrich (St. Louis, MO, USA) and used without further purification, and the relevant information on the selected solvents has been listed in Table 1. All solvents were also used without further purification. The detailed information on the materials used in the present work was shown in Table 1.

Table 1. Detailed information about the materials used.

Chemicals	CAS No.	Source	Mass Fraction Purity	Analysis Method	Molar Volume [c] (cm^3·mol^{-1})
α-LM	5989-81-1	Sigma-Aldrich, St. Louis, MO, USA	$\geq$0.990	GC [a]	235.4967
Methanol	67-56-1	Saan Chemical Technology (Shanghai, China) Co., Ltd.	$\geq$0.995	GC [a]	40.5057
Ethanol	64-17-5	Tianjin Kemao Chemical Reagent Co., Ltd. (Tianjin, China)	$\geq$0.997	GC [a]	58.3904
1-Propanol	71-23-8	Saan Chemical Technology (Shanghai) Co., Ltd. (Shanghai, China)	$\geq$0.995	GC [a]	75.1188
1-Butanol	71-36-3	Adamas-beta, Shanghai Titan Scientific Co., Ltd. (Shanghai, China)	$\geq$0.995	GC [a]	91.5062
Isobutanol	78-83-1	Saan Chemical Technology (Shanghai) Co., Ltd. (Shanghai, China)	$\geq$0.990	GC [a]	92.3064
2-Butanol	78-92-2	Saan Chemical Technology (Shanghai) Co., Ltd. (Shanghai, China)	$\geq$0.990	GC [a]	92.6525
1-Pentanol	71-41-0	Saan Chemical Technology (Shanghai) Co., Ltd. (Shanghai, China)	$\geq$0.990	GC [a]	106.2048
Isoamylol	123-51-3	Saan Chemical Technology (Shanghai) Co., Ltd. (Shanghai, China)	$\geq$0.990	GC [a]	108.8272
1-Hexanol	111-27-3	Saan Chemical Technology (Shanghai) Co., Ltd. (Shanghai, China)	$\geq$0.980	GC [a]	125.0610
1-Heptanol	111-70-6	Saan Chemical Technology (Shanghai) Co., Ltd. (Shanghai, China)	$\geq$0.990	GC [a]	141.3625
1-Octanol	111-87-5	Saan Chemical Technology (Shanghai) Co., Ltd. (Shanghai, China)	$\geq$0.980	GC [a]	158.0461
Propanoic Acid	79-09-4	Saan Chemical Technology (Shanghai) Co., Ltd. (Shanghai, China)	$\geq$0.990	GC [a]	74.8263
Acetonitrile	75-05-8	General-reagent, Shanghai Titan Scientific Co., Ltd. (Shanghai, China)	$\geq$0.990	GC [a]	52.2591
Cyclohexanone	108-94-1	Saan Chemical Technology (Shanghai) Co., Ltd. (Shanghai, China)	$\geq$0.990	GC [a]	102.9832
Isopropanol	67-63-0	Saan Chemical Technology (Shanghai) Co., Ltd. (Shanghai, China)	$\geq$0.999	HPLC [b]	76.4609

[a] Gas chromatography. [b] High-performance liquid chromatography. Both the mass fraction purity and analysis method were provided by corresponding suppliers. [c] Molar volume equals molar mass divided by density. Both the molar mass and density were taken from [17,18].

2.2. Characterization

X-ray powder diffractometer (XRD) was used to verify the crystal forms of α-LM during the experiments, and the tests were carried out using a D-max 2000 VPC diffractometer with Cu Kα radiation (Rigaku, Tokyo, Japan). The diffraction angle is 5~60° with the scanning step of 0.02°. The characteristic peaks of XRD spectrum were located by using MDI Jade 6 software (Materials Data, Inc., Livermore, CA, USA).

The melting temperature (T_m) and fusion entropy ($\Delta_{fus}H$) of α-LM were determined by a differential scanning calorimeter (DSC F204 Phoenix, Netzsch, Selb, Germany) under a nitrogen atmosphere. About 7 mg sample was put in a DSC pan and heated from 423.15 K to 533.15 K with a heating rate of 5 K/min. The measurement was repeated three times. The three replicate DSC measurements were taken from the purchased raw material samples and carried out separately.

2.3. Solubility Measurements

The solubility of α-LM was carried out in 15 mono-solvents (methanol, ethanol, 1-propanol, isopropanol, 1-butanol, 2-butanol, isobutanol, 1-pentanol, isoamylol, 1-hexanol, 1-heptanol, 1-octanol, propanoic acid, acetonitrile, and cyclohexanone) from 274.05 K to 323.05 K according to [19]. For the method, excess α-LM was added to a 250 mL jacketed glass vessel containing about 100 mL of the above solvent. Then, the mixture solution was continuously stirred by a magnetic agitator (HJ-1, Anhui Haixin, China) and the solute was added at regular intervals to ensure that there were always visible solids in the solution. The temperature was kept at a required value by the smart refrigerated and heating circulators with an accuracy of ±0.01 K (FP 51, JULABO, Seelbach, Germany). The actual solution temperature was measured by a calibrated mercury thermometer with an accuracy of ±0.01 K. The mass of α-LM dissolved in unit mass supernatant was measured every hour until the figure accounted to two decimal places maintained unchanged to find out the dissolution equilibrium time. The magnetic agitator was turned off and settled for 7 h at the same temperature and the residual solids were sampled for XRD measurement after drying. Subsequently, the supernatant was filtered and transferred to a pre-weighed weighing bottle (m_1) by a preheated syringe equipped with a 0.45 μm filter. Then, the total weight of the bottle and solution was measured quickly (m_2). The saturated solution was placed in a vacuum oven at 313.15 K until the weight of the sample was constant (m_3). All the above samples were weighed by an analytical balance with an accuracy of ±0.0001 g (Mettler Toledo AL204, Nänikon, Switzerland). To ensure accuracy, all experiments were tested three times and the arithmetic average value was used to calculate the solubility of α-LM.

The mole fraction solubility (x_1) of α-LM was calculated by Equation (1):

$$x_1 = \frac{m_A/M_A}{m_A/M_A + m_B/M_B} \tag{1}$$

where $m_A = m_3 - m_1$, is the mass of α-LM; $m_B = m_2 - m_3$ is the mass of the solvent; M_A and M_B are the molecular weights of α-LM and the solvent, respectively.

3. Thermodynamic Models

The theories of correlation phase equilibrium data mainly include empirical model, state equation model, and activity coefficient model. The state equation model is usually too complicated because of the choice of mixing rules, which requires a large number of thermodynamic parameters in the calculation process, and is seldom used in the actual process. Therefore, this work chose the practical empirical model (Apelblat equation and λh equation) and activity coefficient model (NRTL model and Wilson model) to correlate solubility, which were used to correctly predict the saturation concentration of solute under different conditions.

3.1. Apelblat Equation

The Apelblat equation is a semi-empirical model with three parameters, which can be used to describe the general relationship between solubility and temperature [20–22]. It can be expressed as Equation (2). The Apelblat equation is suitable for interpolation, but does not have the function of extrapolation. Because the model is simple and the number of model parameters is small, if the model is used to correlate and predict the system with a wide range of solubility values, the deviation of the results will increase.

$$\ln x_1 = A + B/(T/K) + C\ln(T/K) \tag{2}$$

where x_1 is the mole fraction solubility of α-LM; T is the absolute temperature; A, B, and C are adjustable constants; C demonstrates the effect of temperature on the fusion enthalpy.

3.2. λh Equation

The λh equation is another empirical model with two parameters (λ and h) proposed by Buchowski et al. in 1981, which can be used to describe the relationship between solubility and temperature [23]. The model is suitable for studying the solvent activity along a saturation line and solubility of hydrogen-bonding solids [24], and the equation can be expressed as Equation (3). When dealing with multicomponent systems, two parameters are still maintained. Good results can also be obtained by treating mixed solvents as virtual unitary solvents. However, it is difficult to use the solubility data of pure solvents to predict the solubility behavior of multicomponent systems.

$$\ln\left[1 + \lambda\frac{1 - x_1}{x_1}\right] = \lambda h\left(\frac{1}{T/K} - \frac{1}{T_m/K}\right) \tag{3}$$

Herein, x_1 is the mole fraction solubility of α-LM; T and T_m are the absolute temperature and melting temperature of the solute, respectively; λ and h are the two parameters of the λh equation, which reflect the non-ideality of the solution and enthalpy of the solution, respectively.

3.3. NRTL Model

Based on the solid–liquid phase equilibrium theory proposed by Renon et al. and the concept of local composition, the NRTL model is used to describe the fluid phase equilibrium and calculate the activity coefficient of the solute [25–27]. Based on the activity coefficient model, the simplified equation can be described as Equation (4). The NRTL model can be applied to partially miscible and immiscible systems. Compared with other thermodynamic models, the regression parameters of NRTL model need a large amount of work, and sometimes the parameters can not be steadily extended from room temperature to a wider temperature range. When there is ionization equilibrium, the correlation of model parameters at different temperatures is more complex.

$$\ln x_1 = \frac{\Delta_{fus}H}{R}\left(\frac{1}{T_m/K} - \frac{1}{T/K}\right) - \ln\gamma_1 \tag{4}$$

Herein, x_1 is the mole fraction solubility of α-LM; γ_1 is the activity coefficient of solute; T is the experimental temperature; T_m and $\Delta_{fus}H$ are the melting temperature and fusion enthalpy of α-LM, respectively.

The γ_1 can be calculated with the NRTL equation, which is expressed as Equations (5)–(8):

$$\ln\gamma_1 = x_2^2\left[\frac{\tau_{21}G_{21}^2}{(x_1 + x_2G_{21})^2} + \frac{\tau_{12}G_{12}}{(x_2 + x_1G_{12})^2}\right] \tag{5}$$

$$G_{ji} = \exp(-\alpha_{ji}\tau_{ji}) \tag{6}$$

$$\alpha_{ij} = \alpha_{ji} = \alpha \tag{7}$$

$$\tau_{ij} = \frac{\Delta g_{ij}}{RT} \tag{8}$$

Herein, γ_1 is the activity coefficient of component i; Δg_{ij} is the Gibbs energy of intermolecular interaction; α_{ij} is an adjustable constant, which usually varied from 0.2 to 0.47.

For model correlation, it can be assumed that the cross-interaction parameters between solvent and solute (τ_{ij}) in the NRTL model have a linear relationship with temperature, which can be expressed as Equation (9) [28]:

$$\tau_{ij} = a_{ij} + \frac{b_{ij}}{T/K} \tag{9}$$

Herein, a_{ij} and b_{ij} are equation parameters independent of composition and temperature.

3.4. Wilson Model

Based on the concept of excess free enthalpy G^F, the Wilson model can describe the activity coefficient more concretely, which can be expressed as Equations (10)–(12) [29,30]. The model can reflect the effect of temperature on activity coefficient, has semi-theoretical physical meaning, and can predict the behavior of multicomponent systems. However, the Wilson model cannot be applied to the liquid phase stratification system, nor can it reflect the solution characteristics in which the activity coefficient has the highest or lowest value.

$$\ln \gamma_1 = -\ln(x_1 + \Lambda_{12}x_2) + x_2\left(\frac{\Lambda_{12}}{x_1 + \Lambda_{12}x_2} - \frac{\Lambda_{21}}{x_2 + \Lambda_{21}x_1}\right) \tag{10}$$

$$\Lambda_{12} = \frac{V_2}{V_1}\exp\left[-\frac{\lambda_{12} - \lambda_{11}}{RT}\right] = \frac{V_2}{V_1}\exp\left[-\frac{\Delta\lambda_{12}}{RT}\right] \tag{11}$$

$$\Lambda_{21} = \frac{V_1}{V_2}\exp\left[-\frac{\lambda_{21} - \lambda_{22}}{RT}\right] = \frac{V_1}{V_2}\exp\left[-\frac{\Delta\lambda_{21}}{RT}\right] \tag{12}$$

Herein, V_1 and V_2 represent the molar volumes of α-LM and the solvents, respectively; x_1 and x_2 denote the mole fractions of α-LM and the solvent, respectively; $\Delta\lambda_{ij}$ represents the energy parameters about cross-interactions between i and j components in the dissolution process; Λ_{ij} represents the binary cross-interaction parameters in the Wilson model, which can be assumed to have a linear relationship with temperature [28]. The Wilson model can be expressed as Equation (13):

$$\Lambda_{ij} = \frac{V_j}{V_i}\exp\left[-\left(a_{ij} + \frac{b_{ij}}{T/K}\right)\right] \tag{13}$$

Herein, a_{ij} and b_{ij} are the parameters of the model, which are independent of composition and temperature.

Finally, relative average deviation (RAD) and the root-mean square deviation ($RMSD$) were used to evaluate the overall correlation effects of the thermodynamic models. The values fitted by the model with smaller RAD or $RMSD$ values mean that they are closer to the experimental values, implying a better model. The two criteria can be described as Equations (14) and (15):

$$RAD = \frac{1}{N}\sum_{i}^{N}\left|\frac{x_i - x_i^{calc}}{x_i}\right| \tag{14}$$

$$RMSD = \left[\frac{\sum_{i=1}^{N}\left(x_i^{exp} - x_i^{calc}\right)^2}{N}\right]^{1/2} \tag{15}$$

Herein, N represents the number of experimental values; x_i^{exp} represents the experimental values; x_i^{calc} represents the model fitted solubility values.

Parameters of four thermodynamic models for solubility correlation and KAT-LSER model regression were calculated by 1stOpt software (Professional Version 1.5) using the Levenberg–Marquardt and Universal Global Optimization (LM–UGO) method.

4. Results and Discussion

4.1. XRD Analysis

Different crystal forms can lead to different solubility. The XRD patterns of α-LM raw material and residual solids of α-LM in the selected solvents are displayed in Figure 2. The characteristic peaks of α-LM raw material are located at $12.60°$, $16.48°$, $19.22°$, $19.66°$, $20.08°$, $20.92°$, $21.30°$, $23.86°$, $26.28°$, and $37.64°$. The residual α-LM solids in 15 solvents have the same crystal forms as the raw material, implying that there is no polycrystalline transformation of the solids in the dissolution process.

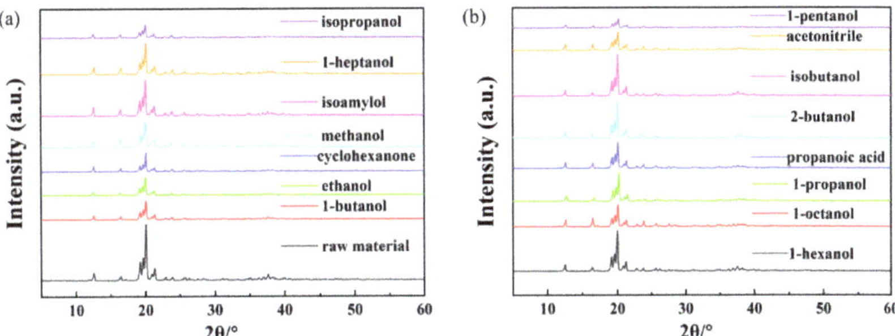

Figure 2. X-ray powder diffraction patterns of α-LM in different solvents: (**a**) the raw material, 1-butanol, ethanol, cyclohexanone, methanol, isoamylol, 1-heptanol, isopropanol; (**b**) 1-hexanol, 1-octanol, 1-propanol, propanoic acid, 2-butanol, isobutanol, acetonitrile, 1-pentanol.

4.2. Melting Properties of α-LM

The melting temperature (T_m) and fusion enthalpy ($\Delta_{fus}H$) were measured by DSC, and the results are shown in Figure 3. An exothermic peak appeared at 447.75 K, which was due to the transformation of amorphous lactose into crystals, and there is still a dehydration peak of α-LM near 418 K that has not been shown according to [31,32]. This is because during the heating process of DSC test, α-LM will preferentially lose the bound H_2O molecule to become α-lactose. Therefore, the strong endothermic melting peak in DSC indicates that the melting of α-lactose at 483.05 K is not α-LM with a corresponding standard uncertainty of $u\,(T_m) = 0.5$ K. The fusion enthalpy $\Delta_{fus}H$ is 99.121 kJ/mol with a relative standard uncertainty of $u_r\,(\Delta_{fus}H) = 0.05$, and the fusion entropy ($\Delta_{fus}S$) of α-lactose is calculated as 205.20 J·mol^{-1}·K^{-1} with Equation (16).

$$\Delta_{fus}S = \frac{\Delta_{fus}H}{T_m/K} \tag{16}$$

In addition, a small exothermic peak was also observed at 499.55 K, which may be attributed to solid-state epimerization and melting of the sample powder caused by the heating and dehydration of α-LM, and about 29.1 ± 0.7% of the sample powder was converted into β-lactose at 463.15 K, and the results are following [32,33].

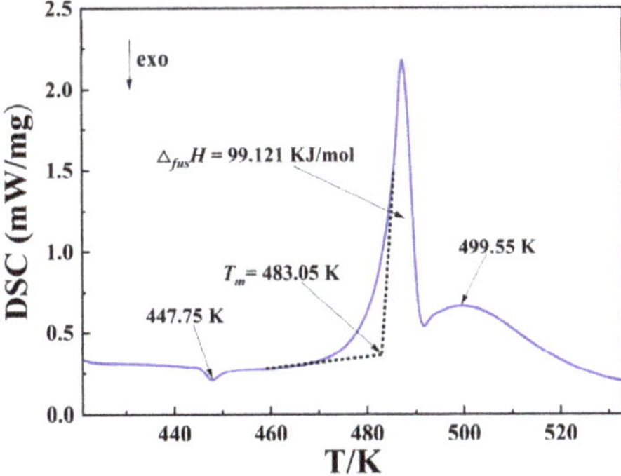

Figure 3. DSC plot of α-LM.

4.3. Solubility Data and Correlation

The experimental mole fraction solubility $x_1^{\exp}$ of α-LM in 1-butanol, ethanol, cyclohexanone, methanol, isoamylol, 1-heptanol, and isopropanol, 1-hexanol, 1-octanol, 1-propanol, propanoic acid, 2-butanol, isobutanol, acetonitrile, and 1-pentanol from 274.05 K to 323.05 K are presented in Table S1. The relationship between temperature and solubility is shown in Figure 4. It can be seen that the solubility of α-LM increased with increasing temperature in the above solvents, implying that the dissolution process is endothermic. The α-LM has the largest solubility in methanol, but the smallest solubility in 1-hexanol.

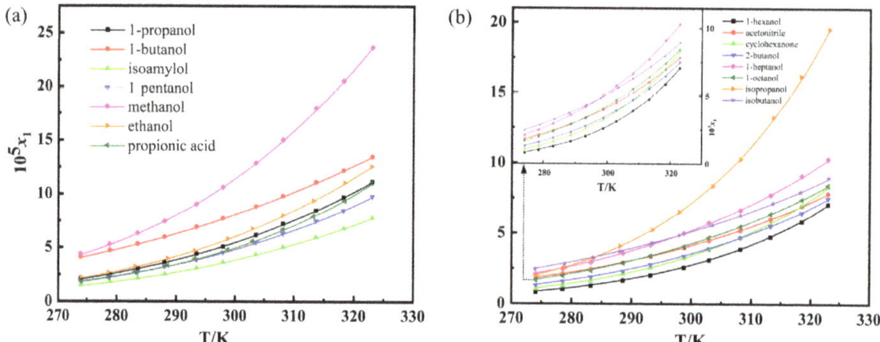

Figure 4. Solubility of α-LM in 15 solvents: (**a**) ($E_T(30) \geq 49.0$): 1-propanol, 1-butanol, isoamylol, 1-pentanol, methanol, ethanol, and propionic acid; (**b**) ($E_T(30) < 49.0$): 1-hexanol, acetonitrile, cyclohexanone, 2-butanol, 1-heptanol, 1-octanol, isopropanol, and isobutanol. The trend lines were fitted with the Apelblat equation.

To evaluate the differences of α-LM solubility in the given solvents, some physical parameters, including polarity index (E_T (30)), dipole moments (μ), dielectric constants (ε) and Hansen solubility parameters (δ_H) are also shown in Table 2. Among them, $E_T(30)$ was also widely used to empirically evaluate the polarity of various molecular liquids and ionic liquids as an important parameter to describe the hydrogen bond and electrostatic interaction of solvents [34–36]. In this study, the solvents were divided into two groups according to the boundary of the values: $E_T(30) \geq 49.0$ and $E_T(30) < 49.0$. It can be observed from Figure 4 that the solubility order of α-LM in the strong polar solvents is: methanol ($E_T(30) = 55.4$) > 1-butanol ($E_T(30) = 49.7$) > ethanol ($E_T(30) = 51.9$) > 1-propanol ($E_T(30) = 50.7$) > propionic acid ($E_T(30) = 55.0$) > 1-pentanol ($E_T(30) = 49.1$) > isoamylol ($E_T(30) = 49.0$). In addition, the solubility of α-LM in weak polar solvents decreases in the sequence: isopropanol (above 283.55 K) > isobutanol > 1-heptanol > acetonitrile ≈ 1-octanol > 2-butanol > cyclohexanone > 1-hexanol below 298.15 K and isopropanol > 1-heptanol > isobutanol > 1-octanol > acetonitrile > cyclohexanone (below 318.45 K) ≈ 2-butanol > 1-hexanol above 298.15 K. In addition, the solubility order of α-LM in 15 pure solvents at 298.15 K is: methanol > 1-butanol > isopropanol > ethanol > 1-propanol > 1-heptanol > isobutanol > propionic acid > 1-pentanol > 1-octanol > acetonitrile > isoamylol > 2-butanol > cyclohexanone > 1-hexanol.

Based on the above results in Table S1 and Table 2, the solubility order of α-LM is not in accordance with the order of polarity of solvents, which deviates from the rule of "like dissolves like". Therefore, the polarity of the solution is not a critical factor that affected the solubility of α-LM, so it is difficult to deduce the phenomenon by a single reason. The solubility of solute is significantly affected by solvent–solvent and solute–solvent interactions [37]. The α-LM contains 8 hydrogen receptor groups (-OH), and hydrogen bonds can be formed between the solute and some solvent molecules. The dissolution of α-LM in different polar solvents can cause various intermolecular forces. In addition, cohesive energy density has been used to describe the binding degree of solvent–solvent [38]. The exact mechanism which led to the complex solubility performance of α-LM is still not clear and more investigation should be performed.

Table 2. Some physical properties of selected solvents.

Solvent	$E_T(30)$ [a]	α [a]	β [a]	π^{*a}	μ [b]	ε [c]	δ_H [d]
Methanol	55.40	0.98	0.66	0.60	1.70	32.60	22.30
Ethanol	51.90	0.86	0.75	0.54	1.70	22.40	19.40
1-Propanol	50.70	0.84	0.9	0.52	1.70	20.10	17.40
Isopropanol	48.40	0.76	0.84	0.48	1.66	18.30	16.40
1-Butanol	49.70	0.84	0.84	0.47	1.66	18.20	15.80
Isobutanol	48.60	0.79	0.84	0.40	1.70	17.70	15.90
2-Butanol	47.10	0.69	0.80	0.40	1.70	16.56	14.50
1-Pentanol	49.10	0.84	0.86	0.40	1.70	13.90	13.90
Isoamylol	49.00	0.84	0.86	0.40	1.80	15.20	13.30
Cyclohexanone	39.80	0.00	0.53	0.68	3.10	18.20	12.70
1-Hexanol	48.80	0.80	0.84	0.40	-	-	13.00
1-Heptanol	-	-	-	-	-	-	11.90
1-Octanol	48.10	0.77	0.81	0.40	1.90	-	6.10
Acetonitrile	45.60	0.19	0.40	0.66	3.20	37.50	5.10
Propinoic acid	55.00	1.12	0.45	0.58	-	-	12.40

[a] Dimroth and Reichardt's polarity parameter, Kamlet–Taft parameter. Taken from [39]. [b] Dipole moment, μ/D. Taken from [40]. [c] Dielectric constant at $T = 293.15$ K. Taken from [40]. [d] Hydrogen bonding cohesion (Hansen) solubility parameter, the unit is MPa$^{1/2}$. Taken from [41]. "-" means the data were not found.

The solubility data of α-LM in different solvents can offer useful information to optimize the crystallization process. In this work, four thermodynamic models were used to correlate the experimental data. The model parameters, including RAD and $RMSD$, are shown in Tables 3–6. The average RAD values of the four models were 0.53% (Apelblat), 0.55% (Wilson), 1.11% (λh), and 0.34% (NRTL). The average values of RAD and $RMSD$ of the NRTL model are the lowest among the four models, implying that this model is more suitable for the data correlation.

Table 3. Parameters and deviations of Apelblat equation for the solubility of α-LM in 15 solvents.

Solvent	A	B	C	$10^3\ RAD$	$10^6\ RMSD$
Methanol	3.0766	−3158.8693	−0.2847	5.3031	0.6003
Ethanol	41.7699	−4985.8779	−6.1120	4.6061	0.2374
1-Propanol	26.4854	−4185.2840	−3.9175	4.1847	0.2885
Isopropanol	−27.8252	−2736.3574	4.8044	6.3433	0.6439
Acetonitrile	−27.5986	−1497.9216	3.9436	3.4318	0.1189
1-Butanol	4.5383	−2459.6923	−1.0101	2.9809	0.2425
Isobutanol	−6.8557	−2120.3304	0.7088	2.4968	0.1839
2-Butanol	4.0985	−3337.5824	−0.5650	4.9549	0.2350
1-Pentanol	17.0290	−3736.0487	−2.5440	5.6961	0.3223
Isoamylol	32.6382	−4461.5797	−4.8957	4.6822	0.1659
1-Hexanol	−47.5650	−1692.9922	7.4855	6.8966	0.2083
1-Heptanol	−2.2769	−2787.9947	0.2990	5.8348	0.3460
1-Octanol	28.3460	−4215.4499	−4.2710	3.7780	0.1634
Cyclohexanone	−27.1953	−2419.8664	4.3772	9.7513	0.3162
Propinoic acid	−43.2062	−1265.0271	6.5779	8.4350	0.4790
Average				5.2917	0.3034

Table 4. Parameters and deviations of λh equation for the solubility of α-LM in 15 solvents.

Solvent	$10^3 \lambda$	h	$10^2\ RAD$	$10^6\ RMSD$
Methanol	4.8545	615,583.7552	4.8535	0.7199
Ethanol	3.1697	997,826.5251	15.6423	1.1342
1-Propanol	2.3316	1,285,742.1272	13.0935	0.8522
Isopropanol	16.0734	267,512.2672	26.7948	1.4094
Acetonitrile	1.0672	2,444,208.9247	5.9051	0.2256
1-Butanol	0.8784	2,233,532.0823	6.6374	0.5483
Isobutanol	0.7550	2,895,562.0914	4.7101	0.2708
2-Butanol	1.7099	1,806,144.9113	5.6122	0.2595
1-Pentanol	1.8496	1,573,562.5892	7.2038	0.5004
Isoamylol	1.4327	2,013,266.8911	8.6628	0.3579
1-Hexanol	4.2654	940,265.8582	18.1818	0.3672
1-Heptanol	1.6977	1,641,263.9352	6.9722	0.3709
1-Octanol	1.4556	1,941,581.3104	9.2550	0.3589
Cyclohexanone	3.9075	965,202.1135	14.0863	0.4350
Propinoic acid	2.7888	1,145,606.1334	5.3089	0.5203
Average			10.1946	0.5554

Table 5. Parameters and deviations of Wilson model for the solubility of α-LM in 15 solvents.

Solvent	a_{12}	b_{12}	a_{21}	b_{21}	$10^3\ RAD$	$10^6\ RMSD$
Methanol	24.4427	−8960.6721	0.4448	34.8474	5.4478	0.6006
Ethanol	25.7710	−8790.9862	0.0104	−0.0075	7.8584	0.4502
1-Propanol	26.3558	−8924.0253	−0.2396	−0.0038	5.5948	0.3651
Isopropanol	17.2970	−7415.4742	7.5370	−1468.9739	6.9079	0.6353
Acetonitrile	28.5466	−8231.7192	−0.2444	−119.7887	2.6844	0.1094
1-Butanol	28.1475	−9769.2383	−0.2111	1.1678	3.2012	0.2580
isobutanol	32.7860	−9600.4299	−1.1306	−0.0058	2.9048	0.1557
2-Butanol	26.4039	−8729.5396	−0.4449	−6.1837	4.7570	0.2359
1-Pentanol	26.8768	−8963.5924	−0.5753	1.8416	4.7443	0.3470
Isoamylol	26.5113	−8946.4676	−0.4400	0.0851	5.5650	0.2588
1-Hexanol	25.6327	−6718.4932	−1.1445	−139.6036	5.7548	0.1595
1-Heptanol	31.3149	−9079.4249	−1.5496	3.4011	5.7054	0.3349
1-Octanol	27.4758	−9001.5085	−0.9517	0.0247	6.3363	0.2515
Cyclohexanone	30.4941	−8406.5104	−1.4374	17.9929	9.1296	0.2281
Propinoic acid	32.0520	−9018.3050	−1.1804	29.1649	6.0851	0.3158
Average					5.5118	0.3137

Table 6. Parameters and deviations of NRTL model for the solubility of α-LM in 15 solvents.

Solvent	α	a_{12}	b_{12}	a_{21}	b_{21}	$10^3\ RAD$	$10^6\ RMSD$
Methanol	7.6935	−38.6535	12,490.0130	23.4391	−8826.6631	0.2460	0.4874
Ethanol	−0.3667	2.8759	−920.7980	21.4235	−7978.7635	4.6061	0.2389
1-Propanol	17.3089	−4.9224	1601.6066	24.3282	−8873.3037	4.0046	0.2632
Isopropanol	1.3652	0.1969	−418.1983	−9.4994	5151.6911	3.2121	0.1504
Acetonitrile	44.7979	−0.2714	84.6165	25.9768	−9283.6565	2.6844	0.1036
1-Butanol	10.5622	−27.8827	9009.6038	26.8760	−9754.0188	2.6124	0.2014
Isobutanol	21.3971	−12.1041	3908.5777	26.7979	−9593.3165	1.8288	0.0764
2-Butanol	−0.0345	−2.9422	872.3605	27.3048	−9624.3411	4.9549	0.2351
1-Pentanol	4.3661	−59.3899	19,189.7345	24.6120	−8920.9197	3.9488	0.1798
Isoamylol	23.2447	−4.4141	1437.1100	24.8075	−8912.0932	2.3763	0.1222
1-Hexanol	35.1965	−1.5530	499.1438	21.9911	−7964.3999	4.7214	0.1074
1-Heptanol	11.0309	−2.0698	688.8884	24.7314	−8983.8417	4.6317	0.3104
1-Octanol	−0.1241	−4.5717	1289.6954	29.2548	−10,195.5144	3.7780	0.1624
Cyclohexanone	7.7270	−3.9109	1279.8161	22.1958	−8097.0602	4.2176	0.1130
Propinoic acid	32.1107	−13.0524	4210.3300	23.8667	−8708.3199	2.9581	0.1232
Average						3.3854	0.1917

4.4. Solvent Effect

Kamlet et al. proposed the KAT-LSER model to analyze the solvent effect to describe complex solubility performance, which divided the intermolecular forces into non-specific ones and specific ones [42,43]. The KAT-LSER model can reasonably explain the effect of various physical properties of the solvent on the solute solubility through multiple linear regression correlation of solute solubility data in different pure solvents [44]. The expression of KAT-LSER model can be expressed as Equation (17):

$$\ln x = c_0 + c_1\alpha + c_2\beta + c_3\pi^* + c_4\left(\frac{V_s\delta_H^2}{100RT}\right) \tag{17}$$

Herein, α and β are the acidity and basicity of hydrogen bonds, respectively; π^* is the dipolarity-polarizability of the solvents; δ_H is the Hansen solubility parameter of some solvents; c_0 is a constant, depending on the solute; c_1, c_2, c_3, and c_4 are all constants, indicating the influence of the four property parameters of solvents on the solubility of α-LM; V_s = 235.4967 cm^3/mol is the molar volume of α-LM; R = 8.314 J/(mol·K) is the molar gas constant; x is the solubility of α-LM at T; T is the experimental temperature around 298.15 K.

The values of α, β, π^* and δ_H of fourteen solvents used in the correlation of KAT-LSER model are listed in Table 3. Multiple linear regression analysis was used to correlate the solubility data of α-LM with the property parameters of solvents according to Equation (17), and the correlation result is shown in Equation (18).

$$\ln x = -11.4635 + 0.2313\alpha + 0.1419\beta + 1.5897\pi^* + 2.1243\left(\frac{V_s\delta_H^2}{100RT}\right) \tag{18}$$
$$n = 14,\ R^2 = 0.9980,\ RMSD = 0.1965,\ RSS = 0.5407,\ \chi^2 = 0.0191$$

Herein, n is the number of solvents used, except 1-heptanol. For the regression effect, R^2 is the square of the correlation coefficient; $RMSD$ is the root-mean square deviation; RSS is the residual sum of squares; χ^2 is the value of the Chi-Squared test. These indicators show a reliable result.

In the fitted KAT-LSER model, c_0 = −11.4635, indicating that the dissolution process of α-LM needs to overcome the strong crystal lattice cohesion energy, so it is difficult to dissolve. However, c_1, c_2, and c_3 are all positive (c_1 = 0.2313, c_2 = 0.1419, c_3 = 1.5897), implying that the solubility of α-LM increases with the rising of hydrogen bond donation ability, electron pair donation ability, and polarity of the solvents. Furthermore, the coefficient of δ_H is positive (c_4 = 2.1243), which indicates that the solvent hydrogen bonding cohesion (Hansen solubility parameter) is the most beneficial to the dissolution of α-LM. In the solvent effect distribution ratio, the four parameters α, β, π^*, and δ_H are 1.49%, 0.91%, 10.22%, and 13.66%, respectively. The total distribution proportion of the solvent effect is 26.28%. As a result, the properties of α-LM have a more significant effect than properties of solvents, which can explain the low solubility of α-LM in this study.

4.5. Thermodynamic Properties of Dissolution

The calculation of the thermodynamics of the dissolution of α-LM in selected solvents will guide its production applications, and the dissolution thermodynamic properties were described by the changes of Gibbs energy (G), enthalpy (S), and entropy (H) of the α-LM in the dissolution process. Such as $\Delta_{dis}H$ can help to determine the energy exchanged in the crystallization system, $\Delta_{dis}S$ can help to determine the degree of confusion in the system, $\Delta_{dis}G$ can help to determine the difficulty of spontaneity and driving force of the process, which can be described as four stages: heating, melting, cooling, and mixing [45,46], expressed as Equation (19).

$$\Delta_{dis}M = x(\Delta_{heat}M + \Delta_{fus}M + \Delta_{cool}M) + \Delta_{mix}M \tag{19}$$

Herein, x is the mole fraction of α-LM in a pure solvent; M can be considered as Gibbs energy (G), entropy (S), and enthalpy (H). The values of S and H in the heating ($_{heat}M$) and cooling ($_{cool}M$) process are lower than those in the fusion ($_{fus}M$) process, so they can be ignored in the calculation of dissolution properties [16].

According to the Lewis–Randall law, the real thermodynamic properties of mixed solutions were composed of ideal mixing properties and excess thermodynamic properties, which can be expressed by Equation (20) [47]:

$$\Delta_{mix}M = M^E + \Delta_{mix}M^{id} \tag{20}$$

Herein, M can be S, H, and G, representing entropy, enthalpy, and Gibbs energy, respectively; M^E represents the excess property; $\Delta_{mix}M^{id}$ is the thermodynamic property of mixing in the ideal solution, which can be calculated as Equations (21)–(23), respectively [19,48].

$$\Delta_{mix}S^{id} = -R(x_1 \ln x_1 + x_2 \ln x_2) \tag{21}$$

$$\Delta_{mix}H^{id} = 0 \tag{22}$$

$$\Delta_{mix}G^{id} = RT(x_1 \ln x_1 + x_2 \ln x_2) \tag{23}$$

Herein, x_1 and x_2 are the mole fraction of α-LM and the solvent, respectively; $\Delta_{mix}S^{\,id}$, $\Delta_{mix}H^{\,id}$, and $\Delta_{mix}G^{\,id}$ refer to the mixing entropy, enthalpy, and Gibbs energy of the deal solution, respectively.

The excess mixing property (S^E, H^E, and G^E) can be calculated as Equations (24)–(26) [49,50], based on the correlation results of the Wilson model.

$$S^E = \frac{H^E - G^E}{T/K} \tag{24}$$

$$H^E = -T^2 \left[\frac{\partial (G^E/T)}{\partial T} \right] = Rx_1x_2 \left(\frac{b_{12}\Lambda_{12}}{x_1 + \Lambda_{12}x_2} + \frac{b_{21}\Lambda_{21}}{x_2 + \Lambda_{21}x_1} \right) \tag{25}$$

$$G^E = -RT(x_1 \ln(x_1 + x_2\Lambda_{12}) + x_2 \ln(x_2 + x_1\Lambda_{21})) \tag{26}$$

Based on the experimental solubility data and the fitted parameters of the Wilson model, the values of dissolution properties ($\Delta_{dis}H$, $\Delta_{dis}S$ and $\Delta_{dis}G$) of α-LM in 15 mono-solvents from 274.05 to 323.05 K were calculated and are listed in Table S2. Positive values of $\Delta_{dis}H$ demonstrate that the dissolution of α-LM is endothermic in selected 15 mono-solvents, and the positive values of $\Delta_{dis}S$ are the degree of confusion, indicating that the dissolution process of α-LM is entropy-driven. In addition, the higher the solubility of α-LM, the higher are the values of $\Delta_{dis}H$ and $\Delta_{dis}S$, which indicates that the heat absorption and entropy increase are also increased during the dissolution of the corresponding solvent. The dissolution of α-LM in these 15 mono-solvents is driven by both heat and entropy. The $\Delta_{dis}G$ of α-LM in 15 mono-solvents are all negative, and the higher the dissolution temperature is, the lower the value is and the greater the decline rate is, implying that the dissolution process of α-LM is spontaneous and favorable for high temperature. Moreover, Figure 5 shows the $\Delta_{dis}G$ of α-LM in 15 solvents. By comparison with Figure 4, it can be seen that the decreasing order of $\Delta_{dis}G$ values in different pure solvents with temperature is the same as that of their solubility increasing with temperature. This shows that both theoretical calculation and experiment section are reliable.

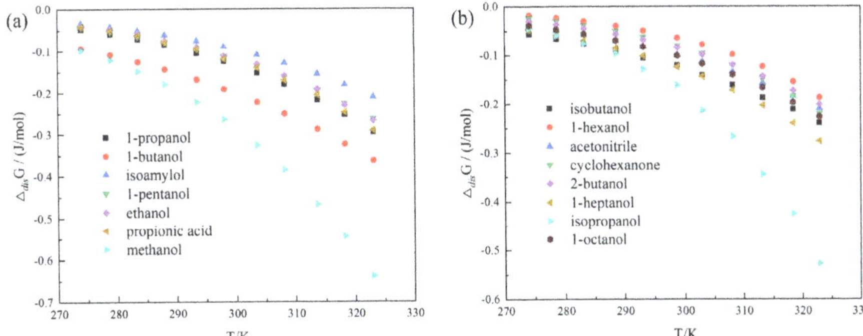

Figure 5. $\Delta_{dis}G$ of α-LM in 15 solvents: (**a**) ($E_T(30) \geq 49.0$): 1-propanol, 1-butanol, isoamylol, 1-pentanol, methanol, ethanol, and propionic acid; (**b**) ($E_T(30) < 49.0$): 1-hexanol, acetonitrile, cyclohexanone, 2-butanol, 1-heptanol, 1-octanol, isopropanol, and isobutanol.

5. Conclusions

In this work, the solubility of α-LM in 15 pure solvents, namely methanol, ethanol, 1-propanol, isopropanol, 1-butanol, 2-butanol, isobutanol, 1-pentanol, isoamylol, 1-hexanol, 1-heptanol, 1-octanol, propanoic acid, acetonitrile, and cyclohexanone, was measured in the temperature range of 274.05 K to 323.05 K under atmospheric pressure by a static gravimetric method. The solubility of α-LM in all selected solvents increased with increasing temperature. At the given temperature, the solubility of α-LM in methanol was the highest and that in 1-hexanol was the lowest. Four thermodynamic models including the Apelblat equation, λh equation, NRTL model and Wilson model were used to correlate the experimental data. The fitting values of the above models were close to the experimental values, and the NRTL model provided the best fitting results. The solvent effect showed that hydrogen bond donation ability, electron pair donation ability, and polarity of the solvents were beneficial for the dissolution of α-LM. In addition, the dissolution thermodynamics ($\Delta_{dis}H$, $\Delta_{dis}S$, and $\Delta_{dis}G$) were calculated. The $\Delta_{dis}H$ and $\Delta_{dis}S$ were positive, but $\Delta_{dis}G$ was negative, implying that the dissolution process was endothermic, entropy-driven, and spontaneous. The effect of the dissolution process of α-LM is important to its recrystallization and purification.

Supplementary Materials: The following supporting information can be downloaded at: https://www.mdpi.com/article/10.3390/pharmaceutics14091774/s1, Table S1: Experimental and Model Fitted Solubility of α-LM in 15 Solvents (P = 0.1 MPa); Table S2: Dissolution Thermodynamic Properties of α-LM in 15 Solvents.

Author Contributions: Conceptualization, Y.G., K.W., Z.Y. and H.J.; data curation, Y.G., K.W. and Z.Y.; formal analysis, Y.G. and K.W.; funding acquisition, K.W., Z.Y. and H.J.; investigation, Y.G., Z.Y. and Y.G.; methodology, Y.G.; project administration, Y.G., Z.Y. and H.J.; resources, Z.Y. and H.J.; software, Y.G.; supervision, Z.Y. and H.J.; validation, Z.Y. and H.J.; visualization, Y.G.; writing—original draft, Y.G. and K.W.; writing—review and editing, Y.G. and H.J. All authors have read and agreed to the published version of the manuscript.

Funding: The work was supported by the National Natural Science Foundation of China (21961160741, 21808247), Guangdong Basic and Applied Basic Research Foundation (2021A1515010260), Natural Science Foundation of Guangdong Province (2020A1515010609), and Doctoral Foundation of Jinggangshan University (JZB2007).

Institutional Review Board Statement: Not applicable.

Informed Consent Statement: Not applicable.

Data Availability Statement: Not applicable.

Conflicts of Interest: The authors declare no conflict of interest.

References

1. Kougoulos, E.; Marziano, I.; Miller, P.R. Lactose particle engineering: Influence of ultrasound and anti-solvent on crystal habit and particle size. *J. Cryst. Growth* **2010**, *312*, 3509–3520. [CrossRef]
2. Singh, R.; Shah, B.; Nielsen, S.; Chambers, J. α-Lactose Monohydrate from Ultrafiltered Whey Permeate in One-step Crystallization Using Ethanol-Water Mixtures. *J. Food Sci.* **2006**, *56*, 777–781. [CrossRef]
3. Lara-Mota, E.E.; Nicolás–Vázquez, M.I.; López-Martínez, L.A.; Espinosa-Solis, V.; Cruz-Alcantar, P.; Toxqui-Teran, A.; Saavedra-Leos, M.Z. Phenomenological study of the synthesis of pure anhydrous β-lactose in alcoholic solution. *Food Chem.* **2021**, *340*, 128054. [CrossRef]
4. Pawar, N.; Agrawal, S.; Methekar, R. Continuous Antisolvent Crystallization of α-Lactose Monohydrate: Impact of Process Parameters, Kinetic Estimation, and Dynamic Analysis. *Org. Process Res. Dev.* **2019**, *23*, 2394–2404. [CrossRef]
5. MacFhionnghaile, P.; Svoboda, V.; McGinty, J.; Nordon, A.; Sefcik, J. Crystallization Diagram for Antisolvent Crystallization of Lactose: Using Design of Experiments to Investigate Continuous Mixing-Induced Supersaturation. *Cryst. Growth Des.* **2017**, *17*, 2611–2621. [CrossRef]
6. Pawar, N.; Methekar, R.; Agrawal, S. Modeling, Simulation, and Parameter Estimation of Antisolvent Crystallization of α-Lactose Monohydrate. In *Global Challenges in Energy and Environment*; Springer: Singapore, 2020; pp. 99–107.
7. Raghavan, S.L.; Ristic, R.I.; Sheen, D.B.; Sherwood, J.N.; Trowbridge, L.; York, P. Morphology of Crystals of α-Lactose Hydrate Grown from Aqueous Solution. *J. Phys. Chem. B* **2000**, *104*, 12256–12262. [CrossRef]
8. Altamimi, M.J.; Wolff, K.; Nokhodchi, A.; Martin, G.P.; Royall, P.G. Variability in the α and β anomer content of commercially available lactose. *Int. J. Pharm.* **2019**, *555*, 237–249. [CrossRef]
9. Jiang, T.; Yan, S.; Zhang, S.; Yin, Q.; Chen, X.; Wu, W. Uniform lactose microspheres with high crystallinity fabricated by micro-fluidic spray drying technology combined with post-treatment process. *Powder Technol.* **2021**, *392*, 690–702. [CrossRef]
10. Khaire, R.A.; Gogate, P.R. Understanding the role of different operating modes and ultrasonic reactor configurations for improved sonocrystallization of lactose. *Chem. Eng. Process.* **2021**, *159*, 108212. [CrossRef]
11. Gajendragadkar, C.N.; Gogate, P.R. Ultrasound assisted intensified recovery of lactose from whey based on antisolvent crystallization. *Ultrason. Sonochem.* **2017**, *38*, 754–765. [CrossRef]
12. Rachah, A.; Noll, D.; Espitalier, F.; Baillon, F. Control of solvated crystallisation of α-lactose monohydrate. *Int. J. Math. Model. Numer. Optim.* **2015**, *6*, 159. [CrossRef]
13. López-Pablos, A.L.; Leyva-Porras, C.C.; Silva-Cázares, M.B.; Longoria-Rodríguez, F.E.; Pérez-García, S.A.; Vértiz-Hernández, Á.A.; Saavedra-Leos, M.Z. Preparation and Characterization of High Purity Anhydrous β-Lactose from α-Lactose Monohydrate at Mild Temperature. *Int. J. Polym. Sci.* **2018**, *2018*, 5069063. [CrossRef]
14. Majd, F.; Nickerson, T.A. Effect of Alcohols on Lactose Solubility. *J. Dairy Sci.* **1976**, *59*, 1025–1032. [CrossRef]
15. Choscz, C.; Held, C.; Eder, C.; Sadowski, G.; Briesen, H. Measurement and Modeling of Lactose Solubility in Aqueous Electrolyte Solutions. *Ind. Eng. Chem. Res.* **2019**, *58*, 20797–20805. [CrossRef]
16. Machado, J.J.B.; Coutinho, J.A.; Macedo, E.A. Solid–liquid equilibrium of α-lactose in ethanol/water. *Fluid Phase Equilib.* **2000**, *173*, 121–134. [CrossRef]
17. Lide, D.R. *CRC Handbook of Chemistry and Physics*, 87th ed.; CRC Press: Boca Raton, FL, USA, 2006.
18. *Vogel's Textbook of Practical Organic Chemistry*, 5th ed.; Addison-Wesley Longman Ltd.: Boston, MA, USA, 2013.
19. Wu, K.; Guan, Y.; Yang, Z.; Ji, H. Solid–Liquid Phase Equilibrium of Isophthalonitrile in 16 Solvents from T = 273.15 to 324.75 K and Mixing Properties of Solutions. *J. Chem. Eng. Data* **2021**, *66*, 4442–4452. [CrossRef]
20. Apelblat, A.; Manzurola, E. Solubilities of o-acetylsalicylic, 4-aminosalicylic, 3,5-dinitrosalicylic, and p-toluic acid, and magnesium-DL-aspartate in water from T = (278 to 348) K. *J. Chem. Thermodyn.* **1999**, *31*, 85–91. [CrossRef]
21. Apelblat, A.; Manzurola, E. Solubilities of L-aspartic, DL-aspartic, DL-glutamic, p-hydroxybenzoic, o-anistic, p-anisic, and itaconic acids in water from T = 278 K to T = 345 K. *J. Chem. Thermodyn.* **1997**, *29*, 1527–1533. [CrossRef]
22. Ahmad, A.; Raish, M.; Alkharfy, K.M.; Alsarra, I.A.; Khan, A.; Ahad, A.; Jan, B.L.; Shakeel, F. Solubility, solubility parameters and solution thermodynamics of thymoquinone in different mono solvents. *J. Mol. Liq.* **2018**, *272*, 912–918. [CrossRef]
23. Buchowski, H.; Ksiazczak, A.; Pietrzyk, S. Solvent activity along a saturation line and solubility of hydrogen-bonding solids. *J. Phys. Chem.* **1980**, *84*, 975–979. [CrossRef]
24. Kodide, K.; Asadi, P.; Thati, J. Solubility and Thermodynamic Modeling of Sulfanilamide in 12 Mono Solvents and 4 Binary Solvent Mixtures from 278.15 to 318.15 K. *J. Chem. Eng. Data* **2019**, *64*, 5196–5209. [CrossRef]
25. Renon, H.; Prausnitz, J.M. Local compositions in thermodynamic excess functions for liquid mixtures. *AIChE J.* **1968**, *14*, 135–144. [CrossRef]
26. Wang, Z.; Zhou, G.; Dong, J.; Li, Z.; Ding, L.; Wang, B. Measurement and correlation of the solubility of antipyrine in ten pure and water + ethanol mixed solvents at temperature from (288.15 to 328.15) K. *J. Mol. Liq.* **2018**, *268*, 256–265. [CrossRef]
27. Liu, B.; Asadzadeh, B.; Yan, W. Solubility Determination and Modeling of EGCG Peracetate in 12 Pure Solvents at Temperatures from 278.15 to 318.15 K. *J. Chem. Eng. Data* **2019**, *64*, 5218–5224. [CrossRef]
28. Shao, D.; Yang, Z.; Zhou, G. Solubility Determination of 1,5-Naphthalenediamine and 1,8-Naphthalenediamine in Different Solvents and Mixing Properties of Solutions. *J. Chem. Eng. Data* **2019**, *64*, 1770–1779. [CrossRef]

29. Wilson, G.M. Vapor-Liquid Equilibrium.XI. New expression for excess free energy of mixing. *J. Am. Chem. Soc.* **1964**, *86*, 127–130. [CrossRef]

30. Kuang, W.; Ji, S.; Wang, X.; Liao, A.; Lan, P.; Zhang, J. Solid–Liquid Equilibrium of Lamotrigine in 12 Pure Solvents from T = 283.15 to 323.15 K: Experimental Determination and Thermodynamic Modeling. *J. Chem. Eng. Data* **2020**, *65*, 169–176. [CrossRef]

31. Figura, L.O. The physical modification of lactose and its thermoanalytical identification. *Thermochim. Acta* **1993**, *222*, 187–194. [CrossRef]

32. GombÁs, Á.; Szabó-Révész, P.; Kata, M.; Regdon, G.; Erős, I. Quantitative Determination of Crystallinity of α-Lactose Monohydrate by DSC. *J. Therm. Anal. Calorim.* **2002**, *68*, 503–510. [CrossRef]

33. Alzoubi, T.; Martin, G.P.; Barlow, D.J.; Royall, P.G. Stability of α-lactose monohydrate: The discovery of dehydration triggered solid-state epimerization. *Int. J. Pharm.* **2021**, *604*, 120715. [CrossRef]

34. Marcus, Y. The Properties of Organic Liquids That Are Relevant to Their Use as Solvating Solvents. *Chem. Soc. Rev.* **1993**, *22*, 409–416. [CrossRef]

35. Cerón-Carrasco, J.P.; Jacquemin, D.; Laurence, C.; Planchat, A.; Reichardt, C.; Sraïdi, K. Solvent polarity scales: Determination of new ET(30) values for 84 organic solvents. *J. Phys. Org. Chem.* **2014**, *27*, 512–518. [CrossRef]

36. Spange, S.; Lienert, C.; Friebe, N.; Schreiter, K. Complementary interpretation of ET(30) polarity parameters of ionic liquids. *Phys. Chem. Chem. Phys.* **2020**, *22*, 9954–9966. [CrossRef]

37. Wu, K.; Li, Y.J. Solid–Liquid Equilibrium of Azacyclotridecan-2-one in 15 Pure Solvents from T = 273.15 to 323.15 K: Experimental Determination and Thermodynamic Modeling. *J. Chem. Eng. Data* **2019**, *64*, 1640–1649. [CrossRef]

38. Gu, C.-H.; Li, H.; Gandhi, R.B.; Raghavan, K. Grouping solvents by statistical analysis of solvent property parameters: Implication to polymorph screening. *Int. J. Pharm.* **2004**, *283*, 117–125. [CrossRef] [PubMed]

39. Marcus, Y. *The Properties of Solvents*; John Wiley & Sons Ltd.: Chichester, UK, 1998.

40. Smallwood, I.M. *Handbook of Organic Solvent Properties*; Wiley: New York, NY, USA, 1996.

41. Hansen, C.M. *Hansen Solubility Parameters: A User's Handbook*, 2nd ed.; CRC Press: Boca Raton, FL, USA, 2007.

42. Kamlet, M.; Abboud, J.-L.; Abraham, M.; Taft, R. Linear solvation energy relationships. 23. A comprehensive collection of the solvatochromic parameters,.pi.*,.alpha., and. beta., and some methods for simplifying the generalized solvatochromic equation. *J. Org. Chem.* **1983**, *48*, 2877–2887. [CrossRef]

43. Taft, R.W.; Abraham, M.H.; Famini, G.R.; Doherty, R.M.; Abboud, J.-L.M.; Kamlet, M.J. Solubility Properties in Polymers and Biological Media 5: An Analysis of the Physicochemical Properties Which Influence Octanol–Water Partition Coefficients of Aliphatic and Aromatic Solutes. *J. Pharm. Sci.* **1985**, *74*, 807–814. [CrossRef]

44. Zheng, M.; Farajtabar, A.; Zhao, H. Solubility of 4-amino-2,6-dimethoxypyrimidine in aqueous co-solvent mixtures revisited: Solvent effect, transfer property and preferential solvation analysis. *J. Mol. Liq.* **2019**, *288*, 111033. [CrossRef]

45. Delgado, D.R.; Romdhani, A.; Martínez, F. Solubility of sulfamethizole in some propylene glycol+water mixtures at several temperatures. *Fluid Phase Equilib.* **2012**, *322-323*, 113–119. [CrossRef]

46. Wang, Y.; Liu, Y.; Xu, S.; Liu, Y.; Yang, P.; Du, S.; Yu, B.; Gong, J. Determination and modelling of troxerutin solubility in eleven mono-solvents and (1,4-dioxane+2-propanol) binary solvents at temperatures from 288.15K to 323.15K. *J. Chem. Thermodyn.* **2017**, *104*, 138–149. [CrossRef]

47. Wang, J.; Yuan, X.; Jaubert, J.-N. 4-Chloro-2-nitroaniline Solubility in Several Pure Solvents: Determination, Modeling, and Solvent Effect Analysis. *J. Chem. Eng. Data* **2020**, *65*, 222–232. [CrossRef]

48. Xu, R.; Xu, A.; Du, C.; Yang, C.; Jian, W. Solubility determination and thermodynamic modeling of 2,4-dinitroaniline in nine organic solvents from T = (278.15 to 318.15)K and mixing properties of solutions. *J. Chem. Thermodyn.* **2016**, *102*, 178–187. [CrossRef]

49. Orye, R.V.; Prausnitz, J.M. Multicomponent Equilibria—The Wilson Equation. *Ind. Eng. Chem. Res.* **1965**, *57*, 18–26. [CrossRef]

50. Jia, Z.; Yin, H.; Zhao, Y.; Zhao, H. Solubility of 3-Bromo-4-Hydroxybenzaldehyde in 16 Monosolvents at Temperatures from 278.15 to 323.15 K. *J. Chem. Eng. Data* **2020**, *65*, 287–295. [CrossRef]

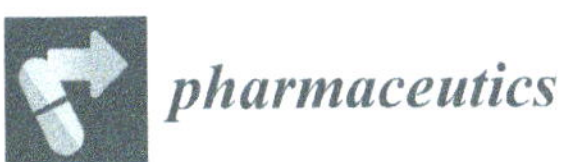

pharmaceutics

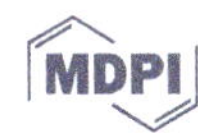

Article

Glasdegib Dimaleate: Synthesis, Characterization and Comparison of Its Properties with Monomaleate Analogue

Boris Peklar [1,2], Franc Perdih [3], Damjan Makuc [4,5], Janez Plavec [4,5], Jérôme Cluzeau [1], Zoran Kitanovski [1] and Zdenko Časar [1,6,*]

1. Lek Pharmaceuticals d.d., Sandoz Development Center Slovenia, Kolodvorska 27, 1234 Mengeš, Slovenia
2. Faculty of Chemistry and Chemical Engineering, University of Maribor, Smetanova ulica 17, 2000 Maribor, Slovenia
3. Faculty of Chemistry and Chemical Technology, University of Ljubljana, Večna pot 113, 1000 Ljubljana, Slovenia
4. Slovenian NMR Centre, National Institute of Chemistry, Hajdrihova 19, 1000 Ljubljana, Slovenia
5. EN-FIST Centre of Excellence, Trg Osvobodilne Fronte 13, 1000 Ljubljana, Slovenia
6. Faculty of Pharmacy, University of Ljubljana, Aškerčeva Cesta 7, 1000 Ljubljana, Slovenia
* Correspondence: zdenko.casar@sandoz.com or zdenko.casar@ffa.uni-lj.si; Tel.: +386-1-5802079

Abstract: Glasdegib is a recently approved drug for the treatment of acute myeloid leukemia. It is formulated and marketed in monomaleate salt form. In our investigation, we were able to prepare a glasdegib dimaleate form, which could, in theory, exist in double-salt form or as a mixture of salt and co-crystal species. Therefore, the obtained crystals of glasdegib dimaleate were characterized via ^{15}N ssNMR and single-crystal X-ray diffraction, which revealed that the obtained glasdegib dimaleate exists in double-salt form. This is a surprising finding based on the pK_a values for glasdegib and maleic acid. Furthermore, we fully characterized the new dimaleate form using thermal analyses (DSC and TGA) and spectroscopy (IR and Raman). Finally, the physicochemical properties, such as solubility and chemical stability, of both forms were determined and compared.

Keywords: glasdegib; salts; X-ray diffraction; ssNMR; stability; solubility

Citation: Peklar, B.; Perdih, F.; Makuc, D.; Plavec, J.; Cluzeau, J.; Kitanovski, Z.; Časar, Z. Glasdegib Dimaleate: Synthesis, Characterization and Comparison of Its Properties with Monomaleate Analogue. *Pharmaceutics* **2022**, *14*, 1641. https://doi.org/10.3390/pharmaceutics14081641

Academic Editor: Hisham Al-Obaidi

Received: 7 July 2022
Accepted: 3 August 2022
Published: 6 August 2022

Publisher's Note: MDPI stays neutral with regard to jurisdictional claims in published maps and institutional affiliations.

1. Introduction

Acute myeloid leukemia (AML) is a cancer disease that affects the blood and bone marrow. It represents a type of acute leukemia that is most commonly found in adults and can progress rapidly without proper treatment [1]. In recent years, several new therapies for the treatment of AML have appeared. These therapies involve kinase inhibitors (FLT3 inhibitors), IDH1/IDH2 inhibitors, BCL-2 inhibitors, hedgehog inhibitors and others [2–15]. Glasdegib (Figure 1), 1-((2R,4R)-2-(1H-benzo[d]imidazol-2-yl)-1-methylpiperidin-4-yl)-3-(4-cyanophenyl)urea (previously also known as PF-04449913), was developed by Pfizer for the treatment of AML [16–19]. Glasdegib inhibits the hedgehog signaling pathway, known to be associated with a broad range of cancers, via the binding to and inhibition of transmembrane protein Smoothened [17,19–23]. It was approved in November 2018 by the U.S. Food and Drug Administration and in June 2020 by the European Medicines Agency for use, in combination with low-dose cytarabine, as a treatment for newly diagnosed AML in patients aged ≥75 and/or unfit for intensive induction chemotherapy [20–23].

Glasdegib was developed as a film-coated tablet for oral use which contains the active pharmaceutical ingredient in the form of a monomaleate salt (Figure 1) [24]. Glasdegib was reported to have pK_a values of 1.7 (benzimidazole nitrogen) and 6.1 (methylpiperidine nitrogen) [24,25], which makes it suitable for the formation of mono-salts with carboxylic acids. Although several salts of glasdegib have been reported in the literature (e.g., maleate, (S)-mandelate and dihydrochloride, which forms a hydrate) [17,26], the monomaleate salt has the most favorable properties in terms of chemical stability, thereby forming the lowest levels of (2*S*,4*R*)-epimer under stress conditions (50 °C and 75% relative humidity over 6 weeks) [26]. Furthermore, glasdegib monomaleate is a moderately soluble drug [27] with an aqueous solubility of 1.7 mg/mL [24,25]. Therefore, there is a need for the development of alternative glasdegib salts with better stability and/or solubility.

In our study we were able to isolate a glasdegib dimaleate form upon treatment of glasdegib monomaleate with an additional amount of maleic acid [28]. Based on the pK_a values of glasdegib [24,25] and maleic acid (pK_{a1} = 1.9 and pK_{a2} = 6.3) [29], the structure of this novel form with regard to the ionization state was not evident. Thus, in this report, we provide full details on the preparation and characterization of the glasdegib dimaleate form. Interestingly, glasdegib dimaleate proved to be a double-salt form, which is surprising. Furthermore, we compare its properties with its monomaleate analogue.

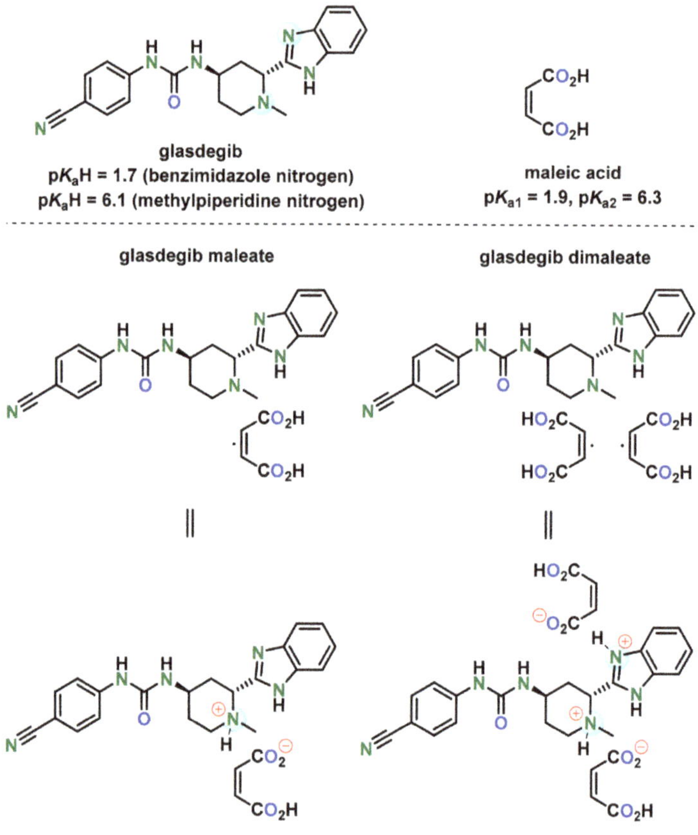

Figure 1. Chemical structure of glasdegib, maleic acid, glasdegib monomaleate and glasdegib dimaleate and their reported p*K*a values [24,25,29].

2. Materials and Methods

2.1. Materials

For the purpose of this study, glasdegib monomaleate (Taros, Dortmund, Germany) was used.

For the purpose of glasdegib dimaleate synthesis, maleic acid, sodium hydroxide, methanol, ethyl acetate and dichloromethane were purchased from Merck KGaA (Darmstadt, Germany). Hydrochloric acid and isopropanol were obtained from FluoroChem (Derbyshire, UK).

2.2. Characterization Methods

2.2.1. Fourier Transform Infrared (FTIR) Measurements

FTIR spectra were collected using a Nicolet™ iS50 FTIR Spectrometer (Thermo Fisher Scientific Inc., Waltham, MA, USA) with a KBr disk.

2.2.2. Raman Measurements

Raman spectra were collected using a Nicolet™ iS50 FTIR Spectrometer (Thermo Fisher Scientific Inc., Waltham, MA, USA) with an iS50 Raman Module.

2.2.3. Differential Scanning Calorimetry (DSC) and Thermogravimetric Analysis (TGA) Measurements

DSC thermograms were acquired using a differential scanning calorimeter DSC 3+ STAR^e System instrument (Mettler Toledo, Columbus, OH, USA), and TGA thermograms were collected using a TGA/DSC 1 STAR^e System instrument (Mettler Toledo, Polaris Parkway, Columbus, OH, USA). The sample was heated in a 40 microliter aluminum pan with a pierced aluminum lid from 30 to 300 °C at a rate of 10 K/min. Nitrogen (purge rate 200 mL/min) was used as a purge gas.

2.2.4. Powder X-ray Diffraction (PXRD) Measurements

Bulk powder samples of glasdegib base, dihydrochloride, monomaleate and dimaleate were analyzed via powder X-ray diffraction using the PANalytical Empyrean diffractometer (Malvern Panalytical GmbH, Kassel, Germany) equipped with a theta/theta coupled goniometer in transmission geometry, Cu-Kα1, 2 radiation (wavelength 0.15419 nm) with a focusing mirror and a solid state PIXcel1D detector. The patterns (Figures S16, S18 and S20–S23) were recorded at a tube voltage of 45 kV and a tube current of 40 mA, applying a step size of 0.026° 2-Theta with 50 s per step in the angular range of 2° to 40° 2-Theta under ambient conditions. Automatic divergence and antiscatter slits were used to irradiate 10 mm of sample length.

2.2.5. Nuclear Magnetic Resonance (NMR) Spectroscopy

All solutions' NMR spectra (Figures S27–S30) were recorded at 298 K using a Bruker Avance III 500 MHz spectrometer (Bruker Biospin, Rheinstetten, Germany). The spectrometer was equipped with a 5 mm BBO, Z-gradient probe operating at a ^{1}H resonance frequency of 500 MHz and a ^{13}C resonance frequency of 125 MHz. Spectra were acquired and processed using Bruker TopSpin software, version 3.1. ^{1}H NMR chemical shifts (δ_H) and ^{13}C NMR chemical shifts (δ_C) are quoted in parts-per-million (ppm) downfield from tetramethylsilane (TMS), and coupling constants (J) are quoted in Hertz (Hz). The abbreviations for NMR data are s (singlet), d (doublet), t (triplet), sept (septet) and m (multiplet).

2.2.6. Solid-State Nuclear Magnetic Resonance (ssNMR) Analysis

ssNMR spectra were acquired using the Agilent Technologies NMR System 600 MHz NMR spectrometer (Varian Inc., Palo Alto, CA, USA) equipped with a 3.2 mm NB dual resonance HX MAS probe. The Larmor frequencies of proton and nitrogen nuclei were 599.39 and 60.75 MHz, respectively. ^{1}H NMR chemical shifts are reported relative to external reference adamantane (δ_H 1.85 ppm), which corresponds to the TMS signal at δ_H 0.0 ppm. ^{15}N NMR chemical shifts are reported relative to ammonium sulfate (δ_N −355.7 ppm), which corresponds to the nitromethane signal at δ_N 0.0 ppm. Samples were spun at 20,000 (^{1}H) and 10,000 Hz (^{15}N). A short excitation time of 200 µs was used to transfer polarization, relaxation delays of 1.5–4.75 s and at least 50,000 repetitions.

2.2.7. X-ray Single-Crystal Analysis

Single-crystal X-ray diffraction data for glasdegib monomaleate and glasdegib dimaleate were collected on an Agilent Technologies SuperNova Dual diffractometer (Yarnton, UK) using an Atlas detector with monochromated Cu-Kα radiation (λ = 1.54184 Å) at

150 K. The data were processed using CrysAlis Pro [30]. Structures were solved via the SHELXT program [31] and refined using a full-matrix least-squares procedure based on F^2 with SHELXL [32] using the Olex2 program suite [33]. All non hydrogen atoms were refined anisotropically. All hydrogen atoms were readily located in difference Fourier maps. Hydrogen atoms bonded to carbon atoms were subsequently treated as riding atoms in geometrically idealized positions with $U_{iso}(H) = kU_{eq}(C)$, where $k = 1.5$ for methyl groups—which were permitted to rotate but not to tilt—and 1.2 for all other H atoms. N–H groups were refined by restraining bonding distances, except for H atoms attached to N4 with $U_{iso}(H) = 1.2U_{eq}(N)$. Hydrogen atoms involved in the intramolecular O–H$\cdots$O interactions in maleate monoanions were refined freely with $U_{iso}(H) = 1.5U_{eq}(O)$. Geometric parameters were calculated using the SHELXL [32] and Platon programs [34]. The crystallographic data are listed in Table 1.

Table 1. Crystallographic data for glasdegib monomaleate and glasdegib dimaleate.

	Glasdegib Monomaleate	Glasdegib Dimaleate
CCDC number	2,180,664	2,180,665
Formula	$C_{25}H_{26}N_6O_5$	$C_{29}H_{30}N_6O_9$
M_r	490.52	606.59
T (K)	150.00(10)	150.00(10)
Crystal system	monoclinic	orthorhombic
Space group	$P2_1$	$P2_12_12_1$
a (Å)	9.7312(3)	10.3645(2)
b (Å)	12.3780(3)	14.5078(3)
c (Å)	10.5764(3)	19.2377(3)
α (°)	90	90
β (°)	113.776(3)	90
γ (°)	90	90
Volume (Å^3)	1165.83(6)	2892.71(10)
Z	2	4
D_c (g/cm^3)	1.397	1.393
μ (mm^{-1})	0.827	0.885
F (000)	516.0	1272.0
Reflections collected	8533	10926
Independent reflections (R_{int})	4415 (0.0196)	5775 (0.0376)
Data/restraints/parameters	4415/3/342	5775/4/419
R, wR_2 [$I > 2\sigma(I)$] [a]	0.0284, 0.0718	0.0436, 0.1047
R, wR_2 (all data) [a]	0.0304, 0.0737	0.0499, 0.1104
GOF, S [b]	1.039	1.052
Largest diff. peak/hole/e Å^{-3}	0.15/−0.16	0.27/−0.21
Flack parameter	−0.10(8)	0.23(13)

[a] $R = \sum||F_o| - |F_c||/\sum|F_o|$, $wR_2 = \{\sum[w(F_o^2 - F_c^2)^2]/\sum[w(F_o^2)^2]\}^{1/2}$. [b] $S = \{\sum[(F_o^2 - F_c^2)^2]/(n/p)\}^{1/2}$, where n is the number of reflections and p is the total number of refined parameters.

2.2.8. Ultra-High-Performance Liquid Chromatography (UHPLC) Method

The solubility of glasdegib and related substances/degradation products were measured using ultra-high-performance liquid chromatography (UHPLC) with UV detection. For that purpose, an Acquity UPLC system (Waters, Millford, MA, USA) equipped with a quaternary solvent manager (QSM), a sample manager (SM), a temperature-controlled column compartment and a tunable UV (TUV) detector was used. The method conditions were as follows: column: Acquity UPLC CSH C18 (1.7 μm, 100 mm × 2.1 mm); mobile phase A: A = ammonium bicarbonate (pH 9.0; 10 mM) pH-adjusted using ammonia solution (25%); mobile phase B: B = 100% ACN; pump flow: 0.4 mL/min; injection volume: 1 μL; column temperature: 30 °C; autosampler temperature: 10 °C; detection wavelength: 270 nm; needle-wash solvent: ACN-water (1:9, *v/v*); purge wash solvent: methanol-water (1:9, *v/v*); sample solvent composition: methanol-water (3:7, *v/v*); gradient: t = 0 min, 15% B; t = 0.5 min, 15% B; t = 11 min, 40% B; t = 11.5 min, 75% B; t = 13 min, 75% B; t = 13.5 min, 15% B; re-equilibration = 4.5 min; and t_R (glasdegib) = 9.0 min (Figure S24).

The concentrations of glasdegib salt for solubility measurements and for the determination of related substances/degradation products were 0.2 and 0.5 mg/mL, respectively.

2.2.9. Chiral High-Performance Liquid Chromatography (HPLC) Method

The chiral purity of glasdegib was determined using an Alliance 2695 Separations Module (Waters, Millford, MA, USA) equipped with a quaternary pump, an autosampler, temperature-controlled column compartment and a 2487 Dual Absorbance Detector (Waters, Millford, MA, USA). The method conditions were as follows: column: Chiralpak IC (5 μm, 250 mm × 4.6 mm; Daicel Corp, Tokyo, Japan); mobile phase A: A = 100% heptane; mobile phase B: B = 2-propanol containing 0.1% (*v/v*) diethylamine; pump flow: 1.5 mL/min; injection volume: 10 μL; column temperature: 25 °C; autosampler temperature: 5 °C; detection wavelength: 270 nm; needle-wash solvent: 100% 2-propanol; sample solvent: 100% methanol; gradient: t = 0 min, 10% B; t = 0.5 min, 10% B; t = 20.5 min, 40% B; t = 27 min, 60% B; t = 28 min, 10% B; re-equilibration = 12 min; t_R (glasdegib) = 8.7 min; and t_R (2S,4R-epimer) = 15.8 min (Figure S25). The concentration of glasdegib salt for the determination of chiral purity was 1.0 mg/mL.

2.2.10. Stress Stability Testing

Preliminary stress stability testing was conducted using dynamic vapor sorption apparatus (ProUmid SPSx-1μ Sorption Test System, Ulm, Germany). Samples of glasdegib monomaleate and glasdegib dimaleate were exposed to a temperature of 40 °C and relative humidity of 75% for 3 months. Samples were taken for analysis after 1, 2 and 3 months and analyzed via UHPLC (purity), chiral HPLC (chiral purity) and PXRD (form purity).

2.2.11. Dissolution and Solubility Testing

Dissolution and solubility were evaluated for both glasdegib monomaleate and glasdegib dimaleate. Dissolution was tested at different pH values using the following buffer solutions: pH 1.2 (United States Pharmacopeia 29), pH 4.0 (European Pharmacopoeia 7.0, ref. 4013800), pH 5.5 (European Pharmacopoeia 7.0, ref. 4002000) and pH 7.0 (European Pharmacopoeia 7.0, ref. 4008200) at 37 °C and 300 rpm using an EasyMax 102 reactor system (Mettler Toledo, Greifensee, Switzerland) using 50 mL reactor and a magnetic stirrer. Experiments were performed by adding excess glasdegib salts into the desired buffer solution already set at 37 °C. Samples were taken after stopping the stirring for 5–10 min (decantation) to avoid the contamination of samples with insoluble particles. Samples were then analyzed via UHPLC to measure glasdegib concentration.

2.3. Synthesis Methods and Characterization Data

To facilitate the ssNMR characterization of glasdegib dimaleate, standards of glasdegib base and glasdegib dihydrochloride were prepared from glasdegib maleate.

2.3.1. Characterization of Glasdegib Monomaleate

DSC (10 °K/min): 195.4 °C onset, 202.2 °C peak; FTIR (KBr): 3424, 3326, 3297, 3275, 3188, 3042, 2975, 2954, 2912, 2882, 2837, 2787, 2750, 2219, 1690, 1602, 1535, 1499, 1463, 1445, 1411, 1387, 1359, 1329, 1319, 1273, 1261, 1240, 1218, 1174, 1143, 1113, 1096, 1070, 1061, 1030, 1016, 1008, 986, 960, 927, 901, 861, 847, 829, 801, 771, 755, 716, 673, 570, 550, 520, 508, 495, 480, 454 and 420 cm^{-1}; Raman: 3118, 3072, 3059, 3029, 3013 2988, 2976, 2955, 2933, 2219, 1691, 1613, 1589, 1535, 1490, 1445, 1432, 1387, 1329, 1320, 1303, 1288, 1273, 1261, 1233, 1208, 1175, 1145, 1113. 1070, 1035, 1023, 1014, 997, 966, 926, 911, 901, 874, 841, 830, 800, 782, 748, 729, 716, 676, 646, 620, 561, 551, 520, 511, 495, 480, 466, 455, 445, 422 and 401 cm^{-1}; ^{1}H NMR (MeOD, 500 MHz): δ 7.68–7.62 (m, 2H), 7.59 (s, 4H), 7.34 (dd, J = 6.1, 3.1 Hz, 2H), 6.30 (s, 2H), 4.57 (d, J = 4.3 Hz, 1H), 4.27–4.22 (m, 1H), 3.61 (d, J = 12.8 Hz, 1H), 3.30–3.23 (m, 1H), 2.67 (s, 3H), 2.48–2.36 (m, 2H), 2.25 (ddt, J = 15.1, 11.1, 4.2 Hz, 1H) and 2.08 (dt, J = 14.9, 4.5 Hz, 1H) ppm; ^{13}C NMR (MeOD, 125 MHz, proton-decoupled): δ 170.80, 156.73, 150.78, 145.62, 138.35, 135.92, 134.25, 124.93, 120.16, 119.50, 119.41, 116.29, 105.46, 59.45, 51.82, 43.35,

42.81, 35.46 and 29.08 ppm; PXRD diffractogram (Figure S16) corresponds to the previously published data [26].

2.3.2. Synthesis of Amorphous Glasdegib Base

Ethyl acetate (60 mL) and 0.5 M sodium hydroxide solution (100 mL) were added to glasdegib monomaleate (2.00 g, 4.08 mmol). The suspension was mixed at 25 °C until no solid particles were observed. The phases were separated, and the organic phase was washed two times with 0.5 M sodium hydroxide solution (2 × 45 mL) and another two times with water (2 × 20 mL). Ethyl acetate phase was dried over sodium sulfate. The solids were filtered off, and the filtrate was concentrated on the rotary evaporator until a solid phase was obtained. The amorphous solid was additionally dried at 40 °C under reduced pressure to obtain 1.30 g (65% yield) of amorphous glasdegib base, which was used directly for the preparation of the crystalline glasdegib base.

2.3.3. Synthesis and Characterization of Crystalline Glasdegib Base

The amorphous glasdegib base (200 mg, 0.534 mmol) was dissolved in mixture of ethyl acetate (40 mL) and methanol (0.6 mL) upon heating to 60 °C using an ultrasonic bath. Clear solution was placed into the vial and stirred at room temperature (25 °C) for about 16 h, with a pierced vial cap to enable slow evaporation of part of the solvent. The resulting solid was filtered and dried at 40 °C under reduced pressure to give to give 110 mg (55% yield) of crystalline glasdegib base (Figure S20). DSC (10 °K/min): 235.5 °C onset, 237.2 °C peak; FTIR (KBr): 3356, 3051, 2982, 2947, 284, 2793, 2219, 1708, 1659, 1622, 1593, 1456, 1431, 1418, 1380, 1369, 1328, 1271, 1177, 1146, 1146, 1112, 1073, 1042, 1002, 991, 896, 834, 778, 767, 744, 677, 639, 617, 569, 549, 513, 467 and 424 cm^{-1}; Raman: 3353, 3066, 3053, 2982, 2951, 2929, 2897, 2224, 2216, 1709, 1661, 1610, 1592, 1543, 1532, 1455, 1321, 1270, 1230, 1206, 1180, 1147, 1114, 1046, 1028, 1003, 982, 926, 890, 850, 830, 751, 714, 643, 625, 617, 552, 514, 503, 469 and 446 cm^{-1}.

2.3.4. Synthesis and Characterization of Glasdegib Dihydrochloride Hydrate

The glasdegib base (100 mg, 0.267 mmol) was dissolved in mixture of ethyl acetate (17 mL) and methanol (3 mL). The suspension was mixed at 50 °C until it became clear. To the solution, 6 N hydrochloric acid in isopropanol (0.1068 mL) was added. After several minutes, a solid phase was observed. The suspension was cooled down to 5 °C, and the solid particles were filtered and dried at 40 °C under reduced pressure to provide 50 mg (42% yield) of crystalline glasdegib dihydrochloride hydrate [17] (Figure S21). DSC (10 °K/min): 159.1 °C onset, 189.4 °C peak and 208.0 °C onset, 210.7 °C peak; FTIR (KBr): 3314, 3100, 3050, 2928, 2853, 2736, 2613, 2224, 1707, 1629, 1595, 1534, 1486, 1471, 1453, 1430, 1414, 1383, 1325, 1288, 1223, 1175, 1151, 1116, 1064, 1023, 989, 968, 930, 896, 876, 836, 759, 750, 668, 638, 620, 546, 518, 495 and 479 cm^{-1}; Raman: 3087, 3078, 3053, 3024, 2993, 2982, 2974, 2945, 2934, 2227, 2215, 1715, 1706, 1610, 1573, 1545, 1528, 1491, 1453, 1430, 1388, 1336, 1317, 1306, 1287, 1266, 1242, 1205, 1176, 1155, 1118, 1101, 1064, 1037, 1019, 1001, 968, 930, 896, 878, 843, 831, 800, 745, 714, 704, 644, 620, 561, 544, 520, 509, 495, 474, 446, 417 and 400 cm^{-1}.

2.3.5. Synthesis and Characterization of Glasdegib Dimaleate

Glasdegib monomaleate (100 mg, 0.22 mmol) and maleic acid (31 mg, 0.27 mmol) were dissolved in a mixture of dichloromethane (1.9 mL) and methanol (0.1 mL) upon heating to 40 °C and with the aid of sonication in an ultrasonic bath. The obtained clear solution was filtered through a 0.45 μm syringe filter into a fresh vial fitted with a stir bar. Under constant mixing, dichloromethane (12 mL) was added to the solution. After 2 h of stirring, a white suspension was formed, which was further stirred at room temperature for approximately 16 h. The precipitate was isolated via filtration, rinsed with dichloromethane (1 mL) and dried for about 16 h at room temperature and under a reduced pressure of about 50 mbar to obtain 60 mg (49% yield) of crystalline the glasdegib dimaleate form (Figure S18). DSC

(10 °K/min): 186.0 °C onset, 190.1 °C peak; FTIR (KBr): 3390, 3326, 3274, 3223, 3183, 3149, 3105, 3047, 2946, 2868, 2704, 2595, 2215, 1699, 1626, 1599, 1536, 1416, 1384, 1355, 1330, 1317, 1291, 1244, 1227, 1176, 1147, 1123, 1096, 1067, 1008, 988, 930, 891, 867, 849, 821, 799, 752, 718, 673, 667, 618, 577, 551, 521, 505, 492, 450 and 427 cm^{-1}; Raman: 3192, 3077, 3049, 2990, 2950, 2216, 1699, 1602, 1562, 1536, 1454, 1381, 1347, 1318, 1292, 1271, 1209, 1176, 1146, 1119, 1110, 1037, 1018, 999, 964, 932, 894, 876, 864, 843, 830. 799, 782, 745, 729, 715, 618 and 486 cm^{-1}; ^{1}H NMR (MeOD, 500 MHz): δ 7.70–7.63 (m, 2H), 7.59 (s, 4H), 7.40–7.32 (m, 2H), 6.31 (s, 4H), 4.71 (dd, J = 8.9, 4.9 Hz, 1H), 4.26 (t, J = 4.6 Hz, 1H), 3.70 (d, J = 12.9 Hz, 1H), 3.37 (ddd, J = 14.1, 11.3, 3.3 Hz, 1H), 2.74 (s, 3H), 2.52–2.41 (m, 2H), 2.28 (ddt, J = 15.0, 11.0, 4.2 Hz, 1H) and 2.11 (dt, J = 15.2, 4.6 Hz, 1H) ppm; ^{13}C NMR (MeOD, 125 MHz, proton-decoupled): δ 169.93, 156.75, 149.89, 145.59, 138.31, 134.24, 133.74, 125.11, 120.16, 119.53, 119.44, 116.36, 105.47, 59.31, 51.86, 43.22, 42.56, 35.16 and 28.83 ppm; PXRD (Cu-Kα): 5.5, 7.5, 9.2, 10.3, 11.0, 11.3, 11.9, 13.8, 14.7, 15.4, 17.0, 17.3, 18.0, 18.6, 19.3, 20.3, 20.8, 22.0, 22.8, 24.6, 25.4, 25.6, 26.0, 26.6, 27.3, 27.9, 29.2 and 29.8° 2θ.

3. Results

3.1. Synthesis of Glasdegib Dimaleate

Initially we conducted an extensive screening of the solid form in order to identify potential novel forms of glasdegib. In the majority of cases, no new solid form was detected. However, when we crystalized glasdegib monomaleate from dichloromethane, we observed that the substance was only partially soluble. Furthermore, after the removal of undissolved material via filtration, a new solid was crystallized from a clear dichloromethane solution. The analyses of the solid via PXRD (Figures 2, S16, S18, S20 and S21) and DSC (Figures S1–S4) suggested that a new form was obtained. Moreover, the solution ^{1}H NMR analysis of the obtained solid indicated that excess maleic acid was present in a novel form. Therefore, subsequent targeted crystallization experiments using glasdegib monomaleate in the presence of additional quantities of maleic acid provided a new form, which was determined to be glasdegib dimaleate based on the solution ^{1}H NMR analysis (Figures S27 and S29). In order to improve the process feasibility, due to the low solubility of glasdegib monomaleate in dichloromethane, we conducted subsequent crystallization experiments from the mixture of dichloromethane and methanol, which provided consistently pure glasdegib dimaleate.

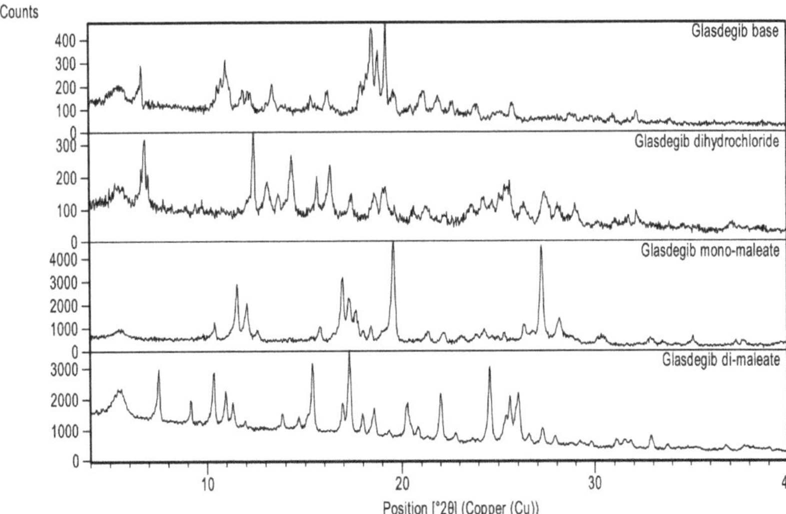

Figure 2. Powder X-ray diffraction patterns of glasdegib derivatives: glasdegib base, glasdegib dihydrochloride, glasdegib monomaleate and glasdegib dimaleate.

3.2. Characterization of Glasdegib Dimaleate

3.2.1. PXRD Analysis

As presented in Figures 2 and S18, glasdegib dimaleate had notably different PXRD signal pattern in the PXRD diffractogram compared to the glasdegib monomaleate, glasdegib base or glasdegib dihydrochloride. The PXRD pattern of glasdegib dimaleate contained several characteristic signals at 2-Theta of 7.5°, 15.4°, 20.3°, 20.8°, 22.0°, 24.6°, 25.4°, 25.6° and 26.0°, which were not observed in the glasdegib monomaleate, glasdegib base or glasdegib dihydrochloride. To obtain a more complete picture on the characteristics of this novel form, we performed additional characterization using IR, Raman, DSC, TGA ssNMR and single-crystal X-ray analysis, which is described below.

3.2.2. Infrared Spectral Analysis

In the IR spectrum of glasdegib monomaleate (Figure 3) and glasdegib dimaleate (Figure 4), the region between 3500 and 2500 cm^{-1} is populated by overlapping N–H, O–H, sp^2 C–H (benzene rings) and sp^3 C–H (CH$_2$ and CH$_3$ groups) stretching vibrations. In the case of the monomaleate form, distinct bands are observed at 3424, 3326, 3275, 3188, 3042, 2975, 2912, 2882, 2787 and 2750 cm^{-1} (Figure 3), while in the case of the dimaleate form, distinct bands are observed at 3326, 3274, 3183, 3105, 3047, 2946, 2868 and 2595 cm^{-1} (Figure 4). The most diagnostic band in the IR spectra is associated with stretching of the nitrile (C≡N) group, which is located at 2219 cm^{-1} for the monomaleate form (Figure 3) and at 2215 cm^{-1} for the dimaleate form (Figure 4). The carbonyl (C=O), alkene (C=C) and aromatic (C=C) stretching vibration regions (ca. 1700–1500 cm^{-1}) are densely populated with bands for the *cis*-alkene group, aromatic double bonds, the urea carbonyl group, the carboxylic acid carbonyl group and the carboxylate anion carbonyl group. In this region the most diagnostic band is located at 1690 cm^{-1} for the monomaleate form (Figure 3) and at 1699 cm^{-1} for the dimaleate form (Figure 4). Similarly, the fingerprint regions or IR spectra for both forms are crowded with a large number of similar absorption bands.

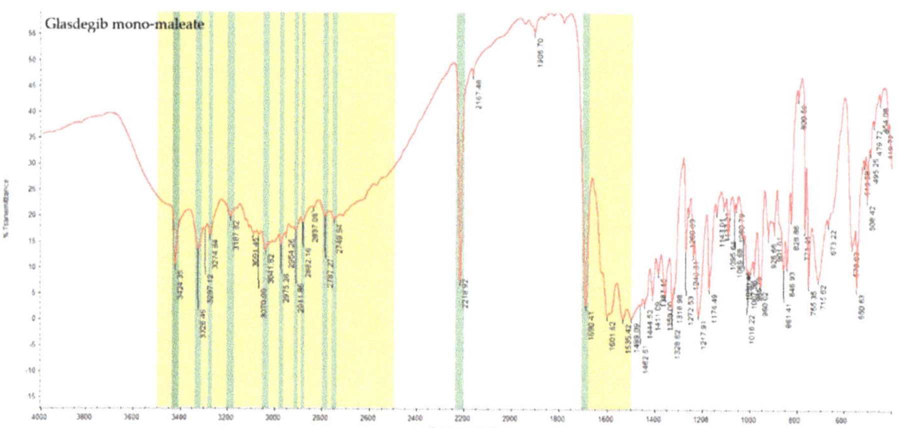

Figure 3. IR spectrum of glasdegib monomaleate with highlighted diagnostic regions and bands.

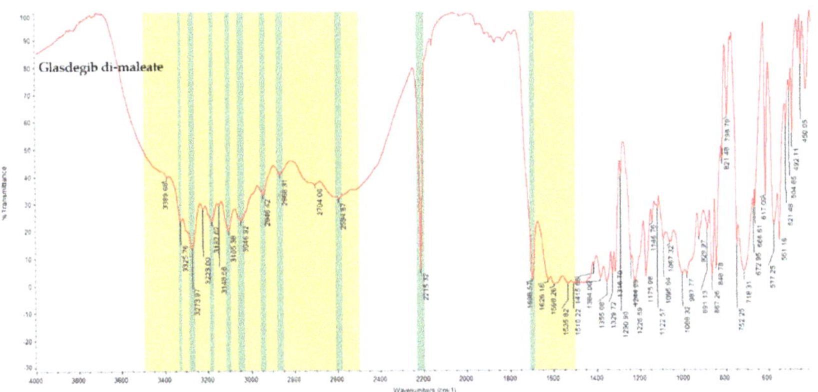

Figure 4. IR spectrum of glasdegib dimaleate with highlighted diagnostic regions and bands.

3.2.3. Raman Analysis

Due to the congested IR spectrum with a large number of overlapping bands in the fingerprint region, we decided to also characterize the glasdegib monomaleate and dimaleate forms using Raman spectroscopy, which should enable better distinction of both forms. The Raman spectrum of glasdegib monomaleate (Figure 5) and glasdegib dimaleate (Figure 6) display CH stretching of unsaturated carbons in the region above 3000 cm^{-1}, while CH stretching of saturated carbons popthe ulates the region from 3000 to 2933 cm^{-1} for monomaleate form, and from 3000 to 2950 cm^{-1} for the dimaleate form. The most diagnostic bands (C$\equiv$N stretch of a nitrile bond) in the Raman spectra are located at 2219 cm^{-1} for the monomaleate form (Figure 5) and at 2216 cm^{-1} for the dimaleate form (Figure 6). Furthermore, a distinct characteristic band is also observed for the carbonyl group (C=O) at 1691 cm^{-1} for the monomaleate form (Figure 5) and at 1699 cm^{-1} for the dimaleate form (Figure 6). In addition, very strong aryl C=C stretches at 1613 cm^{-1} for the monomaleate form (Figure 5) and 1602 cm^{-1} for the dimaleate form (Figure 6) are observed, and are also detected in the glasdegib base (Figure S13).

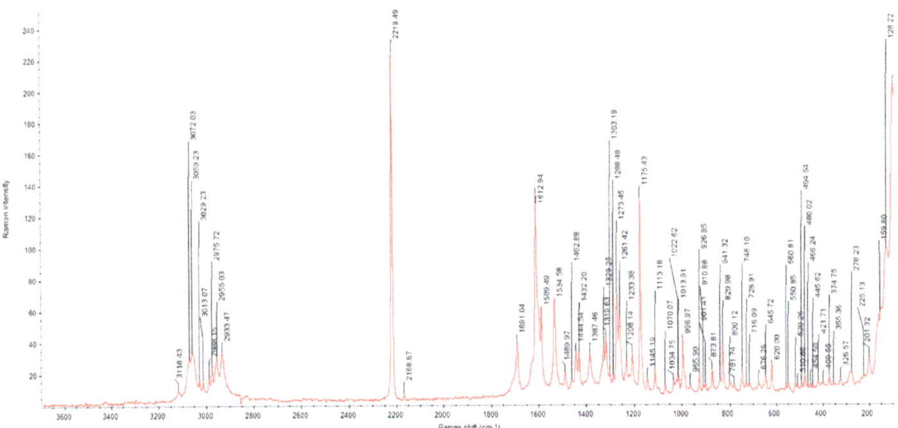

Figure 5. Raman spectrum of glasdegib monomaleate.

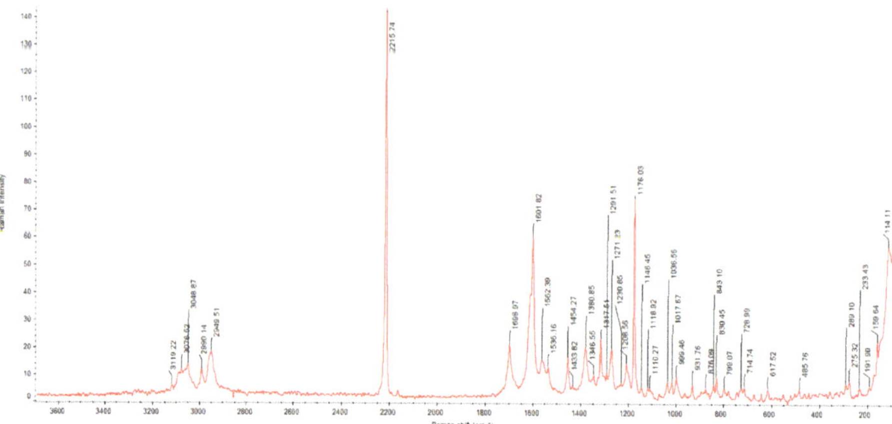

Figure 6. Raman spectrum of glasdegib dimaleate.

3.2.4. DSC and TGA Analysis

The thermal behaviors of the obtained glasdegib dimaleate, glasdegib monomaleate, glasdegib dihydrochloride hydrate [17] and glasdegib base are shown in Figures 7 and S1–S4. It can be observed that the new dimaleate form exhibits distinct thermal behavior compared to the other glasdegib derivatives (Figure 7).

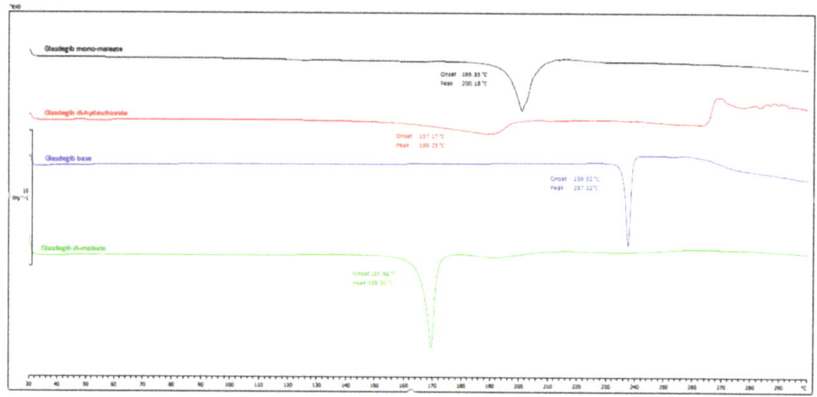

Figure 7. DSC thermograms of glasdegib derivatives. Black: glasdegib monomaleate, red: glasdegib dihydrochloride hydrate; blue: glasdegib base; and green: glasdegib dimaleate.

In the DSC thermogram of glasdegib monomaleate (Figure 7, black line and Figure S1) two endothermic transitions were observed. The first transition at 118.5 °C (onset) and 124.8 °C (peak) is associated with a 2.3% mass loss, as observed in the TGA thermogram above 100 °C (Figure S1), which is probably associated with the partial desolvation of the residual solvent. The second broader peak transition at 195.4 °C (onset) and 200.2 °C (peak) is associated with the melting of the monomaleate form. After both endothermic phenomena, an exothermic transition associated with decomposition was not observed up to 300 °C.

Glasdegib dihydrochloride hydrate (Figure 7, red line and Figure S4) exhibited more complex thermal behavior, where a very broad endothermic peak was observed at 159.1 °C (onset) and 189.4 °C (peak). In this endothermic transition, the TGA thermogram (Figure S4) shows that 10.86% of the mass is lost until 206 °C, which probably corresponds to a loss of one hydrochloric acid and one water (calculated mass loss 11.7%). Subsequently, another endothermic transition is observed at 208.0 °C (onset) and 210.7 °C (peak), which probably corresponds to the melting of the formed hydrochloride form. In the TGA thermogram (Figure S4) it can be observed that additional mass loss starts at temperatures above 215 °C and continues up to the final measured temperature of 300 °C. In this temperature range, the formation of the glasdegib base (see paragraph below) can be observed in the DSC thermogram, which melts at 235.7 °C (onset) and 237.8 °C (peak). Interestingly, at temperatures between 265 and 270 °C, an exothermic transition can be observed, which is not observed in other glasdegib derivatives and is probably associated with decomposition.

The glasdegib base (Figure 7, blue line and Figure S3) has a simple thermogram with a single melting peak at 235.2 °C (onset) and 237.2 °C (peak) and no exothermal transition up to 300 °C. The mass loss for the glasdegib base was observed in the TGA thermogram (Figure S3) above 230 °C and continued until the final measured temperature of 300 °C.

The DSC curve of glasdegib dimaleate (Figure 7, green line and Figure S2) shows no thermal events until the first endothermic peak, with an onset temperature of 165.9 °C and a peak temperature of about 169.3 °C; this indicates the good thermal stability of the glasdegib dimaleate form. Furthermore, no exothermic phenomena are observed in the DSC thermogram up to 300 °C. The TGA thermogram (Figure S2) shows that mass loss for glasdegib dimaleate starts at temperatures above 110 °C.

3.2.5. Solid-State Nuclear Magnetic Resonance Analysis

In order to determine the true ionization state of glasdegib dimaleate, we first conducted an ssNMR study, which involved ^{1}H ssNMR as well as ^{15}N ssNMR measurements using glasdegib monomaleate, glasdegib dihydrochloride and glasdegib bases as key standards for the ionized and unionized state of glasdegib. The glasdegib base presents a reference substance for non-protonated species of glasdegib derivatives, whereas glasdegib dihydrochloride serves as a reference for the protonated double-salt form.

The ssNMR characterization of different glasdegib forms included ^{1}H echo MAS (magic-angle spinning) ssNMR spectra, which showed proton signals between δ_H 14 and 16 ppm for glasdegib (δ_H 14.6 ppm) as well as dihydrochloride (δ_H 15.8 ppm) that are most likely involved in intermolecular hydrogen bonds (Figure S26). The signal of dihydrochloride salt appears broader, which could be attributed to the fact that multiple molecules are present per asymmetric unit, as also observed in ^{15}N ssNMR spectra (vide infra). Glasdegib monomaleate and glasdegib dimaleate showed two sets of signals each: one at δ_H 14–16 ppm and the other at δ_H 20 ppm (Figure S26). The latter suggests the formation of additional hydrogen bonds for monomaleate and dimaleate species. A ^{1}H ssNMR chemical shift of such high value is typical for strong hydrogen-bond interactions.

The glasdegib base showed four groups of signals in the ^{15}N CP-MAS ssNMR spectrum (Figure 8a). The lowest NMR chemical shift was assigned to methylpiperidine nitrogen (δ_N −334.6 ppm). The intense signal at δ_N −285.7 ppm was attributed to both urea nitrogen atoms, followed by two benzimidazole nitrogen atoms in the region between δ_N −266.5 and −272.3 ppm (pyrrole-like NH) and at δ_N −231.0 ppm (pyridine-like N). Similarly, four groups of NMR signals were observed for glasdegib dihydrochloride (Figure 8b). The lowest NMR chemical shift at δ_N −326.2 ppm was assigned to methylpiperidine nitrogen. The signal at δ_N −290.1 ppm was attributed to both urea nitrogen atoms, followed by two benzimidazole nitrogen atoms in the regions between δ_N −268 and −270 ppm (pyrrole-like NH) and between δ_N −210 and −223 ppm (pyridine-like N). Note that some of the NMR signals in the ^{15}N CP-MAS spectra of glasdegib dihydrochloride are doubled, which suggests that more than one molecule is present per asymmetric unit (Figure 8b).

Glasdegib dihydrochloride showed a higher intensity of methylpiperidine nitrogen compared to the glasdegib base. Furthermore, the protonation of the methylpiperidine nitrogen atom showed an NMR chemical shift change of ca. 10 ppm (Figure 8a,b).

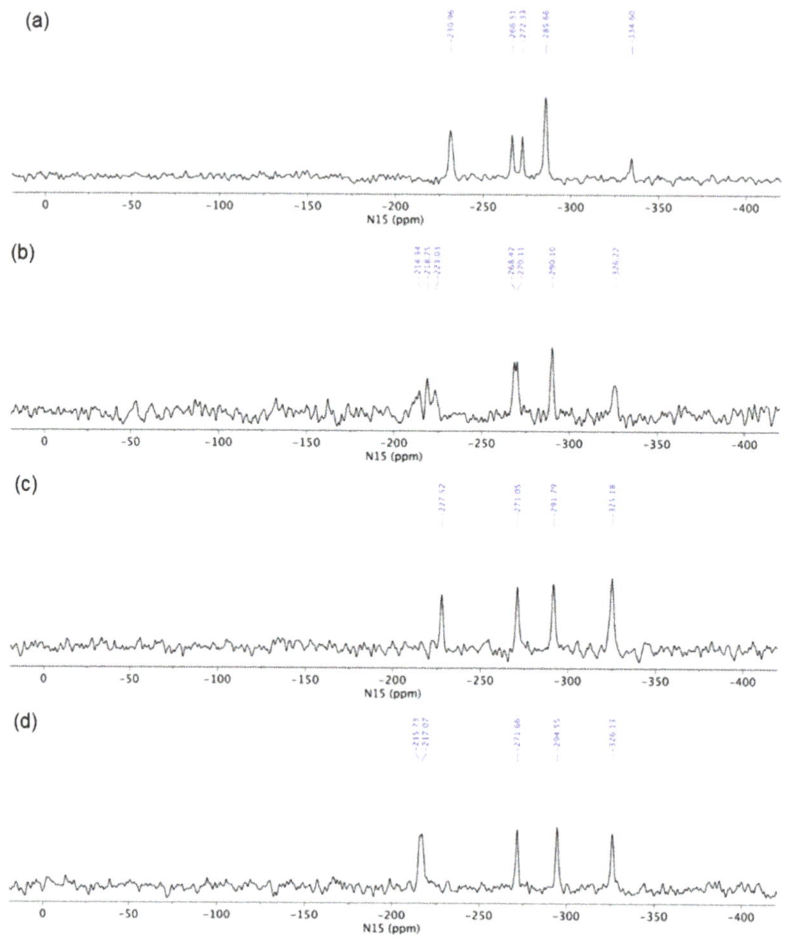

Figure 8. ^{15}N CP MAS ssNMR (^{15}N cross-polarization magic-angle spinning solid-state nuclear magnetic resonance) spectra of (**a**) glasdegib base, (**b**) glasdegib dihydrochloride, (**c**) glasdegib monomaleate and (**d**) glasdegib dimaleate.

The ^{15}N ssNMR spectra of the glasdegib monomaleate and glasdegib dimaleate species were compared to the glasdegib base and dihydrochloride forms (Figure 8). The methylpiperidine nitrogen atoms of both glasdegib monomaleate and glasdegib dimaleate showed ^{15}N chemical shifts similar to glasdegib dihydrochloride, which suggests the protonation of methylpiperidine nitrogen. A chemical shift of the methylpiperidine nitrogen atom was observed at δ_N −325.2 ppm for glasdegib monomaleate species (Figure 8c) and at δ_N −326.1 ppm for glasdegib dimaleate species (Figure 8d). In addition, a small chemical-shift difference was observed for pyridine-like the benzimidazole nitrogen atom when comparing glasdegib monomaleate and glasdegib dimaleate, where dimaleate species showed NMR chemical shifts similar to glasdegib dihydrochloride (compare ^{15}N NMR signals at ca. δ_N −216 ppm).

The ^{15}N LG-CP MAS ssNMR spectra [35–37] were recorded for each glasdegib form, where a short excitation time (200 µs) was used to transfer polarization from the ^{1}H to ^{15}N nuclei. The comparison with the CP MAS spectra of glasdegib derivatives allowed enabled the detection of protonated and unprotonated species (Figure 9). The ^{15}N ssNMR chemical shift of the glasdegib base is consistent with the non-protonated form, as no signal could be observed for the methylpiperidine nitrogen atom at ca. δ_N −335 ppm (Figure 9a). The NMR signals of other nitrogen atoms (urea and benzimidazole nitrogens) were observed at the same chemical shifts as in the ^{15}N CP-MAS spectra (compare Figures 8a and 9a).

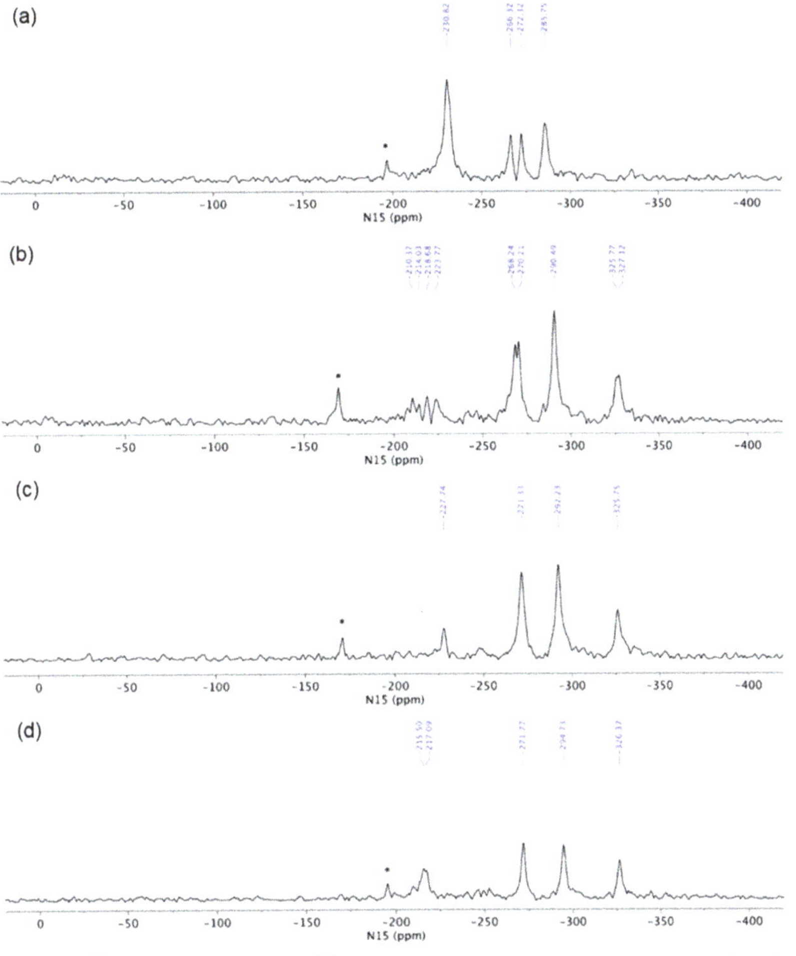

Figure 9. ^{15}N LG-CP MAS ssNMR (^{15}N Lee–Goldburg cross-polarization magic-angle spinning solid-state nuclear magnetic resonance) spectra of (**a**) glasdegib base, (**b**) glasdegib dihydrochloride, (**c**) glasdegib monomaleate and (**d**) glasdegib dimaleate. Note that signals marked with * were attributed to artefacts that correspond to transmitter-frequency offset.

The ^{15}N LG-CP MAS ssNMR spectra confirmed that both monomaleate and dimaleate species correspond to protonated forms of glasdegib (Figures 9c and 9d, respectively). Strong ^{15}N NMR signals were observed for methylpiperidine nitrogen atoms in the case of glasdegib monomaleate at δ_N −325.8 ppm (Figure 9c) as well as in the case of glasdegib dimaleate at δ_N −326.4 ppm (Figure 9d). Furthermore, the pyridine-like benzimidazole nitrogen atom of glasdegib monomaleate species showed a negligible shift when compared to the glasdegib base (δ_N −227.7 ppm; $\Delta\delta_N$ 3 ppm), which suggests that glasdegib monomaleate exists in salt form with its primary protonation site on the methylpiperidine nitrogen atom. Glasdegib dimaleate showed an identical deshielded methylpiperidine nitrogen atom, and interestingly, a remarkable shift in the pyridine-like benzimidazole nitrogen atom (δ_N −216 ppm; $\Delta\delta_N$ 15 ppm) with respect to the glasdegib base.

In essence, the salt/co-crystal properties of glasdegib monomaleate were assessed by comparing its ^{15}N chemical shifts to the glasdegib base and dihydrochloride species. The methylpiperidine nitrogen atoms of glasdegib monomaleate exhibit δ_N −325.8 ppm, which is consistent with the downfield shift of ca. 10 ppm, as observed in the case of glasdegib dihydrochloride. Additionally, the pyridine-like benzimidazole nitrogen atom of the glasdegib monomaleate species showed a negligible shift when compared to the glasdegib base ($\Delta\delta_N$ 3 ppm), which suggests that glasdegib monomaleate exists in salt form with its primary protonation site on the methylpiperidine nitrogen atom. Glasdegib dimaleate showed and identical deshielded methylpiperidine nitrogen atom (δ_N −326.1 ppm), and moreover, a remarkable shift in the pyridine-like benzimidazole nitrogen atom ($\Delta\delta_N$ 15 ppm). The latter implies that despite the low ΔpKa value for the benzimidazole nitrogen/maleic acid pair, the obtained glasdegib dimaleate exists in double-salt form.

3.2.6. X-ray Single-Crystal Determination

We were able to obtain crystals of glasdegib monomaleate and glasdegib dimaleate suitable for the X-ray structural analysis (Figure 10a,b). The crystallographic data are listed in Table 1. In both crystal structures, partially deprotonated maleic acid is present in the form of maleate monoanions with a strong intramolecular O–H···O hydrogen bond (2.386(4)–2.403(2) Å). The C–O distances are within the ranges expected for maleate monoanion.

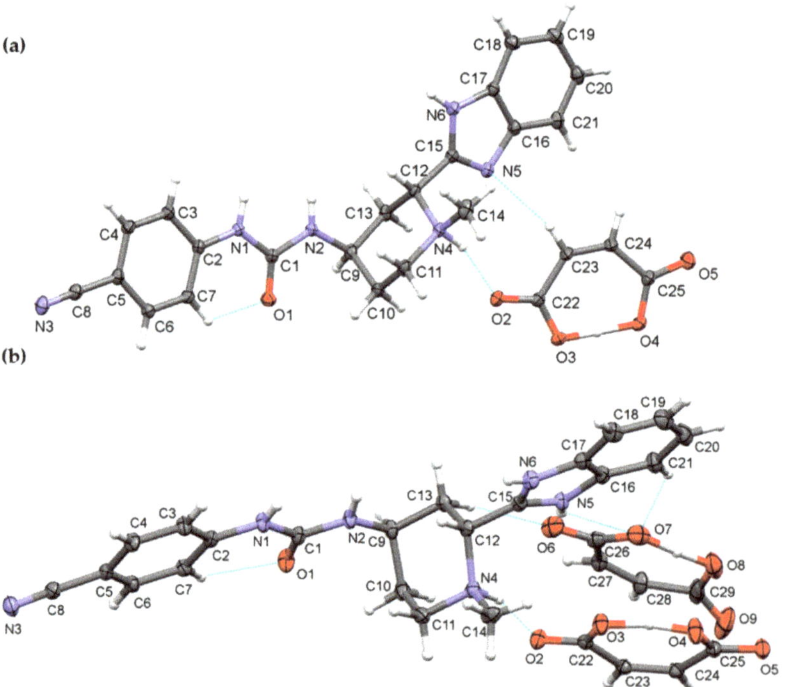

Figure 10. Thermal ellipsoid figures of (**a**) glasdegib monomaleate and (**b**) glasdegib dimaleate drawn at the 30% probability level. The asymmetric unit of glasdegib monomaleate contains one protonated glasdegib molecule and one maleate monoanion. The asymmetric unit of glasdegib dimaleate contains one double-protonated glasdegib molecule and two maleate monoanions. Hydrogen bonds are represented by dashed blue lines.

Compound glasdegib monomaleate crystalizes in monoclinic space group $P2_1$ with one protonated glasdegib molecule and one maleate monoanion in an asymmetric unit (Figure 10a).

The glasdegib molecule is protonated on the methylpiperidine N4 nitrogen atom. In glasdegib monomaleate, a hydrogen-bonded chain is formed along the *c* axis through a series of interactions between a protonated glasdegib molecule and a maleate monoanion (Figure 11). The methylpiperidine NH group of glasdegib is connected to maleate via N4–H4$\cdots$O2 hydrogen bonding and supported by a C23–H23$\cdots$N5 interaction between maleate and a benzimidazole moiety, forming an $R^2_2(9)$ ring motif [38]. Furthermore, glasdegib interacts with the adjacent maleate monoanion through N1–H1$\cdots$O3^i and N6–H6a$\cdots$O5^i interactions with urea and benzimidazole moieties, respectively, supported by C3–H3$\cdots$O2^i and C12–H12$\cdots$O4^i bonding and forming one $R^2_2(12)$ and two $R^2_2(8)$ ring motifs (symmetry code: (i) $x, y, 1 + z$) (Table 2). The chains are connected into layers along the *bc* plane through C18–H18$\cdots$O1^{iii} interactions between the benzimidazole moiety and the urea oxygen atom (symmetry code: (iii) $x, 1 + y, z$) (Figure 11a). Double layers are formed through C11–H11b$\cdots$N3^{ii} interaction, connecting the methylpiperidine moiety of one glasdegib molecule with the cyano-group of the adjacent glasdegib molecule (symmetry code: (ii) $1 - x, \frac{1}{2} + y, 2 - z$) (Figure 11b,c).

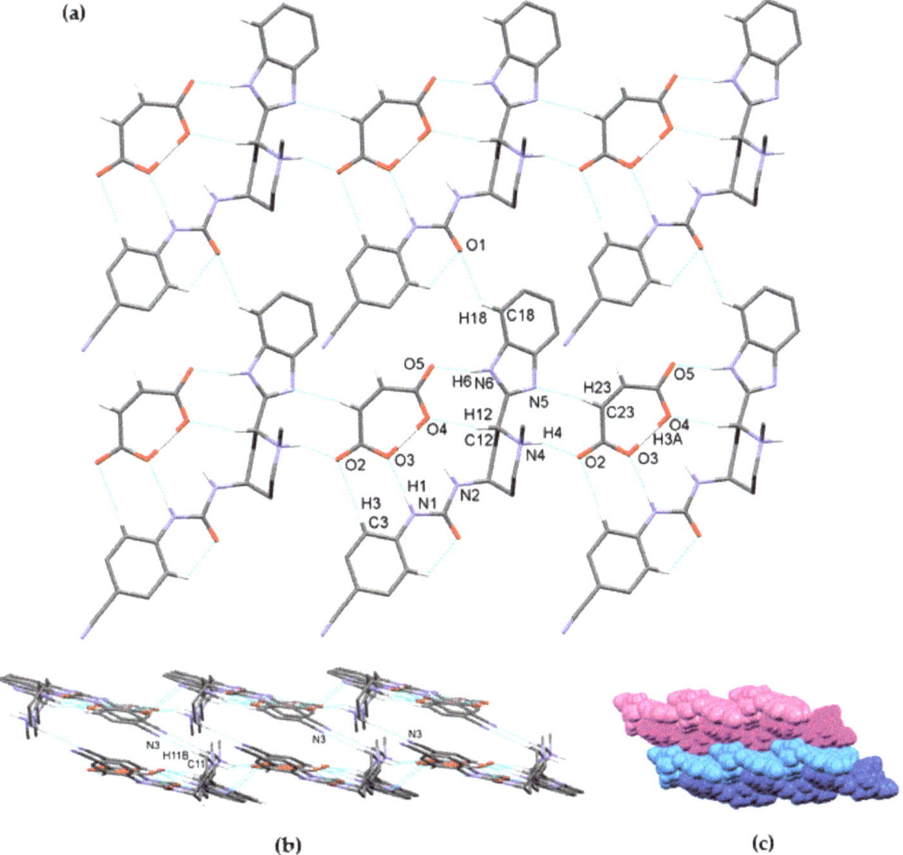

Figure 11. Hydrogen-bond architecture in the glasdegib monomaleate: (**a**) layer formation along *bc* plane; (**b**) formation of double layers via C11–H11b$\cdots$N3 interactions; (**c**) packing of double layers along *a* axis (arbitrary colors; one double layer is presented by light and dark blue and second double layer is represented by light and dark magenta). Hydrogen bonds are represented by dashed blue lines. Hydrogen atoms not involved in the motif shown have been omitted for clarity.

Table 2. Hydrogen bonds for glasdegib monomaleate and glasdegib dimaleate [Å and °].

D–H$\cdots$A	d(D–H)	d(H$\cdots$A)	d(D$\cdots$A)	$\sphericalangle$(DHA)
glasdegib monomaleate				
N1–H1$\cdots$O3^{i}	0.885(13)	2.033(15)	2.892(2)	164(2)
N4–H4$\cdots$O2	0.98(2)	1.78(3)	2.687(2)	151(2)
N6–H6$\cdots$O5^{i}	0.90(3)	1.87(3)	2.762(2)	171(3)
O3–H3A$\cdots$O4	1.16(3)	1.25(3)	2.403(2)	177(3)
C3–H3$\cdots$O2^{i}	0.95	2.54	3.458(3)	162.7
C7–H7$\cdots$O1	0.95	2.25	2.863(3)	121.7
C11–H11B$\cdots$N3^{ii}	0.99	2.42	3.407(3)	172.5
C12–H12$\cdots$O4^{i}	1.00	2.25	3.211(2)	161.9
C18–H18$\cdots$O1^{iii}	0.95	2.56	3.302(3)	135.2
C23–H23$\cdots$N5	0.95	2.54	3.274(3)	134.3
glasdegib dimaleate				
N1–H1$\cdots$O4^{i}	0.891(13)	1.929(14)	2.820(3)	177(4)
N2–H2$\cdots$O5^{i}	0.886(13)	2.122(15)	2.999(3)	170(3)
N4–H4$\cdots$O2	0.99(4)	1.76(4)	2.703(3)	158(3)
N5–H5$\cdots$O6	0.871(13)	1.872(15)	2.736(4)	171(4)
N5–H5$\cdots$O7	0.871(13)	2.56(3)	3.192(4)	130(3)
N6–H6$\cdots$O8^{i}	0.877(13)	2.36(2)	3.153(4)	150(3)
N6–H6$\cdots$O9^{i}	0.877(13)	2.05(3)	2.772(4)	140(3)
O4–H3A$\cdots$O3	1.17(5)	1.23(5)	2.397(3)	170(4)
O8–H7A$\cdots$O7	1.15(5)	1.24(6)	2.386(4)	177(5)
C7–H7$\cdots$O1	0.95	2.22	2.842(4)	122.4
C9–H9$\cdots$O5^{ii}	1.00	2.50	3.326(4)	139.6
C12–H12$\cdots$O5^{i}	1.00	2.45	3.228(4)	134.6
C13–H13B$\cdots$O6	0.99	2.42	3.364(4)	159.0
C21–H21$\cdots$O7	0.95	2.50	3.244(4)	134.8
C28–H28$\cdots$N3^{iii}	0.95	2.60	3.404(5)	142.7

Symmetry codes for glasdegib monomaleate: (i) x, y, $1 + z$; (ii) $1 - x$, $\frac{1}{2} + y$, $2 - z$; (iii) x, $1 + y$, z, and for glasdegib dimaleate: (i) $\frac{1}{2} - x$, $1 - y$, $\frac{1}{2} + z$; (ii) $1 - x$, $-\frac{1}{2} + y$, $\frac{1}{2} - z$; (iii) x, y, $-1 + z$.

Compound glasdegib dimaleate crystalizes in orthorhombic space group $P2_12_12_1$ with one double-protonated glasdegib molecule and two maleate monoanions in an asymmetric unit (Figure 10b). The glasdegib molecule is protonated on the methylpiperidine N4 nitrogen atom as well as on the benzimidazole N5 nitrogen atom. A small structural difference between the monoprotonated vs. diprotonated glasdegib molecule is also evident due to the C15–N5 and C15–N6 distances being 1.315(3) and 1.359(3) Å in glasdegib monomaleate vs. 1.331(4) and 1.328(4) Å in glasdegib dimaleate, respectively. In glasdegib dimaleate, a hydrogen-bonded chain is formed along the c axis through a series of interactions between the double-protonated glasdegib molecule and two maleate monoanions (Figure 12). The methylpiperidine moiety of the glasdegib dication is connected to one maleate anion via N4–H4$\cdots$O2 hydrogen bonding, and this maleate anion is further connected to the adjacent glasdegib dication through N1–H1$\cdots$O4^{i} and N2–H2$\cdots$O5^{i} interactions with the urea moiety supported by a C12–H12$\cdots$O5^{i} interaction with the methylpiperidine moiety, forming $R^2_2(8)$ and $R^1_2(7)$ ring motifs (symmetry code: (i) $\frac{1}{2} - x$, $1 - y$, $\frac{1}{2} + z$) (Figure 12a, Table 2). The benzimidazole moiety interacts with one maleate monoanion through bifurcated N5–H5$\cdots$O6 and N5–H5$\cdots$O7 hydrogen bonding, supported by C13–H13b$\cdots$O6 and C21–H21$\cdots$O7 interactions; thus, each oxygen atom (O6 and O7) is an acceptor of two hydrogen bonds, and $R^1_2(7)$, $R^1_2(6)$ and $R^2_1(4)$ ring motifs are formed. Furthermore, the benzimidazole moiety also interacts with the adjacent maleate monoanion through bifurcated N6–H6$\cdots$O8^{i} and N6–H6$\cdots$O9^{i} hydrogen bonding, forming an $R^2_1(4)$ ring motif. This maleate monoanion also supports the formation of the chain through a C28–H28$\cdots$N3^{iii} interaction with the cyano-group of the adjacent glasdegib dication (symmetry code: (iii) x, y, $-1 + z$). Chain formation is also further supported by almost-parallel $\pi\cdots\pi$ interactions between the phenyl rings of the cyanophenyl and benzimidazole moieties of two adjacent molecules, with a centroid-to-centroid distance of 3.9040(18) Å and ring slippage of 1.413 Å. A supramolecular structure is achieved, connecting the chains via C9–H9$\cdots$O5^{ii} interactions (symmetry code: (ii) $1 - x, -\frac{1}{2} + y, \frac{1}{2} - z$) (Figure 12b,c).

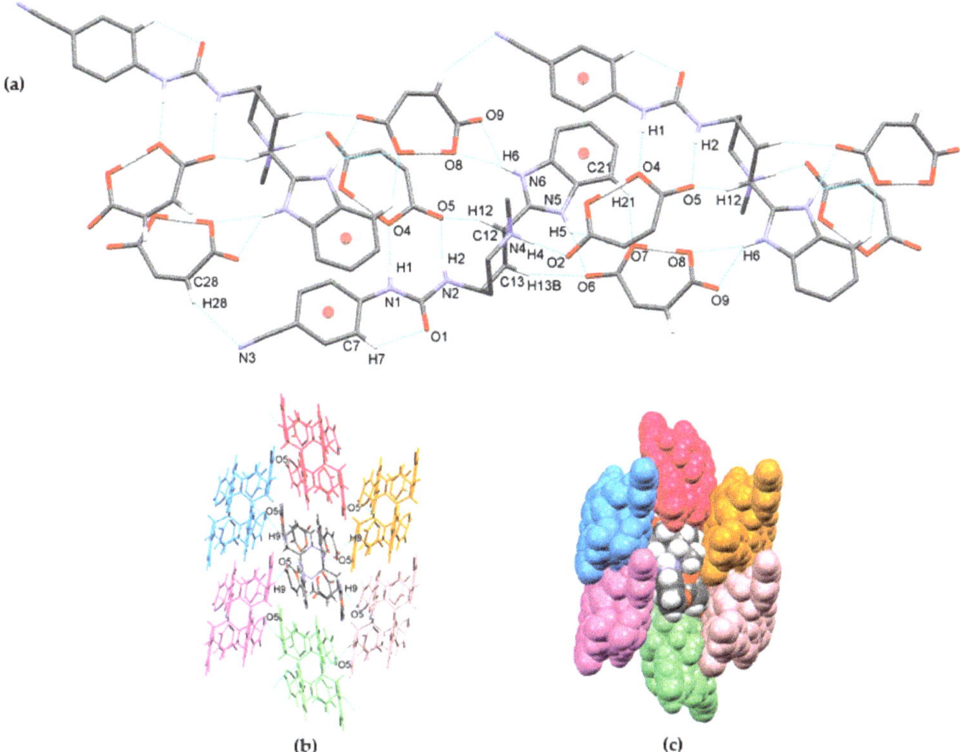

Figure 12. Hydrogen-bond architecture in the glasdegib dimaleate: (**a**) chain formation along *c* axis; (**b**) packing of chains along *ab* plane via C9–H9$\cdots$O5 interactions; (**c**) space-filled presentation of packing of chains (arbitrary colors). Hydrogen bonds are represented by dashed blue lines and $\pi\cdots\pi$ interactions by dashed green lines. Hydrogen atoms not involved in the motif shown have been omitted for clarity.

The crystal structures of glasdegib monomaleate and glasdegib dimaleate differ primarily in their glasdegib:maleate monoanion ratios and in a charge on the glasdegib species. In glasdegib monomaleate, each protonated glasdegib molecule is hydrogen-bonded to two adjacent maleate monoanions, forming a chain along the *c* axis, primarily through N–H$\cdots$O interactions. In glasdegib dimaleate, each double-protonated glasdegib molecule is hydrogen-bonded to four adjacent maleate monoanions, forming a chain along the *c* axis, also primarily through N–H$\cdots$O interactions. Monoprotonated and diprotonated glasdegib species differ in their number of potential NH hydrogen-bond donating sites as well as in their N hydrogen-bond acceptor sites. Different hydrogen-bonding patterns can be observed due to the different behavior of urea NH groups. In glasdegib monomaleate, only one urea NH group is involved in hydrogen bonding, while both urea NH groups are hydrogen-bond donors in glasdegib dimaleate. The urea oxygen atom is in both crystal structures involved only in intramolecular hydrogen bonding. In both structures, the methylpiperidine N atom is protonated and is involved in strong N–H$\cdots$O interactions with maleate monoanion. The main difference regarding hydrogen-bond donor/acceptor sites lies in the benzimidazole group. Nitrogen atom N5 is protonated only in glasdegib dimaleate; thus, the benzimidazole moiety possesses two NH groups as a hydrogen-bond donor. Contrarily, in glasdegib monomaleate, benzimidazole possesses only one NH group acting as hydrogen-bond donor and one N atom acting as hydrogen-bond acceptor. In glasdegib monomaleate, four NH groups form three N–H··· O interactions with maleate monoanion, while in glasdegib dimaleate, five NH groups form seven N–H··· O interactions, with four being bifurcated. A higher number of hydrogen-bonding interactions in the dimaleate form potentially explains the slightly higher stability of this form. Even though in glasdegib dimaleate, two monoanionic maleate ions are present and the glasdegib is double-protonated, as well as possessing a higher number of hydrogen-donating sites, there is an almost negligible difference in the conformation of mono- vs. diprotonated glasdegib species (Figure 13a). Although their conformations are similar, their intermolecular interactions still lead to different packing arrangements; this is already shown by the fact that glasdegib monomaleate and glasdegib dimaleate crystallize in monoclinic and orthorhombic space groups, respectively. In glasdegib monomaleate, the protonated glasdegib molecules are arranged in a head-to-head fashion, while in glasdegib dimaleate, the double-protonated glasdegib molecules are arranged in a head-to-tail fashion (Figure 13b).

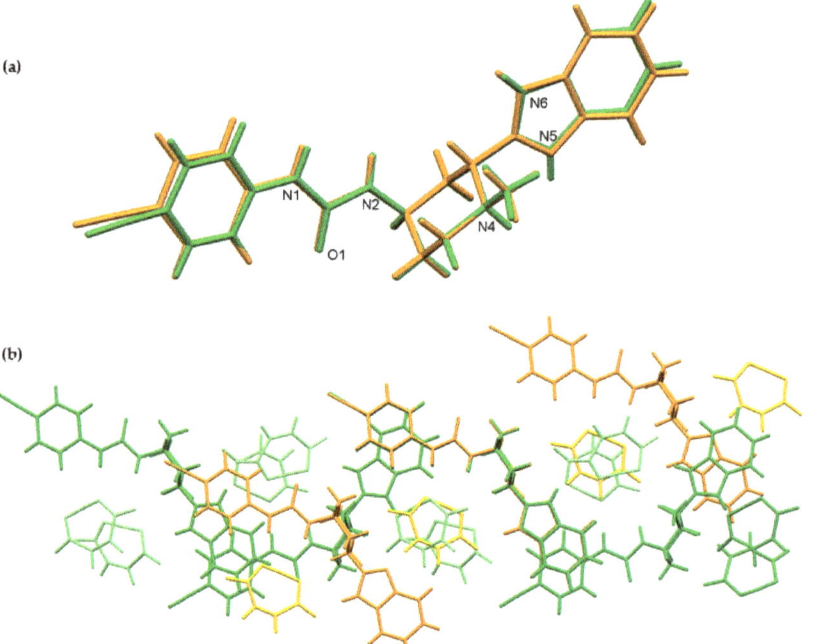

Figure 13. Superposition showing the differences in the conformation of glasdegib monomaleate (orange) and glasdegib dimaleate (green) of (**a**) glasdegib molecule and (**b**) chains along *c* axes, formed primarily by N–H··· O interactions. Maleate monoanions are presented in light orange and light green colors.

3.2.7. Stability Testing

To gain initial insights into the stability of glasdegib dimaleate, we conducted preliminary comparative stress testing with glasdegib monomaleate in a 3-month study. The stress stability testing of both glasdegib monomaleate and glasdegib dimaleate was conducted under storage conditions of 40 °C and 75% RH (open dish). Both samples were analyzed for purity and chiral purity using liquid chromatography methods at four time points: initially (t = 0), and after each month and was completed after 3 months (Table 3). In addition, solid-form purity was also checked wiusingth PXRD.

Table 3. Stability of glasdegib monomaleate and glasdegib dimaleate.

Form Type and Testing Time Point	Chiral Purity [1] [Area%]	Purity [2] [Area%]
glasdegib monomaleate, t = 0	100.00	99.86
glasdegib monomaleate, t = 1 month	99.96	99.81
glasdegib monomaleate, t = 2 months	99.96	99.73
glasdegib monomaleate, t = 3 months	99.96	99.72
glasdegib dimaleate, t = 0	100.00	99.98
glasdegib dimaleate, t = 1 month	100.00	99.97
glasdegib dimaleate, t = 2 months	100.00	99.93
glasdegib dimaleate, t = 3 months	100.00	99.90

[1] Determined via chiral HPLC method. [2] Determined via UHPLC method.

The testing results of both glasdegib monomaleate and glasdegib dimaleate indicated that both forms are stable in terms of chiral purity, indicating that the previously reported epimerization of the dihydrochloride form to (2*S*,4*R*)-epimer [26] does not take place in either maleate form in a solid state. Interestingly, the study showed that the monomaleate form is chemically slightly less stable, as evidenced by the analysis of UHPLC purity, where a slightly higher rise in degradation products was observed for glasdegib monomaleate (purity dropped from a 99.86 area% at the beginning of the testing to a 99.72 area% after 3 months; $\Delta(\Sigma$ impurities) = 0.14%) compared to glasdegib dimaleate (purity dropped from 99.98 area% at the beginning of the testing to 99.90 area% after 3 months; $\Delta(\Sigma$ impurities) = 0.08%). The results obtained using the PXRD measurements indicated that glasdegib dimaleate is fully stable for at least 2 months at 40 °C and 75% RH (Figure S22), while in the case of glasdegib monomaleate, traces of glasdegib dimaleate were already observed after 1 month (Figure S23).

3.2.8. Solubility Testing

The dissolution and solubility of glasdegib monomaleate and glasdegib dimaleate were evaluated at a pH of 1.2, 4.0, 5.5 and 7.0 using the United States Pharmacopeia and European Pharmacopoeia buffers.

At pH = 1.2 (Figure 14), similar dissolution behavior was observed for both the mono and dimaleate form, with solubility slightly rising over the time. After 24 h, glasdegib monomaleate had slightly higher solubility (11.08 mg/mL) compared to the glasdegib dimaleate (10.62 mg/mL).

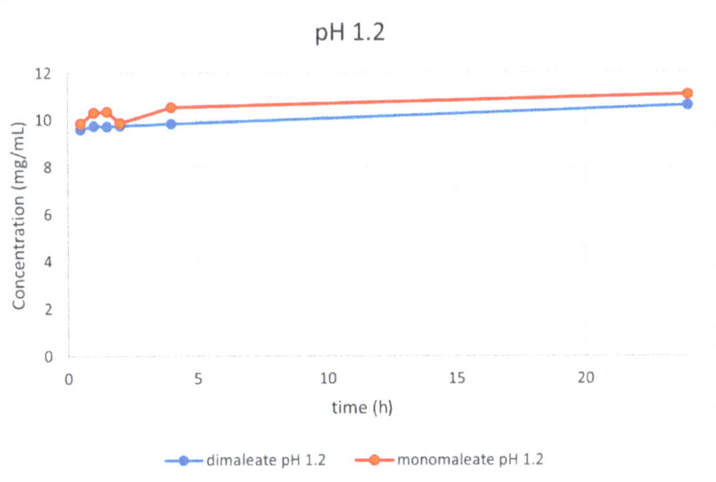

Figure 14. Dissolution testing of glasdegib monomaleate and glasdegib dimaleate at pH = 1.2.

At pH = 4.0 (Figure 15), the dissolution curves were different compared to those obtained at pH = 1.2. In this case, the solubility of both forms was dropping over time. After 24 h, glasdegib monomaleate had higher solubility (2.56 mg/mL) compared to the glasdegib dimaleate (1.68 mg/mL).

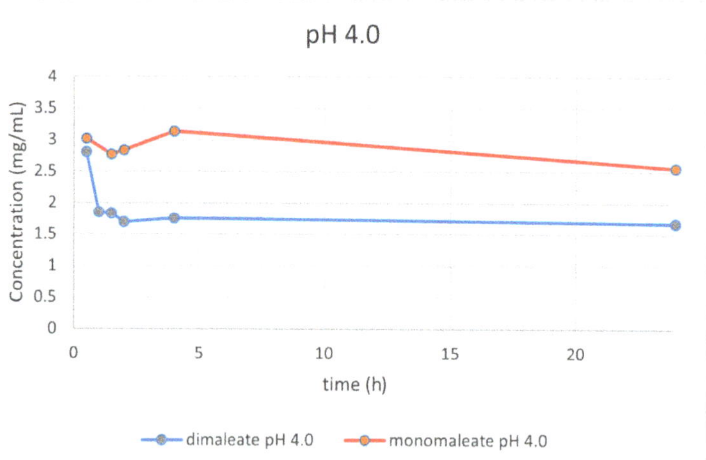

Figure 15. Dissolution testing of glasdegib monomaleate and glasdegib dimaleate at pH = 4.0.

At pH = 5.5 (Figure 16) the dissolution curves were similar compared to those obtained at pH = 1.2, slightly rising over time. After 24 h, glasdegib dimaleate had higher solubility (3.02 mg/mL) compared to the glasdegib monomaleate (2.28 mg/mL).

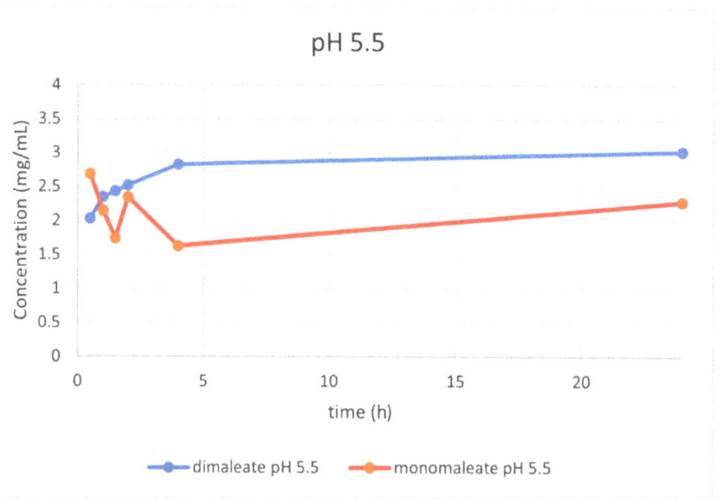

Figure 16. Dissolution testing of glasdegib monomaleate and glasdegib dimaleate at pH = 5.5.

At pH = 7.0 (Figure 17), the dissolution curves revealed that solubility was rising slightly over time after 4 h for both forms. After 24 h, glasdegib monomaleate had slightly lower solubility (0.76 mg/mL) compared to the glasdegib dimaleate (0.79 mg/mL).

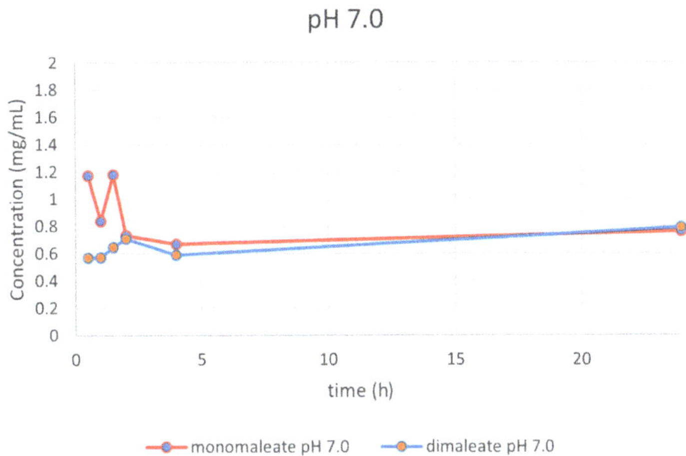

Figure 17. Dissolution testing of glasdegib monomaleate and glasdegib dimaleate at pH = 7.0.

4. Discussion

The formation of novel maleic acid containing a solid form of glasdegib was confirmed via PXRD, IR, Raman and DSC analysis. Indeed, notable differences in the PXRD diffractogram (Figure 2), IR and Raman spectra (Figures 3–6), as well as in the DSC thermograms, were observed (Figure 7) between the known glasdegib monomaleate form and the novel form. As revealed by the solution ^{1}H NMR analysis, the novel solid form had 2:1 stoichiometry between maleic acid and glasdegib. However, the determined stoichiometry of the formed solid brought some ambiguity related to the ionization state of the novel form.

In the past, the pKa difference between base and acid (ΔpKa = pKa $_{\text{protonated base}}$ − pKa $_{\text{acid}}$) was established as one of the key parameters that defines the likelihood of salt formation. In general, it is considered that complexes with ΔpKa > 4 form as salts, while ΔpKa < −1 favors co-crystal formation. In the interim zone where −1 < ΔpKa < 4, both types of species can be formed. Nevertheless, the likelihood of co-crystal formation is higher in the lower part of the scale close to or below ΔpKa = 0 [39]. In the zone where ΔpKa is between 0 and 3, a continuum between neutral and ionized species exits, which can provide acid–base complexes with mixed ionization states [40]. Very recently, such evidence was provided experimentally using ssNMR [41] and single-crystal X-ray determination [42] in the pharmaceutical field on tenofovir alafenamide fumarate.

Glasdegib contains two basic sites that can be protonated by an acid: methylpiperidine nitrogen and benzimidazole nitrogen (Figure 1). The reported pKa values of glasdegib (6.1 for methylpiperidine nitrogen and 1.7 for benzimidazole nitrogen) [24,25] and maleic acid (pK_{a1} = 1.9 and pK_{a2} = 6.3) [29] give ΔpKa values of 4.2 in the case of the methylpiperidine nitrogen/maleic acid pair and −0.2 for the benzimidazole nitrogen/maleic acid pair (more acidic proton in maleic acid is considered; Table 4). The reported pKa values for glasdegib [24,25] do not provide information on which solvent they acquired, which brings some ambiguity to the ΔpKa calculation, because pKa values change in different solvents. Therefore, we also calculated the pKa values for glasdegib and maleic acid using the ChemAxon Marvin Suite [43] in order to obtain solvent bias-free pKa and ΔpKa values. The calculation using the ChemAxon Marvin Suite provided pKa values of 6.67 (methylpiperidine nitrogen) and 3.01 (benzimidazole nitrogen) for glasdegib, while pKa values of 2.85 and 5.75 were obtained for maleic acid. The calculated pKa values were 3.82 in the case of the methylpiperidine nitrogen/maleic acid pair and 0.16 for the benzimidazole nitrogen/maleic acid pair (Table 4). Thus, the calculated pKa data fit well with the measured data, and the obtained ΔpKa values are similar for the reported and calculated values.

Table 4. Calculated ΔpKa values for glasdegib–maleic acid complex considering glasdegib methylpiperidine nitrogen/maleic acid pair and benzimidazole nitrogen/maleic acid pair.

pK_a Protonated Base	pK_{a1} Acid [29]	$\Delta pKa = pKa$ (Protonated Base) $-$ pK_{a1} (Acid) ** [39]
6.1 (methylpiperidine nitrogen) [24,25]	1.9 [29]	4.2
1.7 (benzimidazole nitrogen) [24,25]	1.9 [29]	−0.2
6.67 (methylpiperidine nitrogen) * [43]	2.85 * [43]	3.82
3.01 (benzimidazole nitrogen) * [43]	2.85 * [43]	0.16

* Calculated using ChemAxon Marvin Suite 17.28.0. ** Calculation performed for more acidic proton in maleic acid.

Based on the calculated ΔpKa values for the glasdegib–maleic acid pair, it is obvious that in the case of glasdegib monomaleate, salt will be formed on methylpiperidine nitrogen because ΔpKa = ca. 4 (Table 4). A similar situation can be anticipated in the case of glasdegib dimaleate, where one maleic acid will protonate the methylpiperidine nitrogen, whereas the second maleic acid could either act as a co-former to form a co-crystal, or form a salt with the benzimidazole nitrogen of glasdegib. The calculated probability for the formation of salt on the benzimidazole nitrogen $\mathbf{P(A^-B^+)}$ with the second maleic acid using Cruz-Cabeza equations [39] show that benzimidazole nitrogen should remain unprotonated (the probability of salt formation only 25–31%, Table 5), while the probability of co-crystal formation $\mathbf{P(AB)}$ is three times higher (Table 5). Therefore, the obtained glasdegib dimaleate should be a mixture of salt and co-crystal species: (maleic acid)$^-$·(maleic acid)·(glasdegib)$^+$ = A$^-$AB$^+$, rather than a double-salt form: (maleic acid)$^-$·(maleic acid)$^-$·(glasdegib)$^{++}$ = A$^-$A$^-$B^{++} (Table 5).

Table 5. Calculated probability for salt or co-crystal formation for the protonation of benzimidazole nitrogen with the second maleic acid molecule in the glasdegib–maleic acid 1:2 complex.

	ΔpKa	$\mathbf{P(A^-B^+)}$ [1] (%)	$\mathbf{P(AB)}$ [1] (%)
Reported pKa values.	−0.2	24.6	75.4
Calculated pKa values	0.16	30.7	69.3

[1] Calculated probability (P) value based on Cruz-Cabeza equations [39]: P (AB, %) = $-17 \cdot \Delta pKa + 72$ and P (A$^-$B$^+$, %) = $17 \cdot \Delta pKa + 28$.

To further confirm the structure of glasdegib monomaleate and glasdegib dimaleate, a single-crystal X-ray analysis of both forms was performed. As expected, it confirmed that glasdegib monomaleate exists in salt form with protonated methylpiperidine nitrogen. In the case of glasdegib dimaleate, it affirmed an interesting observation from the ^{15}N ssNMR study that this complex exists as a double salt with protonated methylpiperidine nitrogen and benzimidazole nitrogen.

The confirmed double-salt structure (A$^-$A$^-$B^{++}), instead of a salt-co-crystal species structure (A$^-$AB$^+$), for glasdegib dimaleate by ^{15}N ssNMR and single-crystal X-ray analysis is surprising based on the pKa values of this acid–base pair. This outcome might be attributed to the specific choice of solvents used in the preparation of glasdegib dimaleate, since it is known that the proton transfer process can be solvent-dependent [44] and the choice of solvent plays a very important role in the synthesis of organic salts [45].

Until 2006, the maleate anion was used in 4.2% of marketed drugs containing basic active pharmaceutical ingredients [46]. Similarly, in the period of 2007–2016, the maleate anion was used in 4.3% of drugs that contained basic active pharmaceutical ingredients [47]. Some recent or well-known examples of marketed drugs that contain a maleate anion [48] are afatinib dimaleate (contains two basic sites with pKa values of 8.2 and 5.0) [49], neratinib monomaleate (contains two basic sites with pKa values of 7.65 and 4.66) [50], sunitinib monomaleate (contains one basic site with a p*K*a of 8.95) [51] and enalapril monomalate (contains one basic site with a p*K*a of 5.5) [52]. These data suggest that the maleate anion is used in active pharmaceutical ingredients that contain basic moieties with a p*K*a of 5 or higher, which facilitates salt-species formation. In this respect, glasdegib dimaleate represents and unusual example.

After the determination of the ionization state of glasdegib dimaleate by ^{15}N ssNMR and single-crystal X-ray determination, the physiochemical properties of glasdegib dimaleate were investigated. The stress stability testing at 40 °C and 75% relative humidity demonstrated slightly better chemical and physical stability of glasdegib dimaleate compared to the monomaleate form. Moreover, dissolution testing and solubility determination at pH values of 1.2 (Figure 14) and 7.0 (Figure 17) showed good comparability of both forms, while lower solubility of dimaleate was observed at a pH of 4.0 (Figure 15) and higher solubility was observed at a pH of 5.5 (Figure 16). These properties of glasdegib dimaleate ascertain its suitability for the development of pharmaceutical dosage forms.

5. Conclusions

In summary, for the first time, glasdegib dimaleate was prepared and fully characterized using spectroscopic and thermal analyses, which demonstrated that glasdegib dimaleate exists in double-salt form. This is a surprising finding based on the known pK_a values of glasdegib and maleic acid in the literature. This comparative study of the physicochemical properties of both forms suggested that glasdegib dimaleate has similar aqueous solubility and slightly better stability under stress conditions. These properties affirm the glasdegib dimaleate form as a suitable candidate for the development of pharmaceutical preparation. Finally, the presented study demonstrates how unpredictable the formation of a specific pharmaceutical solid can be in terms of its chemical structure.

6. Patents

This work is based on our International Patent Application WO 2021191278 A1, 30 September 2021.

Supplementary Materials: The following supporting information can be downloaded at: https://www.mdpi.com/article/10.3390/pharmaceutics14081641/s1, Figure S1: DSC and TGA thermogram of glasdegib monomaleate; Figure S2: DSC and TGA thermogram of glasdegib dimaleate; Figure S3: DSC and TGA thermogram of glasdegib base; Figure S4: DSC and TGA thermogram of glasdegib dihydrochloride hydrate; Figure S5: IR spectrum of glasdegib monomaleate, 1800–400 cm^{-1}; Figure S6: IR spectrum of glasdegib dimaleate, 1800–400 cm^{-1}; Figure S7: IR spectrum of glasdegib base, 4000–400 cm^{-1}; Figure S8: IR spectrum of glasdegib base, 1800–400 cm^{-1}; Figure S9: IR spectrum of glasdegib dihydrochloride hydrate, 4000–400 cm^{-1}; Figure S10: IR spectrum of glasdegib dihydrochloride hydrate, 1800–400 cm^{-1}; Figure S11: IR spectrum of maleic acid, 4000–400 cm^{-1}; Figure S12: IR spectrum of maleic acid, 1800–400 cm^{-1}; Figure S13: Raman spectrum of glasdegib base; Figure S14: Raman spectrum of glasdegib dihydrochloride; Figure S15: Raman spectrum of maleic acid; Figure S16: Measured PXRD pattern of glasdegib monomaleate powder; Figure S17: Calculated PXRD pattern from the single-crystal structure of glasdegib monomaleate; Figure S18: Measured PXRD pattern of glasdegib dimaleate powder; Figure S19: Calculated PXRD pattern from the single-crystal structure of glasdegib dimaleate; Figure S20: Measured PXRD pattern of glasdegib base powder; Figure S21: Measured PXRD pattern of glasdegib dihydrochloride powder; Figure S22: Measured PXRD pattern of glasdegib dimaleate powder exposed to stress conditions for 2 months; Figure S23: Measured PXRD pattern of glasdegib monomaleate powder exposed to stress conditions for 1 month; Figure S24: Ultra-high-performance liquid chromatogram of glasdegib for determination of solubility; Figure S25: Chiral high-performance liquid chromatogram for determination of chiral purity; Figure S26: ^{1}H echo MAS NMR spectra of glasdegib base, glasdegib dihydrochloride hydrate, glasdegib monomaleate and glasdegib dimaleate; Figure S27: ^{1}H-NMR spectrum of glasdegib monomaleate in MeOD at 500 MHz; Figure S28: ^{13}C-NMR spectrum of glasdegib monomaleate in MeOD at 125 MHz; Figure S29: ^{1}H-NMR spectrum of glasdegib dimaleate in MeOD at 500 MHz; Figure S30: ^{13}C-NMR spectrum of glasdegib dimaleate in MeOD at 125 MHz; Figure S31: MarvinSketch 17.28 calculated pK_a values for glasdegib; Figure S32: MarvinSketch 17.28 calculated pK_a values for maleic acid. CCDC 2180664 and 2180665 contain the supplementary crystallographic data for this paper. These data can be obtained free-of-charge via www.ccdc.cam.ac.uk/data_request/cif, by emailing data_request@ccdc.cam.ac.uk or by contacting The Cambridge Crystallography Data Centre, 12 Union Road, Cambridge CB2 1EZ, UK; fax: +44-1223-336033.

Author Contributions: Conceptualization, B.P. and Z.Č.; methodology, B.P., D.M., F.P., J.P., Z.K., J.C. and Z.Č.; data curation, B.P., D.M., F.P., Z.K., J.C. and J.P.; funding acquisition, Z.Č.; formal analysis B.P., D.M., F.P., Z.K., J.C. and J.P.; investigation, B.P., D.M., F.P., Z.K., J.C. and J.P.; project administration, Z.Č.; resources, Z.Č.; supervision, Z.Č.; validation, B.P., D.M., F.P., Z.K., J.C. and J.P.; visualization, D.M., F.P., J.P. and Z.Č.; writing—original draft, D.M., F.P., J.P. and Z.Č.; writing—review and editing, B.P., D.M., F.P., J.P., Z.K., J.C. and Z.Č. All authors have read and agreed to the published version of the manuscript.

Funding: This research was funded by Lek a Sandoz company.

Institutional Review Board Statement: Not applicable.

Informed Consent Statement: Not applicable.

Data Availability Statement: Not applicable.

Acknowledgments: The authors gratefully acknowledge Z. Ham for the PXRD measurements; M. Črnugelj for the solution ^{1}H- and ^{13}C-NMR measurements; H. Cimerman and L. Kolenc for the IR, Raman and thermal analysis measurements; K. Gosak for the conducting the synthesis of the analytical standards of glasdegib diastereomeric impurities; and M. Jazbec for their assistance in the glasdegib dimaleate preparation. We thank the EN-FIST Centre of Excellence, Ljubljana, Slovenia, for use of their SuperNova diffractometer.

Conflicts of Interest: The authors declare no conflict of interest. The funders had no role in the design of the study; in the collection, analyses, or interpretation of the data; in the writing of the manuscript; or in the decision to publish the results.

References

1. U.S. Department of Health and Human Services, National Institutes of Health, National Cancer Institute. Acute Myeloid Leukemia Treatment (PDQ®)—Patient Version; National Cancer Institute, Rockville, MD, USA. 2022. Available online: https://www.cancer.gov/types/leukemia/patient/adult-aml-treatment-pdq (accessed on 29 July 2022).
2. Ling, Y.; Zhang, Z.; Zhang, H.; Huang, Z. Protein Kinase Inhibitors as Therapeutic Drugs in AML: Advances and Challenges. *Curr. Pharm. Des.* **2017**, *23*, 4303–4310. [CrossRef] [PubMed]
3. Ferguson, F.; Gray, N. Kinase inhibitors: The road ahead. *Nat. Rev. Drug Discov.* **2018**, *17*, 353–377. [CrossRef] [PubMed]
4. Fiorentini, A.; Capelli, D.; Saraceni, F.; Menotti, D.; Poloni, A.; Olivieri, A. The time has come for targeted therapies for AML: Lights and shadows. *Oncol. Ther.* **2020**, *8*, 13–32. [CrossRef] [PubMed]
5. Yu, J.; Jiang, P.Y.Z.; Sun, H.; Zhang, X.; Jiang, Z.; Li, Y.; Song, Y. Advances in targeted therapy for acute myeloid leukemia. *Biomark. Res.* **2020**, *8*, 17. [CrossRef] [PubMed]
6. Carter, J.L.; Hege, K.; Yang, J.; Kalpage, H.A.; Su, Y.; Edwards, H.; Hüttemann, M.; Taub, J.W.; Ge, Y. Targeting multiple signaling pathways: The new approach to acute myeloid leukemia therapy. *Signal Transduct. Target. Ther.* **2020**, *5*, 288. [CrossRef] [PubMed]
7. Griffiths, E.A.; Carraway, H.E.; Chandhok, N.S.; Prebet, T. Advances in non-intensive chemotherapy treatment options for adults diagnosed with acute myeloid leukemia. *Leuk. Res.* **2020**, *91*, 106339. [CrossRef] [PubMed]
8. Megías-Vericat, J.E.; Martínez-Cuadrón, D.; Solana-Altabella, A.; Montesinos, P. Precision medicine in acute myeloid leukemia: Where are we now and what does the future hold? *Expert Rev. Hematol.* **2020**, *13*, 1057–1065. [CrossRef]
9. Himmelstein, G.; Mascarenhas, J.; Marcellino, B.K. Alternatives to intensive treatment in patients with AML. *Clin. Adv. Hematol. Oncol.* **2021**, *19*, 526–535. Available online: https://www.hematologyandoncology.net/archives/august-2021/alternatives-to-intensive-treatment-in-patients-with-aml/ (accessed on 31 July 2022).
10. Attwood, M.M.; Fabbro, D.; Sokolov, A.V.; Knapp, S.; Schiöth, H.B. Trends in kinase drug discovery: Targets, indications and inhibitor design. *Nat. Rev. Drug Discov.* **2021**, *20*, 839–861. [CrossRef]
11. Yeoh, Z.H.; Bajel, A.; Wei, A.H. New drugs bringing new challenges to AML: A brief review. *J. Pers. Med.* **2021**, *11*, 1003. [CrossRef]
12. Roskoski, R. Properties of FDA-approved small molecule protein kinase inhibitors: A 2021 update. *Pharmacol. Res.* **2021**, *165*, 105463. [CrossRef]
13. Solana-Altabella, A.; Ballesta-López, O.; Megías-Vericat, J.E.; Martínez-Cuadrón, D.; Montesinos, P. Emerging FLT3 inhibitors for the treatment of acute myeloid leukemia. *Expert Opin. Emerg. Drugs* **2022**, *27*, 1–18. [CrossRef]
14. Kayser, S.; Levis, M.J. Updates on targeted therapies for acute myeloid leukaemia. *Br. J. Haematol.* **2022**, *196*, 316–328. [CrossRef]

15. Ayala-Aguilera, C.C.; Valero, T.; Lorente-Macias, A.; Baillache, D.J.; Croke, S.; Unciti-Broceta, A. Small molecule kinase inhibitor drugs (1995–2021): Medical indication, pharmacology, and synthesis. *J. Med. Chem.* **2022**, *65*, 1047–1131. [CrossRef]

16. Jones, C.S.; La Greca, S.; Li, Q.; Munchhof, M.J.; Reiter, L.A. Benzimidazole Derivatives. International Patent Application WO 09004427 A2, 8 January 2009.

17. Munchhof, M.J.; Li, Q.; Shavnya, A.; Borzillo, G.V.; Boyden, T.L.; Jones, C.S.; LaGreca, S.D.; Martinz-Alsina, L.; Patel, N.; Pelletier, K.; et al. Discovery of PF-04449913, a potent and orally bioavailable inhibitor of smoothened. *ACS Med. Chem. Lett.* **2012**, *3*, 106–111. [CrossRef]

18. Peng, Z.; Wong, J.W.; Hansen, E.C.; Puchlopek-Dermenci, A.L.A.; Clarke, H.J. Development of a concise, asymmetric synthesis of a smoothened receptor (SMO) inhibitor: Enzymatic transamination of a 4-piperidinone with dynamic kinetic resolution. *Org. Lett.* **2014**, *16*, 860–863. [CrossRef]

19. Gras, J.G. Hedgehog signaling inhibitor, treatment of myelodysplastic syndrome, treatment of chronic myelomonocytic leukemia, treatment of acute myeloid leukemia, treatment of myelofibrosis. *Drugs Future* **2017**, *42*, 265–274. [CrossRef]

20. Hoy, S.M. Glasdegib: First Global Approval. *Drugs* **2019**, *79*, 207–213. [CrossRef]

21. Goldsmith, S.R.; Lovell, A.R.; Schroeder, M.A. Glasdegib for the treatment of adult patients with newly diagnosed acute myeloid leukemia or high-grade myelodysplastic syndrome who are elderly or otherwise unfit for standard induction chemotherapy. *Drugs Today* **2019**, *55*, 545–562. [CrossRef]

22. Wolska-Washer, A.; Robak, T. Glasdegib in the treatment of acute myeloid leukemia. *Future Oncol.* **2019**, *15*, 3219–3232. [CrossRef]

23. Fersing, C.; Mathias, F. Update on glasdegib in acute myeloid leukemia—Broadening horizons of Hedgehog pathway inhibitors. *Acta Pharm.* **2022**, *72*, 9–34. [CrossRef]

24. Highlights of Prescribing Information. DaurismoTM (Glasdegib) Tablets, for Oral Use. Available online: https://www.accessdata.fda.gov/drugsatfda_docs/label/2018/210656s000lbl.pdf (accessed on 12 May 2022).

25. Product Monograph Including Patient Medication Information, Daurismo®, Glasdegib Tablets. Available online: https://www.pfizer.ca/sites/default/files/202202/Daurismo_PM_EN_250530_21Jan2022.pdf (accessed on 12 May 2022).

26. Hansen, E.C.; Seadeek, C.S. Crystalline Forms of 1-((2R, 4R)-2-(1H-benzo[d]imidazol-2-yl)-1-methylpiperidin-4-yl)-3-(4-cyanophenyl)urea Maleate. International Patent Application WO 2016170451 A1, 27 October 2016.

27. Moreton, C. Poor Solubility—Where do we stand 25 years after the 'rule of five'? *Am. Pharm. Rev.-Rev. Am. Pharm. Bus. Technol.* **2021**, *24*, 16–22.

28. Peklar, B. Dimaleate Form of 1-((2R,4R)-2-(1H-benzo[d]imidazol-2-yl)-1-methylpiperidin-4-yl)-3-(4-cyanophenyl)urea. International Patent Application WO 2021191278 A1, 30 September 2021.

29. Hussain, S.; Pinitglang, S.; Bailey, T.S.; Reid, J.D.; Noble, M.A.; Resmini, M.; Thomas, E.W.; Greaves, R.B.; Verma, C.S.; Brocklehurst, K. Variation in the pH-dependent pre-steady state and steady-state kinetic characteristics of cysteine-proteinase mechanism: Evidence for electrostatic modulation of catalytic site function by the neighboring carboxylate anion. *Biochem. J.* **2003**, *372*, 735–746. [CrossRef] [PubMed]

30. Agilent Technologies Ltd. *CrysAlisPro, Version 1.171.36.28*; Agilent Technologies: Yarnton, UK, 2013. Available online: https://www.agilent.com/cs/library/usermanuals/Public/CrysAlis_Pro_User_Manual.pdf (accessed on 8 May 2022).

31. Sheldrick, G.M. SHELXT—Integrated space-group and crystal-structure determination. *Acta Crystallogr.* **2015**, *A71*, 3–8. [CrossRef]

32. Sheldrick, G.M. Crystal structure refinement with SHELXL. *Acta Crystallogr.* **2015**, *C71*, 3–8. [CrossRef]

33. Dolomanov, O.V.; Bourhis, L.J.; Gildea, R.J.; Howard, J.A.K.; Puschmann, H. OLEX2: A complete structure solution, refinement and analysis program. *J. Appl. Crystallogr.* **2009**, *42*, 339–341. [CrossRef]

34. Spek, A.L.J. Single-crystal structure validation with the program PLATON. *J. Appl. Crystallogr.* **2003**, *36*, 7–13. [CrossRef]

35. Lee, M.; Goldburg, W. Nuclear magnetic resonance line narrowing by a rotating RF field. *Phys. Rev.* **1965**, *140*, 1261–1271. [CrossRef]

36. Ladizhansky, V.; Vega, S. Polarization transfer dynamics in Lee–Goldburg cross polarization under magnetic resonance experiments on rotating solids. *J. Chem. Phys.* **2000**, *112*, 7158–7168. [CrossRef]

37. Van Rossum, B.-J.; de Groot, C.P.; Ladizhansky, V.; Vega, S.; de Groot, H.J.M. A method for measuring heteronuclear (1H–13C) distances in high speed MAS NMR. *J. Am. Chem. Soc.* **2000**, *122*, 3465–3472. [CrossRef]

38. Bernstein, J.; Davis, R.E.; Shimoni, L.; Chang, N.L. Patterns in hydrogen bonding: Functionality and graph set analysis in crystals. *Angew. Chem. Int. Ed.* **1995**, *34*, 1555–1573. [CrossRef]

39. Cruz-Cabeza, A.J. Acid–base crystalline complexes and the pK_a rule. *CrystEngComm* **2012**, *14*, 6362–6365. [CrossRef]

40. Childs, S.L.; Stahly, G.P.; Park, A. The salt-cocrystal continuum: The influence of crystal structure on ionization state. *Mol. Pharm.* **2007**, *4*, 323–338. [CrossRef]

41. Lengauer, H.; Makuc, D.; Šterk, D.; Perdih, F.; Pichler, A.; Trdan Lušin, T.; Plavec, J.; Časar, Z. Co-crystals, salts or mixtures of both? The case of tenofovir alafenamide fumarates. *Pharmaceutics* **2020**, *12*, 342. [CrossRef]

42. Wang, J.-W.; Liu, L.; Yu, K.-X.; Bai, H.-Z.; Zhou, J.; Zhang, W.-H.; Hu, X.; Tang, G. On the single-crystal structure of tenofovir alafenamide mono-fumarate: A metastable phase featuring a mixture of co-crystal and salt. *Int. J. Mol. Sci.* **2020**, *21*, 9213. [CrossRef]

43. ChemAxon Marvin Suite 17.28.0, ChemAxon Home Page. Available online: http://www.chemaxon.com (accessed on 19 June 2022).

44. Clark, J.H.; Jones, C.W. Solvent-dependent proton pransfer in a strongly hydrogen bonded fluoride complex. *J. Chem. Soc. Chem. Commun.* **1990**, *24*, 1786–1787 [CrossRef]
45. Black, S.N.; Collier, E.A.; Davey, R.J.; Roberts, R.J. Structure, solubility, screening, and synthesis of molecular salts. *J. Pharm. Sci.* **2007**, *96*, 1053–1068. [CrossRef]
46. Paulekuhn, G.S.; Dressman, J.B.; Saal, C. Trends in active pharmaceutical ingredient salt selection based on analysis of the orange book database. *J. Med. Chem.* **2007**, *50*, 6665–6672. [CrossRef]
47. Ule, M.; Časar, Z. Analysis of the selection of active pharmaceutical ingredients' salts in medicinal products registered in the USA between 2007 and 2016. *Farm. Vestn.* **2018**, *69*, 175–187.
48. Bharate, S.S. Carboxylic acid counterions in FDA-approved pharmaceutical salts. *Pharm. Res.* **2021**, *38*, 1307–1326. [CrossRef]
49. Australian Public Assessment Report for Afatinib (as Dimaleate). Available online: https://www.tga.gov.au/sites/default/files/auspar-afatinib-dimaleate-140414.pdf (accessed on 31 July 2022).
50. Australian Product Information NERLYNX®(Neratinib) Tablets. Available online: https://www.tga.gov.au/sites/default/files/auspar-neratinib-as-maleate-020512-pi.pdf (accessed on 31 July 2022).
51. Highlights of Prescribing Information. SUTENT®(Sunitinib Malate) Capsules, Oral. Available online: https://www.accessdata.fda.gov/drugsatfda_docs/label/2011/021938s13s17s18lbl.pdf (accessed on 31 July 2022).
52. Loftsson, T.; Thorisdóttir, S.; Fridriksdóttir, H.; Stefánsson, E. Enalaprilat and enalapril maleate eyedrops lower intraocular pressure in rabbits. *Acta Ophthalmol.* **2010**, *88*, 337–341. [CrossRef] [PubMed]

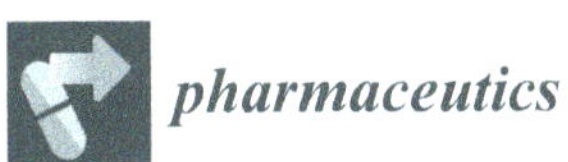 *pharmaceutics*

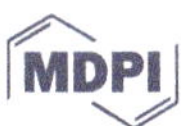

Article

Fabrication and Characterization of Tedizolid Phosphate Nanocrystals for Topical Ocular Application: Improved Solubilization and In Vitro Drug Release

Mohd Abul Kalam [1,2], Muzaffar Iqbal [3,4], Abdullah Alshememry [1,2], Musaed Alkholief [1,2] and Aws Alshamsan [1,2,*]

[1] Nanobiotechnology Unit, Department of Pharmaceutics, College of Pharmacy, King Saud University, Riyadh 11451, Saudi Arabia; makalam@ksu.edu.sa (M.A.K.); aalshememry@ksu.edu.sa (A.A.); malkholief@ksu.edu.sa (M.A.)

[2] Department of Pharmaceutics, College of Pharmacy, King Saud University, Riyadh 11451, Saudi Arabia

[3] Department of Pharmaceutical Chemistry, College of Pharmacy, King Saud University, Riyadh 11451, Saudi Arabia; muziqbal@ksu.edu.sa

[4] Bioavailability Unit, Central Lab, College of Pharmacy, King Saud University, Riyadh 11451, Saudi Arabia

* Correspondence: aalshamsan@ksu.edu.sa

Citation: Kalam, M.A.; Iqbal, M.; Alshememry, A.; Alkholief, M.; Alshamsan, A. Fabrication and Characterization of Tedizolid Phosphate Nanocrystals for Topical Ocular Application: Improved Solubilization and In Vitro Drug Release. *Pharmaceutics* 2022, 14, 1328. https://doi.org/10.3390/pharmaceutics14071328

Academic Editor: Hisham Al-Obaidi

Received: 30 May 2022
Accepted: 21 June 2022
Published: 23 June 2022

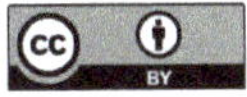

Abstract: Positively charged NCs of TZP (0.1%, w/v) for ocular use were prepared by the antisolvent precipitation method. TZP is a novel 5-Hydroxymethyl-Oxazolidinone class of antibiotic and is effective against many drug-resistant bacterial infections. Even the phosphate salt of this drug is poorly soluble, therefore the NCs were prepared for its better solubility and ocular availability. P188 was found better stabilizer than PVA for TZP-NCs. Characterization of the NCs including the particle-size, PDI, and ZP by Zeta-sizer, while morphology by SEM indicated that the preparation technique was successful to get the optimal sized (151.6 nm) TZP-NCs with good crystalline morphology. Mannitol (1%, w/v) prevented the crystal growth and provided good stabilization to NC_1 during freeze-drying. FTIR spectroscopy confirmed the nano-crystallization did not alter the basic molecular structure of TZP. DSC and XRD studies indicated the reduced crystallinity of TZP-NC_1, which potentiated its solubility. An increased solubility of TZP-NC_1 ($25.9\ \mu gmL^{-1}$) as compared to pure TZP ($18.4\ \mu gmL^{-1}$) in STF with SLS. Addition of stearylamine (0.2%, w/v) and BKC (0.01%, w/v) have provided cationic (+29.4 mV) TZP-NCs. Redispersion of freeze-dried NCs in dextrose (5%, w/v) resulted in a clear transparent aqueous suspension of NC_1 with osmolarity ($298\ mOsm\cdot L^{-1}$) and viscosity (21.1 cps at 35 °C). Mannitol (cryoprotectant) during freeze-drying could also provide isotonicity to the nano-suspension at redispersion in dextrose solution. In vitro release in STF with SLS has shown relatively higher (78.8%) release of TZP from NC_1 as compared to the conventional TZP-AqS (43.4%) at 12 h. TZP-NC_1 was physically and chemically stable at three temperatures for 180 days. The above findings suggested that TZP-NC_1 would be a promising alternative for ocular delivery of TZP with relatively improved performance.

Keywords: tedizolid phosphate; nanocrystals; thermal characterization; in vitro release; stability

1. Introduction

Due to the unique anatomy and physiology of eyes, the development of ocular drug delivery (ODD) is a major challenge to the formulators [1–4]. The aim of ODD is to maximize drug concentration in the ocular sites to achieve maximum beneficial effects at low dosing [5,6]. Some conventional formulations for ODD including the eye drops (solutions, suspensions, emulsions, etc.) containing poorly soluble or low permeable drugs have shown low ocular availability (approximately 1–5% of the applied dose) of the drugs [7,8]. Due to normal physiology of eyes (blinking, precorneal loss, nasolacrimal drainage), the conventional formulations are not fully successful to attain effective therapeutic drug concentrations in the eyes [9,10].

Application of ointments, to some extent, could resolve the poor ocular bioavailability issues though they cause blurring of vision [11]. Due to the unique anatomical structure and natural defense mechanism of eyes, the permeation of applied drugs is hindered and leads to poor ocular bioavailability [8,12,13].

Nanotechnology-based ODD approaches have successfully overcome the problems associated with the conventional dosage forms and enhance the ocular bioavailability of poorly soluble drugs [14]. The technologies including the supercritical assisted (CO_2-mediated) method to produce the nano-formulations (e.g., liposomes) [2,15–17], nanocrystals by top-down or bottom-up techniques [5,7,9,15,18], polymeric micelles [19], polymeric nanoparticles (NPs) [3,20], nanoemulsion [1,21], microemulsion [22], solid lipid nanoparticles [10,23,24], niosomes [25,26], dendrimer nanoparticles [27,28] etc.

Despite having some drawbacks, the nanocarriers in ODD have been explored well. The perspective of nanocrystals (NCs) for ocular use has been comparatively unnoticed because of the availability of numerous established bioadhesive polymeric NPs [8,29]. Therefore, we developed the NCs of tedizolid phosphate (BCS Class-IV) for topical ocular application. The potential application of NCs for oral and parenteral delivery has already been carried-out [9,30–33]. It also shows substantial possibilities for ODD [7]. The application of NCs has not been well explored for ocular applications, hence it opened new opportunities for the cure of ocular diseases [4,9,34,35].

The NCs can be a successful alternative to the pharmaceutical industries as they have achieved commercial success to some extent in oral, parenteral, and ODD of highly lipophilic, poorly soluble, and low permeable drugs [30,36]. We believe that in near future the NCs would support the development of robust and effective therapies for ocular disorders. The NCs-based formulations have received prime interest as a feasible and commercial substitute as evidenced by some product patents based on NCs of poorly soluble drugs [37,38].

The NCs-suspension of poorly soluble drugs such as dexamethasone, hydrocortisone and prednisolone have improved the ocular bioavailability as compared to their microcrystalline suspensions and aqueous solutions [9,39]. The NCs as ODDS can increase ocular retention, transcorneal permeation and hence bioavailability [7,9]. The positively charged formulations may interact electrostatically with the ocular mucin layer which can prolong the retention of the formulation that facilitates the increased transcorneal permeation and improve the ocular bioavailability of the drug [8]. Also, the high absolute zeta-potentials provide potential stability to any colloidal systems.

Above finding encouraged us to develop the NCs for topical ocular application of a highly lipophilic and poorly aqueous soluble drug (TZP). The TZP is a novel 5-Hydroxymethyl-Oxazolidinone class of antibiotic [40] having excellent antibacterial activity against *Mycobacterium tuberculosis* [41], methicillin-resistant *Staphylococcus aureus* (MRSA) and many other Gram-positive bacteria [42] including their infections in the eyes [8]. TZP is a prodrug and converted into tedizolid (TDZ) in vivo by alkaline and acid phosphatases, hence either TZP or TDZ can be chosen for its ocular uses [43]. The chemical structure of TDZ is represented in Figure 1.

The prodrug TDZ was chosen as its phosphate salt has better aqueous solubility [40] and hence, would result in an improved ocular availability of the active moiety. Also, the presence of modified side chains at the C5 site of the oxazolidinone nucleus of TDZ provides an excellent activity against vancomycin-resistant *enterococci* [44] and some linezolid-resistant strains [45].

The antisolvent precipitation method was adopted to develop the NCs of TZP [7]. The PVA and P188 were tried as stabilizers to optimize the NCs. The developed TZP-NCs were characterized and evaluated for their suitability and potential as nanosystems for the ocular delivery of TZP.

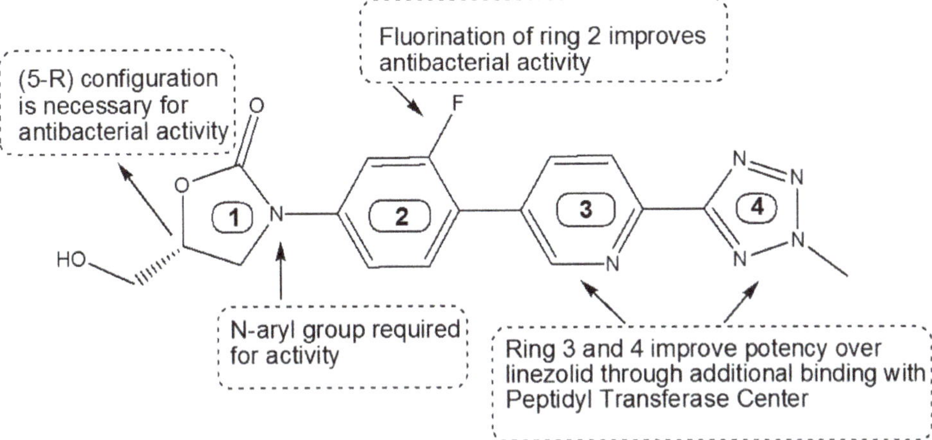

Figure 1. The chemical structure of TDZ, where 1–4 symbolizes the different aromatic rings present in the structure of TDZ. Ring-1 represents the oxazolidinone nucleus; Ring-2 is the meta-fluorine and para-oriented electron withdrawing group; Ring-3 is the pyridine ring and Ring-4 is the tetrazole ring.

2. Materials and Methods

2.1. Materials

Tedizolid base (CAS: 856866-72-3) and tedizolid phosphate ($C_{17}H_{15}FN_6O_6P$; MW 450.32 Da) (CAS: 856867-55-5) with more than 98% purity, were purchased from "Beijing Mesochem Technology Co. Ltd. (Beijing, China)". Tween-80 (CAS: 9005-65-6) and HPLC grade methanol (CAS: 67-56-1) were purchased from "BDH Ltd. (Poole, England)" Polyvinyl alcohol (Mw 16,000) (CAS: 9002-89-5), Poloxamer-188 (Pluronic-F68) (CAS: 9003-11-6), Chloroform (CAS: 67-66-3), Ethanol (CAS: 64-17-5), Dimethyl Sulfoxide (CAS: 67-68-5), Polyvinylpyrrolidone-K30 (CAS: 9003-39-8), Vit-E-TPGS (CAS: 9002-96-4), Sodium Lauryl Sulfate (CAS: 151-21-3), and Benzalkonium chloride (CAS:63449-41-2) were purchased from Sigma Aldrich, St. Louis, MO, USA. Stearylamine (CAS: 124-30-1) was purchased from Alpha Chemika, Mumbai, India. Mannitol (CAS: 69-65-8) was purchased from Qualikems Fine Chem Pvt. Ltd. (Vadodara, India). Purified water was obtained using a Milli-Q® water purifier (Millipore, Molsheim, France). All other chemicals and solvents were of analytical grade and HPLC grade, respectively.

2.2. Methods

2.2.1. Chromatographic Analysis of TZP

A reverse phase (RP) high-performance liquid chromatography (HPLC) with UV-detection (at 251 nm wavelength) was used for the quantification of TZP after slight modification of the reported HPLC method [46]. In brief, the HPLC system (Waters® 1500-series controller, Milford, MA, USA) was used, which was equipped with a UV-detector (Waters® 2489, dual absorbance detector, Milford, MA, USA), a binary pump (Waters® 1525, Milford, MA, USA), automated sampling system (Waters® 2707 Autosampler, Milford, MA, USA). The HPLC system was monitored by "Breeze software". The TZP was analyzed by injecting 30 μL of the supernatant into the analytical column. An RP, C_{18} column (Macherey-Nagel 250 × 4.6 mm, 5 μm) at 40 °C was used. The mobile phase consisted of 65:35 v/v of 0.02 M Sodium acetate buffer (the pH was adjusted to 3.5 by Hydrochloric acid) and acetonitrile was pumped isocratically at 1 mL/min of flow rate. The total run time was 10 min. The standard stock solution of TZP was prepared in methanol (100 μgmL^{-1}) and working standard solutions (0.25–50 μgmL^{-1}) were prepared by serial dilution of the stock solution with 65:35, v/v mixture of mobile phase. The results of the method were briefly explained in Supplementary Materials.

2.2.2. Preparation of Nanocrystals

The antisolvent precipitation method (bottom up technique) was used to prepare the nanocrystals (NCs) of TZP [31,47]. Accurately weighed 10 mg of TZP was dissolved in 1: 1, v/v, mixture of chloroform and ethanol with 0.2 mL of Dimethyl Sulfoxide (DMSO). This solution (2 mL) was added drop-wise (1.5 mL/min) into 20 mL of aqueous phase containing varying concentrations (0.5 to 2.5%, w/v) of stabilizers (P188 and PVA) at continuous magnetic stirring (800 rpm) to obtain a homogenous suspension. The mixture was homogenized (IKA®-WERKE, GMBH & Co., Staufen, Germany) for 5 min at 21,000 rpm, followed by pulsative probe sonication (Sonics & Materials, Inc., Newtown, CT, USA) at 40% power for 60 s (10 s each cycle) on ice bath. The probe sonication during this process provided added stability to the TZP-NCs by minimizing the metastable zone for TZP and its super-saturation level. Organic to aqueous phase ratio was 1:9, v/v. The organic solvents were then evaporated by continuous magnetic stirring (12 h) at room temperature to get the suspension of NCs. The suspended NCs were purified by washing (in triplicate) with Milli-Q® water to get rid of the excess stabilizers, and collected using ultracentrifugation (Preparative ultracentrifuge, WX-series by Hitachi Koki, Ibaraki, Japan) at 4 °C for 20 min and at 30,000 rpm. The obtained pellets of NCs were then resuspended in 10 mL of Milli-Q® water containing different concentrations of mannitol (0, 1, 2.5 and 5%, w/v) as protectant during freeze-drying (FreeZone-4.5 Freeze Dry System, Labconco Corporation, Kansas, MO, USA). The freeze-dried and free flowing product was then stored at −20 °C for further characterization.

2.2.3. Measurement of Average Size, Polydispersity-Index and Zeta-Potential

The particle size (hydrodynamic diameter) and polydispersity-index (PDI) of the NCs were measured by Differential Light Scattering (DLS) technique using Zetasizer Nanoseries, (Nano-ZS, Malvern Instruments, Worcestershire, UK). The results are the mean particle size, which is the intensity versus average diameter/thickness of the NCs majority population, and PDI is the measure of the size distribution width. The suspension of NCs was diluted with Milli-Q® water to get their appropriate concentration and the mean values were calculated from three measurements. The zeta-potential (ZP) of the NCs was measured by the same instrument at ambient temperature in the original dispersion medium of the NCs (aqueous solution of stabilizer with and without mannitol). The installed software (DTS Version 4.1, Malvern, Worcestershire, UK) with this instrument automatically measured the electrophoretic mobility of the NCs and transformed it to zeta potential using the "Helmholtz-Smoluchowski equation".

2.2.4. Scanning Electron Microscopy (SEM)

The morphological characteristics of the NCs were visually observed by micrographs of the samples obtained through SEM (Zeiss EVO LS10, Cambridge, UK) imaging following the gold-sputter technique. In this technique, the dried samples were coated with gold in the "Q-150R Sputter Unit" from "Quorum Technologies Ltd. (East Sus-sex, UK)" in Argon atmosphere at 20 mA for 1 min. Micrographs were at the accelerating voltage of 5 kV and 20–60 KX of magnification.

2.3. Differential Scanning Calorimetry (DSC)

Thermal analysis by DSC was carried out on the pure drug (TZP), Poloxamer-188 (P188), mannitol, physical mixture of TZP, P188, and mannitol (PM) and freeze-dried NC_1 using DSC-8000 (Perkin Elmer Instruments, Shelton, CT, USA) at 10 °C·min^{-1} scan rate. Approximately 2.5–5 mg of weighed samples were hermetically sealed in aluminum pans for this purpose. The DSC was calibrated with pure Indium (having a 156.60 °C melting point and 6.80 cal·g^{-1} heat of fusion). The DSC curves were obtained at 10 °C·min^{-1} scanning rate over 40–280 °C temperature range under the inert atmosphere purged with N_2 at 20 mL·min^{-1} of flow rate. The results from the obtained curves were further analyzed by the installed software Pyris V-11.

2.4. Fourier Transform Infrared Spectroscopy (FTIR)

The FTIR spectra of pure drug (TZP), Poloxamer-188 (P188), mannitol, physical mixture of TZP, P188, and mannitol (PM) and freeze-dried NC_1 using a BRUKER Optik GmBH (Model ALPHA, Ettlingen, Germany) attached with the software OPUS Version-7.8. The analytes were triturated Potassium bromide (KBr) in 1:100 (w/w) ratio using mortar and pestle; thereafter, the mixture was compressed to pellets by hydraulic press. The spectra of the pellets were obtained from 4000 to 500 cm^{-1} wavenumber using 2 cm^{-1} resolutions.

2.5. Powdered X-ray Diffraction (PXRD)

The powder X-ray diffractions of the above-mentioned samples were carried out by Ultima-IV Diffractometer (Rigaku, Inc., Tokyo, Japan) over the $2\theta(°)$ range from 3 to 60 at 0.5 degree/min of scan rate to examine the crystallinity of the samples. The X-ray tube (anode material) was Cu with Ka2 elimination of 0.154 nm, monochromatized with the graphite crystal. The diffraction pattern was obtained at 40 mA of tube current and 40 kV of tube voltage for the generator with step scan mode (step size 0.02° and counting time was 1 s per step).

Furthermore, the crystallite size of NC_1 as compared to TZP-pure was determined using the data obtained by XRD analysis [48] following the Scherrer Equation (1):

$$D = \frac{K\lambda}{\beta cos\theta} \tag{1}$$

where D = average size of crystallite size, K = Scherrer constant "(i.e., 0.68 to 2.08, 0.94 for spherical crystallites with cubic symmetry)", λ = wavelength of X-ray, $CuKa2$ = 1.5406 Å, β = the line broadening at FWHM in radians which describes the transmission characteristics of an optical band-pass filter and θ = Bragg's angle.

2.6. Physicochemical Characterization of Suspension of NCs

The equivalent amount of the freeze-dried NC_1 (freeze-dried with 1%, w/v mannitol) was suspended in 5%, w/v dextrose solution to get a final TZP concentration (0.1%, w/v). Benzalkonium chloride (BKC, 0.01%, w/v) was added to the suspension as preservative [49]. The clarity/transparency of the NC_1 suspension was examined visually under normal light against dark and white. The pH was checked at room temperature and steady state using the pH meter (Mettler Toledo MP-220, Greifensee, Switzerland), which was previously calibrated with standard buffer solutions of pH 4.0, 7.0, and 10.0. Osmolarity, that is the measure of solute concentration (the number of Osmoles of solute/L of a solution (Osml·L^{-1}), was measured by Osmometer (Fiske Associate Inc., Waterford, Pennsylvania, USA) and viscosity of the NC_1 suspension was determined by "Sine-wave VIBRO VISCOMETER, Model SV-10, having range 0.3~10,000 mPa·s or cP, A & D Co. Ltd., Tokyo, Japan)" by the Tuning-fork vibration method. In this method the viscosity with high accuracy is determined through the detection of the driving electric current which resonates the two sensor plates at 30 Hz constant frequency and less than 1 mm of amplitude. The viscosity of the samples was determined at non-physiological ($25 \pm 1\ °C$) and ocular physiological temperatures ($35 \pm 1\ °C$) [50]. All the measurements were performed in triplicate.

2.7. Solubility of Tedizolid Phosphate (TZP)

Solubility of TZP was evaluated by preparing saturated solutions in STF and STF with SLS (0.5%, w/v). The STF was obtained by dissolving 6.8 g of NaCl, 2.2 g of $NaHCO_3$, 1.4 g of KCl and 0.08 g of $CaCl_2·2H_2O$ in 1000 mL of purified water [8,51] to get the STF. The excess amount of pure TZP and NC_1, were put into 1 mL of each medium in triplicate in glass vials. Each mixture was vortexed and put for 72 h in an orbital shaking (100 strokes per min) water bath maintained at $37 \pm 1\ °C$ (Julabo® SW22, Seelbach, Germany). After 72 h, the orbital shaking was stopped and the vials were left for 24 h, then centrifuged at 6000 rpm for 20 min to settle down the undissolved solid remains [52]. Thereafter, supernatants were collected, filtered through 0.45 μ filtration unit (Millipore, Molsheim,

France) and used to quantify the TZP contents by HPLC-UV method [46] as mentioned in the Supplementary Materials.

2.8. In Vitro Release Study

The bioavailability of drugs from any formulation finally depends on the in vitro release of the drug, therefore the release pattern of TZP-NCs was determined. Considering the drug-content the weighed amounts of freeze-dried NC_1 were suspended in 1 mL of dextrose solution (5%, w/v) to get 0.1%, w/v of drug concentration. To evaluate the comparative release profiles, the conventional suspension of TZP (TZP-AqS) was prepared in dextrose solution (5%, w/v) where polyvinyl alcohol (0.5%, w/v) and mannitol (1%, w/v) were added as wetting/suspending and iso-osmotic agents, respectively. The formulation (1 mL of each) was put into the Spectra/Por® Dialysis Membrane (Standard RC Tubing, MWCO 12 KDa). Two ends of dialysis tubing were closed using Spectra/Por® Closures. Formulations containing dialysis tubing were put into beakers (three for each formulation) containing 50 mL release medium (simulated tear fluid (STF, pH 7.4) with 0.5%, w/v, Sodium Lauryl Sulfate (SLS)). The set of beakers were placed in shaking (100 rpm) water-bath maintained at 35 ± 1 °C (ocular physiological temperature). The dissolution and diffusion of TZP from the tubing in the release medium was assayed by taking 1 mL samples at predetermined time points. Same volume of fresh release medium (kept at 35 ± 1 °C) was added back into the beakers after each sampling to maintain the sink condition and constant volume of the medium. The samples were centrifuged for 5 min at 13,500 rpm. The supernatants were collected and analyzed by HPLC-UV [46]. Drug release (%DR) was calculated by the following Equation (2), and the cumulative amount of TZP released (%) from the formulations was plotted against time. Each formulation was analyzed in triplicate ($n = 3$).

$$\%DR = \frac{Conc.\ (\mu g/mL) \times Dilution\ Factor \times Volume\ of\ STF\ (mL)}{Initial\ dose\ of\ TZP\ used\ for\ the\ experiment\ (\mu g)} \times 100 \qquad (2)$$

A model independent mathematical approach was used to compare the release profiles of TZP from NC_1 and TZP-AqS, the percentage dissolution efficiency (%DE) was used in this study. The calculations of %DEs were performed for each formulation. The mean %DE for the products with 95% CI was compared by measuring the differences between the mean %DE and CI of the two formulations. If the differences of average %DEs and 95% CI are within the set limits ($\pm 10\%$) then the dissolution profiles of TZP-AqS and test (TZP-NC_1) are considered as equivalent [53,54]. The "%DE" was calculated by Equation (3). The calculated %DEs were further analyzed statistically by GraphPad Prism V-5 (GraphPad Software, Inc., San Diego, CA, USA)

$$\%DE = \frac{\int_{t1}^{t2} Q.dt}{Q_{100} \times (t_2 - t_1)} \times 100 \qquad (3)$$

where, Q is the percentage of drug dissolved. DE is the area under the dissolution curve between the time points t_1 and t_2, percentage of maximum dissolution Q_{100}. The area under the curve is calculated by a model independent method (trapezoidal) by following Equation (4). Where t_i was the ith time point, Q_i was the percentage of the dissolved drug at time t_i. Furthermore, the calculated

$$AUC = \sum_{i=0}^{i=n} \frac{[t_1 - t_{ti-1}]\ [Q_{i-1} + Q_i]}{2} \qquad (4)$$

For the determination of release kinetics and mechanism of drug release, the in vitro release data were fitted into different kinetic models such as the zero-order, first-order, Korsmeyer-Peppas and Hixson-Crowell models. From the values of slopes and co-efficient of correlations (R^2) of the kinetic plots obtained by different models, the release-exponent (*n*-value) was calculated, which provided the idea about the drug release mechanism.

2.9. Stability Study

The stability study of the NC_1 was performed following published reports about the nanocrystals with an intention to evaluate the stability of NC_1 in terms of average size, PDI, ZP, and drug content [16,32,55]. Freeze-dried NC_1 (10 mg) was packed in different tightly closed amber colored glass containers and stored at $4 \pm 2\,°C$, $25 \pm 1\,°C$ and $37 \pm 1\,°C$ for 180 days. Alteration in the above parameters were evaluated at 7 days, 30 days, 90 days and 180 days for stability testing of the developed nanocrystals. The stored freeze-dried sample (NC_1) was redispersed in 5%, w/v dextrose solution to evaluate the said parameters.

2.10. Statistical Analysis

The results of the experiment were presented as mean with standard deviation ($\pm$SD), unless otherwise indicated. Statistical analysis was performed using GraphPad Prism V-5 (GraphPad Software, Inc., San Diego, CA, USA). The data were compared by Student's *t*-test and statistical significance among them was considered at $p < 0.05$.

3. Results and Discussion

3.1. Formulation Development and Characterization

The process optimization of nano-crystallization was performed by preparing the seven types of TZP-NCs with different stabilizers (Table 1a). Physical characterization (particle-size, polydispersity, and zeta-potential) of the prepared NCs were performed. Considering the required physical characteristics, the batches prepared with PVA and P188 were found better as shown in Table 1a. The better performance of these two stabilizers (P188 and PVA) might be attributed to their higher HLB (>24) values that could avoid the steric barrier between the phases.

Table 1. Physical characterization of the preliminary batches of nanocrystals prepared (using 10 mg of TZP) by homogenization (10 min) at 21,500 rpm with different stabilizers (**a**); and with PVA and POL (**b**).

Batches	Stabilizers (mg)/Concentrations (%, *w/v*)	Physical Characterization		
		Particle Size (nm)	Polydispersity Index	Zeta Potential (mV)
(a) Preliminary trials of NCs * with 1.0 % (*w/v*) stabilizers				
NC-P188	Polxamer-188	495.3 ± 23.5	0.265 ± 0.011	-16.2 ± 2.8
NC-PVA	PVA	514.8 ± 29.4	0.375 ± 0.023	-6.8 ± 1.9
NC-P407	Poloxamer-407 (F127)	614.6 ± 72.5	0.419 ± 0.012	-14.1 ± 3.2
NC-PVP	Polyvinylpyrrolidone K_{30}	596.6 ± 45.2	0.279 ± 0.005	$+5.5 \pm 2.1$
NC-TPGS	Vit-E TPGS	675.2 ± 77.6	0.439 ± 0.018	$+9.7 \pm 2.6$
NC-SLS	Sodium lauryl sulfate	579.5 ± 36.7	0.512 ± 0.029	-1.2 ± 0.8
NC-Tween	Tween-80	563.7 ± 43.6	0.468 ± 0.008	-8.4 ± 2.4
(b) Optimization of NCs * prepared with POL * or PVA * as stabilizers (Mean $\pm$ SD, *n* = 3)				
NC-POL1	100 (0.5%, *w/v*)	715.2 ± 61.7	0.458 ± 0.024	-6.6 ± 3.5
NC-POL2	200 (1.0%, *w/v*)	481.7 ± 58.4	0.252 ± 0.021	-17.2 ± 5.6
NC-POL3	400 (2.0%, *w/v*)	603.0 ± 70.4	0.396 ± 0.006	-18.6 ± 4.0
NC-POL4	500 (2.5%, *w/v*)	600.5 ± 65.2	0.442 ± 0.009	-19.9 ± 6.9
NC-PVA1	100 (0.5%, *w/v*)	745.2 ± 89.1	0.403 ± 0.027	-0.6 ± 2.4
NC-PVA2	200 (1.0%, *w/v*)	613.8 ± 65.7	0.375 ± 0.019	-7.6 ± 3.4
NC-PVA3	400 (2.0%, *w/v*)	556.6 ± 59.5	0.328 ± 0.023	-6.3 ± 4.2
NC-PVA4	500 (2.5%, *w/v*)	507.6 ± 45.9	0.292 ± 0.007	-8.8 ± 3.9

* TZP = Tedizolid phosphate, NCs = Nanocrystals, PVA = Polyvinyl alcohol and POL = Poloxamer-188.

Therefore, two batches, consisting of P188 (NC-POL1 to NC-POL4) and PVA (NC-PVA1 to NC-PVA4), were further processed and the results are presented in Table 1b. Among these formulations, NC-POL2 (1% *w/v*, P188) and NC-PVA4 (2.5% *w/v*, PVA) were found better according to the physical characteristics (Table 1b). The physical characteristics suggested that NCs prepared with 1% w/v, of P188 had better characteristics than those prepared with 2.5% w/v, of PVA. This might be due to the good stabilizing property of P188, which could be able to protect the NCs from any steric hindrance. Therefore, NCs prepared using P188 (1% w/v) were further processed, by changing the durations of homogenization (at 21,500 rpm) and probe sonication (at 40% power) for the optimization purpose. The results of physical characterization and drug content analysis suggested that the NCs-3 batch, which was homogenized for 10 min at 21,500 rpm and sonicated for 60 s (6 cycles, each cycle of 10 s) was the best one (Table 2). The NCs prepared by applying 60 s probe sonication increase their stability by minimizing both the metastable zone and the super-saturation level that is a vital reason for nucleation and crystal growth [47]. Therefore, NCs-3 batch (Table 2) was chosen and freeze-dried with different concentrations of mannitol (as protectant) for further characterization (Table 3). Based on physical characterizations and drug content of the different preparations of NCs-3 batch, the NC_1 (with 1%, w/v mannitol) was selected as the best-optimized nanocrystals for the intended purpose. The freeze-dried NC_1 was further suspended in 5%, w/v dextrose solution for further physicochemical characterization associated with ocular application.

Table 2. Physical characterization of the NCs prepared using P188 at 1%, w/v (200 mg in each case) with varying durations of homogenization and probe sonication (Mean $\pm$ SD, $n = 3$) without mannitol.

Nanocrystals (NCs)	TZP (mg)	Homogenization Time (min) at 21,500 rpm	Sonication Time (s); 10 s Each Cycle	Physical Characterization (Mean $\pm$ SD, $n = 3$)			
				Particle Size (nm)	Polydispersity Index	Zeta Potential (mV)	TZP Content (%)
NCs-1	10	5	40	565.3 $\pm$ 42.7	0.428 $\pm$ 0.073	-5.8 ± 2.3	90.9 $\pm$ 1.5
NCs-2	10	7.5	50	389.5 $\pm$ 58.4	0.401 $\pm$ 0.021	-6.7 ± 3.9	90.1 $\pm$ 2.6
NCs-3	10	10	60	150.4 $\pm$ 18.3	0.231 $\pm$ 0.006	-13.5 ± 1.5	96.7 $\pm$ 1.2
NCs-4	10	15	70	147.5 $\pm$ 11.5	0.249 $\pm$ 0.012	-10.6 ± 9.9	92.4 $\pm$ 2.8

Table 3. Physical characterization and drug content of the different preparations of NCs-3 (TZP 10 mg and P188 at 1%, w/v) with Benzalkonium chloride (0.01%, w/v), stearylamine (0.2%, w/v of total formulation) and varying concentrations of mannitol (Mean $\pm$ SD, $n = 3$).

Nanocrystals (NCs)	Particle Size (nm)		PDI		Zeta Potential (mV)		TZP (%) Contents	
	Freeze Drying		Freeze Drying		Freeze Drying		Freeze Drying	
	Before	After	Before	After	Before	After	Before	After
NC_0 (No mannitol)	150.4 $\pm$ 18.3	153.7 $\pm$ 16.6	0.231 $\pm$ 0.006	0.237 $\pm$ 0.003	+26.3 $\pm$ 5.1	+28.07 $\pm$ 5.0	93.1 $\pm$ 2.8	93.3 $\pm$ 2.8
NC_1 (1%, w/v mannitol)	151.6 $\pm$ 17.5	154.3 $\pm$ 17.9	0.237 $\pm$ 0.005	0.243 $\pm$ 0.009	+29.4 $\pm$ 3.9	+31.64 $\pm$ 3.8	96.2 $\pm$ 2.5	96.4 $\pm$ 2.5
$NC_{2.5}$ (2.5%, w/v mannitol)	157.5 $\pm$ 19.4	161.1 $\pm$ 19.3	0.344 $\pm$ 0.012	0.351 $\pm$ 0.016	+27.5 $\pm$ 5.6	+29.21 $\pm$ 5.6	92.4 $\pm$ 3.0	92.6 $\pm$ 2.9
NC_5 (5%, w/v mannitol)	160.8 $\pm$ 18.7	163.2 $\pm$ 20.7	0.358 $\pm$ 0.016	0.365 $\pm$ 0.019	+28.9 $\pm$ 5.2	+30.87 $\pm$ 5.2	91.2 $\pm$ 2.6	91.6 $\pm$ 2.1

As we noticed, the prepared NCs (Table 2) had shown the negative zeta-potentials which may obstruct its ocular use. Due to repulsive forces between the negative surface charges on the NCs and negatively charged mucin layer on ocular surfaces, the formulation would not retain for a long time. Therefore, stearylamine (0.2%, w/v of total formulation) was added to induce positive charge on the surface of NCs [11]. The obtained formulations have shown high magnitudes of positive zeta potentials ranging from +26.3 to +31.6 mV (Table 3). Such positively charged formulations can interact electrostatically with the ocular mucin layer/mucosa that would prolong the ocular retention of the NCs that facilitate its increased transcorneal permeation and ultimately improve the ocular bioavailability of the active form of the drug (tedizolid, TDZ). Also, the high magnitude of positive zeta-potential would provide potential stability to the colloidal system of the NCs.

In this final formulation BKC (0.01%, w/v) was added as a preservative to avoid any growth of microorganisms introduced unintentionally in the treatment interval. Among different preservatives for ophthalmic preparations, BKC is the frequently used one, especially in multi-dose containers, due to its broad-spectrum antimicrobial property [56]. Apart from preservative action, BKC also stabilizes such ocular NCs. Additionally, being a cationic molecule, BKC resulted in positively charged NCs [7]. Moreover, BKC at 0.1%, *w/v* concentration was found virucidal for different adenovirus types [57]. Recently, the broad-spectrum antiviral activity of BKC (in nanodroplet form) against SARS-CoV-2 and other enveloped viruses was also established [58]. Moreover, BKC belongs to a class of quaternary ammonium compounds, therefore, it induced a positive charge to the NCs which was required to improve the electrostatic repulsion among the dispersed NCs (provided stabilization) and to enhance the electrostatic interaction of the NCs with the negatively charged mucin layer of corneal/ocular surface [7]. This interaction would prolong the precorneal/corneal retention of the NCs to provide a sustained release and transcorneal permeation of the drug. These were the reasons why we chose BKC as a preservative in the present investigation.

The antisolvent precipitation is an example of the Bottom-up technique to prepare the NCs, following the principle of controlled precipitation due to the addition of solvent (organic solution containing drug) antisolvent (aqueous solutions of the stabilizers), and evaporation of the organic solvent. The organic solvents were then evaporated by continuous magnetic stirring (12 h) at room temperature to get the suspension of NCs. The supercritical fluid process (SCF) has an advantage over this process in terms of rapid removal of fluids and solvents without requiring extensive drying steps as compared to other solvent precipitation methods. It works with supercritical carbon dioxide (SCO$_2$, at temperature $\approx$31.1 °C and pressure 73.8 bar) for most pharmaceuticals. Due to the low polarity of SCO$_2$, the solubilization of lipophilic drugs are easy to form the solution and passing of the drug solution through the capillary tube into an ambient surroundings forms the fine/small particles [9,16]. The SCF technology was successful to improve the flurbiprofen loading into soft contact lens (SCL) and consequently its prolonged release from the lens [59]. Also, the SCF assisted liposomes were prepared for the ocular delivery of ampicillin and ofloxacin [17].

The simple and low-cost instrumentation, low energy consumption, and very low generation of heat are a few important features of the antisolvent precipitation technique. Due to low heat generation, this method was used for heat-sensitive/thermolabile drugs also [47]. Through this method, by applying magnetic stirring, homogenization and sonication could produce the particles/crystals in the submicron to nano-range. Here, precipitation occurs in the region of high turbulence and forceful mixing of the two phases during homogenization and sonication. When the two liquid phases mix with each other, the antisolvent causes the precipitation of TZP as fine crystalline structures, which was also reported previously [60]. In this technique, the selection of stabilizer, speed and duration of solvent-antisolvent mixing, ratio of solvent-antisolvent and of course the ratio of powdered drug/stabilizer and any interaction between these, are important process parameters [61]. The stabilizers with high HLB-values are commonly employed for the preparation of NCs of highly lipophilic drugs [62]. Therefore, we tried PVA, PVP-K30, P188, P407, Vit-E-TPGS, SLS and Tween-80 to prepare the NCs of TZP through this technique. Out of these, P188 and PVA were found to produce well-stabilized and comparatively smaller-sized NCs of TZP as evidenced by the size measurement (Table 1b). Out of the two chosen stabilizers (PVA and P188), P188 was found better one as it produced smaller-sized nanocrystals as compared to the same concentrations of PVA, where we found little larger, elongated and rod-shaped NCs as shown in Figure 2a, which might be due to the inherent property of PVA and comparatively its lower HLB value than that of P188. The unusual, larger, and rosette-shaped structures can be seen in the SEM image of pure PVA at low (7.27 KX) magnification (Figure 2b). The results of SEM imaging were in agreement with the average sizes and polydispersity of the NCs as determined by Zetasizer suggesting that the process and formulation variables for the NCs were optimized in the proper way. The SEM images of pure TZP and TZP-NCs prepared at varying duration of homogenization and probe sonication, respectively are also represented in Figure 3. These images endorsed that the increasing homogenization and sonication time could stabilize the crystals due to relatively smaller size and smooth surfaces. It also justifies that the P188 (1%, *w/v*) has better stabilized the NCs in their nano-sized form without changing the crystallinity of TZP, which was also discussed in previous reports [63,64].

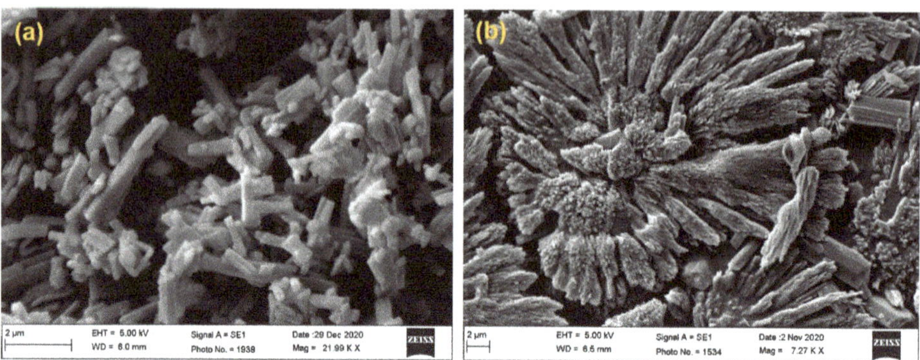

Figure 2. SEM images of elongated and rod-shaped NCs (**a**); unusual, larger, and rosette-shaped NCs (**b**). Both these NCs were stabilized by PVA (1%, w/v) alone.

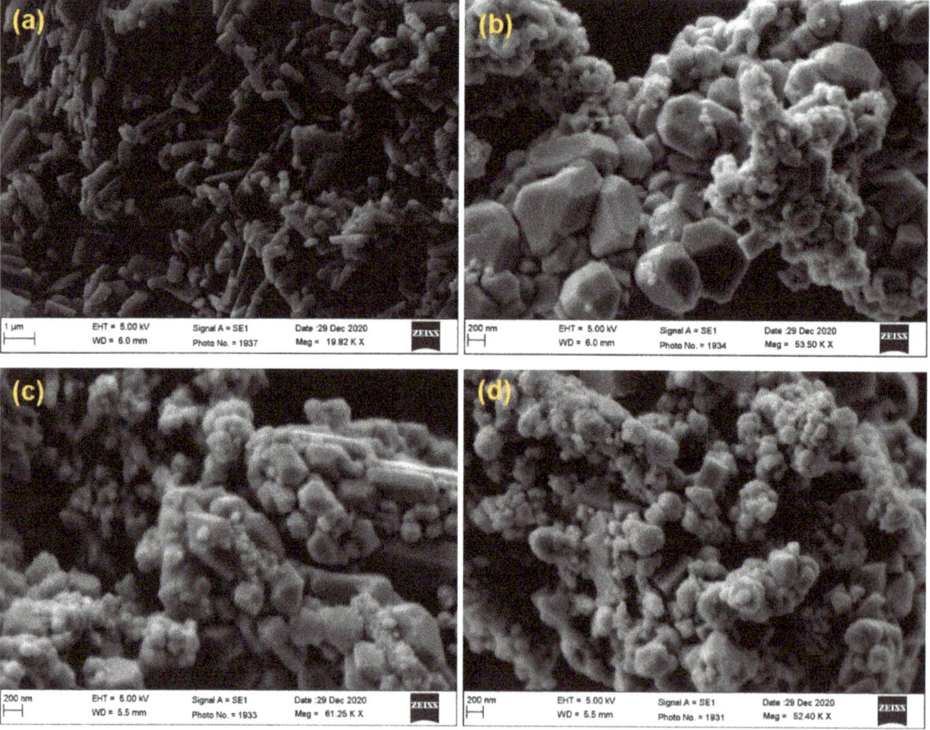

Figure 3. SEM images of pure tedizolid phosphate powder (**a**); and TZP-NCs prepared at varying duration of homogenization and probe sonication, respectively: 5 min and 40 s (**b**); 7.5 min and 50 s (**c**); 10 min and 60 s (**d**).

Solidification/freeze-drying was performed to provide stabilization to the NCs, as we know that solid formulations are more stable than their liquid forms. The freeze-drying of suspensions of NCs would reduce the unstable factors (Ostwald ripening and aggregation) of NCs. Thus, the suspensions of NCs are converted into dried forms and the dried crystals are converted into different dosage forms including sterile powder for injection/ophthalmic, capsules and oral tablets [65]. The aggregation/growth of NCs should be curtailed during freeze-drying. In the suspension of NCs, the use of stabilizers offers spatial or ionic stability to the drug NCs by becoming adsorbed onto their surfaces and preventing the occurrence of any unstable phenomenon (Ostwald ripening or aggregation), thereafter the dried products must exhibit acceptable dispersion ability in case of contact with aqueous phase [66,67]. But, the process of drying may result in the solidification of the stabilizer also, which may cause an irreversible aggregation of the NCs [66]. Therefore, the use of protectants during freeze-drying has become necessary to prevent the occurrence of such unusual phenomenon. Thus, mannitol (1%, w/v) was added as a protectant to the suspension of NC_1 before freeze-drying to get satisfactory re-dispersible freeze-dried NCs [68].

Overall, the results of the present study suggested the antisolvent precipitation method was suitable for the nano-sizing of TZP (a poorly soluble drug) in the range of 150.4–163.2 nm (Table 3). The present method can be applied as an alternative to flash precipitation by CLIJ for the other hydrophobic and poorly soluble drugs such as ibuprofen, salbutamol sulphate, amphotericin-B and cyclosporine-A to get the NCs of sub-micron sizes [47,69,70]. As compared to CLIJ where mixing occurs only once, here if nucleation and crystal growths remain incomplete, secondary crystallization may occur for further growth of the NCs. The antisolvent-precipitation (Bottom-up technique) can further be advanced by employing other "Generally Regarded as Safe" excipients (ophthalmic preparations) for the successful completion and execution of TZP-NCs for ocular use.

3.2. Size, Polydispersity-Index (PDI) and Zeta Potential (ZP)

The physical characterization including the size, PDI and ZP of the preliminary batches of TZP-NCs prepared with varying stabilizers (Table 1a) and their optimization using Poloxamer-188 and PVA (stabilizers) are summarized in Table 1b. Out of different stabilizers the NCs prepared with P188 and PVA have shown relatively lower crystal sizes 495.3 ± 23.5 nm (with PDI and ZP values of 0.265 ± 0.011 and −16.23 ± 2.8 mV) and 514.8 ± 29.4 nm (with PDI and ZP values of 0.375 ± 0.023 and −6.8 ± 1.9 mV), respectively (Table 1a). The optimization of the TZP-NCs with P188 and PVA indicated that the NCs coded as NC-POL2 (with 200 mg of P188) have shown (Table 1b) comparatively smaller size (481.7 ± 58.4 nm) with a low value of PDI (0.252 ± 0.021) and slightly high negative ZP (−17.2 ± 5.6 mV).

Further optimization of the NCs prepared with Poloxamer-188 (1%, w/v) at varying durations of homogenization (21,500 rpm) and probe sonication without mannitol further reduced the size of the NCs (Table 2). The characterization of the four optimal NCs (NCs−1 to NCs−4), suggested that the smallest NCs (150.4 ± 18.3 nm) were obtained by homogenization for 10 min at 21,500 rpm followed by probe sonication for 60 s (NCs−3 in Table 2). The PDI of NCs−3 was lower (0.231 ± 0.006) and zeta potential was relatively higher (−13.5 ± 1.5 mV) with the highest drug content (96.7 ± 1.2%).

3.3. Effect of Homogenization and Probe Sonication Time Duration on Size and PDI

The homogenization and probe sonication time duration had a determinant effect on the crystal size. Initially, the crystal size was 565 nm prepared by homogenization (5 min) and probe sonication for 40 s with a PDI of 0.428. Increasing the homogenization and probe sonication to 7.5 min and 50 s, respectively, the size was reduced to 389 nm with PDI of 0.401 and at 10 min and 60 s homogenization and sonication, the smaller sized crystals (150 nm) were obtained with the lowest value of PDI (0.231). Further increase in time duration for homogenization and sonication to 15 min and 70 s, respectively, could not cause a significant reduction in the crystal sizes (147 nm), although a slight but not significant increase in PDI (0.239) was observed. Thus, the homogenization for 10 min followed by probe sonication for 60 s, was sufficient to get the required sized NCs of TZP without any agglomeration and crystal growth.

3.4. Effect of Mannitol Concentrations on Size, ZP and PDI

The hydrophobic interaction during the freeze-drying may agglomerate the NCs. Hence, for proper re-dispersion of the NCs after freeze-drying, the addition of the cryoprotectant was needed. Here, we have used different concentrations of mannitol (1–5%, w/v) as shown (Table 3). Although no significant changes in the size, ZP and PDI of NC_1 were observed at all concentrations of mannitol, but the highest drug content remained almost constant (96%) with slightly increased negative ZP at 1%, w/v mannitol. The slight increase in size of NC_1 at most of the concentrations was due to the aggregation of the crystals. Such aggregation was attributed to occurrence of the capillary forces (as per the capillary pressure theory) during the process of freeze-drying. Thus, mannitol (1%, w/v) was optimal to prevent the aggregation/crystal growth and provided stabilization to NC_1 during freeze-drying.

Thus, the NCs-3 batch was freeze-dried with different concentrations of mannitol (Table 3). Out of four formulations listed in Table 3, the NC_1 (freeze-dried with mannitol) was considered as the best optimized nanocrystals for ocular use. The smallest size (154.3 nm), low PDI (0.243) and highest positive (due to stearylamine and BKC) ZP (+31.6 mV) of NC_1 even after freeze-drying encouraged us to choose the NC_1 for further studies including the physicochemical characterizations for ophthalmic products. The low PDI indicated the unimodal distribution and its highest ZP could provide the best colloidal stability to the suspended NCs (NC_1). The size and zeta potential distributions of the different NCs and the optimal formulation (NC_1) were represented in Figure 4.

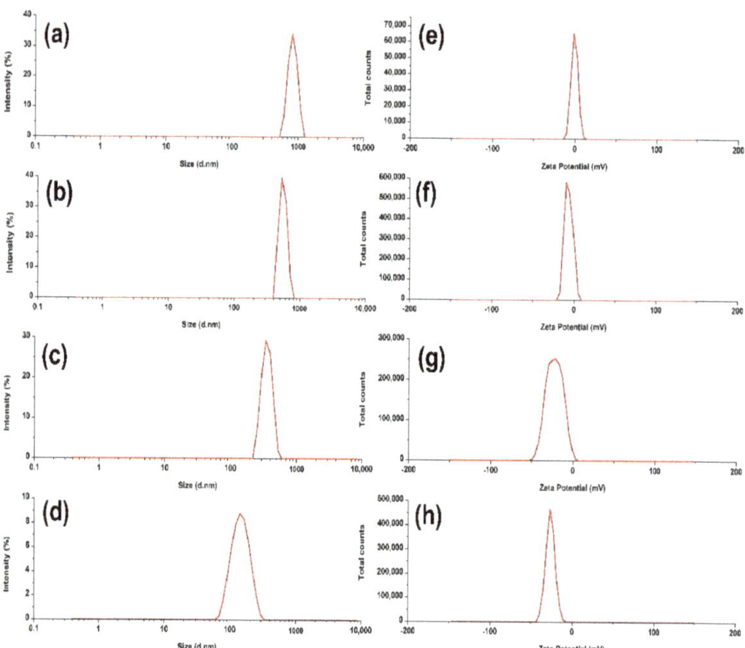

Figure 4. The size distributions of NCs−1, NCs-2, NCs−3 and the optimized NCs−3 as NC_1 ((**a–d**), respectively). Zeta potential distributions of NCs−1, NCs−2, NCs−3 and the optimized NCs−3 as NC_1 ((**e–h**), respectively).

3.5. DSC Analysis

The DSC curves obtained for pure TZP and other components with their PM and NC_1 were represented in Figure 5. The curve of TZP (Figure 5a) exhibited a sharp endothermic peak at 206.3 °C, which corresponds to its melting point and is considered typical for any crystalline and anhydrous molecule [71]. The curve of P188 (Figure 5b) has shown a very broad endothermic peak at 66 °C, which was around its reported melting point [64,72]. In the curve of mannitol (Figure 5c), a slightly broad endothermic peak was seen at 177.5 °C which was near its reported melting point [73]. In the curve of physical mixture of TZP, P188 and mannitol (Figure 5d), three separate and almost unchanged endothermic peaks were located near their respective melting points as described above which were indicating the crystalline nature of the individual component in the investigation.

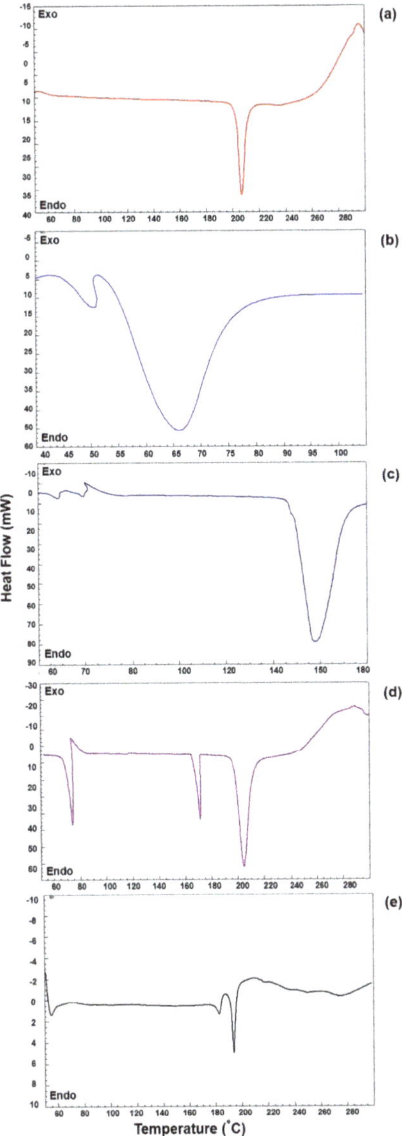

Figure 5. DSC−endotherms of TZP (**a**), P188 (**b**), mannitol (**c**), physical mixture (PM) of TZP, P188, and mannitol (**d**) and lyophilized NC$_1$ (**e**).

In the curve of NC_1 (Figure 5e), the endothermic peak of TZP appeared slightly at a lower temperature (199.6 °C) compared to the melting temperature of pure TZP (206.33 °C), indicating the crystalline character of TZP was not altered during its nano-crystallization by homogenization followed by sonication. The reduced melting temperature of TZP in NC_1 is attributed to its nano-crystallization (reduced crystal-size) and decrease in the crystal lattice energy of TZP. The decrease in the enthalpies was the consequence of the interaction and incorporation of TZP molecules in the hydrophobic territory of micelles created by high HLB (HLB-29) of P188 [74], which was also reported during the nano-crystallization of atorvastatin using Poloxamer-188 as stabilizer [64]. Moreover, a less intense endothermic peak was appeared (near to 177.5 °C) in the DSC curve of NC_1, which was very near to the melting temperature of mannitol, indicating the presence of mannitol in the nanocrystals (NC_1) and no endothermic peak around the melting temperature of P188 was observed, which confirmed the proper washing of the NC_1 to remove the extra surfactants. The results of DSC validate the decreased crystallinity of TZP in NC_1 form which potentiates its solubility. The increased solubility would improve the transcorneal permeation and hence would increase the ocular bioavailability of the drug.

3.6. FTIR Analysis

The FTIR spectrum of TZP (Figure 6a) has significant vibrations of C-H wagging at 877.8 cm^{-1}, C=C stretching as well as C-C stretching of Phenyl ring at 1620.1 cm^{-1}, symmetric C-H stretching in Phenyl ring of (Pyridine-3-yl) Phenyl-3-Fluoro structure at 3256.4 cm^{-1}, C-O stretching vibrations at 1209.2 cm^{-1}, C-H wagging at 1325.5 cm^{-1}, C-H wagging as well as C-N-C bending vibrations at 1407.3 cm^{-1}, C=O stretching vibrations) in the 1,3-oxazolidin-2-one structure at 1746.4 cm^{-1} and C-H wagging in Pyridine ring and C-C-N bending vibrations in the (Pyridine-3-yl) Phenyl-3-Fluoro structure at 1147.8 cm^{-1} and O-H (at 5C position of Oxazolidinone ring) stretching at 3256.4 cm^{-1} [71,75].

The spectrum of P188 (Figure 6b) has shown characteristic and principal absorption peaks of C-H stretching of aliphatic structure at 2875.2 cm^{-1}, in-plane O-H bending vibration at 1344.1 cm^{-1} and C-O stretching at 1099.3 cm^{-1}. An overlapping and unnoticed shifting of distinct C-O stretching of P188 at 1078.2 cm^{-1} was noted in PM, indicating no change in its functional group during the preparation of PM. The FTIR spectrum of mannitol (Figure 6c), has shown the characteristic absorption bands of C-H stretching at 1413 cm^{-1} and C-O stretching at 1011.6 cm^{-1} as well as at 1075.1 cm^{-1}. The distinguished absorption band of mannitol was as observed at 1011.6 cm^{-1} and 1075.1 cm^{-1} for C-O stretching which were also noted at 1012.8 cm^{-1} as well as at 1078.2 cm^{-1} (slightly shifted to higher frequency) in the PM, indicating no change in its molecular structure. The presence of major absorption peaks of TZP, P188, and mannitol in the PM of the excipients with TZP as shown in Figure 6d, indicates that the crystalline behavior of the molecules was not changed in the preparation of PM, which was also reported previously [76]. Figure 6e, has shown the FTIR spectrum of NC_1. Among the distinguish bands obtained for the pure TZP (as shown in Figure 6a), the spectrum of the NC_1 did not show any shifting or less intense bands (except at 3256.4 cm^{-1}) at 877.8 cm^{-1}, 1105.4 cm^{-1}, 1208.4 cm^{-1}, 1406.8 cm^{-1}, 1464.1 cm^{-1}, 1619.8 cm^{-1} and 1746.4 cm^{-1} (characteristic of the molecular structure of 1,3-Oxazolidinone) and (Pyridine-3-yl) Phenyl-3-Fluoro of TZP (Figure 5e). These characteristic bands were predominantly associated with the stretching vibrations of the C-C, C-O and C-F sigma bonds as well as the C-H wagging [75].

However, there was a shifting of O-H (at 5C position of Oxazolidinone ring) stretching (at 3256.4 cm^{-1}) as present in the spectrum of TZP. It was shifted towards a lower frequency (2880.2 cm^{-1}) in the spectrum of NC_1. The reason for this might be due to the formation of hydrogen bonding between hydrogen and oxygen molecules of TZP, P188 and mannitol, which was also reported during the complexation of TZP with β-cyclodextrin [71] and preparation of solid dispersion of aceclofenac with mannitol and hydroxyl β-cyclodextrin.

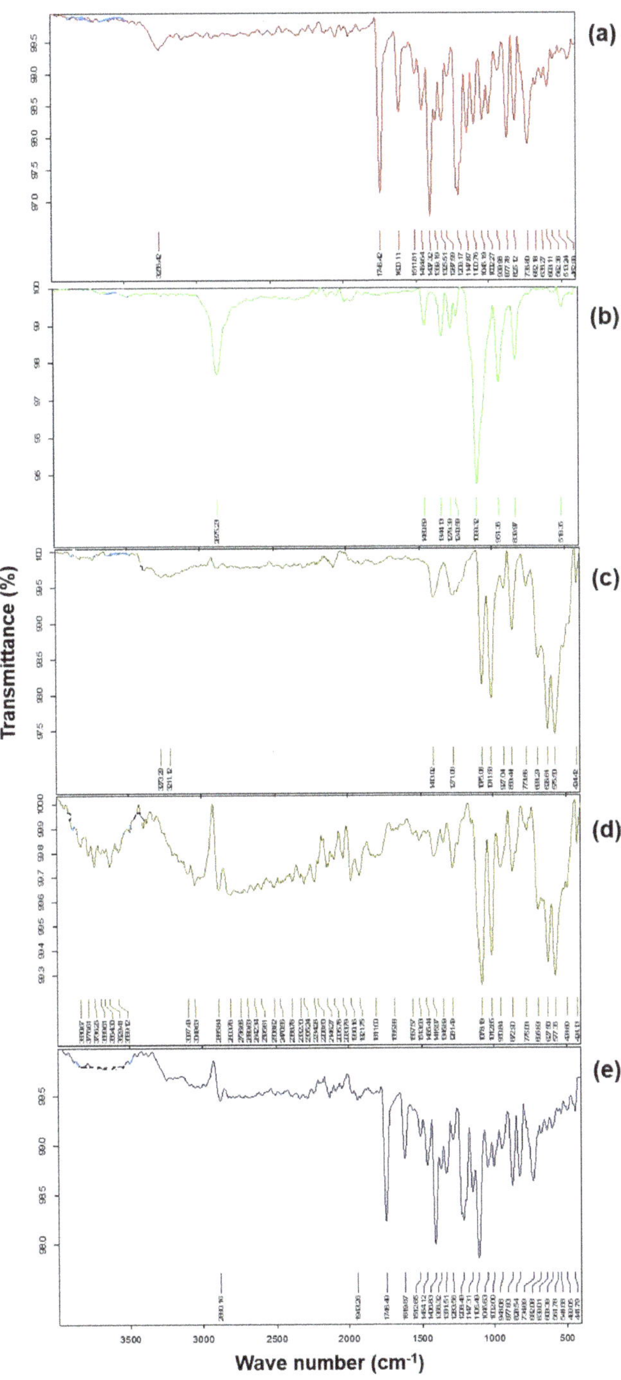

Figure 6. FTIR−Spectra of pure TZP (**a**), P188 (**b**), mannitol (**c**), PM of TZP, P188, and mannitol (**d**) and lyophilized NC$_1$ (**e**).

The characteristic in-plane O-H bending vibration at 1344.1 cm^{-1} and C-O stretching at 1099.3 cm^{-1} for P188 were not present in the final formulation (NC$_1$), which was due to the proper washing of the NC$_1$ by Milli-Q water by centrifugation to remove the extra surfactants. Finally, the results of FTIR spectroscopy confirm that the nano-crystallization of TZP, did not alter the basic molecular structure of TZP during the preparation of NC$_1$ in presence of a high HLB-value (HLB-29) of P188.

3.7. XRD Analysis

The overlay X-ray diffractograms of TZP, P188, Mannitol, Physical mixture of drug, P188 and Mannitol (PM), and the optimized formulation (NC$_1$) were represented in Figure 7. The diffractogram of unprocessed and pure TZP (Figure 7a) has shown some characteristic sharp diffraction peaks at 2θ values of 14.4°, 23.8°, 38.1° and 44.3° having intensities of 3490 cps (with Bragg's or d-value 6.145 and I/I$_0$ 100), 2526 cps (with d-value 3.735 and I/I$_0$ 73), 2492 (with d-value 2.4 and I/I$_0$ 72) and 1036 (with d-value 2.04 and I/I$_0$ 30) clearly indicating the crystallinity of the drug. The diffractogram of P188 (Figure 7b) has characteristic intense diffraction peaks at 2θ values 19.4° and 23.5° with intensities of 3434 cps (with d-value 4.6 and I/I$_0$ 96) and 3583 cps (with d-value 3.8 and I/I$_0$ 100) suggesting its crystallinity. In Figure 7c, the diffractogram of mannitol is representing the peaks at 2θ values 15.0°, 19.1°, 21.4°, 23.8°, 29.8° and 39.0° with intensities 1814 cps (with d-value 5.9 and I/I$_0$ 36), 4060 cps (with d-value 4.6 and I/I$_0$ 80), 1861 cps (with d-value 4.1 and I/I$_0$ 37), 5092 cps (with d-value 3.7 and I/I$_0$ 100), 1177 cps (with d-value 2.9 and I/I$_0$ 24) and 1037 cps (with d-value 2.308 and I/I$_0$), suggesting the crystalline nature of mannitol. The diffractogram of PM (Figure 7d) has shown sharp diffraction peaks at 2θ of 14.4°, 19.3°, 23.8° and 26.4° with intensities 1586 cps (with d-value 6.1 and I/I$_0$ 46), 3472 cps (with d-value 4.6 and I/I$_0$ 100), 2978 cps (with d-value 3.8 and I/I$_0$ 86) and 512 cps (with d-value 3.7 and I/I$_0$ 15), indicating the crystallinity of the individual constituent in their physical mixture.

The diffractogram of NC$_1$ (Figure 7e) has sharp diffraction peaks at approximately the same 2θ values for the pure drug (TZP) with slightly lower intensities 1348 cps (with d-value 9.1 and I/I$_0$ 89), 1531 cps (with d-value 4.3 and I/I$_0$ 100), 626 cps (with d-value 4.1 and I/I$_0$ 41), 608 cps (with d-value 3.6 and I/I$_0$ 40), 392 cps (with d-value 2.4 and I/I$_0$ 26) and 369 cps (with d-value 2.2 and I/I$_0$ 25).

The presence of characteristic diffraction peaks of TZP in the diffractogram of NC$_1$ suggests that the formulation factors (homogenization followed by sonication) could not alter the crystallinity of TZP, which were also observed in previous studies [64,76–78]. However, reduction in the peak intensities were noted around the same 2θ values suggesting the reduced crystalline characters of TZP in NC$_1$ form, which might be associated with the surface coverage and modification of TZP in presence of P188. Also, some extra sharp diffraction peaks were found with the diffractogram of NC$_1$, those were due to the presence of P188 and the use of mannitol (cryoprotectant) during freeze-drying of the NC$_1$.

The crystalline sizes of TZP-NC$_1$ and TZP-pure were calculated by the Scherrer equation as mentioned above using the software Origin© V-7.0 (OriginLab Corp., Northampton, MA, USA). Considering the morphology of TZP-crystals elongated rod shaped, the Scherrer constant value was 0.68 used for the calculation. The crystal size of TZP-NC$_1$ was 113.4 ± 25.2 nm. Which were almost similar to the size measurement by zeta-sizer as mentioned above. The results of XRD studies confirm the decreased crystallinity of TZP in NC$_1$ form which was substantiated by the increased saturation solubility of the NC$_1$, in simulated tear fluid with SLS.

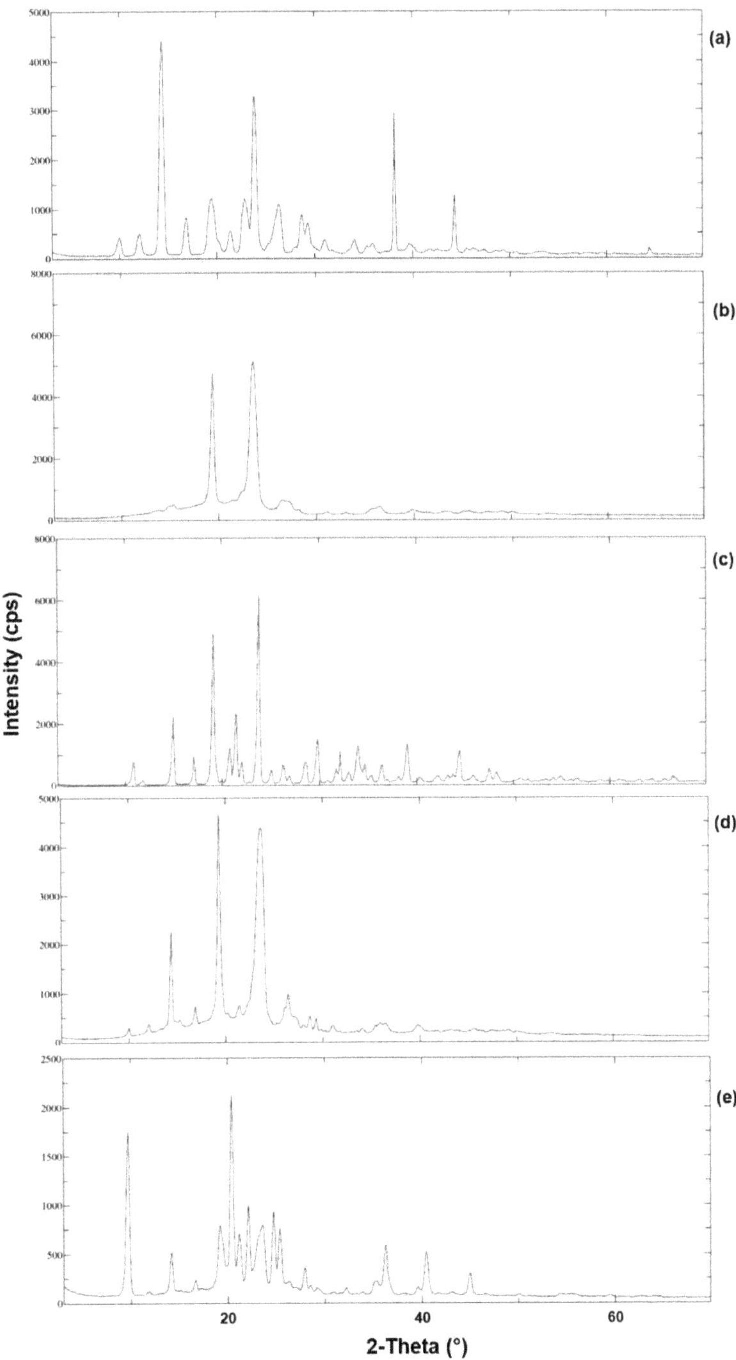

Figure 7. XRD patterns of pure TZP (**a**), P188 (**b**), mannitol (**c**), PM of TZP, P188 and mannitol (**d**) and lyophilized NC_1 (**e**).

3.8. Physicochemical Characterization

The results of physicochemical characterization for NC_1 are presented in Table 4. The visual examination of NC_1 suspension under normal light against a dark and white background was found clear and transparent. So, the formulation will not cause any blurring of vision and will be appropriate for ocular application. The pH of human tear fluids ranged from 6.5 to 7.6 with a mean value of 7.0 as measured by Abelson [79]. In the present investigation the pH of NC_1 was found 7.0 ± 0.4 which falls within the normal range. The rate of tear turnover and the chemical buffering action/capacity of tear fluids can easily bring the pH of the formulation (NC_1) to its own pH by the neutralization process of tear fluids. So, the formulation will not cause any discomfort to the eyes even at unstable tear-film due to bacterial lysis of long-chain components of Meibomian lipids (as stable composition of cholesterol and cholesteryl esters) to free fatty acids that cause irritation to the tear film and the corneal surfaces [80].

Table 4. Physicochemical characterization of redispersed NC_1 and conventional TZP-AqS (mean $\pm$ SD, $n = 3$).

Formulations	Clarity at 25 °C	pH	Osmolarity (mOsm·L^{-1})	Drug Content (%)	Viscosity (cPs) at	
					20 ± 1 °C	35 ± 1 °C
* TZP-NC$_1$ (1%, *w/v* mannitol)	Clear and transparent	7.0 ± 0.4	298.0 ± 5.0	96.4 ± 2.6	28.5 ± 1.2	21.1 ± 1.1
** TZP-AqS	Cloudy and translucent	6.2 ± 0.5	304.0 ± 4.0	98.4 ± 1.8	29.4 ± 2.1	23.1 ± 1.8

* TZP-NC$_1$ = Tedizolid phosphate nanocrystals freeze-dried with 1%, *w/v* of mannitol) and ** TZP-AqS = Conventional aqueous suspension of tedizolid phosphate prepared in-house.

The osmolarity of the NC_1 suspension was found around 298 ± 5 mOsm·L^{-1}, which was almost equivalent to the osmolarity of normal tear fluid. The normal tear fluid has an osmolarity of 300–302 mOsm·L^{-1} (iso-osmotic) [80], but it may increase up to 320–340 mOsm·L^{-1} (hyperosmolarity) in some ocular conditions. Such as bacterial infections or in dry eye conditions, the tear film has shown an increased osmolarity (hyperosmolarity) [81]. Therefore, the topically applied ophthalmic preparations for such diseased conditions should be formulated as hypotonic to counteract the increased osmolarity of the tears/tear film [82]. The conversion of freeze-dried samples of NC_1 to aqueous suspension using dextrose solution (5%, *w/v*) as a vehicle did not alter the drug content of the optimized nanocrystals significantly ($p < 0.05$). This indicated a temporary stability of the drug in its aqueous suspension form. The viscosity of NC_1 suspension at 20 ± 1 °C was 28.5 ± 2.4 cPs and at ocular physiological temperature (35 ± 1 °C), it was 21.1 ± 1.1 cPs. The viscosity of the optimized formulation falls within the limit of desired viscosity for ophthalmic preparations (25–50 cPs). A slight decrease in viscosity at 35 ± 1 °C (attributed to high shear stress at increased temperature), suggesting that the suspension of NC_1 could easily be distributed throughout the ocular surface without any irritation/discomfort in or around the eyes of the patient even during blinking of eyes [83]. Thus, NC_1 would be convenient and stress-free for its ocular application.

3.9. Solubility Determination

The saturation solubility of pure TZP was 10.8 ± 2.4 µgmL^{-1} and 16.1 ± 3.8 µgmL^{-1} in STF and STF with 0.5%, *w/v* of SLS, respectively, while a notable increased solubilization of TZP was found from nanocrystals (NC_1) form, which was 18.4 ± 2.4 µgmL^{-1} and 25.9 ± 3.1 µgmL^{-1} in STF and STF with 0.5%, *w/v* of SLS, respectively. The results of this study revealed that particles/crystals in nano-size have shown a significant ($p < 0.05$) increase in the saturation solubility of TZP. The improved solubilization of the drug was attributed to the fact that nano-sizing (using P188) of the particles lead to an increase in the overall surface area to interact with the aqueous phase. Thus, the point of contact for the drug particles with the solvents (STF and 0.5%, *w/v* of SLS) were increased, which facilitated the wetting and dispersibility of drug particles [84] and hence increased the solubilization of TZP in NC_1. This finding correlates with the well-known "Noyes Whitney Equation" that defines the reliance on comparative saturation solubility of different particles with varying radii and concentration of the dissolved solute [85].

Furthermore, the augmented solubilization of TZP was due to a strong affinity between TZP and P188 to produce "molecular dispersion" which is accountable for altering the solubility equilibrium and saturation solubility of TZP. This finding was substantiated by a previous report on the nano-sizing of poorly aqueous soluble atorvastatin with Poloxamer-188 [64]. The improved solubilization of TZP in STF with SLS would facilitate the in vitro release profiling of the drug. Also, an increased solubility of TZP would improve the oral or ocular bioavailability of the active form of TZP (i.e., tedizolid).

3.10. In Vitro Release Study

In vitro drug release study confers the practical consideration about the possible in vivo performance of any developed formulation. Therefore, this experiment was carried out in simulated tear fluid (STF) with SLS (0.5%, w/v) for the release of TZP from the freeze dried NC_1 and TZP-AqS. The SLS was added in STF to increase the solubility of the poorly soluble drug (TZP). The release profile of the two formulations is represented in Figure 8. The assessment of the obtained release profiles clearly shows a significant ($p < 0.05$) enhancement in the release rate of NC_1. The TZP-nanocrystals (NC_1) have shown a fast release of ~15.3% at 1 h and ~49.2% drug was released within 4 h, followed by delayed release till 12 h (~78.8%). While the pure TZP from AqS has shown only ~6.3% at 1 h and ~24.2% drug was released within 4 h and ~43.1% till 12 h. Initially, the increased rate of drug release from the nanocrystals was contributed by the smaller sized (151.6 to 154.3 nm) NC_1 that provided an overall increased surface area. Due to increased surface area, a large portion of the nanocrystals could come in contact with the release medium, causing higher solubilization and dissolution of the TZP which in turn provided its higher saturation solubility [55].

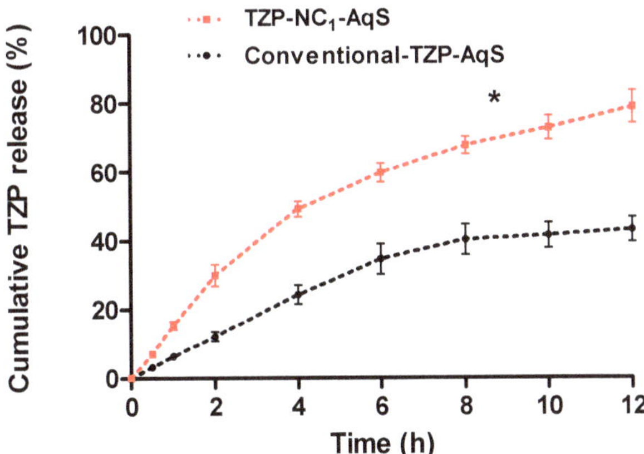

Figure 8. In vitro release of TZP from the freeze dried TZP–NC_1–AqS and conventional TZP–AqS in STF (pH 7.0) with SLS (0.5%, w/v). Results are the mean with $\pm$ SD of three measurements and "*" $p < 0.05$; TZP–NC_1 versus TZP–AqS.

Moreover, the stable smaller size of TZP-nanocrystals prevented their aggregation and facilitated the surface wetting ability because of the presence of traces of P188 and hence the dispersibility of the drug [64]. The presence of P188 at the interface of TZP and STF with SLS (0.5%, w/v) also facilitated the reduction in their interfacial tension by the interaction of ether-oxygen (R–O–R′) of hydrophilic PEO-blocks of P188 through H-bonding with water molecules [86]. On the other hand, the linearity in release profile (till 12 h) of TZP from NC_1 might be endorsed due to the multimolecular micellar formation of P188, which was also reported in the in vitro release of atorvastatin (a poorly aqueous soluble drug) in the nanocrystal states [64]. The central PPO-block of P188 that is the hydrophobic part of the micellar structure might interact with TZP through Van-der Waals intermolecular forces and decrease the partitioning and diffusion of TZP from the core of multimolecular micellar structures [87].

From the dissolution data, the calculation of %DE with their respective 95% CI are illustrated in Figure 9. The average %DE for TZP-NC$_1$ and TZP-AqS were found to be 70.6 ± 3.4% and 56.2 ± 3.5% with mean dissolution times 2.9 ± 0.2 h and 4.3 ± 0.3 h, respectively. The 95% CI was found in the range of 13.3 to 15.8 (>±10%), indicating the differences in the dissolution/release profiles of the drug from the two formulations. Calculation of %DE provides information for the quantitative comparisons between the products. It is easier to interpret the data obtained through %DE than that of the difference and similarity factors [53]. Conclusively, the %DE is a better substitute for the single point dissolution measurement for the dissolved drugs during in vitro release study.

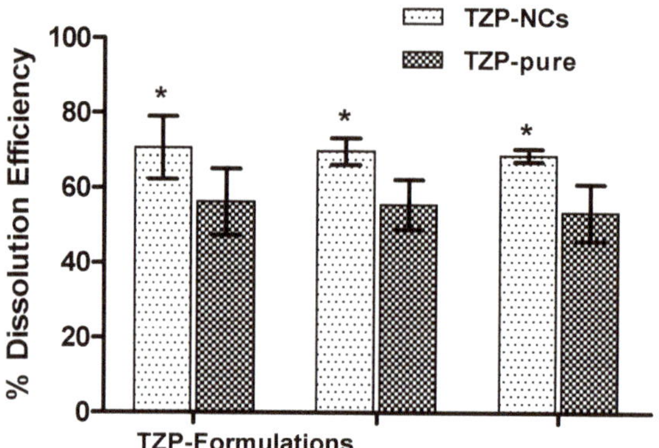

Figure 9. Dissolution efficiencies (%DE) with 95% confidence intervals of TZP-NCs versus TZP−AqS, where * $p < 0.0005$ was indicating the significant difference between the %DE of the two formulations.

Application of some kinetic models on the in vitro release data we found that the in vitro release of TZP from both the formulations followed the first-order release kinetics. Although the release kinetics of the drug from the formulations was the same, but the release of TZP was linear till 12 h from the NC$_1$ while it was linear up to 8 h from the TZP-AqS, thereafter the drug release remained almost the same till 12 h. Among the applied kinetic equations or release models the highest correlation coefficients (R^2) were 0.9875 and 0.9645 (for TZP-NC$_1$ and AqS of TZP-pure, respectively) (Figure S1), which were associated with the first order model. The release kinetic parameters for the two formulations after applying the kinetic models, were mentioned in Table 5. By taking the R^2 values and slope of the tried kinetic equations, the diffusion-exponents (n-value) were obtained. The n-values (0.0238 and 0.0081 for TZP-NC$_1$ and AqS of TZP-pure, respectively) indicate the Fickian-Diffusion type of release mechanism.

Table 5. Obtained parameters after applying the release kinetic models.

Release Models	Kinetic Parameters	TZP-NC$_1$-AqS	Conventional TZP-AqS
Zero order (Fraction drug released vs. time)	R^2	0.9157	0.8309
	n-value	0.2631	0.0138
	k_0 (μgh^{-1})	1.11×10^{-1}	0.53×10^{-1}
First order (Log% Drug remaining vs. time)	R^2	0.9875	0.9728
	n-value	0.0238	0.0081
	k_1 (h^{-1})	2.28	2.37×10^{-1}
Korsmeyer-Peppas (Log Fraction drug released vs. log time)	R^2	0.9685	0.9645
	n-value	0.3221	0.3534
	$k_{K\text{-}P}$ (h^{-n})	4.52×10^{-1}	2.39×10^{-1}
Hixon-Crowell (M$_o^{1/3}$–M$_t^{1/3}$ vs. time)	R^2	0.9699	0.8386
	n-value	0.0141	0.0054
	$k_{H\text{-}C}$ (μg$^{1/3}$h^{-1})	4.79×10^{-1}	4.77×10^{-1}

R^2 = Coefficient of correlation and n-value = Release or diffusion exponent.

3.11. Stability Studies

The optimized nanocrystals (NC$_1$) were evaluated at stipulated time points for the physical and chemical stabilities of NC$_1$ to ascertain the stability limits in support of its storage at $4 \pm 2\,°C$, $25 \pm 1\,°C$ and $37 \pm 1\,°C$ for 180 days. The results were summarized in Table 6. The results of physical stability did not show notable alteration in PDI, zeta-potential, TZP content and cumulative amount of drug released. No significant alteration in the selected parameters were observed at $4 \pm 2\,°C$, but a slight increase in size at 90 days and 180 days, was observed in the samples stored at $25 \pm 1\,°C$ and $37 \pm 1\,°C$. Similarly the increased size was also reported for the stability of liposomes stored at different temperatures for 150 days [16]. The crystal growth in the aqueous environment is generally attributed due to the "Ostwald ripening", where the smaller crystals in the aqueous medium might get dissolved and deposited on to the larger crystals to minimize the surface/area ratio for achieving the thermodynamic stability [64,88]. But the size growth of NC$_1$ in the present investigation stored in freeze-dried state at slightly higher temperatures was not because of the "Ostwald ripening" phenomenon, rather it might be due to dehydration of the stabilizer (P188) and the protectant (mannitol) and consequent loss of NC$_1$ protection [89]. Unremarkable alterations in the PDI, ZP and drug content was noticed even at higher temperature for 180 days. The drug content analysis indicated that the TZP content was around 94.9% up to 180 days, demonstrating that the optimized freeze-dried TZP-nanocrystals (NC$_1$) remained stable without any significant degradation of the drug. Moreover, the results obtained for drug content suggested that the homogenization (at 21,000 rpm) followed by probe sonication (at 40% power for 60 s) processes to obtain the NC$_1$ did not affect the chemical stability of TZP [90,91]. Overall, the TZP-NC$_1$ were physically (size, polydispersity-index and zeta potential) and chemically (drug content) stable at all three storage temperatures ($4\,°C$, $25\,°C$ and $37\,°C$). Thus, the product can be stored at these storage temperatures without significant alterations in the above-mentioned physical and chemical parameters for up to 180 days.

Table 6. Stability results of TZP-NC$_1$. All data were presented as mean $\pm$ SD, $n = 3$.

Stability of TZP-NC$_1$	Values at Different Time Points (Mean $\pm$ SD, $n = 3$)				
	Initially (0 Day)	**At 7 Days**	**At 30 Days**	**At 90 Days**	**At 180 Days**
At $4 \pm 2\,^\circ$C					
Particle size (nm)	154.3 ± 17.9	157.2 ± 14.7	159.8 ± 15.2	161.8 ± 15.6	164.1 ± 15.8
Polydispersity index	0.242 ± 0.009	0.244 ± 0.008	0.245 ± 0.008	0.247 ± 0.009	0.249 ± 0.011
Zeta potentials (mV)	$+31.6 \pm 3.8$	$+31.4 \pm 3.7$	$+30.8 \pm 3.8$	$+30.2 \pm 3.7$	$+29.4 \pm 3.5$
Drug content (%)	96.2 ± 3.1	96.17 ± 2.56	95.8 ± 2.8	95.2 ± 3.4	$94.5 + 3.6$
At $25 \pm 1\,^\circ$C					
Particle size (nm)	154.3 ± 17.9	159.1 ± 14.9	161.6 ± 15.1	174.2 ± 16.4	190.0 ± 17.8
Polydispersity index	0.242 ± 0.009	0.247 ± 0.008	0.248 ± 0.008	0.251 ± 0.009	0.253 ± 0.008
Zeta potentials (mV)	$+31.6 \pm 3.8$	$+31.0 \pm 3.7$	$+30.6 \pm 3.6$	$+29.4 \pm 3.4$	$+29.1 \pm 3.4$
Drug content (%)	96.2 ± 3.1	96.1 ± 2.8	95.6 ± 3.2	95.4 ± 3.5	94.9 ± 3.4
At $37 \pm 1\,^\circ$C					
Particle size (nm)	154.3 ± 17.9	161.0 ± 15.2	162.8 ± 15.3	176.4 ± 16.6	192.1 ± 18.0
Polydispersity index	0.242 ± 0.009	0.247 ± 0.007	0.249 ± 0.008	0.252 ± 0.009	0.255 ± 0.008
Zeta potentials (mV)	$+31.6 \pm 3.8$	$+30.6 \pm 3.8$	$+30.3 \pm 3.6$	$+29.0 \pm 3.4$	$+28.6 \pm 3.4$
Drug content (%)	96.2 ± 3.1	95.8 ± 2.9	95.6 ± 3.1	95.3 ± 3.5	94.2 ± 3.2

4. Conclusions

The positively charged (+29.4 mV) TZP-NCs prepared by antisolvent precipitation method including the homogenization followed by sonication, resulted in considerably smaller sized ($\approx$151.6 nm) nanocrystals (suitable for ocular use). The NCs were well stabilized by Poloxamer-188 at 1% (w/v) concentration. Mannitol (as cryoprotectant at 1%, w/v) prevented the crystal growth and stabilized the TZP-NC$_1$ during freeze-drying. The SEM study indicated good crystalline morphology of the optimal NCs. The FTIR spectroscopy revealed that the basic molecular structure of TZP was not altered, while the DSC and XRD studies showed a reduction in the crystallinity of the drug in NC$_1$ form. Due to reduced crystallinity and nano-sizing of TZP, the solubility of the drug was increased by 1.4-times as compared to pure-TZP in STF with SLS (0.5%, w/v). The increased solubility of TZP-NC$_1$ would definitely improve the transcorneal permeation which in turn would increase the ocular bioavailabity of the active form of the drug (TDZ) if applied in vivo. The redispersion of freeze-dried NC$_1$ in dextrose solution (5%, w/v) with mannitol (1%, w/v) ensued in a clear transparent iso-osmotic nano-suspension with $\approx$298 mOsm$\cdot$L^{-1} osmolarity and $\approx$21.1 cps viscosity at 35 $^\circ$C. Relatively higher drug release ($\approx$78.8%) was found from NC$_1$ at 12 h as compared to TZP-AqS ($\approx$43.4%) during in vitro release study. %DE determination indicated a different release profile of the drug from the two formulations. The TZP-NC$_1$ were physically (size, PDI and ZP) and chemically (drug content) stable at all three storage temperatures (4 $^\circ$C, 25 $^\circ$C and 37 $^\circ$C) for 180 days. Based on the above findings, the TZP-NC$_1$ would be a promising and viable alternative for the ocular delivery of TZP in vivo. Further studies including in vitro antimicrobial study in vivo ocular irritation and pharmacokinetics in rabbits have been performed to ensure the efficacy, safety, and drug bioavailability but these are out of the scope of the present article.

Supplementary Materials: The following supporting information can be downloaded at: https://www.mdpi.com/article/10.3390/pharmaceutics14071328/s1. Figure S1. Different kinetic model plots for TZP-NC1 (a, b, c and d) and the plots for conventional aqueous suspension of TZP-pure (a', b', c' and d').

Author Contributions: Conceptualization, M.A.K. and M.A.; methodology, M.A.K.; software, M.I.; validation, M.A.K., A.A. (Abdullah Alshememry), A.A. (Aws Alshamsan) and M.I.; formal analysis, M.A.K.; investigation, M.I.; resources, M.A.K and M.A.; data curation, M.A.K. and M.I.; writing-original draft preparation, M.A.K.; writing-review and editing, A.A. (Aws Alshamsan) and A.A. (Abdullah Alshememry); visualization, M.A.K.; supervision, A.A. (Aws Alshamsan); project administration, M.A.K., A.A. (Aws Alshamsan) and M.A.; funding acquisition, M.A.K., M.A. and A.A. (Aws Alshamsan). All authors have read and agreed to the published version of the manuscript.

Funding: This project was funded by the National Plan for Science, Technology and Innovation (MAARIFAH), King Abdulaziz City for Science and Technology, Kingdom of Saudi Arabia, Award Number (2-17-03-001-0035).

Institutional Review Board Statement: Not applicable.

Informed Consent Statement: Not applicable.

Data Availability Statement: This study did not report any data related animal study.

Acknowledgments: Authors are thankful to the National Plan for Science, Technology and Innovation (MAARIFAH), King Abdulaziz City for Science and Technology, Kingdom of Saudi Arabia, for the grant.

Conflicts of Interest: The authors declare no conflict of interest.

Abbreviations

BCS	Biopharmaceutics Classification Systems
PVA	Polyvinyl alcohol
TZP	Tedizolid phosphate
TDZ	Tedizolid
NCs	Nanocrystals
DMSO	Dimethyl Sulfoxide
GRAS	Generally Regarded As Safe
P188	Poloxamer-188
HLB	Hydrophilic Lipophilic Balance
ZP	Zeta Potential
PDI	Polydispersity Index
SEM	Scanning Electron Microscopy
CLIJ	Confined Liquid Impinging Jets
FTIR	Fourier Transform Infrared Spectroscopy
DSC	Differential Scanning Calorimetry
XRD	X-Ray Diffraction; Å = Angstrom
FWHM	Full-Width Half-Maximum
STF	Simulated Tear Fluid
SLS	Sodium Lauryl Sulfate
BKC	Benzalkonium chloride
AqS	Aqueous Suspension
SCO_2	Supercritical Carbon-dioxide
Vit-E-TPGS	D- α-Tocopheryl Polyethylene Glycol-1000 Succinate
PPO	Polypropylene oxide
PEO	Polyethylene oxide
H-bonding	Hydrogen bonding
DE	Dissolution Efficiency
CI	Confidence intervals

References

1. Ammar, H.O.; Salama, H.A.; Ghorab, M.; Mahmoud, A.A. Nanoemulsion as a potential ophthalmic delivery system for dorzolamide hydrochloride. *AAPS Pharmscitech* **2009**, *10*, 808–819. [CrossRef] [PubMed]
2. Lopez-Cano, J.J.; Gonzalez-Cela-Casamayor, M.A.; Andres-Guerrero, V.; Herrero-Vanrell, R.; Molina-Martinez, I.T. Liposomes as vehicles for topical ophthalmic drug delivery and ocular surface protection. *Expert Opin. Drug Deliv.* **2021**, *18*, 819–847. [CrossRef] [PubMed]

3. Kalam, M.A.; Alshamsan, A. Poly (d, l-lactide-co-glycolide) nanoparticles for sustained release of tacrolimus in rabbit eyes. *Biomed. Pharmacother.* **2017**, *94*, 402–411. [CrossRef] [PubMed]

4. Zhang, J.; Jiao, J.; Niu, M.; Gao, X.; Zhang, G.; Yu, H.; Yang, X.; Liu, L. Ten Years of Knowledge of Nano-Carrier Based Drug Delivery Systems in Ophthalmology: Current Evidence, Challenges, and Future Prospective. *Int. J. Nanomed.* **2021**, *16*, 6497–6530. [CrossRef]

5. Araújo, J.; Gonzalez, E.; Egea, M.A.; Garcia, M.L.; Souto, E.B. Nanomedicines for ocular NSAIDs: Safety on drug delivery. *Nanomed. Nanotechnol. Biol. Med.* **2009**, *5*, 394–401. [CrossRef]

6. Gan, L.; Wang, J.; Jiang, M.; Bartlett, H.; Ouyang, D.; Eperjesi, F.; Liu, J.; Gan, Y. Recent advances in topical ophthalmic drug delivery with lipid-based nanocarriers. *Drug Discov. Today* **2013**, *18*, 290–297. [CrossRef]

7. Romero, G.B.; Keck, C.M.; Muller, R.H.; Bou-Chacra, N.A. Development of cationic nanocrystals for ocular delivery. *Eur. J. Pharm. Biopharm.* **2016**, *107*, 215–222. [CrossRef]

8. Kalam, M.A.; Iqbal, M.; Alshememry, A.; Alkholief, M.; Alshamsan, A. Development and Evaluation of Chitosan Nanoparticles for Ocular Delivery of Tedizolid Phosphate. *Molecules* **2022**, *27*, 2326. [CrossRef]

9. Sharma, O.P.; Patel, V.; Mehta, T. Nanocrystal for ocular drug delivery: Hope or hype. *Drug Deliv. Transl. Res.* **2016**, *6*, 399–413. [CrossRef]

10. Abul Kalam, M.; Sultana, Y.; Ali, A.; Aqil, M.; Mishra, A.K.; Aljuffali, I.A.; Alshamsan, A. Part I: Development and optimization of solid-lipid nanoparticles using Box-Behnken statistical design for ocular delivery of gatifloxacin. *J. Biomed. Mater. Res. Part A* **2012**, *101*, 1813–1827.

11. Kalam, M.A.; Sultana, Y.; Ali, A.; Aqil, M.; Mishra, A.K.; Chuttani, K. Preparation, characterization, and evaluation of gatifloxacin loaded solid lipid nanoparticles as colloidal ocular drug delivery system. *J. Drug Target.* **2009**, *18*, 191–204. [CrossRef] [PubMed]

12. Lang, J.C. Ocular drug delivery conventional ocular formulations. *Adv. Drug Deliv. Rev.* **1995**, *16*, 39–43. [CrossRef]

13. Hao, L.; Wang, X.; Zhang, D.; Xu, Q.; Song, S.; Wang, F.; Li, C.; Guo, H.; Liu, Y.; Zheng, D.; et al. Studies on the preparation, characterization and pharmacokinetics of Amoitone B nanocrystals. *Int. J. Pharm.* **2012**, *433*, 157–164. [CrossRef] [PubMed]

14. Loscher, M.; Hurst, J.; Strudel, L.; Spitzer, M.S.; Schnichels, S. Nanoparticles as drug delivery systems in ophthalmology. *Der Ophthalmol.* **2018**, *115*, 184–189. [CrossRef] [PubMed]

15. Franco, P.; De Marco, I. Nanoparticles and nanocrystals by supercritical CO_2-assisted techniques for pharmaceutical applications: A review. *Appl. Sci.* **2021**, *11*, 1476. [CrossRef]

16. Trucillo, P.; Ferrari, P.; Campardelli, R.; Reverchon, E.; Perego, P. A supercritical assisted process for the production of amoxicillin-loaded liposomes for antimicrobial applications. *J. Supercrit. Fluids* **2020**, *163*, 104842. [CrossRef]

17. Campardelli, R.; Trucillo, P.; Reverchon, E. Supercritical assisted process for the efficient production of liposomes containing antibiotics for ocular delivery. *J. CO2 Util.* **2018**, *25*, 235–241. [CrossRef]

18. Joshi, K.; Chandra, A.; Jain, K.; Talegaonkar, S. Nanocrystalization: An Emerging Technology to Enhance the Bioavailability of Poorly Soluble Drugs. *Pharm. Nanotechnol.* **2019**, *7*, 259–278. [CrossRef]

19. Binkhathlan, Z.; Alomrani, A.H.; Hoxha, O.; Ali, R.; Kalam, M.A.; Alshamsan, A. Development and Characterization of PEGylated Fatty Acid-Block-Poly(ε-caprolactone) Novel Block Copolymers and Their Self-Assembled Nanostructures for Ocular Delivery of Cyclosporine A. *Polymers* **2022**, *14*, 1635. [CrossRef]

20. Aksungur, P.; Demirbilek, M.; Denkbaş, E.B.; Vandervoort, J.; Ludwig, A.; Ünlü, N. Development and characterization of Cyclosporine A loaded nanoparticles for ocular drug delivery: Cellular toxicity, uptake, and kinetic studies. *J. Control. Release* **2011**, *151*, 286–294. [CrossRef]

21. Dhahir, R.K.; Al-Nima, A.M.; Al-Bazzaz, F.Y. Nanoemulsions as Ophthalmic Drug Delivery Systems. *Turk. J. Pharm. Sci.* **2021**, *18*, 652–664. [CrossRef] [PubMed]

22. Vandamme, T.F. Microemulsions as ocular drug delivery systems: Recent developments and future challenges. *Prog. Retin. Eye Res.* **2002**, *21*, 15–34. [CrossRef]

23. Seyfoddin, A.; Shaw, J.; Al-Kassas, R. Solid lipid nanoparticles for ocular drug delivery. *Drug Deliv.* **2010**, *17*, 467–489. [CrossRef] [PubMed]

24. Abul Kalam, M.; Sultana, Y.; Ali, A.; Aqil, M.; Mishra, A.K.; Chuttani, K.; Aljuffali, I.A.; Alshamsan, A. Part II: Enhancement of transcorneal delivery of gatifloxacin by solid lipid nanoparticles in comparison to commercial aqueous eye drops. *J. Biomed. Mater. Res. Part A* **2012**, *101*, 1828–1836. [CrossRef] [PubMed]

25. Abdelbary, G.; El-Gendy, N. Niosome-encapsulated gentamicin for ophthalmic controlled delivery. *AAPS Pharmscitech* **2008**, *9*, 740–747. [CrossRef]

26. Durak, S.; Esmaeili Rad, M.; Alp Yetisgin, A.; Eda Sutova, H.; Kutlu, O.; Cetinel, S.; Zarrabi, A. Niosomal Drug Delivery Systems for Ocular Disease-Recent Advances and Future Prospects. *Nanomaterials* **2020**, *10*, 1191. [CrossRef]

27. Kambhampati, S.P.; Kannan, R.M. Dendrimer nanoparticles for ocular drug delivery. *J. Ocul. Pharmacol. Ther.* **2013**, *29*, 151–165. [CrossRef]

28. Lancina, M.G.; Yang, H. Dendrimers for Ocular Drug Delivery. *Can. J. Chem.* **2017**, *95*, 897–902. [CrossRef]

29. Kalam, M.A. Development of chitosan nanoparticles coated with hyaluronic acid for topical ocular delivery of dexamethasone. *Int. J. Biol. Macromol.* **2016**, *89*, 127–136. [CrossRef]

30. Muller, R.H.; Keck, C.M. Twenty years of drug nanocrystals: Where are we, and where do we go? *Eur. J. Pharm. Biopharm.* **2012**, *80*, 1–3. [CrossRef]

31. Mohammad, I.S.; Hu, H.; Yin, L.; He, W. Drug nanocrystals: Fabrication methods and promising therapeutic applications. *Int. J. Pharm.* **2019**, *562*, 187–202. [CrossRef] [PubMed]

32. Gigliobianco, M.R.; Casadidio, C.; Censi, R.; Di Martino, P. Nanocrystals of Poorly Soluble Drugs: Drug Bioavailability and Physicochemical Stability. *Pharmaceutics* **2018**, *10*, 134. [CrossRef] [PubMed]

33. Sun, B.; Yeo, Y. Nanocrystals for the parenteral delivery of poorly water-soluble drugs. *Curr. Opin. Solid State Mater. Sci.* **2012**, *16*, 295–301. [CrossRef] [PubMed]

34. Sahoo, S.K.; Dilnawaz, F.; Krishnakumar, S. Nanotechnology in ocular drug delivery. *Drug Discov. Today* **2008**, *13*, 144–151. [CrossRef]

35. Weng, Y.; Liu, J.; Jin, S.; Guo, W.; Liang, X.; Hu, Z. Nanotechnology-based strategies for treatment of ocular disease. *Acta Pharm. Sin. B* **2016**, *7*, 281–291. [CrossRef]

36. Chen, Z.; Wu, W.; Lu, Y. What is the future for nanocrystal-based drug-delivery systems? *Ther. Deliv.* **2020**, *11*, 225–229. [CrossRef]

37. Pathi, S.L.; Chennuru, R.; Bollineni, M. Olaparib Co-Crystals and Process of Preparation Thereof. WO2021044437A1, 11 March 2021.

38. Rey, A.W.; Souza, F.E.S.; Bhattacharyya, A.; Khalili, B. Crystalline form of Olaparib. U.S. Patent 10662178B2, 26 May 2020.

39. Kassem, M.A.; Abdel Rahman, A.A.; Ghorab, M.M.; Ahmed, M.B.; Khalil, R.M. Nanosuspension as an ophthalmic delivery system for certain glucocorticoid drugs. *Int. J. Pharm.* **2007**, *340*, 126–133. [CrossRef]

40. Im, W.B.; Choi, S.H.; Park, J.Y.; Choi, S.H.; Finn, J.; Yoon, S.H. Discovery of torezolid as a novel 5-hydroxymethyl-oxazolidinone antibacterial agent. *Eur. J. Med. Chem.* **2011**, *46*, 1027–1039. [CrossRef]

41. Ruiz, P.; Causse, M.; Vaquero, M.; Casal, M. In Vitro Activity of Tedizold against Mycobacterium tuberculosis. *Antimicrob. Agents Chemother.* **2019**, *63*, e01939-18. [CrossRef]

42. Das, D.; Tulkens, P.M.; Mehra, P.; Fang, E.; Prokocimer, P. Tedizolid phosphate for the management of acute bacterial skin and skin structure infections: Safety summary. *Clin. Infect. Dis.* **2013**, *58* (Suppl. S1), S51–S57. [CrossRef]

43. Yang, Z.; Tian, L.; Liu, J.; Huang, G. Construction and evaluation in vitro and in vivo of tedizolid phosphate loaded cationic liposomes. *J. Liposome Res.* **2017**, *28*, 322–330. [CrossRef] [PubMed]

44. Ferrandez, O.; Urbina, O.; Grau, S. Critical role of tedizolid in the treatment of acute bacterial skin and skin structure infections. *Drug Des. Dev. Ther.* **2016**, *11*, 65–82. [CrossRef]

45. Kisgen, J.J.; Mansour, H.; Unger, N.R.; Childs, L.M. Tedizolid: A new oxazolidinone antimicrobial. *Am. J. Health-Syst. Pharm.* **2014**, *71*, 621–633. [CrossRef] [PubMed]

46. Moaaz, E.M.; Abdel-Moety, E.M.; Rezk, M.R.; Fayed, A.S. Stability-Indicating Determination of Tedizolid Phosphate in the Presence of its Active Form and Possible Degradants. *J. Chromatogr. Sci.* **2021**, *60*, 51–60. [CrossRef] [PubMed]

47. Chan, H.-K.; Kwok, P.C.L. Production methods for nanodrug particles using the bottom-up approach. *Adv. Drug Deliv. Rev.* **2011**, *63*, 406–416. [CrossRef] [PubMed]

48. Langford, J.I.; Wilson, A. Scherrer after sixty years: A survey and some new results in the determination of crystallite size. *J. Appl. Crystallogr.* **1978**, *11*, 102–113. [CrossRef]

49. Iwasawa, A.; Ayaki, M.; Niwano, Y. Cell viability score (CVS) as a good indicator of critical concentration of benzalkonium chloride for toxicity in cultured ocular surface cell lines. *Regul. Toxicol. Pharmacol.* **2013**, *66*, 177–183. [CrossRef]

50. Efron, N.; Young, G.; Brennan, N.A. Ocular surface temperature. *Curr. Eye Res.* **1989**, *8*, 901–906.

51. Alkholief, M.; Kalam, M.A.; Almomen, A.; Alshememry, A.; Alshamsan, A. Thermoresponsive sol-gel improves ocular bioavailability of Dipivefrin hydrochloride and potentially reduces the elevated intraocular pressure in vivo. *Saudi Pharm. J.* **2020**, *28*, 1019–1029. [CrossRef]

52. Kalam, M.A.; Alshehri, S.; Alshamsan, A.; Haque, A.; Shakeel, F. Solid liquid equilibrium of an antifungal drug itraconazole in different neat solvents: Determination and correlation. *J. Mol. Liq.* **2017**, *234*, 81–87. [CrossRef]

53. Kassaye, L.; Genete, G. Evaluation and comparison of in-vitro dissolution profiles for different brands of amoxicillin capsules. *Afr. Health Sci.* **2013**, *13*, 369–375. [CrossRef] [PubMed]

54. Anderson, N.H.; Bauer, M.; Boussac, N.; Khan-Malek, R.; Munden, P.; Sardaro, M. An evaluation of fit factors and dissolution efficiency for the comparison of in vitro dissolution profiles. *J. Pharm. Biomed. Anal.* **1998**, *17*, 811–822. [CrossRef]

55. Ige, P.P.; Baria, R.K.; Gattani, S.G. Fabrication of fenofibrate nanocrystals by probe sonication method for enhancement of dissolution rate and oral bioavailability. *Colloids Surf. B Biointerfaces* **2013**, *108*, 366–373. [CrossRef] [PubMed]

56. Freeman, P.D.; Kahook, M.Y. Preservatives in topical ophthalmic medications: Historical and clinical perspectives. *Expert Rev. Ophthalmol.* **2009**, *4*, 59–64. [CrossRef]

57. Romanowski, E.G.; Yates, K.A.; Shanks, R.M.Q.; Kowalski, R.P. Benzalkonium Chloride Demonstrates Concentration-Dependent Antiviral Activity Against Adenovirus In Vitro. *J. Ocul. Pharmacol. Ther.* **2019**, *35*, 311–314. [CrossRef]

58. Pannu, J.; Ciotti, S.; Ganesan, S.; Arida, G.; Costley, C.; Fattom, A. Nanodroplet-Benzalkonium Chloride Formulation Demonstrates In Vitro and Ex Vivo Broad-Spectrum Antiviral Activity Against SARS-CoV-2 and Other Enveloped Viruses. *bioRxiv* **2020**. [CrossRef]

59. Yanez, F.; Martikainen, L.; Braga, M.E.; Alvarez-Lorenzo, C.; Concheiro, A.; Duarte, C.M.; Gil, M.H.; de Sousa, H.C. Supercritical fluid-assisted preparation of imprinted contact lenses for drug delivery. *Acta Biomater.* **2011**, *7*, 1019–1030. [CrossRef]

60. Reverchon, E.; De Marco, I.; Torino, E. Nanoparticles production by supercritical antisolvent precipitation: A general interpretation. *J. Supercrit. Fluids* **2007**, *43*, 126–138. [CrossRef]

61. Srivalli, K.M.R.; Mishra, B. Drug nanocrystals: A way toward scale-up. *Saudi Pharm. J.* **2014**, *24*, 386–404. [CrossRef]
62. Saengsorn, K.; Jimtaisong, A. Determination of hydrophilic–lipophilic balance value and emulsion properties of sacha inchi oil. *Asian Pac. J. Trop. Biomed.* **2017**, *7*, 1092–1096. [CrossRef]
63. Liu, F.; Park, J.-Y.; Zhang, Y.; Conwell, C.; Liu, Y.; Bathula, S.R.; Huang, L. Targeted cancer therapy with novel high drug loading nanocrystals. *J. Pharm. Sci.* **2010**, *99*, 3542–3551. [CrossRef] [PubMed]
64. Sharma, M.; Mehta, I. Surface stabilized atorvastatin nanocrystals with improved bioavailability, safety and antihyperlipidemic potential. *Sci. Rep.* **2019**, *9*, 16105–16111. [CrossRef] [PubMed]
65. Wang, Y.; Zheng, Y.; Zhang, L.; Wang, Q.; Zhang, D. Stability of nanosuspensions in drug delivery. *J. Control. Release* **2013**, *172*, 1126–1141. [CrossRef] [PubMed]
66. Medarević, D.; Ibrić, S.; Vardaka, E.; Mitrić, M.; Nikolakakis, I.; Kachrimanis, K. Insight into the formation of glimepiride nanocrystals by wet media milling. *Pharmaceutics* **2020**, *12*, 53. [CrossRef]
67. Medarevic, D.; Djuris, J.; Ibric, S.; Mitric, M.; Kachrimanis, K. Optimization of formulation and process parameters for the production of carvedilol nanosuspension by wet media milling. *Int. J. Pharm.* **2018**, *540*, 150–161. [CrossRef] [PubMed]
68. Li, J.; Wang, Z.; Zhang, H.; Gao, J.; Zheng, A. Progress in the development of stabilization strategies for nanocrystal preparations. *Drug Deliv.* **2020**, *28*, 19–36. [CrossRef] [PubMed]
69. Chiou, H.; Chan, H.-K.; Heng, D.; Prud'homme, R.K.; Raper, J.A. A novel production method for inhalable cyclosporine A powders by confined liquid impinging jet precipitation. *J. Aerosol Sci.* **2008**, *39*, 500–509. [CrossRef]
70. Kumar, V.; Adamson, D.H.; Prud'homme, R.K. Fluorescent polymeric nanoparticles: Aggregation and phase behavior of pyrene and amphotericin B molecules in nanoparticle cores. *Small* **2010**, *6*, 2907–2914. [CrossRef]
71. Paczkowska-Walendowska, M.; Rosiak, N.; Tykarska, E.; Michalska, K.; Plazinska, A.; Plazinski, W.; Szymanowska, D.; Cielecka-Piontek, J. Tedizolid-Cyclodextrin System as Delayed-Release Drug Delivery with Antibacterial Activity. *Int. J. Mol. Sci.* **2020**, *22*, 115. [CrossRef]
72. Liao, J.B.; Liang, Y.Z.; Chen, Y.L.; Xie, J.H.; Liu, W.H.; Chen, J.N.; Lai, X.P.; Su, Z.R. Novel patchouli alcohol ternary solid dispersion pellets prepared by poloxamers. *Iran. J. Pharm. Res.* **2015**, *14*, 15–26.
73. Gombás, Á.; Szabó-Révész, P.; Regdon, G.; Erős, I. Study of thermal behaviour of sugar alcohols. *J. Therm. Anal. Calorim.* **2003**, *73*, 615–621. [CrossRef]
74. Hardiningtyas, S.D.; Wakabayashi, R.; Ishiyama, R.; Owada, Y.; Goto, M.; Kamiya, N. Enhanced potential of therapeutic applications of curcumin using solid-in-water nanodispersion technique. *J. Chem. Eng. Jpn.* **2019**, *52*, 138–143. [CrossRef]
75. Michalska, K.; Mizera, M.; Lewandowska, K.; Cielecka-Piontek, J. Infrared, Raman and ultraviolet with circular dichroism analysis and theoretical calculations of tedizolid. *J. Mol. Struct.* **2016**, *1115*, 136–143. [CrossRef]
76. Sharma, A.; Jain, C.P.; Tanwar, Y.S. Preparation and characterization of solid dispersions of carvedilol with poloxamer 188. *J. Chil. Chem. Soc.* **2013**, *58*, 1553–1557. [CrossRef]
77. Rachmawati, H.; Al Shaal, L.; Muller, R.H.; Keck, C.M. Development of curcumin nanocrystal: Physical aspects. *J. Pharm. Sci.* **2013**, *102*, 204–214. [CrossRef]
78. Srivalli, K.M.R.; Mishra, B. Preparation and pharmacodynamic assessment of ezetimibe nanocrystals: Effect of P-gp inhibitory stabilizer on particle size and oral absorption. *Colloids Surf. B Biointerfaces* **2015**, *135*, 756–764. [CrossRef]
79. Abelson, M.B.; Udell, I.J.; Weston, J.H. Normal human tear pH by direct measurement. *Arch. Ophthalmol.* **1981**, *99*, 301. [CrossRef]
80. Tomlinson, A.; Khanal, S.; Ramaesh, K.; Diaper, C.; McFadyen, A. Tear film osmolarity: Determination of a referent for dry eye diagnosis. *Investig. Ophthalmol. Vis. Sci.* **2006**, *47*, 4309–4315. [CrossRef]
81. Potvin, R.; Makari, S.; Rapuano, C.J. Tear film osmolarity and dry eye disease: A review of the literature. *Clin. Ophthalmol.* **2015**, *9*, 2039–2047. [CrossRef]
82. Troiano, P.; Monaco, G. Effect of hypotonic 0.4% hyaluronic acid drops in dry eye patients: A cross-over study. *Cornea* **2008**, *27*, 1126–1130. [CrossRef]
83. Zhu, H.; Chauhan, A. Effect of viscosity on tear drainage and ocular residence time. *Optom. Vis. Sci.* **2008**, *85*, 715–725. [CrossRef] [PubMed]
84. Salmani, J.M.M.; Lv, H.; Asghar, S.; Zhou, J. Amorphous solid dispersion with increased gastric solubility in tandem with oral disintegrating tablets: A successful approach to improve the bioavailability of atorvastatin. *Pharm. Dev. Technol.* **2015**, *20*, 465–472. [CrossRef] [PubMed]
85. Hattori, Y.; Haruna, Y.; Otsuka, M. Dissolution process analysis using model-free Noyes–Whitney integral equation. *Colloids Surf. B Biointerfaces* **2013**, *102*, 227–231. [CrossRef] [PubMed]
86. Kim, M.; Heinrich, F.; Haugstad, G.; Yu, G.; Yuan, G.; Satija, S.K.; Zhang, W.; Seo, H.S.; Metzger, J.M.; Azarin, S.M.J.L. Spatial Distribution of PEO–PPO–PEO Block Copolymer and PEO Homopolymer in Lipid Bilayers. *Langmuir* **2020**, *36*, 3393–3403. [CrossRef] [PubMed]
87. Zana, R.; Marques, C.; Johner, A. Dynamics of micelles of the triblock copolymers poly(ethylene oxide)-poly(propylene oxide)-poly(ethylene oxide) in aqueous solution. *Adv. Colloid Interface Sci.* **2006**, *123–126*, 345–351. [CrossRef]
88. Al-Kassas, R.; Bansal, M.; Shaw, J. Nanosizing techniques for improving bioavailability of drugs. *J. Control. Release* **2017**, *260*, 202–212. [CrossRef]
89. Verma, S.; Kumar, S.; Gokhale, R.; Burgess, D.J. Physical stability of nanosuspensions: Investigation of the role of stabilizers on Ostwald ripening. *Int. J. Pharm.* **2011**, *406*, 145–152. [CrossRef]

90. Ezquer-Garin, C.; Ferriols-Lisart, R.; Martinez-Lopez, L.M.; Sangrador-Pelluz, C.; Nicolas-Pico, J.; Alos-Alminana, M. Stability of tedizolid phosphate-sodium rifampicin and tedizolid phosphate-meropenem admixtures in intravenous infusion bags stored at different temperatures. *Die Pharm.* **2020**, *75*, 172–176. [CrossRef]

91. Gora, S.; Mustafa, G.; Sahni, J.K.; Ali, J.; Baboota, S. Nanosizing of valsartan by high pressure homogenization to produce dissolution enhanced nanosuspension: Pharmacokinetics and pharmacodyanamic study. *Drug Deliv.* **2016**, *23*, 940–950. [CrossRef]

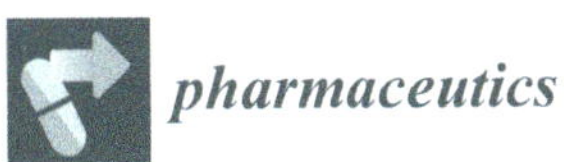 *pharmaceutics*

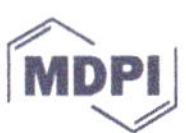

Article

Simultaneous Improvement of Dissolution Behavior and Oral Bioavailability of Antifungal Miconazole via Cocrystal and Salt Formation

Ksenia V. Drozd, Alex N. Manin, Denis E. Boycov and German L. Perlovich *

G.A. Krestov Institute of Solution Chemistry of the Russian Academy of Sciences, 1 Akademicheskaya St., 153045 Ivanovo, Russia; ksdrozd@yandex.ru (K.V.D.); anm@isc-ras.ru (A.N.M.); denboycov11@gmail.com (D.E.B.)
* Correspondence: glp@isc-ras.ru

Abstract: Miconazole shows low oral bioavailability in humans due to poor aqueous solubility, although it has demonstrated various pharmacological activities such as antifungal, anti-tubercular and anti-tumor effects. Cocrystal/salt formation is one of the effective methods for solving this problem. In this study, different methods (liquid-assisted grinding, slurrying and lyophilization) were used to investigate their impact on the formation of the miconazole multicomponent crystals with succinic, maleic and dl-tartaric acids. The solid state of the prepared powder was characterized by differential scanning calorimetry, powder X-ray diffraction and scanning electron microscopy. It was found that lyophilization not only promotes partial amorphization of both salts but also allows obtaining a new polymorph of the miconazole salt with dl-tartaric acid. The lyophilized salts compared with the same samples prepared by two other methods showed better dissolution rates but low stability during the studies due to rapid recrystallization. Overall, it was determined that the preparation method of multicomponent crystals affects the solid-state characteristics and miconazole physicochemical properties significantly. The in vivo studies revealed that the miconazole multicomponent crystals indicated the higher peak blood concentration and area under the curve from 0 to 32 h values 2.4-, 2.9- and 4.6-fold higher than the pure drug. Therefore, this study demonstrated that multicomponent crystals are promising formulations for enhancing the oral bioavailability of poorly soluble compounds.

Keywords: antifungal; miconazole; dicarboxylic acids; grinding; slurry; lyophilization; dissolution; bioavailability

Citation: Drozd, K.V.; Manin, A.N.; Boycov, D.E.; Perlovich, G.L. Simultaneous Improvement of Dissolution Behavior and Oral Bioavailability of Antifungal Miconazole via Cocrystal and Salt Formation. *Pharmaceutics* **2022**, *14*, 1107. https://doi.org/10.3390/pharmaceutics14051107

Academic Editor: Hisham Al-Obaidi

Received: 25 April 2022
Accepted: 19 May 2022
Published: 22 May 2022

Publisher's Note: MDPI stays neutral with regard to jurisdictional claims in published maps and institutional affiliations.

1. Introduction

Miconazole (MCL, Figure 1) is a first-generation synthetic imidazole that displays a broad spectrum of antifungal activity against many Candida species [1,2]. MCL is also known to be active against Mycobacterium tuberculosis [3], and exhibits anti-tumor effects in the treatment of breast cancer [4]. Miconazole is a weak base with an extremely low solubility in water (less than $1\mu g \cdot mL^{-1}$). Along with poor oral absorption and rapid clearance [5], it is one of the main reasons for its poor systemic activity against fungal infections [6]. Thus, the oral bioavailability of MCL in humans is 25–30% [7] compared with 55% for itraconazole [8] or 90% for fluconazole [9]. Hence, the MCL-based preparations are currently used only topically and are available in various topical formulations, including cream, lotion, spray liquid or suppository [10]. The active pharmaceutical ingredient (API) used in these preparations is applied as a nitrate salt [11]. Although the aqueous solubility of the MCL nitrate salt is much better than that of its base [12], its gastrointestinal side effects prevent the use of the salt form as solid oral dosage form [13,14]. However, even with topical use of MCL-based preparations, side effects may often occur on the application site, such as burning, redness, and swelling [15]. The use of nitrate as a counterion is one of the reasons for the presence of these side effects [13]. One possible solution to this problem is to obtain new MCL pharmaceutical salts with counterions, which can be used without limitations and not cause side effects, including from the gastrointestinal tract. This would make it possible, in the future, to use MCL preparations orally.

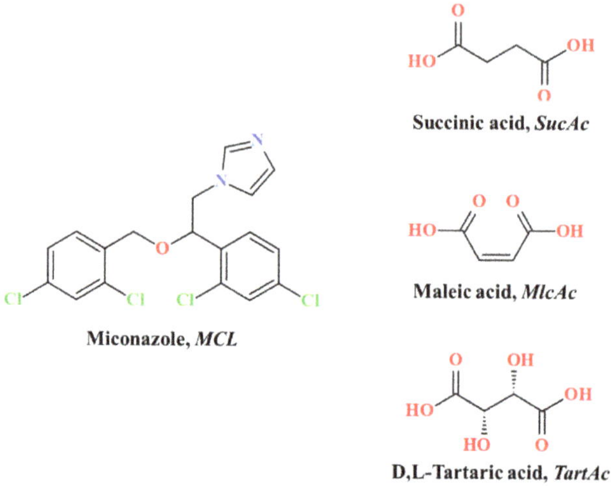

Succinic acid, *SucAc*

Miconazole, *MCL*

Maleic acid, *MlcAc*

D,L-Tartaric acid, *TartAc*

Figure 1. Chemical structures of miconazole and dicarboxylic acids used in this study.

Previously, in an attempt to simplify counterion choice for the preparation of pharmaceutical salts, counterions suitable for oral or parenteral delivery have been divided into three classes in accordance with their GRAS (Generally Recognized as Safe) status and Accepted Daily Intake values [16,17]. According to this classification, the most preferred for the preparation of pharmaceutical salts counterions, belonging to the first class, contain physiologically ubiquitous ions and/or ions that occur as metabolites in biochemical pathways [17]. Hydrochloride and sodium are the most common counterions that have been used to prepare pharmaceutical salts in the past 20 years [18]. However, the study of the impact of different salt formers is necessary to select an optimal salt form, since the influence of a given counterion on the API's physicochemical properties and pharmacodynamics is still difficult to predict without appropriate experiments. In addition to the above salt formers, the first class also includes some carboxylic acids, in particular aliphatic dicarboxylic acids. Previously, we have already screened MCL with a number of dicarboxylic acids, as a result of which the formation of a new two-component solid phases (salts or cocrystals) was confirmed for seven out of ten acids [19]. At the same time, according to the analysis of the Cambridge Structural Database, crystal structures have not been deciphered for all of them due to the difficulty of obtaining single crystals, as in the case of the itraconazole multicomponent crystals [20,21]. However, this is no reason not to carry on further studies of new multicomponent crystals, including the study of bioavailability in comparison with the original API, if new forms are promising [22]. From this list, three multicomponent solid forms of MCL can be selected based on the frequency of use of dicarboxylic acids in pharmaceutical formulations: cocrystal with succinic acid (SucAc) and two salts with maleic (MlcAc) or dl-tartaric (TartAc) acids (Figure 1) [17], which can become a modern alternative to the commercial form of this API. In this work, we were able to show the influence of not only a specific dicarboxylic acid on the API dissolution process but also methods used for preparing the MCL multicomponent crystals.

A great number of techniques are known today for obtaining multicomponent crystals [23]. However, researchers rarely investigate the effect of different preparation methods of multicomponent crystals on the API's physicochemical properties and pharmacokinetics [24,25]. Researchers typically use one of the most common methods for preparing multicomponent crystals, such as grinding, while the preparation method has a great influence on the characteristics of the solid state of a chemical (crystallinity, porosity, particle size, surface area) and its physicochemical properties, respectively [23]. In this work, the MCL multicomponent solid forms were obtained via multiple methods (liquid-assisted grinding (LAG), slurrying and lyophilization) and characterized comprehensively. Lyophilization, unlike the first two methods, is used extremely rarely for the preparation of multicomponent crystals [26–30], considering that this method makes it possible to obtain a fine powders. In addition, the in vivo pharmacokinetic study of the three MCL multicomponent crystals was conducted for the first time in rabbits in order to evaluate their pharmaceutical applicability, which will lay a solid foundation for the further development of new dosage forms of miconazole.

2. Materials and Methods

2.1. Materials

The miconazole base was purchased from abcr GmbH. The dicarboxylic acids (succinic acid, maleic acid and dl-tartaric acid) were procured from Merck (Kenilworth, NJ, USA), Sigma-Aldrich (St. Louis, MO, USA) or Acros Organics (Geel, Belgium), respectively, and were used as received. All solvents used (tert-butanol, methanol, acetonitrile) were of analytical or chromatographic grade.

2.2. Sample Preparation

2.2.1. Liquid-Assisted Grinding (LAG)

Physical mixtures (50–60 mg) of MCL with a dicarboxylic acid in a 2:1 (for the [MCL + SucAc] cocrystal) or 1:1 (for the [MCL + MlcAc] and [MCL + TartAc] salts) molar ratios were added to a 12 mL agate grinding jars with 10 agate balls. The mixtures were ground along with 50 μL methanol for 30 min at a rate of 500 rpm using a Fritsch planetary micro mill (Pulverisette 7).

2.2.2. Slurry Experiments

Physical mixtures (120–140 mg) of MCL and dicarboxylic acid in a 2:1 (for the MCL + SucAc] cocrystal) or 1:1 (for the [MCL + MlcAc] and [MCL + TartAc] salts) molar ratios were slurred in methanol for 12 h under ambient conditions. The resulting samples were filtered and dried for 4 h.

2.2.3. Lyophilization

Firstly, the physical mixtures of MCL and dicarboxylic acid (10–12 mg) were dissolved on stirring in 10 mL of aqueous solution, comprising 30 to 90% (w/v) of tert-butanol (TBA). The resulting solution was kept in a freezer at $-40\ ^\circ$C for 10–12 h. Then, the flasks containing the frozen MCL solution with dicarboxylic acid were quickly transferred into a precooled chamber ($-50\ ^\circ$C) of the INEY LS-500/80 freeze-dryer (Prointeh-bio, Pushchino, Russia). Primary drying was performed at a temperature $-50\ ^\circ$C and a pressure $p < 50$ mTorr for 24 h. After that, the temperature in a chamber was increased up to 30 $^\circ$C and held at this level for the next 4–6 h. All samples after the experiment were characterized by PXRD and DSC.

2.3. Powder X-ray Diffraction (PXRD)

PXRD analysis of the MCL multicomponent crystals was performed on a D2 Phaser diffractometer (Bruker AXS, Karlsruhe, Germany) with Cu-Kα radiation at 30 kV and 10 mA, equipped with a Lynxeye XE-T high-resolution position sensitive detector. The PXRD patterns were recorded over the range of 5–30° (2θ) with a step size of 0.02° and a dwell time of 1 s.

2.4. Differential Scanning Calorimetry (DSC)

DSC thermograms of the MCL multicomponent crystals were recorded using a DSC 4000 (Perkin Elmer, Waltham, MA, USA). Samples tested were placed in an aluminum crucible and heated from 20 °C to 250 °C at a constant rate of 10 °C·min^{-1} under a nitrogen flow of 20 mL·min^{-1}.

2.5. Scanning Electron Microscopy (SEM)

The particle sizes and surface morphology of the powder samples were investigated by a Quattro S scanning electron microscope (Thermo Fisher Scientific, Černovice, Czech Republic). The analysis was carried out using the secondary electron mode, line-average scanning with a work distance of 10.4 mm and acceleration voltage of 5.00 kV.

2.6. Powder Dissolution Experiments

During the powder dissolution experiments, an excess amount of solid sample (100 mg of MCL or an MCL-equivalent amount of cocrystal or salts) was suspended in 15 mL of a pH 6.8 phosphate buffer as dissolution medium at 37.0 ± 0.1 °C. An aliquot of the suspension was withdrawn at predetermined time points (5, 10, 15, 20, 30, 45, 60, 90, 120, 180, 240, 360 min) and filtered through a 0.2 μm syringe filter (Rotilabo® PTEF). The filtrate was diluted, and the MCL concentration was determined by HPLC. All dissolution experiments were performed in triplicate. After the powder dissolution experiments, the undissolved solids were filtered, dried and analyzed by PXRD.

2.7. In Vivo Pharmacokinetic Study

The in vivo study was conducted with prior permission from the Ministry of Health of the Russian Federation (order no. 267 from 19 June 2003). The experimental protocol followed the ethical Guidelines of the animal research ethics and Rules of laboratory practice in conducting preclinical research in the Russian Federation (GOST 51000.3-96 and 51000.4-96). Albino rabbits with a body weight 2 ± 0.3 kg were fasted for 24 h before commencing experiments. All animals had free access to water throughout the experimental period. Powder samples of MCL and its multicomponent crystals were administrated to rabbits using a gavage vehicle at a single dose corresponding 50 mg·kg^{-1} of MCL. Blood samples (about 0.5 mL) were collected from the marginal ear vein at 0.5, 0.75, 1, 1.5, 2, 3, 4, 8, 12, 24 and 32 h after oral administration. Normal heparin was used as an anticoagulant. The blood was centrifuged at 1600 rpm for 15 min and saved at −70 °C until analysis. The MCL concentration in plasma was determined by HPLC. Pharmacokinetic parameters were determined by PKSolver [31] software based on a noncompartmental model. All results were expressed as mean ± SD.

2.8. High-Performance Liquid Chromatography (HPLC)

The MCL concentrations were determined by an LC-20AD Shimadzu Prominence equipped with a PDA detector and a Luna C18 column with a 5 μm particle size, 150 mm length and 4.6 mm inner diameter. The mobile phase was a mixture of acetonitrile and a 0.1% aqueous solution of trifluoroacetic acid (40:60, *v/v*) with a flow rate of 1.0 mL·min^{-1} at 40 °C. The PDA detector was set at 223 nm.

3. Results and Discussion

3.1. Solid State Analysis

It is known that MCL forms seven multicomponent crystals (cocrystals and salts) with a number of aliphatic dicarboxylic [11,19]. In this work, one cocrystal and two salts of MCL with C4-dicarboxylic acids were selected from the list of previously known multicomponent crystals based on the GRAS status of coformers: [MCL + SucAc] cocrystal (2:1), [MCL + MlcAc] salt (1:1) and [MCL + TartAc] salt (1:1). These MCL multicomponent crystals were prepared via multiple methods: liquid-assisted grinding, slurry and lyophilization. In each case, all MCL multicomponent forms, regardless of the preparation method, were characterized by DSC and PXRD methods. In contrast to the first two methods for the preparation of the MCL multicomponent solid forms, the conditions were described previously [19] and reproduced in this work without any difficulties (Figure S1), the lyophilization experiments for these systems were carried out for the first time.

Lyophilization (or freeze-drying) is a unique method of processing drug compounds to obtain high-porous powders with a low density and much better solubility [32,33]. Due to the extremely low solubility of MCL base in water, binary mixtures of cosolvent (tert-butanol) and water were used for lyophilization of its multicomponent crystals. TBA is one of the most frequently used cosolvents for freeze-drying due to a number benefits, including high freezing temperature, very short sublimation time, low sublimation enthalpy, high equilibrium vapor/solid pressure values, and low toxicity [34]. To select the optimal conditions for obtaining the MCL multicomponent forms by lyophilization method, organic solvent-water (TBA/H_2O) mixtures with different contents of TBA (30%, 60% and 90% (w/v)) were tested during the trial experiments for each system. Freeze-drying of pure MCL was also carried out, in order to analyze the effect of the cocrystal and salts obtained by this method on the API's physicochemical properties. In contrast to multicomponent crystals, MCL is completely passed into a liquid state during lyophilization, namely a melt. It is related to the fact that the secondary drying of all the samples was carried out at 30 °C, which is almost 28 °C above the glass transition temperature of amorphous MCL (Figure S2). Thus, it is impossible to obtain the lyophilized MCL under these experimental conditions.

Photos of the obtained powders of the MCL cocrystal and salts as a result of freeze-drying are presented in Figure 2. The photographs clearly demonstrate the influence of both the preparation method and the composition of the organic solvent-water mixture on the appearance of lyophilized substances. Moreover, the mass of the samples obtained, regardless of the composition of TBA/H_2O mixture, was the same in all cases. Based on the appearance of the lyophilized [MCL + SucAc] cocrystal (2:1), it can be assumed that sample amorphization does not occur as a result of lyophilization in spite of the composition of the TBA/H_2O mixture. At the same time, it can be claimed that the cocrystallization of MCL with SucAc during the freeze-drying process leads to the stabilization of the system compared to the pure API. For the [MCL + MlcAc] salt (1:1), we observed a significant increase in powder volume due to a decrease in its density with increasing TBA content in the TBA/H_2O mixture. For the [MCL + TartAc] salt (1:1), lyophilization contributed to the production of bulk powders identical to each other in spite of TBA content. In this regard, all the powders obtained as a result of lyophilization were further analyzed using the PXRD method. The PXRD patterns of the lyophilized powders for each MCL multicomponent system are shown in Figure S3. For the [MCL + SucAc] cocrystal (2:1), the PXRD patterns, regardless of the composition of the TBA/H_2O mixture, were identical to each other, which fully corresponded to the calculated single-crystal diffraction pattern of the cocrystal without peaks corresponding to the starting components. The crystallinity of the lyophilized cocrystal was equal to 90% (Table S1). The PXRD patterns for the MCL lyophilized salts, depending on the TBA/H_2O mixture composition, were significantly different. In both cases, we observed both a spreading of the peaks and a reduction in their intensities, which, in turn, indicated a decrease in the degree of crystallinity of the studied samples. Thus, the lowest value of the crystallinity degree for the [MCL + MlcAc] powder (79.4%) was observed when using the maximum amount of TBA, which is consistent with the change in the density of lyophilized powders for this salt (Figure 2). The lowest crystallinity degree for the [MCL + TartAc] salt (46.0%) was achieved using 60% (w/v) of TBA in the TBA/H_2O mixture. Moreover, based on the comparison of the PXRD patterns of the lyophilized [MCL + TartAc] salt (1:1) with that of the crystalline sample, it was found that the peaks did not correspond to the peaks of either the original components or the crystalline salt (Figure S3). Thus, it can be assumed that a new polymorphic form of the [MCL + TartAc] salt (1:1) was obtained by the lyophilization method.

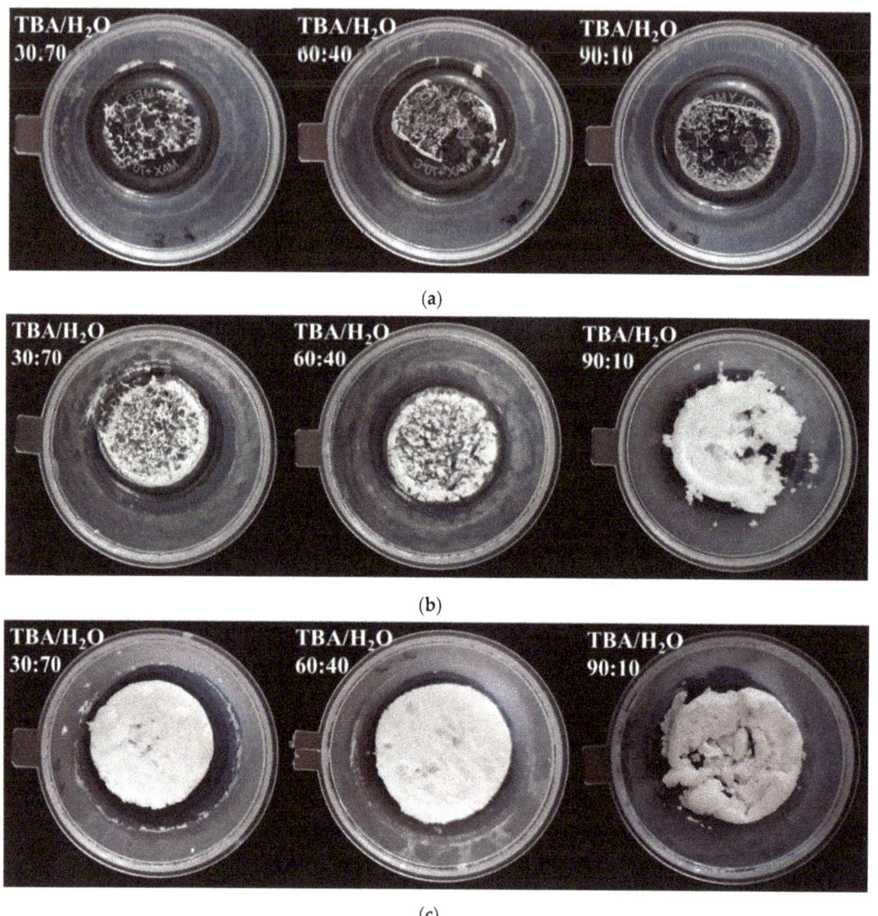

Figure 2. Comparison of the freeze-dried powders of (**a**) [MCL + SucAc] cocrystal (2:1), (**b**) [MCL + MlcAc] salt (1:1) and (**c**) [MCL + TartAc] salt (1:1) obtained from TBA/H_2O mixtures with different TBA content.

Based on the data obtained, to produce the required mass of the MCL cocrystal or salts by lyophilization, the compositions of the TBA/H_2O mixtures were used, at which the crystallinity degree of the powders was the least. We expect that it will contribute to the higher solubility of the investigated MCL multicomponent forms. As for the [MCL + SucAc] cocrystal (2:1), we used an aqueous solution comprising 60% (*w/v*) of TBA, because the experimental conditions we used did not affect the crystallinity degree of the lyophilized powders.

According to the previously published data, melting points of the MCL multicomponent crystals studied in this work are known: 119.7 ± 0.2 °C for the [MCL + SucAc] cocrystal (2:1), 140.3 ± 0.2 °C for the [MCL + MlcAc] salt (1:1) and 171.4 ± 0.2 °C for the [MCL + TartAc] salt (1:1) [19]. The DSC curves for the MCL cocrystal and salts obtained by the various methods are shown on Figure 3. Table S2 provides a comparison of the melting points and the melting enthalpy values of the MCL multicomponent crystals with the literature data. For the [MCL + SucAc] cocrystal (2:1), regardless of the preparation method, we observed one sharp endothermic peak on the DSC curve at a temperature corresponding to the melting temperature of the cocrystal. This is consistent with the identity of the PXRD patterns of the MCL cocrystal prepared via different methods. Moreover, the absence of additional endo/exo effects on the DSC curves additionally confirms the high purity of the samples under investigation. As for the [MCL + MlcAc] salt (1:1) prepared by the various techniques, we also observed similar DSC curves, which is consistent with previously published data [11,19]. However, the melting point of the salt samples prepared by LAG and lyophilization were almost 5 ± 0.2 °C lower than for the sample prepared by the slurry method. The DSC curves of the [MCL + TartAc] salt prepared by LAG and slurrying show one sharp endothermic peak, corresponding to the melting of the powder samples. The melting temperature of the lyophilized [MCL + TartAc] salt was 15.6 ± 0.2 °C lower than the melting temperature of the salt samples prepared by the other two methods. Moreover, the melting enthalpy of the lyophilized salt was almost 2-times less than the melting enthalpy of salt samples prepared by LAG or slurry methods. Additional peaks corresponding to the melting of individual compounds or desolvation were not found on the DSC curves. Such a difference in the melting temperatures of the [MCL + TartAc] salt (1:1) produced by the various methods, coupled with the presence of new peaks in the PXRD pattern for the lyophilized sample, additionally confirms our assumption about obtaining a new polymorph of the MCL salt via freeze-drying. As a result, based on the obtained data (PXRD and DSC), it can be argued that any of the methods used by us for the preparation of the MCL multicomponent crystals makes it possible to obtain high-purity powder samples, differing in the degree of crystallinity.

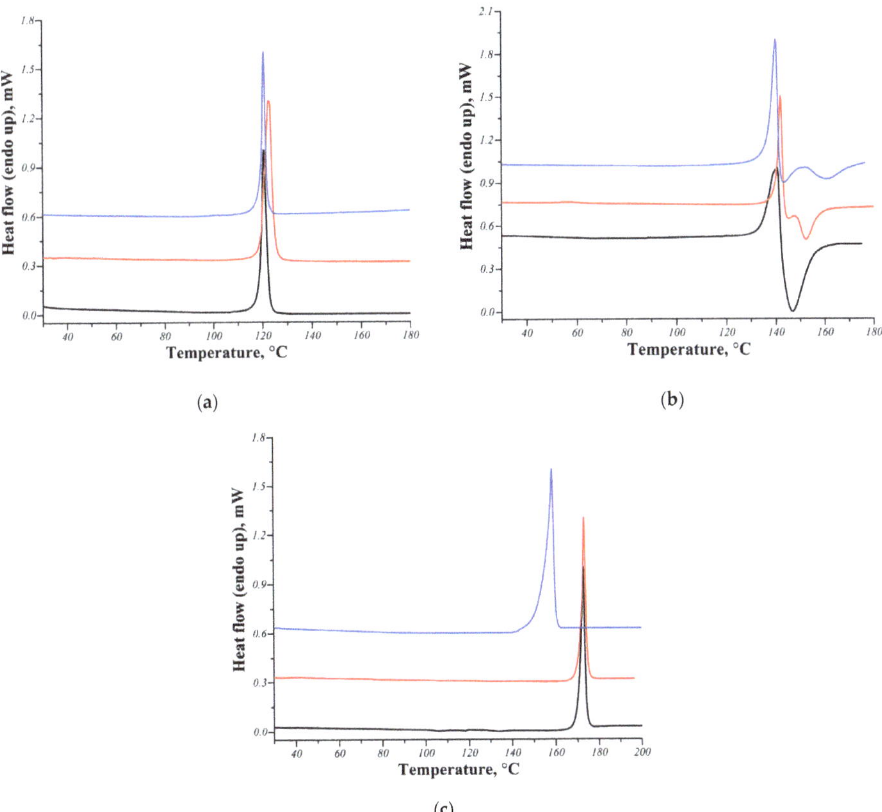

Figure 3. DSC curves of the MCL multicomponent crystals: (**a**) [MCL + SucAc] cocrystal (2:1), (**b**) [MCL + MlcAc] salt (1:1), (**c**) [MCL + TartAc] salt (1:1) prepared via LAG (black line), slurrying (red line) and freeze-drying (blue line).

3.2. Surface Morphology

Morphology and particle size have a significant impact on the API's physicochemical properties, including solubility and dissolution rate [35,36]. SEM analysis of the MCL multicomponent crystals produced by the different methods was carried out to study the influence of the preparation method on the morphology of the powders obtained. As a result of comparing the acquired SEM images for each MCL cocrystal/salt produced by LAG, slurrying and lyophilization, the morphological differences can be seen (Figure 4). The powder samples prepared by LAG had a much broader particle size distribution compared to the other two preparation methods. Particles of the [MCL + SucAc] cocrystal (2:1) and [MCL + MlcAc] salt (1:1) have an irregular shape, the size of which varies on average in the range from 50 to 400 μm. The rough surface of the particles obtained is the result of mechanochemical processing. In contrast to the other two multicomponent forms, the [MCL + TartAc] salt (1:1) obtained by LAG showed pronounced agglomeration of needle-shaped crystals. The average size of the agglomerates exceeded 400 μm. In contrast to the first preparation method of the MCL multicomponent crystals, the slurry method makes it possible to obtain sufficiently homogeneous phases with constant particle morphology. Moreover, the particles have a much smoother surface and smaller size: 5–10 μm for the [MCL + SucAc] cocrystal (2:1) and the [MCL + MlcAc] salt (1:1), and 2–5 μm for the [MCL + TartAc] salt (1:1). The shape of the [MCL + TartAc] salt (1:1) particles is strikingly different from the shape of the other two multicomponent systems, which, in turn, can also affect the difference in the dissolution parameters of the powders. The SEM image of the [MCL + SucAc] cocrystal (2:1) prepared by lyophilization confirms that the powder has a high degree of crystallinity. The cocrystal crystallized as large aggregates with many crystalline features, including a rough surface and irregular edges. The diameter of the aggregates varied over a wide range, and in some cases exceeded 500 μm. The morphology of the lyophilized MCL salts differed significantly compared with the cocrystal. The powders of the lyophilized MCL salts are porous agglomerates formed by perforated flat particles, the size of which did not exceed 1 μm. Thus, it can be assumed that the lyophilized MCL salts will show the greatest increase in API solubility based on the data obtained as a result of the morphology and particle size analysis.

3.3. Physical Stability

Considering that the lyophilized MCL salts were partially amorphous (Table S1), it was necessary to evaluate their relative stability during storage under ambient conditions. The physical stability of the lyophilized MCL salts was examined by PXRD analysis. The crystallization of the samples stored at room temperature was monitored at regular intervals. The PXRD patterns of the [MCL + MlcAc] and [MCL + TartAc] salts produced by lyophilization before and after storage in comparison with the PXRD patterns corresponding to their crystalline forms are presented in Figure 5.

It should be noticed that the traces of recrystallization for all lyophilized MCL salts began to appear after one day of storage, as evidenced by the appearance of some diffraction peaks (Figure 5). The intensity of the diffraction peaks increased over time, which directly affected the increase in the crystallinity degree of the analyzed samples. At the same time, the peaks for the lyophilized [MCL + TartAc] salt on the PXRD patterns do not correspond to the peaks of the crystalline salt prepared by LAG or slurry methods. Thus, the new polymorphic form of the [MCL + TatAc] salt (1:1) is stable during recrystallization. The crystallinity degree of the lyophilized salts after 1 week of storage increased from 79.4% to 86.1% for [MCL + MlcAc] and from 46.0% to 62.7% for [MCL + TartAc].

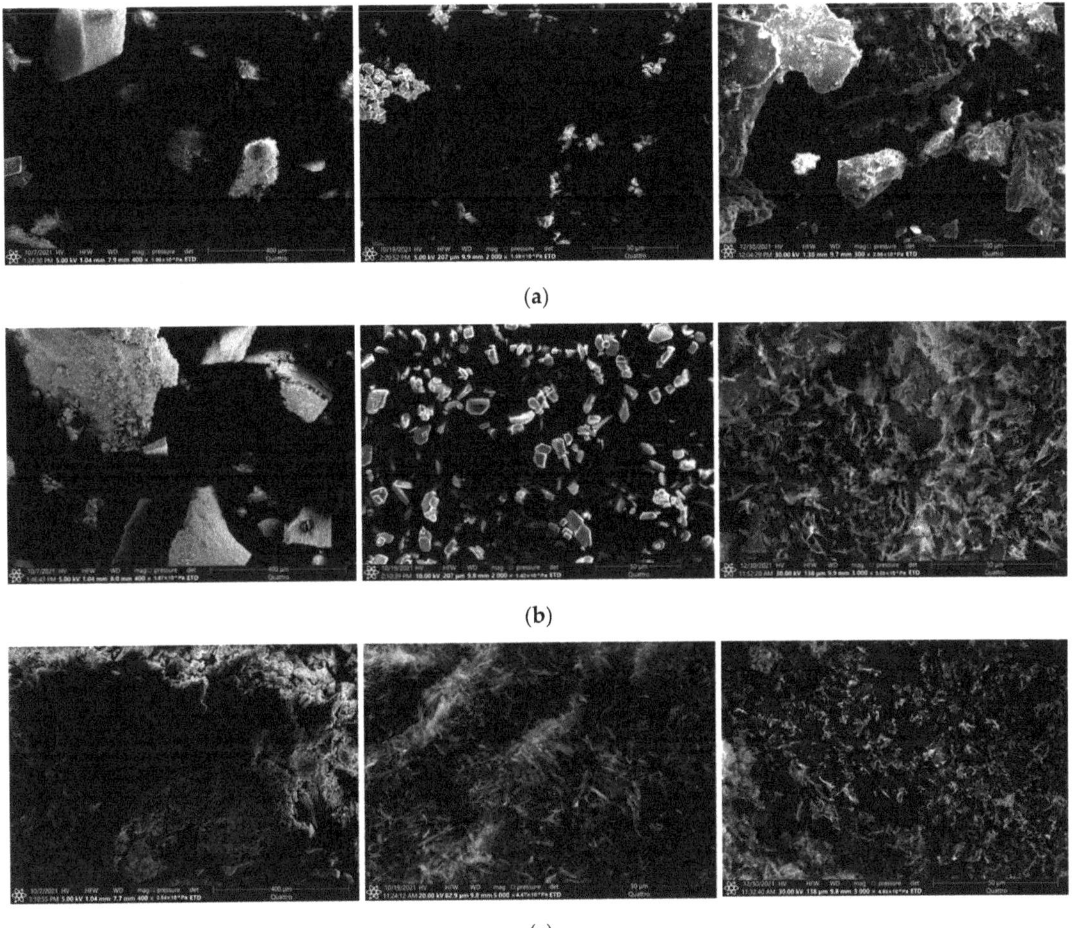

Figure 4. SEM images of the MCL multicomponent crystals: (**a**) [MCL + SucAc] cocrystal (2:1), (**b**) [MCL + MlcAc] salt (1:1) and (**c**) [MCL + TartAc] salt (1:1), prepared by LAG, slurring and freeze-drying (from left to right).

The results obtained showed that the physical stability of both lyophilized salts is extremely low, and they can easy recrystallize during storage under ambient conditions. Moreover, it can be assumed that the lyophilized MCL salts will also be the least stable during dissolution in an aqueous solution compared to their crystalline samples prepared by LAG or slurrying. Therefore, the in vitro powder dissolution experiments with the lyophilized MCL salts were performed only on the freshly prepared samples. In the future, in order to obtain more storage stable MCL salts, we will not exclude the use of various stabilizers; however, we did not set this goal in our work.

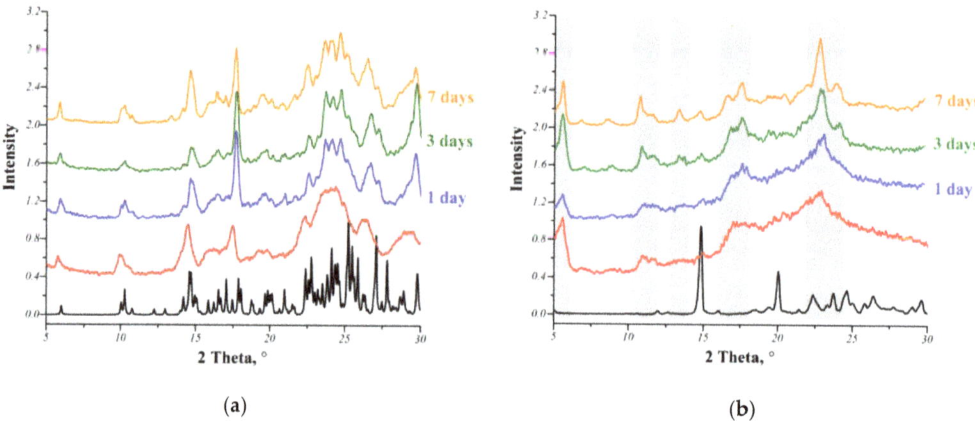

Figure 5. PXRD patterns for the MCL salts: (**a**) [MCL + MlcAc] (1:1) and (**b**) [MCL + TartAc] (1:1) in crystalline forms (black line) and freeze-dried samples (red line) studied as a function of storage time. Grey stripes highlight some unique peaks different from the peaks of the crystalline [MCL + TartAc] salt.

3.4. In Vitro Dissolution Studies

After oral administration, drugs must dissolve well in the intestinal fluid in order to enter the bloodstream. Poor solubility is one of the main reasons for limiting the API amount that is effectively absorbed. As is known, the MCL base is practically insoluble in water ($\sim 0.4 \times 10^{-2}$ $\mu g \cdot mL^{-1}$ [19]). However, we have previously shown the effectiveness of cocrystallization and salt formation on the MCL hydrophilic nature, despite that fact that these multicomponent crystals dissociate in water over time [19]. In the present work, the in vitro dissolution of the MCL multicomponent crystals prepared by multiple methods was studied to evaluate the effect of a particular dicarboxylic acid and preparation method on the level and duration of drug supersaturation in water. The powder dissolution experiments of the MCL multicomponent crystals were made in aqueous solution at pH 6.8 and 37 °C. The time profiles of the MCL dissolved concentrations for each multicomponent form are shown in Figure 6, and the results are summarized in Table 1. The absence of a dissolution profile for the original MCL was due to the fact that the solubility of MCL in the studied medium was so low that it was not possible to determine it correctly.

Table 1. Dissolution results of the MCL multicomponent crystals prepared by the multiple methods in aqueous solution pH 6.8 at 37 °C.

MCL Multicomponent Crystal	Preparation Method	Dissolution Profile				Residue Form at 24 h
		T_{max}, h	C_{max}, $\mu g \cdot mL^{-1}$	C_{6h}, $\mu g \cdot mL^{-1}$	AUC_{0-6}, $\mu g \cdot mL^{-1} \cdot h$	
[MCL + SucAc] (2:1)	LAG	0.7 ± 0.2	0.80 ± 0.02	$(1.78 \pm 0.23) \times 10^{-2}$	1.42	cocrystal, $MCL \cdot H_2O$
	slurry	1.2 ± 0.4	0.89 ± 0.03	0.34 ± 0.06	3.36	
	freeze-drying	0.7 ± 0.3	0.39 ± 0.03	$(0.85 \pm 0.03) \times 10^{-2}$	0.90	
[MCL + MlcAc] (1:1)	LAG	1.3 ± 0.5	3.82 ± 0.17	0.41 ± 0.07	10.6	cocrystal, $MCL \cdot H_2O$
	slurry	1.4 ± 0.5	4.30 ± 0.20	0.48 ± 0.09	11.9	
	freeze-drying	0.2 ± 0.1	13.43 ± 0.38	7.67 ± 0.26	48.2	
[MCL + TartAc] (1:1)	LAG	3.2 ± 0.6	17.45 ± 0.40	10.13 ± 0.50	73.3	cocrystal, $MCL \cdot H_2O$
	slurry	1.7 ± 0.5	85.26 ± 3.05	17.71 ± 0.60	248.2	
	freeze-drying	0.1 ± 0.05	548.60 ± 24.31	41.84 ± 2.10	769.7	

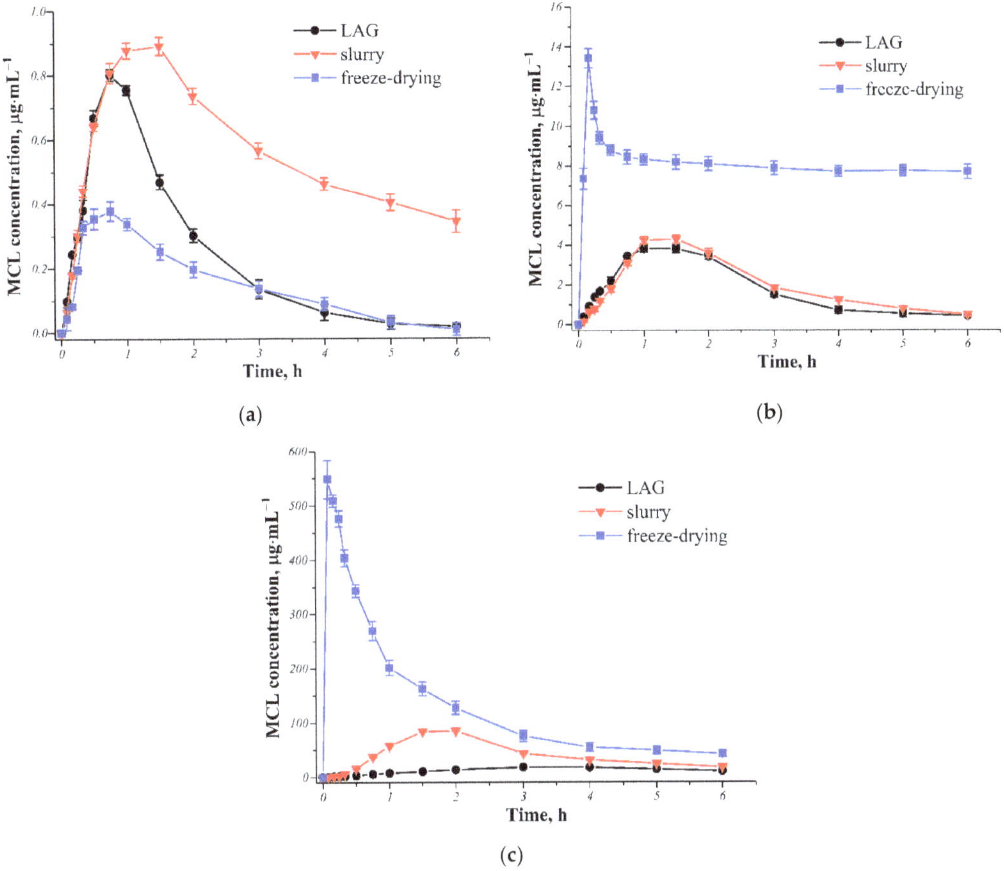

Figure 6. Time profiles of the MCL dissolved concentrations from its multicomponent crystals prepared via different methods in aqueous solution pH 6.8 at 37 °C: (**a**) [MCL + SucAc] (2:1), (**b**) [MCL + MlcAc] (1:1), (**c**) [MCL + TartAc] (1:1).

According to the obtained dissolution profiles, all MCL multicomponent forms, regardless of the preparation method, are metastable in an aqueous solution, as evidenced primarily by the presence of a "spring and parachute" type effect in each case. This statement was also confirmed by PXRD analysis of the solid state after the experiment (Figure S4). However, if for both salts in the bottom phase there was only a crystalline MCL hemihydrate, then in the case of [MCL + SucAc] (2:1), along with the traces of the crystalline MCL hemihydrate, the traces of the initial cocrystal were also present, even after 24 h of the sample being in the buffer solution.

As expected, the preparation method of the MCL multicomponent crystals made a significant contribution to the difference in dissolution profiles for a particular system. The lyophilized salts showed a much higher initial dissolution rate compared to their crystalline forms obtained by LAG or slurry methods. The MCL maximum concentration (C_{max}) was reached in 0.2 ± 0.1 h for the [MCL + MlcAc] (1:1) or 0.1 ± 0.05 h for [MCL + TartAc] (1:1) (T_{max} values are presented in Table 1). The C_{max} value for the lyophilized [MCL + TartAc] salt (1:1) was more than 40 times higher than for the [MCL + MlcAc] salt (1:1). However, the increased MCL concentration for these salts was not maintained and decreased rapidly over time. After 6 h, the MCL concentration decreased by almost 2 times for [MCL + MlcAc] and

13 times for [MCL + TartAc]. This increase in solubility and dissolution rate of MCL was facilitated precisely by the fact that the obtained powders of the MCL salts via lyophilization had a porous structure, which thereby led to an increase in the contact surface of the drug substance with the solvent. The MCL salts prepared by LAG and slurry methods had a much lower dissolution rate. C_{max} values of MCL were achieved after 1.3 ± 0.5 or 1.4 ± 0.5 h for [MCL + MlcAc] and 3.2 ± 0.6 or 1.7 ± 0.5 h for [MCL + TartAc], respectively (Table 1). A subsequent decrease in the MCL concentration for these salts was much more gradual than for the lyophilized forms, thus providing a more comfortable window of the period required for API release [37]. In contrast to the [MCL + TartAc] salt, the dissolution profiles for the [MCL + MlcAc] salt produced by both LAG and slurry methods were almost identical, as evidenced by the AUC_{0-6} (area under the curve) values of 10.6 and 11.9 µg·mL^{-1}·h, respectively. The values of C_{max} and AUC_{0-6} for the [MCL + TartAc] salt prepared by slurrying were almost 5- and 3.5-times higher, respectively, compared to the same salt prepared by LAG. This difference in the dissolution parameters may be due precisely to significant differences in the morphology of the powders obtained using these methods (Figure 4). We believe that the crystal agglomeration, characteristic of the grinded salt, is one of the reasons preventing the MCL release from the salt form. Nevertheless, the level of the MCL supersaturation in the aqueous solution was the highest for the [MCL + TartAc] salt (1:1), regardless of its preparation method.

The influence of the different preparation methods on the [MCL + SucAc] cocrystal (2:1) dissolution was not as significant as for the two MCL salts. The highest C_{max} and AUC_{0-6} values of the API are achieved for the cocrystal produced by slurry method, and the lowest values for the lyophilized sample. We assume that this may be related to the influence of the cocrystal preparation method on the particle size of the powder samples.

3.5. In Vivo Pharmacokinetic Study

After satisfactory in vitro dissolution studies, the in vivo pharmacokinetic investigations of the pure MCL and its cocrystal and salts were carried out for the first time to evaluate whether the in vitro dissolution advantages of the MCL multicomponent crystals can translate into in vivo oral bioavailability advantages. In vivo studies have been performed on rabbits, which are often used as an animal model for pharmacokinetic studies.

Based on the dissolution profiles, as well as the physical stability of the powders during storage and in aqueous media of the MCL multicomponent crystals prepared by the multiple methods, the in vivo studies were carried out for the samples produced by slurry method. The time profiles of the MCL plasma concentration after oral administration of the pure API or its multicomponent crystals to rabbits are shown in Figure 7. Calculated pharmacokinetic parameters, such as maximum MCL plasma concentration (C_{max}), time to reach C_{max} (T_{max}) and area under the MCL plasma concentration versus time cure (AUC_{0-32}), are summarized in Table 2.

Table 2. Main pharmacokinetic parameters of pure MCL and its multicomponent crystals in rabbits.

	MCL	[MCL + SucAc] (2:1)	[MCL + MlcAc] (1:1)	[MCL + TartAc] (1:1)
C_{max}, ng·mL^{-1}	120 ± 20	261 ± 37	365 ± 23	379 ± 30
T_{max}, h	2 ± 0.6	1.3 ± 0.6	2.2 ± 0.5	6.2 ± 0.6
AUC_{0-32}, ng·mL^{-1}·h	1372 ± 418	3296 ± 537	4017 ± 617	6349 ± 661

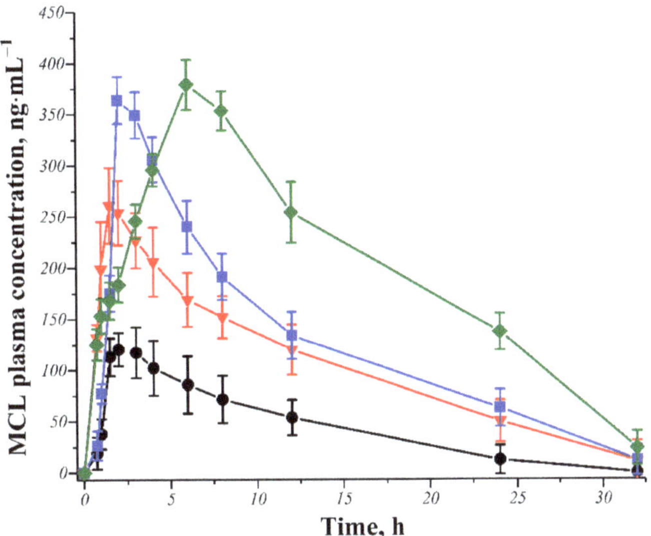

Figure 7. Mean plasma concentration-time profiles of the MCL and its multicomponent crystals after oral administration to rabbits. Key: ●—pure MCL, ▼—[MCL + SucAc] (2:1), ■—[MCL + MlcAc] (1:1), ◆—[MCL + TartAc] (1:1).

For the pure MCL, the C_{max} и AUC_{0-32} values are only 120 ± 20 ng·mL^{-1} and 1372 ± 420 ng·h·mL^{-1}, indicating poor oral absorption due to its extremely low intrinsic solubility. However, the MCL cocrystal and salts showed significantly higher absorption compared to pure API, which is consistent with previously in vitro data. The C_{max} values for [MCL + SucAc], [MCL + MlcAc] и [MCL + TartAc] were 2.2, 3- and 3.2-times higher, respectively, than the pure MCL. Due to that, the AUC_{0-32} values also increased several times compared to the original API, namely 2.4 times for the cocrystal, 2.9 and 4.6 times for the salts. Moreover, while the C_{max} value of the [MCL + TartAc] salt (1:1) is only 14 ng·mL^{-1} higher that of the [MCL + MlcAc] salt (1:1), the AUC_{0-32} value for it is almost 40% higher. It is associated with a much more gradual decrease in the MCL concentration over time for the [MCL + TartAc] salt. T_{max} for the [MCL + TartAc] salt was also far different and is 6 h instead of 1.5–2 h for pure MCL or two other MCL multicomponent crystals, referring to the prolonged effect of the salt. Thus, the MCL multicomponent crystals with C4-dicarboxylic acids studied in this work are promising for the development of new oral forms of MCL.

4. Conclusions

In this work, the influence of the preparation methods (liquid-assisted grinding, slurrying and lyophilization) on the solid state and dissolution of the miconazole multicomponent crystals with succinic, maleic and dl-tartaric acids was studied. It was found that the preparation method significantly affects both the morphology and size of the particles. It was revealed that the lyophilization of both miconazole salts leads to their partial amorphization, in contrast to the cocrystal. However, while the dissolution rate and the miconazole maximum concentration value in the aqueous solution for the lyophilized salts was many times higher than for the same samples prepared by grinding and slurrying, their physical stability was extremely low. The in vivo pharmacokinetic study of the miconazole cocrystal and salts was carried out for the first time. It was found that the improved dissolution parameters of miconazole are successfully converted into improved in vivo pharmacokinetic profiles. It justified the promise of the miconazole multicomponent forms in the development of new oral dosage forms based on it.

Supplementary Materials: The following supporting information can be downloaded at: https://www.mdpi.com/article/10.3390/pharmaceutics14051107/s1, Figure S1: Overlay of the experimental PXRD patterns of the MCL multicomponent crystals prepared by LAG (red line) and slurry (blue line) and calculated PXRD (black line) form the X-ray crystal structure for: (a) [MCL + SucAc] (2:1), (b) [MCL + MlcAc] (1:1) and (c) [MCL + TartAc] (1:1), Figure S2: DSC profiles of MCL indicating its transformation from crystalline to the glassy state by cooling sample from the melt, Figure S3: Overlay of the experimental PXRD patterns of the freeze-dried powders of (a) [MCL + SucAc] cocrystal (2:1), (b) [MCL + MlcAc] salt (1:1) and (c) [MCL + TartAc] salt (1:1) obtained from TBA/H_2O mixtures with different TBA content, Figure S4: Results of PXRD analysis of the residual materials collected at the end of the dissolution experiments: (a) [MCL + SucAc] cocrystal (2:1), (b) [MCL + MlcAc] salt (1:1) and (c) [MCL + TartAc] salt (1:1), Table S1: Crystallinity percentage of the freeze-dried powders of the MCL multicomponent crystals calculated on basis of PXRD analysis. Table S2: Thermophysical data of the MCL multicomponent crystals prepared by the multiple methods.

Author Contributions: Conceptualization, G.L.P.; investigation, K.V.D., A.N.M. and D.E.B.; writing—original draft preparation, K.V.D. and A.N.M.; writing—review and editing, G.L.P.; supervision, G.L.P.; project administration, G.L.P. All authors have read and agreed to the published version of the manuscript.

Funding: This work was supported by the Russian Science Foundation, Grant No. 19-13-00017.

Institutional Review Board Statement: Not applicable.

Informed Consent Statement: Not applicable.

Data Availability Statement: The results obtained for all experiments performed are shown in the manuscript and Supplementary Materials, the raw data will be provided upon request.

Acknowledgments: We thank "the Upper Volga Region Centre of Physicochemical Research" for the assistance with powder X-ray diffraction and scanning electron microscopy experiments.

Conflicts of Interest: The authors declare no conflict of interest.

References

1. Quatresooz, P.; Vroome, V.; Borgers, M.; Cauwenbergh, G.; Piérard, G.E. Novelties in the multifaceted miconazole effects on skin disorders. *Expert Opin. Pharmacother.* **2008**, *9*, 1927–1934. [CrossRef] [PubMed]
2. Isham, N.; Ghannoum, M.A. Antifungal activity of miconazole against recent Candida strains. *Mycoses* **2010**, *53*, 434–437. [CrossRef] [PubMed]
3. Kim, S.; Cho, S.-N.; Oh, T.; Kim, P. Design and synthesis of 1H-1,2,3-triazoles derived from econazole as antitubercular agents. *Bioorg. Med. Chem. Lett.* **2012**, *22*, 6844–6847. [CrossRef] [PubMed]
4. Chengzhu, W.U.; Gao, M.; Shen, L.; Bohan, L.I.; Bai, X.; Gui, J.; Hongmei, L.I.; Huo, Q.; Tao, M.A. Miconazole triggers various forms of cell death in human breast cancer MDA-MB-231 cells. *Pharmazie* **2019**, *74*, 290–294. [CrossRef] [PubMed]
5. Lewi, P.J.; Boelaert, J.; Daneels, R.; De Meyere, R.; Van Landuyt, H.; Heykants, J.J.P.; Symoens, J.; Wynants, J. Pharmacokinetic profile of intravenous miconazole in man. *Eur. J. Clin. Pharmacol.* **1976**, *10*, 49–54. [CrossRef]
6. Jain, S.; Jain, S.; Khare, P.; Gulbake, A.; Bansal, D.; Jain, S.K. Design and development of solid lipid nanoparticles for topical delivery of an anti-fungal agent. *Drug Deliv.* **2010**, *17*, 443–451. [CrossRef]
7. Heel, R.C.; Brogden, R.N.; Pakes, G.E.; Speight, T.M.; Avery, G.S. Miconazole: A preliminary review of its therapeutic efficacy in systemic fungal infections. *Drugs* **1980**, *19*, 7–30. [CrossRef]
8. Sahoo, B.M.; Banik, B.K.; Mahato, A.K.; Shanthi, C.N.; Mohantad, B.C. 23-Microwave-assisted synthesis of antitubercular agents: A novel approach. In *Green Approaches in Medicinal Chemistry for Sustainable Drug Design*; Banik, B.K., Ed.; Advances in Green and Sustainable Chemistry; Elsevier: Amsterdam, The Netherlands, 2020; pp. 779–818, ISBN 978-0-12-817592-7.
9. Brammer, K.W.; Farrow, P.R.; Faulkner, J.K. Pharmacokinetics and tissue penetration of fluconazole in humans. *Rev. Infect. Dis.* **1990**, *12*, S318–S326. [CrossRef]
10. Abdel-Rashid, R.S.; Helal, D.A.; Alaa-Eldin, A.A.; Abdel-Monem, R. Polymeric versus lipid nanocapsules for miconazole nitrate enhanced topical delivery: In vitro and ex vivo evaluation. *Drug Deliv.* **2022**, *29*, 294–304. [CrossRef]
11. Tsutsumi, S.; Iida, M.; Tada, N.; Kojima, T.; Ikeda, Y.; Moriwaki, T.; Higashi, K.; Moribe, K.; Yamamoto, K. Characterization and evaluation of miconazole salts and cocrystals for improved physicochemical properties. *Int. J. Pharm.* **2011**, *421*, 230–236. [CrossRef]
12. Shahzadi, I.; Masood, M.; Chowdhary, F.; Anjum, A.; Nawaz, M.; Maqsood, I.; Zaman, M.; Qadir, A.; Road, J.; Lahore, P.; et al. Microemulsion Formulation for Topical Delivery of Miconazole Nitrate. *Int. J. Pharm. Sci. Rev. Res.* **2014**, *24*, 30–36.
13. Berge, S.M.; Bighley, L.D.; Monkhouse, D.C. Pharmaceutical salts. *J. Pharm. Sci.* **1977**, *66*, 1–19. [CrossRef] [PubMed]

14. Tong, W.-Q. Salt Screening and Selection: New Challenges and Considerations in the Modern Pharmaceutical Research and Development Paradigm. In *Developing Solid Oral Dosage Forms*; Qiu, Y., Chen, Y., Zhang, G.G.Z., Liu, L., Porter, W.R., Eds.; Academic Press: San Diego, CA, USA, 2009; pp. 75–86, ISBN 978-0-444-53242-8.
15. Kenechukwu, F.C.; Attama, A.A.; Ibezim, E.C.; Nnamani, P.O.; Umeyor, C.E.; Uronnachi, E.M.; Momoh, M.A.; Akpa, P.A.; Ozioko, A.C. Novel Intravaginal Drug Delivery System Based on Molecularly PEGylated Lipid Matrices for Improved Antifungal Activity of Miconazole Nitrate. *Biomed. Res. Int.* **2018**, *2018*, 3714329. [CrossRef] [PubMed]
16. Serajuddin, A.T.M.; Pudipeddi, M. Salt selection strategies. In *Handbook of Pharmaceutical Salts: Properties, Selection and Use*; Stahl, P.H., Wermuth, G.H., Eds.; Wiley-VCH: Weinheim, Germany, 2002; pp. 135–160.
17. Williams, H.D.; Trevaskis, N.L.; Charman, S.A.; Shanker, R.M.; Charman, W.N.; Pouton, C.W.; Porter, C.J.H. Strategies to address low drug solubility in discovery and development. *Pharmacol. Rev.* **2013**, *65*, 315–499. [CrossRef]
18. Stahl, P. Preparation of Water-Soluble Compounds Through Salt Formation. In *The Practice of Medicinal Chemistry*; Wermuth, C., Aldous, D., Raboisson, P., Rognan, D., Eds.; Academic Press: Cambridge, MA, USA, 2003; pp. 601–615. ISBN 9780127444819.
19. Drozd, K.V.; Manin, A.N.; Voronin, A.P.; Boycov, D.E.; Churakov, A.V.; Perlovich, G.L. A combined experimental and theoretical study of miconazole salts and cocrystals: Crystal structures, DFT computations, formation thermodynamics and solubility improvement. *Phys. Chem. Chem. Phys.* **2021**, *23*, 12456–12470. [CrossRef]
20. Shevchenko, A.; Miroshnyk, I.; Pietilä, L.-O.; Haarala, J.; Salmia, J.; Sinervo, K.; Mirza, S.; van Veen, B.; Kolehmainen, E.; Nonappa; et al. Diversity in Itraconazole Cocrystals with Aliphatic Dicarboxylic Acids of Varying Chain Length. *Cryst. Growth Des.* **2013**, *13*, 4877–4884. [CrossRef]
21. Vasilev, N.A.; Surov, A.O.; Voronin, A.P.; Drozd, K.V.; Perlovich, G.L. Novel cocrystals of itraconazole: Insights from phase diagrams, formation thermodynamics and solubility. *Int. J. Pharm.* **2021**, *599*, 120441. [CrossRef]
22. Karashima, M.; Sano, N.; Yamamoto, S.; Arai, Y.; Yamamoto, K.; Amano, N.; Ikeda, Y. Enhanced pulmonary absorption of poorly soluble itraconazole by micronized cocrystal dry powder formulations. *Eur. J. Pharm. Biopharm.* **2017**, *115*, 65–72. [CrossRef]
23. Kumar Bandaru, R.; Rout, S.R.; Kenguva, G.; Gorain, B.; Alhakamy, N.A.; Kesharwani, P.; Dandela, R. Recent Advances in Pharmaceutical Cocrystals: From Bench to Market. *Front. Pharmacol.* **2021**, *12*, 780582. [CrossRef]
24. Pi, J.; Wang, S.; Li, W.; Kebebe, D.; Zhang, Y.; Zhang, B.; Qi, D.; Guo, P.; Li, N.; Liu, Z. A nano-cocrystal strategy to improve the dissolution rate and oral bioavailability of baicalein. *Asian J. Pharm. Sci.* **2019**, *14*, 154–164. [CrossRef]
25. Hossain Mithu, M.D.S.; Ross, S.A.; Hurt, A.P.; Douroumis, D. Effect of mechanochemical grinding conditions on the formation of pharmaceutical cocrystals and co-amorphous solid forms of ketoconazole—Dicarboxylic acid. *J. Drug Deliv. Sci. Technol.* **2021**, *63*, 102508. [CrossRef]
26. Eddleston, M.D.; Patel, B.; Day, G.M.; Jones, W. Cocrystallization by Freeze-Drying: Preparation of Novel Multicomponent Crystal Forms. *Cryst. Growth Des.* **2013**, *13*, 4599–4606. [CrossRef]
27. Wang, L.; Wen, X.; Li, P.; Wang, J.; Yang, P.; Zhang, H.; Deng, Z. 2:1 5-Fluorocytosine-acesulfame CAB cocrystal and 1:1 5-fluorocytosine-acesulfame salt hydrate with enhanced stability against hydration. *CrystEngComm* **2014**, *16*, 8537–8545. [CrossRef]
28. Gao, H.; Wang, Q.; Ke, X.; Liu, J.; Hao, G.; Xiao, L.; Chen, T.; Jiang, W.; Liu, Q. Preparation and characterization of an ultrafine HMX/NQ co-crystal by vacuum freeze drying method. *RSC Adv.* **2017**, *7*, 46229–46235. [CrossRef]
29. Gao, H.; Du, P.; Ke, X.; Liu, J.; Hao, G.; Chen, T.; Jiang, W. A Novel Method to Prepare Nano-sized CL-20/NQ Co-crystal: Vacuum Freeze Drying. *Propellants Explos. Pyrotech.* **2017**, *42*, 1–8. [CrossRef]
30. Ogienko, A.G.; Myz, S.A.; Ogienko, A.A.; Nefedov, A.A.; Stoporev, A.S.; Mel'gunov, M.S.; Yunoshev, A.S.; Shakhtshneider, T.P.; Boldyrev, V.V.; Boldyreva, E. V Cryosynthesis of Co-Crystals of Poorly Water-Soluble Pharmaceutical Compounds and Their Solid Dispersions with Polymers. The "Meloxicam-Succinic Acid" System as a Case Study. *Cryst. Growth Des.* **2018**, *18*, 7401–7409. [CrossRef]
31. Zhang, Y.; Huo, M.; Zhou, J.; Xie, S. PKSolver: An add-in program for pharmacokinetic and pharmacodynamic data analysis in Microsoft Excel. *Comput. Methods Programs Biomed.* **2010**, *99*, 306–314. [CrossRef]
32. Dixit, M.; Kini, A.G.; Kulkarni, P.K. Enhancing the aqueous solubility and dissolution of olanzapine using freeze-drying. *Braz. J. Pharm. Sci.* **2011**, *47*, 743–749.
33. Alqurshi, A.; Chan, K.L.A.; Royall, P.G. In-situ freeze-drying-forming amorphous solids directly within capsules: An investigation of dissolution enhancement for a poorly soluble drug. *Sci. Rep.* **2017**, *7*, 2910. [CrossRef]
34. Vessot, S.; Andrieu, J. A Review on Freeze Drying of Drugs with tert-Butanol (TBA) + Water Systems: Characteristics, Advantages, Drawbacks. *Dry. Technol.* **2012**, *30*, 377–385. [CrossRef]
35. Chu, K.R.; Lee, E.; Jeong, S.H.; Park, E.-S. Effect of particle size on the dissolution behaviors of poorly water-soluble drugs. *Arch. Pharm. Res.* **2012**, *35*, 1187–1195. [CrossRef] [PubMed]
36. Mosharraf, M.; Nyström, C. The effect of particle size and shape on the surface specific dissolution rate of microsized practically insoluble drugs. *Int. J. Pharm.* **1995**, *122*, 35–47. [CrossRef]
37. Bavishi, D.D.; Borkhataria, C.H. Spring and parachute: How cocrystals enhance solubility. *Prog. Cryst. Growth Charact. Mater.* **2016**, *62*, 1–8. [CrossRef]

MDPI

St. Alban-Anlage 66

4052 Basel

Switzerland

Tel. +41 61 683 77 34

Fax +41 61 302 89 18

www.mdpi.com

Pharmaceutics Editorial Office

E-mail: pharmaceutics@mdpi.com

www.mdpi.com/journal/pharmaceutics

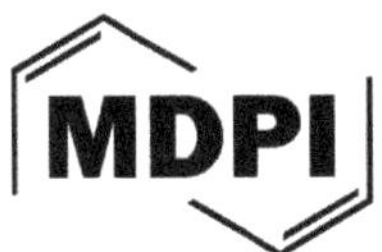

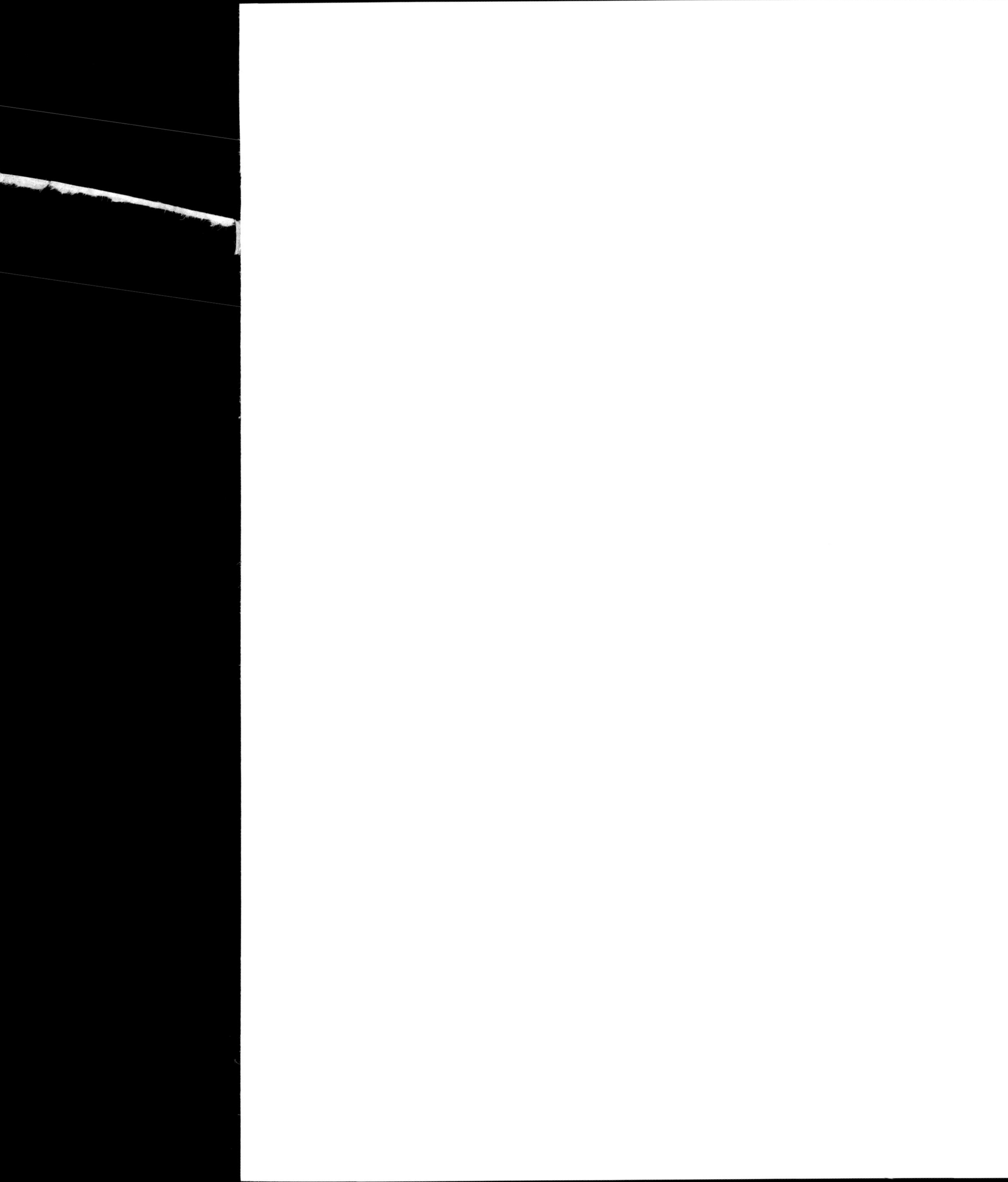